Dermatologic Nursing Essentials:
A Core Curriculum
2nd Edition

Marcia J. Hill, MSN, RN

Editor

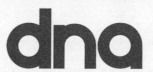

Dermatology Nurses' Association

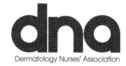

Dermatology Nurses' Association

Copyright © 2003
Dermatology Nurses' Association
East Holly Avenue/Box 56, Pitman, New Jersey 08071-0056

Publication Management by
Anthony J. Jannetti, Inc., East Holly Avenue/Box 56, Pitman, New Jersey 08071-0056

Library of Congress Control Number: 2002117724
ISBN 0-9655310-5-8
Second Edition

Printed in the United States of America

Notice: Any procedure or practice described in this book should be applied by the health-care practitioner under appropriate supervision in accordance with professional standards of care used with regard to the unique circumstances that apply in each practice situation. Care has been taken to confirm the accuracy of information presented and to describe generally accepted practices. However, the authors, editor, and publisher cannot accept any responsibility for errors or omissions or for any consequences from application of the information in this book and make no warranty, expressed or implied, with respect to the contents of the book.

Every effort has been made to ensure drug selections and dosages are in accordance with current recommendations and practice. Because of ongoing research, changes in government regulations, and the constant flow of information on drug therapy, reactions, and interactions, the reader is cautioned to check the package insert for each drug for indications, dosages, warnings, and precautions, particularly if the drug is new or infrequently used.

Dermatologic Nursing Essentials: A Core Curriculum (2nd edition) was funded, in part, through generous educational grants from the following companies:

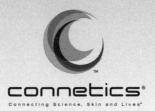

Beiersdorf Inc.

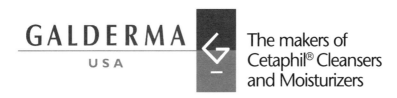

DERMIK®

Fujisawa Healthcare, Inc.

GALDERMA USA — The makers of Cetaphil® Cleansers and Moisturizers

Genentech

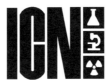

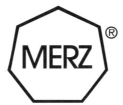

OrthoNeutrogena

For more information about these corporate sponsors, see page 487.

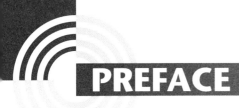

PREFACE

Dermatology Nursing Essentials: A Core Curriculum is written to provide the reader with core knowledge about the specialty of Dermatology Nursing. It is with great pride that I present the second edition of this work. Since the first edition was published in 1998, there has been considerable growth in the knowledge base needed by dermatology nurses. Therefore the authors in this edition committed themselves to providing the most current and factual information available. Many chapters have been expanded and three new chapters were added.

Disorders of the Glands, Benign Neoplasms/Hyperplasia, and Disorders of Oral Mucosa were added to give a more complete picture of the disease entities that may be seen in dermatology practice. The decision was made to rename the chapter on Diseases of Epidermal Proliferation to Diseases of the Epidermis. This allows for the addition of disease entities that may not have been due to proliferation. It also allowed for the separation of dermatitis and eczema into a new chapter for more comprehensive information. A change was also made to Chapter 17, previously Dermatologic Considerations in Black Skin. It was changed to Dermatologic Considerations in Ethnic Skin, thus allowing for information on all different skin types.

Although the first edition was a 2-year project, this edition was completed in just over a year. This is due in part to those individuals who committed to the first edition and did a wonderful job at including current information. Integral to this second edition becoming a reality were the authors who spent many hours writing and rewriting and the reviewers who gave such meaningful and excellent feedback. In addition, the continued commitment to excellence by the staff at Anthony J. Jannetti, Inc. was invaluable.

My hope is that this edition will give you a knowledge base that is current and factual and will serve as an excellent reference not only for certification but your day-to-day interaction with patients. If it stimulates some to research disease entities further then it has more than accomplished its purpose.

I want to personally thank all those individuals who were part of this endeavor. Without your insight and hard work this text would not have been so successful.

Marcia J. Hill, MSN, RN
Editor

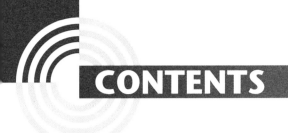

CONTENTS

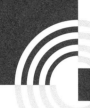

CONTENTS

> **Notice:** *The study questions at the end of each chapter have been provided for the readers to assess their comprehension of the material. However, the questions should not be considered all-inclusive. While the core curriculum is a primary reference to help nurses prepare for the dermatology nursing certification examination, readers are encouraged to use other sources during their course of study. A bibliography is offered at the end of each chapter to provide additional sources.*

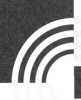

CONTRIBUTORS

EDITOR: *Marcia J. Hill, MSN, RN*

CHAPTER AUTHORS

Lynn A. Babin, MSN, RN, CNS, AAS
Instructor/Clinical Nurse Specialist
Cincinnati State Technical and Community College
Cincinnati, Ohio

Melissa Cooper, RN, CWOCN, DNC
Dermatology Nurse
VA Palo Alto HCS
Palo Alto, California

Janice Zeigler Cuzzell, MA, RN
Director, Wound Care Program
Island Health Care, Inc.
Savannah, Georgia

Bonita Drones, MSN, RN, C, CS
Chief Nurse, Dermatology Clinic
Veterans Affairs Medical Center
Houston, Texas

Maryann Forgach, BSN, RN
Clinical Supervisor
Washington University School of Medicine
St. Louis, Missouri

Marcia J. Hill, MSN, RN
Senior Research Nurse
Department of Dermatology
MD Anderson Cancer Center
Houston, Texas

Lauren L. Johannsen, RN
Clinical Administrator
Affiliated Dermatology & Cosmetic Surgery Center, Inc.
Dublin, Ohio

Janis S. Johnson, BSN, RN, C, DNC
Dermatology Nursing Supervisor
Mayo Clinic Scottsdale
Scottsdale, Arizona

Elizabeth Bevan (Betty) Kasper, MS, ARNP-C
Family Nurse Practitioner
Bradenton Dermatology and Laser Center
Bradenton, Florida

Sue Ann McCann, MSN, RN, DNC
Photopheresis Nurse Coordinator
University of Pittsburgh Medical Center
Pittsburgh, Pennsylvania

Noreen Heer Nicol, MS, RN, FNP
Chief Clinical Officer
National Jewish Medical and Research Center
Denver, Colorado

Marrise M. Phillips, BS, RN, CCRC, DNC
Director of Clinical Trials
Mid-Charlotte Dermatology and Research
Charlotte, North Carolina

Sherrill Jantzi Rudy, MSN, RN, CRNP
Pediatric Nurse Practitioner
Children's Hospital of Pittsburgh
Pittsburgh, Pennsylvania

Anne Marie Ruszkowski, BSN, RN, DNC
Director of Nursing
Columbia University Department of Dermatology
New York, New York

Margaret Sabatini, MS, BSN, RN
HIV/Sexuality Education Specialist
Rhode Island Department of Education
Providence, Rhode Island

Sharon M. Simpson, BS, RN, DNC
Dermatology Surgical & Laser Nurse
Office of Drs. Ashinoff & Levine
New York University Faculty Practice
New York, New York

Nancy Vargo, RN, DNC
Clinic Manager
Oregon Health & Science University
Department of Dermatology
Portland, Oregon

Robin Weber, MN, RN, FNP-C
Nurse Practitioner in Dermatology
VA Medical Center
Portland, Oregon

Bonita Weyrauch, RN, CWS, CCT
Clinical Coordinator
Medical Consulting Services Corp.
Boothwyn, Pennsylvania

Kelly N. White, MS, ARNP
Family Nurse Practitioner
Orlando, Florida

REVIEWERS

Zach N. Anderson, LPN
Director of Compliance and Clinical Relations
Medical Hair Restoration/Leavitt Management Group, Inc.
Orlando, Florida

Edna Atwater, RN
Administrative Director, Wound Management Institute
Duke University Health System
Durham, North Carolina

Laura Beck-Wilson, MSN, RN
Adult Nurse Practitioner
VA Medical Center/Metro Dermatology
Cleveland, Ohio

Barbara Bielan, BSN, RN, ANPC
Nurse Practitioner
San Francisco, California

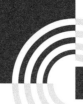

CONTRIBUTORS

Janice T. Chussil, MSN, RN, C, ANP, DNC
Dermatology Nurse Practitioner
Dermatology Associates, PC
Portland, Oregon

Janet T. Crawford, MSN, APN, BC, DNC
Clinical Nurse Specialist-Burns
John H. Stroger Hospital of Cook County
Chicago, Illinois

James Hicks, MS, ARNP-C
Nurse Practioner
Advanced Dermatology, PA
Manhattan, Kansas

Jeanette C. Jones, BSN, RN
Nurse Coordinator
Dermatology Consultants, PC
Nashville, Tennessee

Julie M. Loehr, RN
Medical Practice Manager
Laser & Dermatologic Surgery Center
St. Louis, Missouri

Sue Ann McCann, MSN, RN, DNC
Photopheresis Nurse Coordinator
University of Pittsburgh Medical Center
Pittsburgh, Pennsylvania

Karen Murphy-Lind, RN
Dermatology Staff Nurse/Unit Nurse Leader, Specialties
Massachusetts General Hospital/Charlestown Health Care Center
Charlestown, Massachusetts

Noreen Heer Nicol, MS, RN, FNP
Chief Clinical Officer
National Jewish Medical and Research Center
Denver, Colorado

Marrise M. Phillips, BS, RN, CCRC, DNC
Director of Clinical Trials
Mid-Charlotte Dermatology and Research
Charlotte, North Carolina

Stevelynn J. Pogue, MSN, RN, APRN, BC
Geriatric Nurse Practitioner
Parkland Health and Hospital Systems
Dallas, Texas

Carolita T. Sheetz, MSN, BSN, DNC
ARNP Dermatology Clinic
University of Iowa Health Care Center
Iowa City, Iowa

Barbara Sinni-McKeehen, MSN, ARNP, DNC
Dermatology Clinical Advisor
Bay Pines VA Medical Center
Bay Pines, Florida

Hope Sylvain, MSN, APRN-BC, DNC
Adult Nurse Practitioner
Wilson Dermatology Clinic
Wilson, North Carolina

Marianne C. Tawa, MSN, RN, NP
Nurse Practitioner Dermatology and Cutaneous Oncology
Dana Farber Cancer Institute
Boston, Massachusetts

Darlene M. Thomay, BA, RN, DNC
Clinical Coordinator of the Derm/MED Specialties Outpatient Clinic
Metro Health
Cleveland, Ohio

Robin Weber, MN, RN, FNP-C
Nurse Practioner in Dermatology
VA Medical Center
Portland, Oregon

Melodie Young, MSW, RN, A/GNP
Nurse Practitioner Texas Dermatology Associates
Dallas, Texas
Adjunct Clinical Instructor
The University of Texas at Arlington

ANTHONY J. JANNETTI, INC. STAFF

MANAGING EDITOR
Kenneth J. Thomas
Anthony J. Jannetti, Inc.
Pitman, New Jersey

ASSOCIATE MANAGING EDITOR
Elise A. Denmon
Anthony J. Jannetti, Inc.
Pitman, New Jersey

ART DIRECTOR
Jack M. Bryant
Anthony J. Jannetti, Inc.
Pitman, New Jersey

LAYOUT AND DESIGN
Darin Peters
Anthony J. Jannetti, Inc.
Pitman, New Jersey

DERMATOLOGY NURSES' ASSOCIATION STAFF

EXECUTIVE DIRECTOR
Cynthia R. Nowicki, EdD, RN
Dermatology Nurses' Association
Pitman, New Jersey

EDUCATION DIRECTOR
Sally S. Russell, MN, RN, C
Dermatology Nurses' Association
Pitman, New Jersey

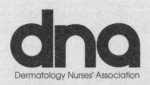

Dermatology Nurses' Association

The Dermatology Nurses' Association (DNA) was established in 1981 as a not-for-profit specialty nursing organization. It serves its members through a national structure, and locally through chapters. DNA also extends its services to its international members. Registered nurses, licensed practical nurses, licensed vocational nurses, and individuals involved or interested in the care of the dermatology patient are eligible for membership in the association.

PHILOSOPHY

The DNA believes that the patient is the fundamental focus of health care. We believe the quality of patient care is greatly enhanced through the promotion of education for nurses in the specialty of dermatology. We believe the advancement of dermatology nursing clinical practice is based on research and we are committed to encouraging the testing and sharing of new ideas. We further believe that a sense of professional pride evolves with an expanded knowledge base, increased opportunity for interdisciplinary collaboration, and the recognition of superior achievement within our membership. We believe in dermatology nurse certification as a means of validating knowledge and expertise in the specialty practice of dermatology nursing.

MISSION

The mission of the DNA is to develop and promote education and nursing leadership in dermatologic care.

DNA accomplishes its mission by:
- Developing and fostering the highest standards of dermatology nursing care.
- Enhancing professional growth through education and research.
- Facilitating communication among its members.
- Providing a support system for its members.
- Promoting interdisciplinary collaboration.
- Providing a forum for learning and sharing.
- Serving as a resource for dermatology nursing information for health care professionals.

DERMATOLOGY NURSES' ASSOCIATION

East Holly Avenue   Box 56   Pitman, New Jersey 08071-0056
Phone: (856) 256-2330; 1-800-454-4DNA (4362)
Fax: (856) 589-7463; (856) 256-2349
E-mail: dna@ajj.com
Web site: www.dnanurse.org

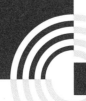

DERMATOLOGY NURSING
SCOPE OF PRACTICE

Acknowledgements

Appreciation is extended to the following individuals who wrote, reviewed, and consulted with DNA in the development and revision of the *Dermatology Nursing Standards of Clinical Practice.*

Agnes Beachman, BSN, RN
Dorothea Caldwell-Brown, MPH, RN
Janice T. Chussil , MSN, RN,C, ANP, DNC
Dorothy J. del Bueno, EdD, RN

Christine M. Hickey, BS, RN
Linda LoPresti, BSN, RN
Ann Marie Mlinaric, BSN, RN
Noreen Heer Nicol, MS, RN, FNP

Marrise M. Phillips, BS, RN, CCRC, DNC
Marie Santiago, RN, Ob/Gyn NP
Doreen B. Siegel, MS, RN,C, FNP
Robin Stupa, BSN, RN

The Dermatology Nurses' Association (DNA), the professional organization of dermatology nurses, is responsible for defining and establishing the scope of professional dermatology nursing practice. In doing so, the DNA, as a member of the Nursing Organizations Alliance (NOA), acknowledges the role of the American Nurses Association (ANA) in defining the scope of practice for the nursing profession as a whole.

The DNA supports the ANA *Social Policy Statement.* This statement charges specialty nursing organizations with defining their individual scope of practice and identifying the characteristics within their unique specialty area.

The Dermatology Nurses' Association *Scope of Practice* document uses the same framework as the ANA's *Social Policy Statement:* core, dimensions, boundaries, and intersections.

The *core* of dermatology nursing addresses the essence of professional dermatology nursing practice, health promotion, the environment in which it occurs and the consumers of care throughout the life cycle.

The dimensions of professional dermatology nursing practice specify those roles, behaviors, and processes inherent in the range of diverse individual practice and identify those characteristics unique to the specialty.

The *boundaries* of dermatology nursing have both internal and external limits; with the flexibility to respond to changes mandated by social needs. *Intersections* describe the interface of dermatology nursing with other professional groups for the enhancement of the delivery of competent quality health care. Dermatology nursing is distinguished at the intersections by its unique knowledge, environment, and focus.

At this time in our society, there are ongoing changes with expanding complexity of today's health care system. There appears to be a transition from the disease-oriented system to a health-oriented system of care. The needs of the consumer in today's health care system demonstrated the need for dermatology nurses to facilitate care and educate clients in the prevention/treatment of dermatologic problems. This turmoil within the current health care system has necessitated a statement clarifying the scope of professional dermatological nursing practice. Given the rapid changes in health care delivery trends and technologies, the task of defining this scope is complex. This document allows for flexibility in recognition of developing issues, methodologies, and technologies in the approach to health care and the practice of dermatology nursing.

Core

The scope of dermatology nursing practice includes an emphasis on health promotion, accountability, assessment, education, infection control, safety, psychosocial support, administration, and research. Holistic care augmented with a multidisciplinary approach is utilized to assist the client, family, and/or significant other(s) to attain the optimal functioning ability.

Professional dermatology nursing practice incorporates both medical and nursing standards of care to formulate an individualized plan of nursing care, implement the plan of care according to the priority of the identified needs, and evaluate the process and outcomes of the nursing interventions. The techniques of assessment, diagnosis, planning, treatment, and evaluation of perceived, actual, or potential physical or psychosocial problem(s) that may result from a dermatologic problem are employed. The dermatology nurse applies measurable outcomes and nursing interventions that are individualized and prioritized to meet the need(s) of the client, families, and/or significant other(s) in his or her society.

Dermatology nurses strive to include the client, family, and/or significant other(s) in developing measurable client-centered outcomes of care using the nursing process. Recognition of the client's needs and uniqueness as well as significance of the potential for psychosocial problems within the client's relationships with significant others, society, and the medical community is included within the framework of the plan. This ongoing practice identifies the client's response to nursing and medical interventions.

Continuity of care is promoted by building collaborative inpatient and/or ambulatory programs of care and by sharing dermatologic nursing expertise with the client, family, significant other(s), other members of the health care team, and the community. The goal of the nurse-client interaction is to promote wellness and to progress from illness to wellness along the health care continuum. Individual professional accountability, incorporation of research advances, and participation in continuing education and professional development activities are the nucleus of the professional dermatology nurses' daily practice.

The unique knowledge base regarding dermatologic illness and wellness promotion, the respective individualized interventions, the physiological and psychological responses to these interventions, and the psychosocial consequences of dermatologic disease are incorporated into the daily practice of the professional dermatology nurse. Dermatology nurses are committed to problem solving, creativity, self-direction, and accountability for their own actions. To this end we hold the beliefs and values that support the contribution of nurses to health care, education, research, and community service.

The environment includes but is not limited to:
- Ambulatory Care Settings
- Inpatient Settings
- Day Treatment Centers
- The Community

Dimensions

Dermatology nursing is multidimensional. These dimensions include the responsibilities, functions, roles, tasks, and skills that involve a specific body of knowledge and are manifested through dermatology nursing processes and behaviors. Characteristics unique to dermatology nursing practice are:

1) *Inquiry Phase* — The dermatology nursing role focuses on identifying potential or actual physical and/or emotional problems that the client, family, and/or significant other(s) exhibit in his/her society and environment. Needs related to health promotion are identified. The client may be a "community" and/or an individual or group. Data are collected from clients, their family and/or significant other(s), appropriate health care personnel, and from results of laboratory and diagnostic tests. Information for the decision making process is gathered through interview and assessment techniques.

2) *Identification Phase* — The role of the dermatology nurse during this phase focuses on the identified data and evaluates the relevance of the data collected. Tentative nursing problems or diagnoses are either accepted or rejected based on the information reviewed. The nursing problem list or nursing diagnosis delineates the client's health needs and problems that require nursing intervention.

3) *Planning Phase* — The role of the dermatology nurse during this phase focuses on problem solving; identifying potential interventions that include health promotion, health maintenance, self-care, and health teaching while promoting the optimal function of the client, family, and/or significant other(s) throughout the health care continuum. For each of the nursing diagnoses or nursing problems identified in the preceding step, the dermatology nurse specifies the desired resolution or goal collaboratively with the client, family, and/or significant other(s). The goals are converted into measurable client-centered outcomes using the nursing process. These are defined as observable client behaviors, but may also be other client characteristics, such as decreased redness of the skin.

4) *Education Phase* — The role of the dermatology nurse in this phase focuses on preparing the client, family,

and/or significant other(s) to care for self, or to be cared for. The client, family, and/or significant other(s) are taught the knowledge, skills, and/or behaviors necessary to initiate health and wellness promotion, for self-care and/or making informed choices. Teaching, counseling, referral to other health care professionals or self-help groups, physical care, and/or other therapeutic behaviors are techniques used in this phase.

5) *Implementation Phase* — The role of the dermatology nurse during this phase focuses on actualization of the nursing care plan. The dermatology nurse may implement the plan of care alone or delegate parts of it to the client, another health care provider, or a member of the client's family or significant other(s).

6) *Analysis Phase* — During this phase the dermatology nurse focuses on examining the effectiveness of the mutually chosen interventions that identify the client's, family's, and/or significant other(s) response to nursing and medical intervention(s). Nursing diagnoses or problem list and strategies for achieving nursing goals are modified, and the overall quality of nursing care is judged based on evaluation of outcome criteria.

Nursing's roles include those of community, client/family and/or significant other(s), environmental assessment, consultation, case management, research, administration, supervision, education, consultation, and consumer advocacy. The specialty practice of dermatology nursing is defined through the implementation of specific role functions that are outlined in the *Dermatology Nursing Standards of Practice.*

Dermatology nursing practice is systematic in nature and includes nursing process decision making, analytical and scientific thinking, and inquiry.

Professional behaviors inherent in dermatology nursing practice are the acquisition and application of specialized knowledge and skills, accountability and responsibility, communication, autonomy, and collaborative relationships with others.

Boundaries

The scope of dermatology nursing practice has both internal and external boundaries. Internal boundaries include recognized forces within the practice of professional nursing such as *ANA Standards of Clinical Nursing Practice,* the ANA guidelines for practice such as the *Social Policy Statement, the Scope of Nursing Practice,* and *the Dermatology Nursing Standards of Practice.* Other actions that influence our own professional practice are quality improvement monitoring activities and risk management activities.

The external boundaries include state and federal legislation and/or regulation, societal needs, economic changes, and health care delivery trends. Individual state nurse practice acts are examples of legal boundaries used to provide the basis for interpretation of safe nursing practice. Rules and regulations that evolve from these acts are used as guidelines by state boards of nursing to issue licenses and ensure the public safety.

Examples of the legislative/regulatory factors are federal and state health codes and mandated reporting requirements, the Joint Commission for Accreditation of Health Care Organizations (JCAHO), and the Professional Standards Review Organization (PSRO). The current trend toward an ambulatory community-based setting for service delivery is an example of economic change as a response to societal needs. The rapidly worsening financial climate has driven the health care delivery system to reduce costs while providing team care, collaboration, and consultation. Health care delivery trends, such as an increased number of ambulatory care centers, client participation in health maintenance organizations (HMOs), and preferred provider organizations (PPOs) all influence the delivery of dermatologic care.

Intersections

The dermatology nurse interacts with a variety of professions for the common purpose of advancing dermatologic care through education, administration, consultation, and collaboration in practice, research, and policy making. Within these roles, dermatology nurses communicate, network, and share resources, information, research, technology, and expertise. This is done to address common concerns such as ethical issues, humanism, psychosocial needs of clients, trends, management of client care, and alternative care modalities.

The dermatology nurse, via the DNA, collaborates with other professional groups within the province of nursing such as the American Nurses Association (ANA), the National League for Nursing (NLN), and the many specialty groups represented in the Nursing Organizations Alliance (NOA). The DNA also maintains a collaborative relationship with the American Academy of Dermatology, American Society for Dermatologic Surgery, Society for Investigative Dermatology, and American College of Mohs Micro-graphic Surgery and Cutaneous Oncology. Intersection is not limited to these groups, however, and may occur with any group.

These health care professions interact with a common overall mission to positively influence the provisions of dermatologic care rendered to society. Dermatology nurses bring their unique knowledge, focus, and perspective to unite all participants in the process and outcome of these intersections.

Summary

The intent of this document is to conceptualize practice and provide education to practitioners, educators, researchers, and administrators, and to inform other health professionals, legislators, and the public about the participation in and contribution to health care by dermatology nursing. Through articulation of the elements of care, dimensions, boundaries, and intersection, the *Dermatology Nursing Scope of Practice* document defines the specialty practice of dermatology nursing.

Bibliography

American Academy of Ambulatory Care Nursing. (2000). *Ambulatory care nursing administration and practice standards.* Pitman, NJ: Author.

American Nephrology Nurses' Association. (1999). *Standards and guidelines of clinical practice for nephrology nursing.* Pitman, NJ: Author.

American Nurses Association. (1988). *Code of ethics with interpretative statements.* Kansas City, MO: Author.

American Nurses Association. (1995). *Nursing's social policy statement.* Washington, DC: Author.

DERMATOLOGY NURSING
STANDARDS OF CLINICAL PRACTICE

Introduction to Dermatology Nursing Standards

Dermatology nursing practice shall be based on individualized client care utilizing prevailing accepted medical/nursing standards of care while incorporating advances in research and education into daily practice. Dermatology nurses are therefore encouraged to be involved in problem solving, creative, self-directed, and accountable for their own actions. To this end, DNA holds beliefs and values that support the contribution of nurses to health care, education, research, and community service.

The purpose of these standards is to provide definitive direction for the provision of care and professional role activities of dermatology nurses while building upon the broad *American Nurses' Association Standards of Clinical Nursing Practice.*

The Dermatology Nursing Standards of Clinical Practice are intended to provide a framework upon which the dermatology nurse shall build his/her practice with assessment, measurable outcomes, and nursing interventions that are customized to meet the need(s) of the individual in his/her society. These *Dermatology Nursing Standards of Clinical Practice* differentiate and articulate the dermatology nurse's specialized practice to provide quality dermatologic client centered care. Professional nurses who practice dermatology nursing shall use these standards of practice to define the desired outcomes of client care for the practice of dermatology nursing and to clarify the standards of professional practice essential to provide a basis on which to build an understanding of dermatology client needs.

Dermatology nurses strive to include the client/family/significant others in developing measurable client centered outcomes of care based on the nursing process. This ongoing practice identifies the client's response to nursing as well as medical intervention(s). Continuity of care is promoted by building collaborative inpatient and/or ambulatory programs of care and by sharing our expertise with the client, family, significant others, other members of the health care team, and the community. The goal of the nurse-client interface is to promote wellness and to progress along the health care continuum from illness to wellness.

The language used to compose the *Dermatology Nursing Standards of Clinical Practice* is intended to focus on global nursing care approaches related to the dermatologic client. Specific nursing approaches and interventions will need to be individualized and prioritized to meet the needs of specific clients, families, and/or significant others. Dermatology Nursing Standards outlined are directed at delineation of outcome behaviors.

Key Terms

Definitions of key terms will assist in using this document. Other definitions are found in the glossary at the end of this document.[1]

Assessment: A systematic, dynamic process by which the nurse, through interaction with the client, significant others, and health care providers, collects and analyzes data about the client. Data may include the following dimensions: physical, psychological, psychosocial, cultural, spiritual, cognitive, functional abilities, developmental, economic, and lifestyle.

Diagnosis: A clinical judgment about the client's response to actual or potential health conditions or needs. Diagnoses provide the basis for determining a plan of care to achieve expected outcomes.

Evaluation: The process of determining the client's progress toward the attainment of expected outcomes and the effectiveness of nursing care.

Implementation: May include any or all of these activities: intervening, delegating, and coordinating. Client, significant others, or health care providers may be designated to implement interventions within the plan of care.

Outcomes: Measurable expected client focused goals.

Plan of Care: Comprehensive outline of care to be delivered to attain expected outcomes.

Client: Recipient of nursing actions. When the client is an individual, the focus is on the health state, problems, or needs of a single person. When the client is a family or group, the focus is on the health state of the unit as a whole or the reciprocal effects of an individual's health state on the other members of the unit. When the client is a community, the focus is on personal and environmental health and the health risks of population groups. Nursing's actions toward clients may focus on disease or injury prevention, health promotion, health restoration, or health maintenance.

Health Care Providers: Individuals with special expertise who provide health care services or assistance to clients. They may include nurses, physicians, psychologists, social workers, nutritionists/dietitians, and various therapists. Providers may also include service organizations and vendors.

Significant Others: Family members and/or those significant to the client.

The Dermatology Nursing Scope of Practice and the Standards of Clinical Practice were revised in 2002.

[1] *Definitions adapted from Standards of Clinical Nursing Practice, 1998. American Nurses Association, Washington, DC.*

I. ASSESSMENT

Standard of Care
The dermatology nurse collects client health data.

Measurement Criteria
The dermatology nurse:
1. Initiates the identification of the client's needs/problems utilizing a logical and/or scientific process, in a timely, organized, systematic, and ongoing manner. Nursing data base may include:
   a) Biophysical assessment.
   b) Personal and family health history.
   c) Psychosocial assessment to include the client/family/ significant other(s).
   d) Patterns of coping with skin manifestations of disease process; patterns of social interaction.
   e) Self-care abilities.
   f) Client's perception of health status and their health goals.
   g) Input from client/family/significant others, as appropriate.
   h) Environmental factors.
   i) Discharge planning factors.
2. Prioritizes data collection as determined by the immediate health care problems of the client to determine current health status, past medical history, and family and social history that require nursing intervention.
3. Determines the scope of data collection as determined by the health status of the client as it relates to the individual's illness, reaction to illness, and/or wellness promotion.
4. Collects data from the client, family, significant others, health care personnel, or individuals in the community and systemically records all pertinent data in the client's permanent medical record in a format that is accessible, retrievable, and confidential.

II. DIAGNOSIS

Standard of Care
The dermatology nurse analyzes the assessment data in determining diagnoses.

Measurement Criteria
The dermatology nurse:
1. Derives diagnoses from the assessment data.
2. Validates the identified problems as they relate to the individual's illness, reaction to illness, and wellness promotion with the client/family/significant others, as appropriate.
3. Communicates client problems as either nursing diagnoses or client care needs.
4. Records findings in a manner that facilitates the determination of client outcome goals, planning, and intervention.
5. Collaborates with other professionals to validate diagnoses.

III. OUTCOME IDENTIFICATION

Standard of Care
The dermatology nurse identifies expected individualized outcomes for the client.

Measurement Criteria
The dermatology nurse:
1. Derives client outcome(s) goals from the diagnosis.
2. Formulates mutual client outcome(s) goals with input from the client/family/significant others and other members of the health care team.
3. Articulates client outcome(s) which:
   a) Are clearly written and measurable.
   b) Are prioritized.
   c) Include a time estimate for attainment.
   d) Provide direction for continuation of care.
   e) Are recorded and communicated to appropriate persons.
4. Derives client outcome(s) goals that are realistic in context with the individual's present and potential capabilities and the human and material resources available.

IV. PLANNING

Standard of Care
The dermatology nurse develops a plan of care that defines interventions to attain expected outcomes.

Measurement Criteria
The dermatology nurse:
1. Formulates a client care plan based on the analysis of collected data to identify individualized needs of the client/family/significant others utilizing the nursing process.
2. Engages the client/family/significant others and other health care team members in mutual planning for diagnostic testing, treatments, home care, psychosocial support, followup care, and any other appropriate intervention(s).
3. Documents a plan of care for all clients.
4. Participates in client centered multidisciplinary discharge planning or follow-ups, as appropriate.
5. Collaborates with other health care providers, as appropriate, to help define and implement client education and information needs that may include some or all of the following:
   a) The client's disease process.
   b) The client's therapeutic regimen.
   c) Nursing responsibilities.
   d) The client's and family's responsibilities and options.
   e) Recommendations for ongoing and/or followup care.
   f) Wellness promotion.
   g) Available support groups and other resources.
   h) Financial concerns.

V. IMPLEMENTATION

Standard of Care
The dermatology nurse implements nursing interventions that are consistent with the identified plan of care.

Measurement Criteria
The dermatology nurse:
1. Implements interventions which may encompass biophysical and psychosocial manifestations of skin disease.
2. Implements interventions in a safe and timely manner.
3. Documents the implementation of nursing intervention in the medical record.

VI. EVALUATION
Standard of Care
The dermatology nurse evaluates the client's progress toward the attainment of mutually set goals and outcomes.

Measurement Criteria
The dermatology nurse:
1. Evaluates in a systematic and ongoing basis.
2. Collaborates with the client/family/significant others and other health care team members in the evaluation process and revises the plan of care, as appropriate.
3. Provides ongoing evaluation of client/family/significant others' knowledge of the client's illness, diagnostic and treatment plans, anticipated outcomes, and self-care activities and revises the plan of care, as appropriate.
4. Evaluates the client/family/significant others' perceptions and appraisals of the care he/she receives.
5. Documents client progress toward treatment goal(s) and makes revisions to the diagnosis and plan of care.
6. Evaluates systematically the quality, timeliness, and cost effectiveness of care in relation to client outcomes and nursing process.
7. Participates in evaluation of care for groups of clients, which is conducted as part of a quality improvement program.

STANDARDS OF PROFESSIONAL PERFORMANCE

I. QUALITY OF CARE
Standard of Professional Performance
The dermatology nurse systematically evaluates the quality and effectiveness of nursing practice.

Measurement Criteria
The dermatology nurse:
1. Participates in quality improvement activities as appropriate for her/his position and practice environment. Such activities may include:
   a) Identification of the indicators[2] to be monitored such as high-risk and high-volume client populations.
   b) Collection of quality improvement data.
   c) Participation with multidisciplinary teams that evaluate clinical practice or health services that affect client care.
2. Utilizes the results of quality improvement activities to initiate appropriate modification of their

practice to create/maintain a safe, comfortable, and therapeutic environment for clients, visitors, and staff.
3. Collaborates with other disciplines and services as appropriate, to assure that the facility is constructed, equipped, and operated in a manner that protects clients, visitors, and personnel from:
   a) Fire hazard.
   b) Electrical hazard.
   c) Exposure to hazardous chemicals.
   d) Exposure to infectious agents.
4. Reports and documents hazardous situations and intervenes.
5. Contributes to the development of a comprehensive infection control program, as appropriate to their position and practice environment, that requires:
   a) Written policies and procedures for the prevention and control of infection among clients, personnel, and visitors.
   b) Compliance with local, state, and federal agency regulations.
   c) Ongoing system for reporting, reviewing, and evaluating infections within the practice setting.

II. PERFORMANCE APPRAISAL
Standard of Professional Performance
The dermatology nurse evaluates her/his nursing practice in relation to professional practice standards.

Measurement Criteria
The dermatology nurse:
1. Participates in a formal mechanism of performance appraisal on a regular basis which may include self-review/peer review to identify areas of strength as well as areas for professional/practice development.
2. Seeks constructive feedback regarding own practice.
3. Takes action to achieve the goals identified during ongoing and formal performance appraisal.
4. Participates in peer performance evaluations.

III. EDUCATION
Standard of Professional Performance
The dermatology nurse acquires and maintains current knowledge of Dermatology Nursing practice.

Measurement Criteria
The dermatology nurse:
1. Seeks to update her/his knowledge and skills on an ongoing basis to ensure clinical competence. Such activities may include:
   a) Attending dermatology nursing education offerings and/or other professional meetings.
   b) Reading the *Dermatology Nursing* journal as well as other nursing/professional journals which pertain to the practice of dermatology nursing.

[2]Those treatment(s) and/or procedure(s) that may cause harm to a client that may alter the desired outcome of care.

c) Participating in other pertinent continuing education activities.
2. Attains knowledge and skills as needed to deliver culturally competent care.
3. Communicates with colleagues and others about new or updated knowledge, skills, and health promotional behavior.
4. Promotes dermatology nursing as a specialty nursing practice.
5. Promotes public awareness of the specialty of dermatology nursing.
6. Acquires certification to validate knowledge and expertise in dermatology nursing.

IV. COLLEGIALITY
Standard of Professional Performance
The dermatology nurse contributes toward the professional development of peers, colleagues, and other members of the health care team.

Measurement Criteria
The dermatology nurse:
l. Shares clinical expertise with colleagues and other members of the health care team.
2. Provides colleagues constructive feedback regarding their professional practice.
3. Contributes to dermatologic learning experiences for nursing students and other health care providers in all areas of practice (hospital, community, etc.).

V. ETHICS
Standard of Professional Performance
The dermatology nurse's decisions and actions on behalf of the client will be provided in an environment that is respectful and in accord with professional codes of ethics related to delivery of health care.

Measurement Criteria
The dermatology nurse:
1. Provides care that is consistent with American Nurses Association Ethical Code for Nurses (ANA, 1976).
2. Maintains client privacy and confidentiality.
3. Respects the client's right to be an active partner in health care decision-making and preserves client autonomy, dignity, and rights.
4. Respects differences in values, lifestyle, coping skills, and health care practices; care to be delivered in a nonjudgmental and nondiscriminatory manner.
5. Serves as a client advocate and may act as a liaison for the client with other members of the health care team and the community, as appropriate.
6. Seeks available resources to help formulate ethical decisions.

VI. COLLABORATION
Standard of Professional Performance
The dermatology nurse collaborates with the client, significant others, and health care providers in providing client care.

Measurement Criteria
The dermatology nurse:
1. Communicates with the client, significant others, and health care providers regarding client care and nursing role in the provision of care.
2. Consults with health care providers for client care as needed.
3. Makes referrals including provisions for continuity of care as needed.

VII. RESEARCH
Standard of Professional Performance
The dermatology nurse uses research findings in practice.

Measurement Criteria
The dermatology nurse:
1. Uses interventions substantiated by research as appropriate to the individual's position, education, and practice environment.
2. Participates in research activities, as appropriate to the individual's position, education, and practice environment. Such activities may include:
a) Identification of clinical problems suitable for nursing research.
b) Participation in data collection.
c) Participation in a unit, organization, or community research committee or program.
d) Sharing of research activities with others.
e) Conducting research.
f) Critiquing research for application to practice.
g) Using research findings in the development of policies, procedures, and guidelines for client care.
3. Encourages and supports nursing colleagues and other professionals engaged in dermatology research.
4. Acts to protect the rights of human subjects.

VIII. RESOURCE UTILIZATION
Standard of Professional Performance
The dermatology nurse considers factors related to safety, effectiveness, and cost in planning and delivering client care.

Measurement Criteria
The dermatology nurse:
1. Considers and evaluates multiple factors related to effectiveness, safety, and cost in planning, delegating, and/or delivering care for the client/family/significant others.
2. Assigns tasks or delegates care based on the individualized client needs and the knowledge and skills of the provider selected.
3. Assists the client and significant others in identifying and securing appropriate services available to address health-related needs.

Glossary[1]

Continuity of Care: An interdisciplinary process that includes clients and significant others in the development of a coordinated plan of care. This process facilitates the client's transition between settings, based on changing needs and available resources.

Criteria: Relevant, measurable indicators of the standards of clinical nursing practice.

Guidelines: Describe a process of client care management which has the potential of improving the quality of clinical and consumer decision making. They are systematically developed statements based on available scientific evidence and expert opinion.

Nursing: The diagnosis and treatment of human responses to actual or potential health problems (*ANA, Nursing's Social Policy Statement*).

Standard: Authoritative statement enunciated and promulgated by the profession by which the quality of practice, service, or education can be judged.

Standards of Nursing Practice: An authoritative statement that describes a level of care or performance common to the profession of nursing by which the quality of nursing practice can be judged. Standards of clinical nursing practice include both standards of care and standards of professional performance.

Standards of Care: Authoritative statements that describe a competent level of clinical nursing practice demonstrated through assessment, diagnosis, outcome identification, planning, implementation, and evaluation.

Standards of Professional Performance: Authoritative statements that describe a competent level of behavior in the professional role, including activities related to quality of care, performance appraisal, education, collegiality, ethics, collaboration, research, and resource utilization.

References

American Nurses Association. (1998). *Standards of clinical nursing practice* (2nd ed.). Washington, DC: Author.

American Nurses Association. (1995). *Nursing's social policy statement.* Washington, DC: Author.

American Nurses Association. (1976). *Ethical code for nurses.* Washington, DC: Author.

[1]Adapted from *Standards of Clinical Nursing Practice,* 1998, American Nurses Association, Washington, DC.

Anatomy and Physiology of the Skin

Noreen Heer Nicol, MS, RN, FNP

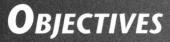

OBJECTIVES

At the end of this chapter, the reader will be able to:
- Define the functions of the skin.
- List the layers of the skin.
- List specialized cells in the epidermis and dermis.
- Delineate the functions of the glands of the skin.

KEY POINTS

- The skin is the largest organ of the body.
- Alterations in the skin will affect the overall well-being of an individual.
- Knowledge of the anatomy and physiology of the skin is essential to accurate patient assessment.

Anatomy and Physiology of the Skin

Noreen Heer Nicol, MS, RN, FNP

FUNCTIONS OF THE SKIN

I. OVERVIEW

A conceptual framework for recognizing and understanding diseases of the skin relies on principles of diagnosis common to general medicine, namely, historical factors, physical examination, and laboratory techniques. To relate these principles of diagnosis to clinicopathologic events in dermatology, it is important to start with an overview of the skin as an organ system. A skin disease may localize exclusively in the epidermis, dermis, or subcutaneous fat; alternatively, more than one or all of these sites may be affected simultaneously. The more common skin conditions take into account a diverse spectrum of clinical pathology, which may be characterized by inflammation (noninfectious), pigmentary abnormalities, infection and infestation, benign and malignant cellular proliferations, as well as disease where the basic mechanisms are relatively obscure. To conceptualize skin disorders effectively, it is essential to consider the changes in the structure and function of the skin, and to understand the specific clinical pathology related to the changes.

A. **Protection.**
   1. An intact stratum corneum provides a physical barrier against foreign substances and bacteria.
   2. Mechanical strength is provided by intercellular bonding in the epidermis; and collagen, elastin, and ground substance in the dermis.
   3. Subcutaneous tissue acts as a shock absorber.
   4. Melanin screens and absorbs ultraviolet radiation.

B. **Homeostasis.**
   1. Prevents dehydration through loss of internal fluids and electrolytes.
   2. Limits absorption of external fluids and gases.

C. **Excretion.**
   1. Functions as minor organ of excretion of urea, lactic acid, bile, sodium chloride, and sweat.

D. **Temperature regulation.**
   1. Body temperature is controlled by:
      a. Conduction of heat from the skin to the air or other objects.
      b. Radiation of heat from the body surface.
      c. Convection of heat by air currents.
      d. Evaporation of perspiration.
   2. The cutaneous vasculature plays an important role in body temperature regulation. Blood vessels:
      a. Dilate when the external environment is warm to promote heat loss.

   b. Constrict in a cold environment to conserve heat.

E. **Vitamin D production.**
   1. Ultraviolet light converts 7-dehydrocholesterol to vitamin D in the epidermis.

F. **Sensory perception.**
   1. Transmits touch, pressure, temperature, pain, and itch through mechanoreceptors and unmyelinated nerve fibers.

G. **Psychosocial.**
   1. Serves function of sexual attraction, general well-being, and influences self-image. Outward expressions of anxiety, fear, and anger visible through sweating, pallor, and flushing.

H. **Wound healing.**
   1. The skin regenerates itself and functions in wound repair.

II. STRUCTURE OF THE SKIN

A. **Epidermis (see Figures 1a and 1b).**
   1. The epidermis is the outermost structure of the skin. It:
      a. Contains multiple layers of cells (stratified).
      b. Is approximately 0.1 mm thick, depending on the site.
      c. Is without lymphatic and vascular channels, and connective tissue; therefore it derives its nutritional support from the underlying dermis.
   2. Keratinization.
      a. The epidermis rejuvenates itself through the process of keratinization. Epidermal keratinization is the process of morphological and biochemical differentiation of the keratinocyte, beginning in the basal cell layer and ending in the stratum corneum as a horn or cornified cell.
   3. Keratin.
      a. Keratin, the major product of the cornified cell, is a highly resistant, insoluble, fibrous protein. It represents the end product of a differentiated epidermal keratinocyte.
      b. Keratinization also involves synthesis of several other proteins and additional substances such as keratohyalin granules which act as glue.
   4. Layers of the epidermis.
      a. There are five layers in the epidermis.
      b. The layers are named to reflect the stage the keratinocytes are in during the process of keratinization.
      c. These layers are not independent of each

Figure 1a.
The Epidermis

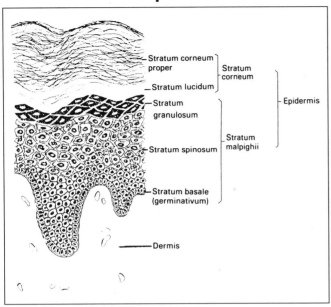

Figure 1b.
The Epidermis

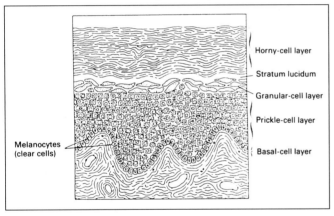

From Rosen, T., Lanning, M., & Hill, M. (1983). *Nurse's atlas of dermatology.* Boston: Little, Brown & Company, p. 2.

Figure 2.
Life Cycles of the Epidermal Cell

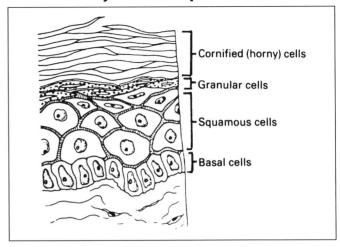

other, but rather are interrelated and continuous phases of the life of a keratinocyte (see Figure 2).

(1) Basal cell layer (stratum germinativum): the basal cell layer is the innermost layer of the epidermis. It consists of a single layer of elongated cells. Each cell divides (mitosis) into two daughter cells. One remains as "basal cell," the other migrates upward through the remainder of the epidermis.

(2) Prickle cell layer (stratum spinosum): the prickle cell layer consists of many rows of flattened polygonal cells that are held together by "prickles" or "spines." These

prickles are desmosomes which are small thickenings in an intracellular bridge.

(3) Granular cell layer (stratum granulosum): the granular cell layer is most prominent on the palms and soles. It consists of one to three layers of flattened, irregularly shaped cells that have large numbers of keratohyalin granules. Keratohyalin granules comprise particulate material that have a high sulfur-protein content. Keratinocytes lose their nucleus in this layer, thereby becoming nonviable.

(4) Stratum lucidum: the stratum lucidum is made up of one or more rows of distended irregular cells. It is an even, colorless, translucent, or shiny band. The stratum lucidum is probably present everywhere, but is most prominent on palms and soles.

(5) Horny cell layer (stratum corneum): the horny cell layer consists of anucleated, cornified cells. They are also known as horn cells. The nucleus and other cytoplasmic organelles have been totally degraded. The remaining material is predominantly keratin. Other substances include water, water-insoluble proteins, amino acids, sugars, urea, minerals, and lipids. These act as buffers and lubricants.

(a) Cells of the epidermis are continuously being shed or desquamated from the stratum corneum.

(b) It takes approximately 14 days for the keratinocyte to travel from the basal cell layer to the stratum corneum. Once in the stratum corneum it takes another 14 days before it is shed.

   (c) New cells are formed in the basal cell layer at the same rate cells are shed in the stratum corneum.

5. Functions of the horny cell layer.
   a. The stratum corneum serves many functions for the epidermis and the skin in general.
      (1) It functions as the body's major barrier by being relatively impermeable to water and electrolytes.
      (2) It resists damaging chemicals, provides physical toughness, impedes passage of electrical currents, and retards the proliferation of microorganisms through its relatively dry surface.
      (3) The stratum corneum also functions as a reservoir for topical medications.
   b. Although the stratum corneum is an effective barrier to most substances, some are able to pass through. Substances can be transported through the skin by three pathways:
      (1) Through adnexal orifices (pilosebaceous unit) and sweat glands.
      (2) Through the intercellular spaces between the cornified cells.
      (3) Directly through the cornified cells.

B. Cells in the epidermis.
   1. Keratinocyte cells.
      a. Keratinocytes account for 90% of the cellular components of the epidermis. They have the specialized function of producing keratin. During keratinization the keratinocytes change shape (flatten), lose organelles, form fibrous protein (keratin), become dehydrated, and thicken their cell membrane.
   2. Melanocyte cells.
      a. Embryonic development: melanocytes are the pigment-producing cells of the epidermis. Embryonically they are derived from the neural crest and by the 8th week of development, melanocytes enter the epidermis. In the fetal epidermis, melanocytes are found at suprabasal levels. When the fetus is fully developed they are located in the basal cell layer. Failure of the melanocyte to migrate to the basal cell layer results in entities such as blue nevus and mongolian spots.
      b. Regional variation: melanocytes are present on all parts of the body with regional variation. There are more melanocytes on the face than on the abdomen. Ratios of melanocytes to keratinocytes vary from 1:4

to 1:10. Advancing age leads to a greater shift favoring keratinocytes.
   c. Melanosome/Melanin: within the cytoplasm of melanocytes are special organelles called melanosomes. Melanin is stored in the melanosome and is synthesized through the conversion of the colorless amino acid, tyrosine. There are two types of melanin. Eumelanins account for brown and black colors. Pheomelanins account for yellow to reddish brown colors.
   d. Epidermal melanin unit: Melanocytes are dendritic cells. Their dendrites extend for long distances in the epidermis. This allows one melanocyte to be in contact with many keratinocytes. The interaction of the melanocyte and keratinocyte forms a biologic unit called the epidermal melanin unit. Melanosomes are transferred from the dendrite of the melanocyte to keratinocytes by a process called apocopation. The keratinocyte phagocytizes the melanin-filled tips of the melanocytes. Once transferred to the keratinocyte, the fully melanized melanosomes are partially degraded by lysosomal enzymes or desquamated with cornified cells.
   e. Melanin production: melanin production is controlled by genetics, hormones, and the environment. The number of melanocytes in the epidermis is the same regardless of race or sex.
      (1) It is the amount of melanin in the keratinocyte that determines skin color. The difference in the races comes from the number, size, distribution, degree of melanization, and rate of degradation of the melanosome within the keratinocyte.
      (2) There is also evidence that tyrosinase activity also plays a role in melanization. Dark-skinned people produce melanosomes that are larger than light-skinned people, resulting in more melanin synthesis. Tyrosinase activity is also increased in blacks.
      (3) The size of melanosomes is the principal factor in determining how they will be distributed in the keratinocyte. The larger melanosomes of dark-skinned people are packaged individually in a membrane within the cytoplasm of the keratinocyte. In light-skinned people, smaller melanosomes are package in membrane-bound complexes in the keratinocyte.
   f. Hormonal influence: hormones profoundly influence melanin pigmentation, but their

precise action at the cellular level is unknown. It is presently believed the melanocyte stimulating hormone (MSH) causes a dispersion of melanosomes within melanocytes. Regional variations exist in the sensitivity of the epidermal melanin units to specific hormones.

(1) In pregnancy there is increased pigmentation of the nipples and areolae, and to a lesser extent, an increased pigmentation of facial skin, midline of the abdomen, and genitalia. This is due to an increase in the number of active melanocytes. The hormones primarily responsible for the color changes are estrogen, progesterone, and possibly MSH.

(2) The same phenomena occurs in women taking birth control pills.

g. Pigment variation: areas of leukoderma or "whitening" of the skin can be caused by different phenomena.

(1) In vitiligo, the affected skin becomes white because melanocytes are destroyed, leading to a decrease in their number.

(2) There are different types of albinism in which there is partial or complete absence of pigment in the skin, hair, and eyes. Albinism results from defects in the production and distribution of melanin. These defects can be found in the enzyme tyrosinase, melanosome development, or in the type of melanin produced.

(3) Local areas of increased pigmentation are due to a variety of causes.

(a) The typical freckle is caused by localized increased production of pigment by a normal number of melanocytes.

(b) Nevi are benign proliferations of melanocytes.

(c) Melanomas are the malignant counterparts of nevi.

h. Ultraviolet light: the most important function of melanin is to shield the skin from the sun's ultraviolet rays by absorbing its radiant energy. The absorption spectrum of melanin encompasses the entire range of ultraviolet and visible light.

(1) Melanosomes function to scatter and absorb ultraviolet light.

(a) Exposure to ultraviolet light expedites the transfer of melanosomes to keratinocytes.

(b) When the skin is tanned by ultraviolet light, an increased number of melanosomes are manufactured and available for transfer to the keratinocyte.

(c) In light-skinned people, chronic sun exposure also "tricks" the melanocyte into producing larger melanosomes.

(d) The pattern of distribution of the melanosome in the keratinocyte then resembles that of dark-skinned people.

3. Langerhans' cells.

a. Another dendritic cell found in the epidermis is the Langerhans' cell. They are found in the granular, spinous, and basal cell layers of the epidermis. Occasionally they are seen in the normal dermis. Langerhans' cells are derived from bone marrow precursor cells.

b. The Langerhans' cell population is self-maintaining. There is a relatively constant number of these cells being maintained by intra-epidermal mitosis and migration from the connective tissue. Langerhans' cells account for approximately 4% of the epidermal cell population.

(1) Function of Langerhans' cells.

(a) They are immunocompetent cells involved in the uptake, processing, and presentation of antigen to lymphocytes.

(b) It is believed that Langerhans' cells act as special kinds of macrophages which function as the initial receptors for the cutaneous response to external antigens.

(c) Experimental evidence shows that Langerhans' cells are directly involved in allergic contact hypersensitivity.

(d) There is a decreased number of Langerhans' cells in patients with skin diseases such as psoriasis and sarcoidosis.

(e) Langerhans' cells are also functionally impaired by ultraviolet radiation. UVB and PUVA treatments lead to morphologic, antigenic, and enzymatic changes within the Langerhans' cell. Research is under way to learn the implications of this information.

4. Merkel cells.

a. Also found in the basal cell layer are Merkel cells. They are collected in specialized structures called tactile discs or touch domes. The most distal part of the Merkel cell is embedded in the dermis. Merkel cells

Dermatologic Nursing Essentials: A Core Curriculum 2nd Edition © DNA 2003

are present in the nonhairy or smooth skin of the digits, lips, regions of the oral cavity, and outer root sheath of hair follicles.

(1) Embryonic development.

    (a) Merkel cells originate from either the neural crest or ectoderm. They are joined to kertinocytes by "spines" or desmosomes which project from their cytoplasm.

    (b) Merkel cells have characteristic organelles. They are membrane-bound granules that contain neurotransmitter substances. Distal to the granules is an unmyelinated neurite or terminal neuraxon.

  b. Function.

    (1) The function of Merkel cells is that of slowly adapting mechanoreceptors. The exact mechanism of action remains uncertain.

    (2) The contacting membrane of the Merkel cell and the dendrite resemble pre and postsynaptic units. It is therefore thought that the Merkel cell acts as a receptor that transmits a stimulus to the neurite via a chemical synapse.

    (3) The Merkel cell may also serve a trophic (concerned with nourishment) role as well as serving as a common contact point for several associated keratinocytes.

    (4) Merkel cells respond to maintained deformation of the skin surface and are involved in sensing touch and pressure.

C. **Basement membrane zone.**

  1. The basement membrane zone is found at the junction of the epidermis and dermis. It runs along the base of the epidermal rete ridges as well as the sweat glands, hair shafts, and sebaceous glands.

    a. Structure.

      (1) Basement membrane zone structures are formed from basal keratinocytes and dermal fibroblasts. There are several components of the basement membrane zone that are seen with the electron microscope. The plasma membrane is the most distal surface of the basal keratinocyte.

      (2) Hemidesmosomes are specialized attachment plates between the basal keratinocyte and the lamina densa. The lamina densa is immediately above the dermis and comprises a collagen that provides structure and flexibility. The lamina densa also functions as a barrier/filter by the selective restriction of molecules.

      (3) The lamina lucida appears as a clear zone and is found between the plasma membranae and the lamina densa.

      (4) Anchoring fibrils, dermal microfibrils, and collagen fibers below the lamina densa compose the fibrous component of the basement membrane zone.

    b. Function.

      (1) The basement zone serves as a porous, semi-permeable filter. It:

        (a) Permits exchange of cells and fluid between the epidermis and dermis.

        (b) Functions as a structural support for the epidermis and helps hold the epidermis and dermis together.

    c. Diseases of the basement membrane zone.

      (1) Many genetic diseases involve structural alterations in the basement membrane zone. Separation of the epidermis and dermis results in blistering. This is seen in disorders such as epidermolysis bullosa letalis, generalized atrophic benign epidermolysis bullosa, bullous pemphigoid, and recessive dystrophic epidermolysis bullosa.

D. **Dermis (see Figure 3).**

  1. The dermis is the principal mass of the skin. It is composed of collagen bundles and is 1 to 4 mm thick. It encloses the appendages of the epidermis and supports the nerve and vascular network.

    a. Function.

      (1) Functions of the dermis include preventing mechanical trauma and maintenance of homeostasis. The dermis:

        (a) Binds large amounts of water and thereby represents a water storage organ.

        (b) Is also involved with thermoregulation and sensory innervation.

    b. Composition.

      (1) The dermis comprises connective tissue, water, and ground substance. There are three types of connective tissue: collagen, elastic fiber, and reticulum.

        (a) Collagen — constitutes the majority of fibers in the dermis.

          i. it is the major structural protein for the entire body.

          ii. collagen is a fibrous protein synthesized by fibroblasts and degraded by the proteolytic enzyme, collagenase. Scleroderma is an example of a collagen disease that involves abnormal synthesis or

Figure 3.
The Dermis and its Appendages

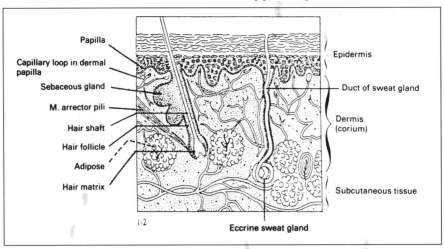

From Rosen, T., Lanning, M., & Hill, M. (1983). *Nurse's atlas of dermatology.* Boston: Little, Brown & Company, p. 5.

degradation of collagen molecules.

iii. collagen is the most important stress-resistant material of the skin. It provides us with both tensile strength and the ability to resist stretching.

iv. individual collagen bundles become thinner in atrophic scars and thicker in keloids.

(b) Elastic fibers — represent 5% to 9% of dermal fibers. They:

   i. differ structurally and chemically from collagen.

   ii. are made up of protein filaments and elastin.

   iii. function to restore the collagen network to a normal position following deformation, stress, or stretching. The skin's resiliency and elegant feel are attributed to the elastic fibers. There is a loss of elastic fibers in stria.

(c) Reticular fibers — are young finely formed collagen fibers.

   i. they are similar in diameter than mature collagen.

   ii. large numbers are found in the papillary dermis where they serve as anchoring fibrils for the basal lamina.

(d) Ground substance — constitutes the interstitial component of the dermis. Ground substance:

   i. is a viscoelastic gel.

   ii. molds to irregular objects.

   iii. is a small fraction of the dermal weight, but accounts for a substantial portion of the volume.

   iv. has a great capacity to bind water.

c. Papillary dermis.

(1) The dermis is divided into two areas — the papillary and reticulum dermis.

   (a) The papillary dermis is the uppermost area of the dermis beginning at the basement membrane zone.

      i. the papillary dermis contains thin, haphazardly arranged collagen fibers, numerous reticular fibers, and delicate branching elastic fibers. There is abundant ground substance and numerous capillaries that extend from the superficial plexus.

      ii. the papillary dermis and the epidermis form a morphologic and functional unit. This is evident as the papillary dermis molds to the contour of the epidermal rete ridges. This relationship is seen in common inflammatory diseases when both areas show alteration.

d. Reticular dermis.

(1) The reticular dermis represents the bulk of the dermis. It:

(a) Extends from the base of the papillary dermis to the subcutaneous tissue.

(b) Carries most of the physical stress of the skin.

(c) Is characterized by thick collagen bundles arranged parallel to the skin surface. Coarse elastic fibers are found around collagen bundles.

(d) Is thicker than the capillary dermis. Proportionally, there are fewer reticular fibers, fibroblasts, and blood vessels and less ground substance in the reticular dermis, as compared to the papillary dermis.

E. **Cells in the dermis.**
1. Fibroblast.
    a. The principal cell of the dermis is the fibroblast. It produces collagen, elastic fibers, reticular fibers, and ground substance. Collagen fibrils are broken down and degraded by collagenase and gelatinase, both of which are also synthesized in the fibroblast.
    b. Fibroblasts have indistinct cytoplasm and spindle-shaped nuclei. They are found among and on the surface of fiber bundles.
2. Mast cell.
    a. Mast cells are secretory cells most commonly found near the superficial plexus and in the subcutaneous fat.
        (1) The cytoplasm of mast cells contain secretory and lysosomal granules. Mediators in the granules are produced that are either vasoactive, stimulate smooth muscle contraction, or function to attract neutrophils and eosinophils.
        (2) The secretory granules contain histamine and heparin.
        (3) The lysosomal granules are nonsecretory but degrade intracellular proteoglycans and complex glycolipids.
    b. Mast cells respond to a number of physical stimuli: light, cold, heat, acute trauma, vibration, and sustained pressure, as well as chemical and immunologic stimuli.
        (1) When stimulated, the mast cell releases histamine and heparin. Once released, vasodilation and dermal edema result.
        (2) Secondly, there is an infiltration of neutrophils, eosinophils, and basophils.
        (3) Immediate hypersensitivity reactions in the skin are due to mast cells.
        (4) Subacute and chronic inflammatory disease can also be related to the mast cell.
3. Macrophages.
    a. Originates in the bone marrow. It initially

circulates as a monocyte in the blood.
    b. Macrophages in the dermis function in the immune response.
    c. Langerhans' cells, along with macrophages, are capable of processing and presenting antigens to immunocompetent lymphocytes.
    d. Defend against microorganisms through phagocytosis.
    e. Important to wound healing cascade.
4. Histiocytes.
    a. Histiocytes are cells found in the dermis which function as scavengers. They engulf hemosiderin, melanin, lipid, and debris.

F. **Dermal vasculature.**
1. Superficial plexus.
    a. The superficial plexus (subpapillary plexus) courses at the junction of the papillary and reticular dermis. It supplies capillaries, end arterioles, and venules to the dermal papillae.
2. Deep plexus.
    a. The deep plexus is located in the base of the reticular dermis. The two plexuses are connected by blood vessels that run perpendicular to the skin surface. The communicating vessels originate from arteries and veins in the subcutaneous tissue.
3. Functions.
    a. Thermoregulation is the most important function of the skin's vascular system. Blood flow through the dermis varies in response to changes in the core temperature of the body, as well as the temperature of the external environment.
    b. Blood pressure: the cutaneous vasculature plays a role in blood pressure regulation. Sympathetic stimulation leads to a constriction of cutaneous blood vessels, thereby, reducing blood flow to the skin. This results in increased venous return, increased cardiac output, and increased blood pressure.
    c. Nutrition is also a function of the dermal vasculature. In the capillaries and venules, oxygen, water, nutrients, and hormones are distributed from the blood to the tissues. Carbon dioxide and other products of skin metabolism are diffused for transmission to the excretory organs.
    d. Inflammation: blood vessels in the dermis also play a role in inflammation. The microcirculatory units of the papillary dermis dilate in skin diseases characterized by erythema.

G. **Lymphatics.**
1. A lymphatic network is also found in the

Figure 4.
Vasculature of the Subcutaneous Tissue

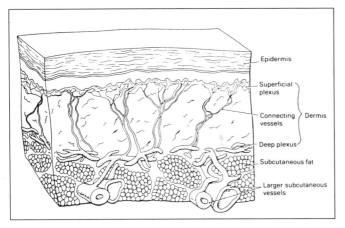

dermis. It parallels the vascular plexuses. The lymphatics act to filter and transport a large amount of capillary transudate or lymph, and return it back to the venous system.

H. Nerves.
1. Autonomic motor.
    a. Autonomic nerves are sympathetic in nature and can be divided into andrenergic and cholinergic fibers.
        (1) Adrenergic fibers regulate vasoconstriction, the apocrine gland, and arrector pili muscles.
        (2) Eccrine sweat secretion is controlled by cholinergic fibers.
2. Somatic sensory.
    a. Somatic sensory nerves are either free nerve endings or corpuscular receptors. Either together or alone they convey touch, pressure, pain, temperature, and itch from every part of the body.
        (1) There is variation in intensity of these senses at different parts of the body. This is because the density and type of receptors are regionally variable and specific.
    b. Corpuscular receptors: Meissner and Pacini corpuscles are two mechanoreceptors in the skin conveying touch and pressure. The Meissner corpuscles are found in the papillary dermis, especially on the palms and soles. Pacini corpuscles are located in the deeper dermis of weight-bearing surfaces.
    c. Free nerve endings: temperature, pain, and itch are transmitted by unmyelinated nerve fibers which terminate in the papillary dermis and around the hair follicles. These impulses are conveyed to the central nervous system through the dorsal root ganglion.

d. Dermatome: the sensory nerves are arranged in dermatomal patterns. A dermatome is the cutaneous area supplied by a single spinal nerve. On the trunk, the dermatomes are horizontal; on the arms and legs they are more vertical and irregularly distributed. Herpes zoster is an example of a disease in a dermatomal pattern.

I. Subcutaneous tissue (see Figure 4).
1. The third layer of the skin is the subcutaneous tissue. It consists of fat cells or lipocytes (adipocyte). The lobules are separated by fibrous walls (septa) of collagen and large blood vessels. Dermal collagen is continuous with the collagen found in the subcutaneous tissue.
2. The thickness of the subcutaneous tissue varies in different parts of the body. It is nearly absent in the eyelids, penis, scrotum, nipple, and overlying the tibia. It is thick in the waist, especially in middle-aged people. Distribution of subcutaneous tissue is controlled by circulating sex hormones, heredity, age, and eating habits.
3. The subcutaneous tissue has three main functions. It:
    a. Insulates the underlying tissue from extreme hot and cold.
    b. Functions as a mechanical shock absorber.
    c. Is a storehouse of energy (calories) used in times of nutritional deprivation.

III. APPENDAGES OF THE SKIN

A. Nail.
1. The nails are keratinized cells cemented together. They are of epidermal origin and are formed from metabolically active tissue. Nails serve as protective coverings for the distal aspects of the fingers and toes, and aide in picking up small objects. The cosmetic aspects of the nails are becoming increasingly important (see Chapter 18, Hair and Nails, for complete descriptions).

B. Hair (see Chapter 18, Hair and Nails, for complete descriptions).
1. Function.
    a. The hair on the human body serves no vital function, but it does have physiologic functions. These include:
        (1) Insulation.
        (2) Social and sexual display.
        (3) Camouflage.
        (4) Tactile perception.
        (5) Thermoregulation.
        (6) Protection from UV light.

2. Distribution.
   a. The entire body is covered by hair follicles except the palms, soles, interspaces of the digits, glans penis, clitoris, and mucocutaneous junctions.
   b. Most of the hair follicles of an adult are present at birth.
   c. As the body surface increases in size, the hair density decreases.

C. **Sebaceous glands.**
   1. Sebaceous glands are found on all areas of the body except the palms, soles, and dorsum of the feet.
   2. Their density varies markedly with location, being most numerous on the face, scalp, upper chest, and back.
   3. Most sebaceous glands are associated with hair follicles (pilosebaceous units). Exceptions to this are the sebaceous glands in the following:
      a. Buccal mucosa.
      b. Vermillion border of the lip.
      c. Areola.
      d. Prepuce.
      e. Eyelids.
   4. Embryonic development.
      a. Embryonically, sebaceous glands are formed as an outgrowth of the upper portion of the hair follicle. They are fully developed at birth and secrete much of the lipid of the vernix caseosa. They atrophy after birth until puberty. Sebaceous glands are usually larger in men than women.
   5. Anatomy.
      a. Germinative cells: sebaceous glands consist of one or more lobules of pale-staining cells called germinative cells. Differentiation of the germinative cells is similar to that of the keratinocyte in the epidermis. As the cells differentiate, lipid droplets accumulate, eventually filling the cytoplasm of the cell. These cells eventually rupture, discharging sebum into the sebaceous duct. Sebum is made up of cellular debris and lipids.
      b. Sebaceous duct: the sebaceous duct is the short, narrow, common excretory duct connecting several sebaceous lobules with the wider follicular infundibulum. This follicular canal is very wide throughout the entire length. It is filled not only with sebum, but keratinous materials, bacteria, and yeast.
   6. Hormonal effects.
      a. There are hormonal effects on the sebaceous gland.
         (1) Sebaceous gland development is one of the earliest signs of puberty. Androgens are the principal hormonal stimulus. Testicular androgens maintain sebum

production in the male and ovarian androgens in the female. Adrenal androgens also play a role.
         (2) Estrogen decreases the size of the sebaceous gland and decreases the production of sebum.
   7. Sebum production.
      a. The actual production of sebum varies in relation to age and sex.
         (1) It is low in children until the time of puberty.
         (2) In adults sebum production is higher in men than women.
         (3) In older men, production falls off slightly.
         (4) In women, production significantly decreases after 50 years of age.
   8. Functions.
      a. Functions of the sebaceous gland include:
         (1) Waterproofing of the hair and skin.
         (2) Promoting the absorption of fat-soluble substances.
         (3) Lubrication and possibly assistance in the synthesis of vitamin D.

D. **Apocrine gland.**
   1. The apocrine glands are found in the:
      a. Axilla.
      b. Umbilical region.
      c. Areolae.
      d. Anogenital region.
      e. External auditory canal (ceruminous gland).
      f. The eyelid (Moll's gland).
   2. Function.
      a. The apocrine gland in man has no proven function.
   3. Anatomy.
      a. Apocrine secretory gland.
         (1) The coiled secretory gland is located either in the lower dermis or in the subcutaneous tissue.
         (2) It consists of secretory cells and myoepithelial cells.
         (3) Collagen and elastic fibers are found in the surrounding dermis.
      b. Apocrine duct.
         (1) The apocrine duct is the straight duct that merges with the infundibular portion of the hair follicle.
         (2) The apocrine duct consists of an inner periluminal cuticle and two to three layers of cuboidal cells. It has no myoepithelial lining.
   4. Secretion composition.
      a. Apocrine gland secretions are milky in color, odorless, and sterile. The exact chemical consistency is uncertain as there is difficulty in obtaining uncontaminated specimens.

(1) Bacteria that are present in the infundibular canal of the hair follicle, as well as bacteria on the skin surface, act upon the apocrine secretion to produce odiferous substances.

(2) The odiferous substances contain, in part, short-chain fatty acids and ammonia.

(3) A moist environment, conducive for bacterial proliferations, is provided by the axillary eccrine gland.

5. Stimulation.
   a. The mode of secretion of the apocrine gland is assumed to be due to the contraction of the myoepithelial cells surrounding the secretory cells.
   b. Myoepithelial contraction and the resulting emptying of the secretory coil are induced by emotional stress that leads to sympathetic nervous discharge.
   c. The apocrine gland is stimulated by both epinephrine and norepinephrine.
   d. Once the gland has been emptied, a refractory period ensues until the secretory gland and duct refill.

E. **Eccrine sweat gland.**
   1. The eccrine sweat glands are present everywhere on the body except in the ear canal, glans penis, labia minora, prepuce, lips, and nail beds. They are concentrated on the palms and soles, head, trunk, and extremities.
      a. There are a total of two to five million eccrine sweat glands on the body.
      b. No new glands develop after birth.
      c. Each gland weighs approximately 30 to 40 mcg, the total mass equaling 100 gm.
   2. Anatomy.
      a. Eccrine duct: in the epidermis, the eccrine duct spirals on itself. It is lined by modified epidermal cells thought to be derived from upward migration of the dermal duct cells. There is a straight duct lying in the center of the dermis. The coiled segment of the duct is continuous with the secretary coil. It is approximately one-third the length of the coil.
         (1) The eccrine duct consists of two layers of cuboidal cells:
            (a) Luminal cells: the luminal cells have a periluminal filamentous zone comprising a dense layer of tonofilaments. This adds to the rigidity of the duct.
            (b) Basal ductal cells: the basal cells have increased mitochondria and Na-K-ATPase (pump) activity.
      b. Eccrine secretory coil: the secretory coil has a larger diameter than the duct and is 2 to 5 mm in length. It makes up one-half of the basal coil and lies in the lower one-third of the dermis, at the dermal subcutaneous border. The secretory coil consists of three types of cells:

      (1) The mucoid or dark cells secrete a dense granule glycoprotein.
      (2) The clear or secretory cells are generally believed to be responsible for water and electrolyte secretion. The ATP-dependent NA+ pump is located within this cell. Where two or more clear cells abut, intercellular canaliculi are formed which open into the lumen of the gland.
      (3) The myoepithelial cells lie between the secretory cells and the basement membrane. These add support to the gland. They do not expel sweat as do those in the apocrine glands.

   3. Stimulation.
      a. There are three types of stimuli that promote eccrine gland secretion.
         (1) Thermal is the most important stimulus. Sweating occurs over the trunk face and sometimes the entire body. The preoptic area of the anterior hypothalamus is the heat regulating center, and it responds to changes in the core temperature. Afferent input from skin temperature also controls thermal sweating, but is not as important as core temperature.
         (2) Mental stimuli usually cause sweating on the palms, soles, and axilla, but sometimes cause generalized sweating. The frontal region of the brain is involved, but the exact pathway is unknown.
         (3) Gustatory produces sweating seen after eating hot or spicy foods. It is controlled by an unknown pathway.

   4. Physiology of sweating.
      a. The physiology of sweating involves a complex process. Very basically, sweating begins in the clear secretory cells.
         (1) The intercellular canaliculi transports the solution secreted by the clear cells into the secretory coil. There is then reabsorption of sodium, chloride, and other electrolytes from the lumen of the duct.
         (2) The eccrine sweat is then secreted. It is an odorless, colorless, hypotonic solution. It has a specific gravity of approximately 1.005 and a pH between 4.5 and 5.5.
      b. Sweat contains:
         (1) Sodium.
         (2) Chloride.

(3) Potassium.
(4) Urea.
(5) Lactate.
(6) Bicarbonate.
(7) Ammonia.
(8) Calcium.
(9) Phosphorus.
(10) Magnesium.
(11) Iodine.
(12) Sulfate.
(13) Iron.
(14) Zinc.
(15) Amino acids.
(16) Proteins.
(17) Immunoglobins.
c. The sweat rate determines the concentration of the solutes.
(1) Increased rates of sweating produce sweat with high pH, increased concentrations of sodium and chloride, and decreased concentrations of potassium, lactate, and urea.
(2) Sweat lactate and urea may be important in controlling desquamation of the stratum corneum and may act as natural skin moisturizers.
(3) The body may produce sweat at the rate of 2 to 4 liters an hour. It may produce up to 12 liters in 24 hours.

IV. IMMUNOLOGY OF THE SKIN

A. **Humoral immunity.**
1. Humoral immunity is regulated by B-lymphocytes that, when stimulated by antigen, form plasma cells that produce antibodies.
2. Antibodies can be divided into five classes:
   a. Immunoglobulin G (IgG)
   b. Immunoglobulin A (IgA)
   c. Immunoglobulin M (IgM)
   d. Immunoglobulin D (IgD)
   e. Immunoglobulin E (IgE)
3. Antibodies, with varying degrees of efficiency can:
   a. Fix complement (IgG, IgM).
   b. Aid macrophages in cytotoxicity or cell killing and phagocytosis (IgG).
   c. Interact with antigen at mucosal surfaces (IgA).
   d. Trigger release of mediators from mast cells of immunoreactive (IgE).
4. Antibodies can react to self as well as foreign antigen to cause inflammation, which in the pathogenic state can be harmful.

B. **Cellular immunity.**
1. Cellular immunity involves T-lymphocytes.
2. T-lymphocytes divide into at least three subtypes:
   a. T-helper cells (CD4 cells).
      (1) T-helper cells activate B cells to produce antibody and activate T-cytotoxic cells.
      (2) Act as killer cells against invading organisms.
      (3) Can be classified as Th1 and Th2 based on cytokine profile.
      (4) Secrete cytokines that increase the number of T-cells, B-cells, natural killer cells and macrophages.
   b. T-cytotoxic cells (CD8).
      (1) T-cytotoxic cells kill target cells by binding with antigens on target cell.
      (2) Cause lysis of antigen-bearing cells.
   c. T-memory cells (CD45RO).
      (1) Play major role in inflammation seen in allergy and atopy.
      (2) Involved in contact and delayed hypersensitivity.
3. Much T-cell function is accomplished by production of soluble proteins called lymphokines.

C. **Complement system.**
1. A complex set of proteins that, when activated in the complement cascade can:
   a. Lyse cells.
   b. Aid in phagocytosis by macrophages.
   c. Cause mast cells to release histamines.
   d. Be chemotactic for neutrophils.
2. Complement can be activated by:
   a. Antibodies.
   b. Immune complexes through the classic pathway.
3. Complement can also be activated by:
   a. Bacteria.
   b. Fungi.
   c. Immunoglobulins and their fragments.
   d. Immune complexes.
   e. Lymphocytes.
   f. Endotoxins.

V. IMMUNITY AND SKIN DISEASE

A. **Diseases in the skin can be caused by an immune response in three ways, and in some skin diseases a combination of the three:**
1. Immune response to foreign antigen.
2. Response to self-antigen (autoimmunity).
3. Lack of appropriate immune response (immunodeficiency).

B. **Response to an antigen (either foreign or self) is divided into four types of hypersensitivity reactions, according to the Gel and Coombs' classification:**
1. Type I — allergic reaction.
   a. Anaphylaxis or immediate hypersensitivity.
   b. An IgE-mediated response.
2. Type II — cytotoxicity reaction.

a. Binding antibodies to cell membranes.
3. Type III — immune complex reaction.
   a. Mediated by circulating immune complexes.
4. Type IV — delayed reactions.
   a. Delayed hypersensitivity.
   b. Cell-mediated response.
   c. Immunodeficiency involves defects in any one or combination of the four types of immunity.

Bibliography
Charlesworth E.N., & Beck L. (1996). *Cutaneous allergy: The skin as an immune organ.* Cambridge, MA: Blackwell Science.
Parslow, T.G., Stites, D.P., Terr, A.I., & Imboden, J.B. (Eds.). (2001). *Medical immunology* (10th ed.). McGraw-Hill.
Chapel, H., Haeney, M., Misbah, S., & Snowden, N. (1999). *Essentials of clinical immunology* (4th ed.). Malden, MA: Blackwell Science.
Fitzpatrick, T.B., Eisen, A.Z., Wolff, K., Friedberg, I.M., & Austin, K.F. (Eds.). (1989). *Dermatology in general medicine* (3rd ed.). New York: McGraw-Hill.
Fleckman, P. (1985). Anatomy and physiology of the nail. *Dermatologic Clinics - The Nail, 3*(3).
Goldsmith. (1983). *Biochemistry and physiology of the skin.* Oxford: Oxford University Press.
Guyton, A. (1987). *Textbook of medical physiology* (5th ed.). Philadelphia: Saunders.
Habif, T. (1990). *Clinical dermatology - a color guide to diagnosis and therapy* (2nd ed.). St. Louis: Mosby.
Hill, M. (1990). The skin: Anatomy and physiology. *Dermatology Nursing, 2*(1), 13-17.
Moschella, S.L., & Sorenson, K. (1985). *Dermatology* (Vol. 2, 2nd ed.). Philadelphia: Saunders.
Thompson, J.M., McFarland, G.K., Hirsch, J.E., Tucker, S.M., & Bowers, A.C. (1986). *Clinical nursing.* St. Louis: Mosby.

1. The outermost layer of the skin is the:
    a. Basal cell layer.
    b. Stratum lucidum.
    c. Horny cell layer.
    d. Granular cell layer.
    e. Prickle cell layer.

2. Body temperature is controlled by:
    a. Evaporation.
    b. Radiation.
    c. Convection.
    d. a & c.
    e. a, b & c.

3. Functions of the dermis include:
    a. Prevention of mechanical trauma.
    b. Thermoregulation.
    c. Maintenance of homeostasis.
    d. a & c.
    e. a, b, & c.

4. Functions of the skin include:
    a. Temperature regulation.
    b. Wound repair.
    c. Vitamin D production.
    d. Sensory perception.
    e. a, b, c, & d.

5. Melanin production is not controlled by:
    a. Number of melanocytes.
    b. Genetics.
    c. Hormones.
    d. Environment.
    e. Any of the above.

6. The principal cell of the epidermis is the:
    a. Keratinocyte
    b. Macrophage.
    c. Mast cell.
    d. Fibroblast.
    e. None of the above.

7. Type 1 hypersensitivity classically involves which of the following:
    a. IgM.
    b. IgE.
    c. Mast cells.
    d. Macrophages.
    e. IgD.

Answers to Study Questions

1.	e	5.	a
2.	e	6.	a
3.	d	7.	b
4.	e		

CE Answer/Evaluation Form

Chapter 1.
Anatomy and Physiology of the Skin

Please photocopy this test page and return.

COMPLETE THE FOLLOWING:

Name: _____

Address: _____

City: _____ State: _____ Zip: _____

Preferred telephone: (Home)_____ (Work) _____

State where licensed and license number: _____

CE application fee: DNA member $10.00
                       Nonmember $13.00

POSTTEST INSTRUCTIONS

1. To receive continuing education credit for individual study after reading the article, complete the answer/evaluation form below.
2. Photocopy and send the answer/evaluation form along with a check or money order payable to **Dermatology Nurses' Association** to: **DNA**, East Holly Avenue Box 56, Pitman, NJ 08071-0056.
3. Test returns must be postmarked by December 31, 2008. Upon completion of the answer/evaluation form, a certificate for 3.0 contact hour(s) will be awarded and sent to you.

This chapter was reviewed and formatted for contact hour credit by Marcia J. Hill, MSN, RN, Core Curriculum Editor; and Sally Russell, MN, RN,C, DNA Education Director.

ANSWER FORM

1. Name one new detail (item, issue, or phenomenon) that you learned by completing this activity.

    _____

    _____

    _____

2. How will you apply the information from this learning activity to your practice?
    a. Patient education.
    b. Staff education.
    c. Improve my patient care.
    d. In my education course work.
    e. Other: Please describe _____

    _____

Evaluation

	Strongly disagree				Strongly agree
3. The offering met the stated objectives.					
a. Define the functions of the skin.	1	2	3	4	5
b. List the layers of the skin.	1	2	3	4	5
c. List specialized cells in the epidermis and dermis.	1	2	3	4	5
d. Delineate the functions of the glands of the skin.	1	2	3	4	5
4. The content was current and relevant.	1	2	3	4	5
5. The content was presented clearly.	1	2	3	4	5
6. The content was covered adequately.	1	2	3	4	5
7. I am more confident of my abilities since completing this material.	1	2	3	4	5

8. The material was (check one) ☐ new, ☐ review for me.

Comments _____

_____

9. Time required to complete reading assignment: _____ minutes

This independent study is provided by the Dermatology Nurses' Association (DNA) for 3.0 contact hours. DNA is accredited as a provider of continuing education in nursing by the American Nurses Credentialing Center's Commission on Accreditation. DNA is approved as a provider of continuing education by the California Board of Registered Nursing Provider #CEP5708.

CHAPTER TWO

Skin Assessment and Diagnostic Techniques

Lauren L. Johannsen, RN
Anne Marie Ruszkowski, BSN, RN, DNC

OBJECTIVES

At the end of this chapter, the reader will be able to:

- Identify what subjective and objective data are necessary for a diagnosis.
- Recognize the appropriate terminology used for primary and secondary lesions.
- Determine how lesion location and distribution help indicate specific diagnoses.
- Identify various diagnostic methods available for use during assessments.
- Recognize which surgical treatment option is optimal and choose a favorable method of documentation.

KEY POINTS

- The history given by the patient (subjective data) and the findings of the physical exam (objective data) give the majority of information needed to make a diagnosis.
- Using proper dermatologic vocabulary when assessing patients gives the physician a better understanding of the patient's problem.
- During the assessment, don't underestimate the significance of pruritus, or the changes in the hair and nails.
- Various in-office tests can help diagnose specific diseases.
- Being familiar with surgical options, how they are performed, and their potential for scarring is advantageous when teaching patients.

Skin Assessment and Diagnostic Techniques
Part I. Skin Assessment

Lauren L. Johannsen, RN

I. OVERVIEW (see Table 1)

The physical assessment of the skin consists of a general inspection and a lesion-specific exam. To insure the physical assessment is done in a systematic way, the general inspection should precede the lesion-specific exam. The general examination of the skin considers normal variants and general changes in the skin. A wide range of normal variations exist in the skin. These may be due to age, genetic factors, and environmental influences.

General changes can alter color (jaundice, cyanosis, pallor), turgor, thickness, temperature, and vascularity (purpura, petechiae, flushing). General findings can suggest a possible association with systemic disease. The lesion-specific examination follows the general assessment and also requires a systematic approach. A good exam requires "visual literacy." Natural lighting in the exam room improves visualization of most skin changes.

Lesions can be defined as primary or secondary. Primary lesions are structural changes in the skin that have specific, visual characteristics and develop without any preceding skin changes. A lesion that has changed due to natural progression or due to physical change is a secondary lesion. Special, or "other" lesions are those that occur in the skin only, in the skin most often, or can be perceived most easily on the skin.

Specific terminology is used to describe the characteristics of skin lesions (color, configuration, distribution, type of lesion, and the lesion pattern which can then be documented) (see Tables 2 & 3). These descriptive clues aid in diagnosing and managing the patient by doctors and nurses. It is important to use generally accepted descriptive terminology for verbal and written documentation to ensure continuity. It assists health care providers interpret the findings.

II. PATIENT HISTORY (Subjective Data)

A. Begin a patient history using the patient's own words regarding his/her skin condition. This gives the nurse a sense of direction as to which triage questions to ask (see Table 4).

B. Information regarding other family members with similar symptoms, past medical history, previous and current drug therapy (including herbs, vitamins, and over-the-counter medications), occupation, and social history are all important parts of the initial interview.

   1. Conditions such as psoriasis, eczema, or even

Table 1.
Structure of Well Skin

Epidermis	Function	Cellular Layers
Pain receptors	Water loss barrier	Stratum corneum
Touch receptors	Sensory organ	Stratum lucidum (on palms and soles only)
Keratin production	Ultraviolet protection	Stratum granulosum
Melanin production	Infection barrier	Stratum spinosum
Immune system afferent limb	Excretion	Stratum germinativum
Dermis		
Temperature receptors	Temperature regulation	Papillary dermis
Deep pressure and touch receptors	Immunoregulatory function	Reticular dermis
Hair shaft and follicles	Vitamin D production	Connective tissue and collagen bundles
Lymphatic vessels	Integument strength	
Sebaceous and sweat glands	Elastic tone	
Nerves		
Arrector pili muscles		
Subcutaneous Fat Layer		**Considered Continuation of Dermal Layer**
Bulb and matrix of hair follicle	Insulation	Adipose tissue
Larger arteries and veins	Shock absorption	Loose connective tissue
Pleuripotential cells	Energy storage and fat metabolism	
	Body topography	

Table 2.
Labeling of Skin Lesions by Configuration and Distribution

Configuration	—	The arrangement or pattern of lesions in relation to other lesions
Distribution	—	The arrangement of lesions over an area of skin
Annular	—	Ring-shaped
Iris lesions	—	Concentric rings; "Bulls eyes"
Gyrate	—	Ring spiral shape
Linear	—	In a line
Nummular, Discoid	—	Coin-like
Polymorphous	—	Occurring in several forms
Punctate	—	Marked by points or dots
Serpiginous	—	Snake-like
Solitary	—	A single lesion
Satellite	—	Single lesion in close proximity to a large grouping
Grouped	—	Cluster lesions
Confluent	—	Merging together
Diffuse	—	Widely distributed, spreading
Discrete	—	Separate from other lesions
Generalized	—	Distributed diffusely
Localized	—	Limited areas of involvement which are defined clearly
Symmetrical or Asymmetrical	—	Distributed bilaterally or unilaterally
Zosteriform	—	Band-like distributions along dermatome

Table 3.
Special Lesions/Other

Telangiectasias	—	Permanently dilated superficial vessels.
Petechia	—	Hemorrhages from superficial blood vessels, less than 5 mm.
Purpura	—	Hemorrhages from superficial blood vessels, 5 mm to 5 cm.
Ecchymosis	—	Bleeding into the tissue affecting large areas.
Lichenification	—	Thickening of the skin with exaggerated markings due to prolonged rubbing or scratching.
Induration	—	Dermal hypertrophy causing the skin to become thicker and firmer. The skin markings remain unchanged.
Sclerosis	—	Circumscribed or diffuse hardening or induration of the skin resulting from dermal or subcutaneous edema, cellular infiltration or collagen proliferation.
Maceration	—	Thickening and whitening of the horny cell layer caused by excessive moisture.
Excoriation	—	A linear or "dug out" traumatized area, usually self-inflicted.
Cyst	—	A sac containing liquid or semisolid material.
Furuncle	—	Deep form of folliculitis with pus accumulation.
Abscess	—	Localized accumulation of purulent material deep within the dermis.
Burrow	—	A characteristic linear lesion caused by tunneling in the stratum corneum produced by an animal parasite.
Comedo	—	Mass of keratin and sebum within the dilated orifice of a hair follicle.

keratosis pilaris have a genetic tendency. Patients may claim another family member shares similar symptoms.

2. The past medical history is significant, for example, if the patient presents with diffuse hair loss, or perhaps an unusual rash that may be due to an unresolved strep infection.

3. When obtaining information regarding current drug therapy or medicines recently used, don't overlook topicals, systemic steroids, alcohol, or home and over-the-counter remedies.

4. Consider an occupational skin disease when patients have symptoms that improve over a weekend or resolve while on vacation.

5. Social and psychological factors in a patient's life may influence whether or not he/she will have a favorable or unfavorable response to treatment of a chronic skin disease. If, for example, the person prefers the added attention and sympathy the condition brings, improvement may be slow.

Table 4.
Sample Triage Questions

How long has it been there?
Does it itch?
What are you using on it?
When did it start?
What did it first look like?
Has it changed?
Have you been out of the country lately?
Does it come and go?
Have you recently started any changes in your daily medicines?
Have you recently started any new medicines?
Any history of similar symptoms?
Do any family members have the same or similar symptoms?
Have you used or done anything that seems to make it better?

Table 5.
Normal Findings

Areas of Concern	Normal Adult Findings	Variations in Children	Variations in Older Adults
Skin Color tone	Deep to light brown in blacks; whitish pink to ruddy with olive or yellow overtones in whites.	Newborn reddish first 8 to 24 hours, then pale pink with transparent tone; slight jaundice starting 2nd or 3rd day of life; mottled appearance of hands and feet in newborns disappears with warming; in black newborns melanotic pigmentation not intense with exception of nail beds and scrotom.	Skin of white persons tends to look paler and more opaque.
Uniformity	Sun-darkened areas; areas of lighter pigmentation in dark-skinned persons (palms, lips, nail beds); labile pigmentation areas associated with use of hormones or pregnancy; callused areas appear yellow; crinkled skin areas darker (knees and elbows); dark-skinned (Mediterranean origin) persons may have lips with bluish hue; vascular flush areas (cheeks, neck, upper chest, or genital area) may appear red, especially with excitement or anxiety; skin color masked through use of cosmetics or tanning agents.	Upper and lower extremities similar in color.	More freckles; uneven tanning; pigment deposits; hypopigmented patches.
Moisture	Minimum perspiration or oiliness felt; dampness in skin folds; increased perspiration associated with warm environment of activity; wet palms, scalp, forehead, and axilla associated with anxiety.	Perspiration present in all children over 1 month of age.	Increased dryness, especially of extremities; decreased perspiration.
Surface temperature	Cool to warm.		
Texture	Smooth, even, soft; some roughness on exposed areas (elbows and soles of feet).	Smooth, soft, flexible, dryness and flakiness of skin in infants less than 1 month of age (shedding of vernix caseosa), may appear as white cheesy skin; presence of milia; small white papules over nose and cheeks (plugged sebaceous glands) may remain for 2 months.	Flaking and scaling associated with dry skin, especially on lower extremeties.
Thickness	Wide body variation, increased thickness in areas of pressure or rubbing (hands and feet).	Varying degrees of adipose tissue; dimpling of skin over joint areas.	Thinner skin, especially over dorsal surface of hands and feet, forearms, lower legs, and bony prominences.

Table 5. (continued)
Normal Findings

Areas of Concern	Normal Adult Findings	Variations in Children	Variations in Older Adults
Turgor	Skin moves easily when lifted and returns to place immediately when released.	Skin moves easily when lifted but falls quickly when released; skin over extremities taut.	General loss of elasticity; skin moves easily when lifted but does not return to place immediately when released; skin appears lax; increased wrinkle pattern more marked in sun-exposed areas, in fair skin, and in expressive areas of face; pendulous parts sag or droop (under chin, earlobes, breasts, and scrotum).
Hygiene	Clean, free of odor.		
Alterations	Striae (stretch marks) usually silver or pinkish; freckles (prominent in sun-exposed areas); some birthmarks.	Cafe'-au-lait spots (light, cream-colored spots on darkened back-ground); some nevi; stork bites (small red or pink spots on back of neck, upper lip, or upper eyelid; usually disappear by 5 years of age).	Nevi often become lighter or disappear, seborreic keratoses (pigmented raised, warty, slightly greasy lesions most often found on trunk or face); senile (actinic) keratoses on exposed surfaces, first seen as small reddened areas and then as raised, rough, yellow to brown lesions; senile sebaceous adenomas (yellowish flat papules with central depressions); cherry adenomas (tiny, bright, ruby red, round); may become brown with age.
Nails Configuration	Nail edges smooth and rounded; nail base angle 160 degrees; nail surface flat or slightly curved.	Nails generally longer than wide.	Toenails may be thickened and distorted.
Consistency	Smooth, hard surface; uniform thickness.	Soft nails in infants and small children; become hardened with age; vernix may be found under nails of newborns.	Fingernails may be more brittle or may peel.
Color	Variations of pink; pigment deposits in nail beds of dark-skinned individuals.	Postmature infants may show yellow staining.	Toenails may lose translucence and luster and may become yellow.
Adherence to nail bed	Nail base feels firm when palpated.		
Hair Surface characteristics	Scalp smooth; hair shiny; vellus hair short, fine, inconspicuous, and unpigmented; terminal hair coarser, thicker, more conspicuous, and usually pigmented.	Scalp smooth and soft.	Sebaceous hyperplasia may extend into scalp.

Dermatologic Nursing Essentials: A Core Curriculum 2nd Edition © DNA 2003

Table 5. (continued)
Normal Findings

Areas of Concern	Normal Adult Findings	Variations in Children	Variations in Older Adults
Distribution and configuration	"Normal" varies with individual; hair present on scalp, lower face, nares, ears, axillae, anterior chest around nipples, arms, legs, back, buttocks; female pubic configuration is upright triangle with hair extending up linea alba; male public configuration is upright triangle with hair extending up linea alba umbilicus.	Newborn displays lanugo (fine hair over body, mostly over shoulders and back; will disappear during first 3 months of life); pubic hair begins to develop between 8 and 12 years old; smooth hair at first, changing to coarse, curly hair, followed approximately 6 months later by facial hair in boys.	Increased facial hair (especially in women), bristly quality; men may have coarse hair in ears, nose, and eyebrows; decreasd scalp hair; symmetric balding in men (most often frontal or occipital); decreased pubic and axillary hair.
Texture	Scalp hair may be fine or coarse; fine vellus hair over body; coarse terminal hair pubic and axillary areas.	Scalp hair soft and fine; as child grows, hair takes on adult characteristic.	Facial hair coarse; body hair fine.
Color	Wide variation from pale to black; color may be masked or changed with rinses or dyes.	Irregularity of pigmentation.	Graying; whitening; hairs that do not lose pigment often become darker.
Quantity	"Normal" varies with individuals; gradual symmetric balding of scalp hair in some men.		General disease of body and scalp hair.

From Thompson, June M., et al. (1989). *Mosby's manual of clinical nursing* (2nd ed.). St. Louis: The C.V. Mosby Co.; modified from Borners, A., & Thompson, J. (1984). *Clinical manual of health assessment.* St. Louis: The C.V. Mosby Co.

III. VISUAL EXAM (Objective Data) (see Table 5)

A. Using a good source of light is the best way to effectively examine the skin (and mouth). There are many dermatologic maladies where examining the patient from head to toe is both necessary and beneficial.

B. Examinations should be done in an orderly manner to insure important diagnostic clues are not missed. Don't overlook the hair, nails, and mouth.

C. Include gentle palpation of lesion areas to distinguish diagnostic characteristics.
   1. Palpable lesions can be located in the epidermis, or extend deep in to the dermis or subcutaneous tissue.
   2. Papules, nodules, and tumors may be smooth or rough, soft or firm, fixed or movable.
   3. Manipulation may elicit tenderness or detect localized heat.

D. Alterations in normal skin color are best observed on the lips, ear lobes, oral mucous membranes, nails (fingers and toes), and extremities.
   1. Natural skin color variances occur not only with the amount of melanin present in the skin but also the blood supply (from pallor to flush).
   2. Abnormal conditions of hypopigmentation or hyperpigmentation may be seen in all skin colors.

E. Skin temperature depends upon the amount of vasoconstriction or vasodilation. Whereby localized inflammation causes dilatation of blood vessels and heat sensation, vasoconstriction occurs as the body tries to conserve heat.

F. When assessing for abnormality, evaluate the skin for moisture, turgor, texture, and elasticity.

G. The pattern, distribution, texture, and quality of hair on both the scalp and body are indicators of a person's general state of health.

H. Nails change with age and ill health. Pale nailbeds can indicate circulatory impedance, whereas red inflamed nail cuticles can be a sign of psoriasis, or even bacterial or fungal infection.

IV. PRIMARY LESIONS (see Table 6)

Primary lesions are caused directly by the disease process. Pay attention to the shape, morphology, distribution, and quality of the lesion(s). Also

Table 6.
Primary Skin Lesions

A primary lesion is a visually recognized structural change in the skin. It has specific characteristics and develops without any preceding skin change.

Primary Skin Lesions Description	Differential Diagnosis	Differential Diagnosis

Macule
A circumscribed, flat discoloration, which may be brown, blue, red, or hypopigmented.
	Brown
	    Becker's nevus
	    Cafe'-au-lait spot
	    Erythrasma
	    Fixed drug eruption
	    Freckle
	    Junction nevus
	    Lentigo
	    Lentigo maligna
	    Melasma
	    Photoallergic drug eruption
	    Phototoxic drug eruption
	    Stasis dermatitis
	    Tinea nigra palmaris
	Blue
	    Ink (tattoo)
	    Maculae ceruleae (lice)
	    Mongolian spot
	    Ochronosis
		Red
		    Drug eruptions
		    Juvenile rheumatoid arthritis
		        (Still's disease)
		    Rheumatic fever
		    Secondary syphilis
		    Viral exanthems
		Hypopigmented
		    Idiopathic guttate hypomelanosis
		    Nevus anemicus
		    Piebaldism
		    Postinflammatory psoriasis
		    Radiation dermatitis
		    Tinea versicolor
		    Tuberous sclerosis

Papule
An elevated solid lesion up to 0.5 cm in diameter; color varies; papules may become confluent and form plaques.
	Flesh colored, yellow, or white
	    Adenoma sebaceum
	    Basal cell epithelioma
	    Closed comedones (acne)
	    Flat warts
	    Granuloma annulare
	    Lichen nitidus
	    Lichen sclerosis et atrophicus
	    Milium
	    Molluscum contagiosum
	    Nevi (dermal)
	    Neurofibroma
	    Pearly penile papules
	    Sebaceous hyperplasia
	    Skin tags
	    Syringoma
	
	Brown
	    Dermatofibroma
	    Keratosis follicularis
	    Melanoma
	    Nevi
	    Seborrheic keratosis
	    Urticaria pigmentosa
	    Warts
		Red
		    Acne
		    Atopic dermatitis
		    Cholingeric urticaria
		    Chondrodermatitis nodularis
		        chronic helicus
		    Eczema
		    Folliculitis
		    Insect bites
		    Keratosis pilaris
		    Leukocytoclastic vasculitis
		    Miliaria
		    Polymorphic light eruption
		    Psoriasis
		    Scabies
		    Urticaria
		
		Blue or violaceous
		    Angiokeratoma
		    Blue nevus
		    Lichen planus
		    Lymphoma
		    Kaposi's sarcoma
		    Melanoma
		    Mycosis fungoides
		    Venous lake

Plaque A circumscribed, elevated, super-ficial, solid lesion more than 0.5 cm in diameter, often formed by the confluence of papules.	**Eczema** Mycosis fungoides Papulosquamous (papular and scaling) lesions Discoid lupus erythematosus Lichen planus Pityriasis rosea Psoriasis	

Table 6. (continued)
Primary Skin Lesions

Primary Skin Lesions Description	Differential Diagnosis	Differential Diagnosis
	Eczema Seborrheic dermatitis Syphilis (secondary) Tinea corporis Tinea versicolor	
Nodule A circumscribed, elevated, solid lesion more that 0.5 cm in diameter; a large nodule is referred to as a tumor.	Basal cell carcinoma Erythema nodosum Furuncle Hemangioma Kaposi's sarcoma Keratoacanthoma Lipoma Lymphoma Melanoma	Metastatic carcinoma Mycosis fungoides Neurofibromatosis Prurigo nodularis Sporotrichosis Squamous cell carcinoma Warts Xanthoma
Wheal A firm edematous plaque resulting from infiltration of the dermis with fluid; wheals are transient and may last only a few hours.	Angioedema Dermatographism Hives Insect bites Urticaria pigmentosa (mastocytosis)	
Pustule A circumscribed collection of leukocytes and free fluid that varies in size.	Acne Candidiasis Dermatophyte infection Dyshidrosis Folliculitis Gonococcemia Hidradenitis suppurativa	Herpes simplex Herpes zoster Impetigo Psoriasis Pyoderma gangrenosum Rosacea Varicella
Vesicle A circumscribed collection of free fluid up to 0.5 cm in diameter.	Herpes simplex Herpes zoster Contact dermatitis Dyshidrosis Impetigo Chicken pox	
Bulla A circumscribed collection of free fluid more that 0.5 cm in diameter.	Bullous pemphigoid Pemphigus vulgaris	Bullous impetigo Bullous lichen planus

Reproduced with permission from Habif, T.P. (1996). *Clinical dermatology: A color guide to diagnosis and therapy* (3rd ed.) (pp. 3-11). St. Louis: Mosby-Yearbook, Inc.

important is an accurate and precise description of the evolution of the disease condition. Some common descriptive terms follow.

A. Macule — A circumscribed, flat discoloration that varies widely in size, color, and shape. Examples are a freckle, vitiligo spot, or petechiae. A macule cannot be palpated.

B. Papule — A solid, elevated palpable lesion on the skin that is usually less than 1 cm. It is round and sometimes pointed, usually red but can be white, yellow, brown, or black. Examples are measles, eczema, and acne lesions.

C. Nodule — A solid palpable mass that is larger than 1 cm. Sometimes considered a small tumor, nodules are located in the epidermis or extend deeper to the dermis or subcutaneous tissue.

Table 7.
Secondary Skin Lesions
A secondary lesion is a lesion that has changed due to its natural evolution or due to physical
change (scratching, irritation, or secondary infection).

Secondary Skin Lesions Description	Differential Diagnosis
Scales Excess dead epidermal cells that are produced by abnormal keratinization and shedding.	**Fine to stratified** Erythema craquele Ichthyosis (quadrangular) Lupus erythematosus (carpet tack) Pityriasis rosea (collarette) Psoriasis (silvery) Scarlet fever (fine, on trunk) Seborrheic dermatitis Syphilis (secondary) Tinea (dermatophytes) Xerosis (dry skin) **Scaling in sheets** Scarlet fever (hands and feet) Staphyloccal scalded skin syndrome
Crusts A collection of dried serum and cellular debris; a scab.	Acute eczematous inflammation Atopic (face) Impetigo (honey colored) Pemphigus foliaceus Tinea capitis
Erosions A focal loss of epidermis; erosions do not penetrate below the dermo-epidermal junction and therefore heal without scarring.	Candidiasis Dermatophyte infection Eczematous diseases Intertrigo Petieche Senile skin Toxic epidermal necrolysis Vesiculobullous diseases
Ulcers A focal loss of epidermis and dermis; ulcers heal with scarring.	Aphthae Chancroid Decubitus Factitial Ischemic Necrobiosis lipoidica diabeticorum Neoplasms Pyoderma gangrenosum Radiodermatitis Syphilis (chancre) Stasis ulcers
Fissure A linear loss of epidermis and dermis with sharply defined, nearly vertical walls.	Chapping (hands, feet) Eczema (fingertip) Intertrigo Petieche
Atrophy A depression in the skin resulting from thinning of the epidermis or dermis.	Aging Dermatomyositis Discoid lupus erythematosus Lichen sclerosis et atrophicus Morphea

Dermatologic Nursing Essentials: A Core Curriculum 2nd Edition © DNA 2003

Table 7. (continued)
Secondary Skin Lesions

Atrophy	Necrobiosis lipoidica diabeticorum Radiodermatitis Striae Topical and intralesional steroids
Scar An abnormal formation of connective tissue implying dermal damage; after injury or surgery scars are initially thick and pink but with time become white and atrophic	Acne Burns Herpes zoster Hidradenitis suppurativa Porphyria Varicella

Reproduced with permission from Habif, T.P. (1996). *Clinical dermatology: A color guide to diagnosis and therapy* (3rd ed.), pp. 12-16. St. Louis: Mosby-Yearbook, Inc.

Examples are keratoacanthomas, verrucae, or some malignant melanoma lesions.

D. Plaque — A slightly raised lesion that covers more than 1 cm of surface skin. Often formed by closely clustered papules, as seen in psoriasis, lichen planus, or mycosis fungoides.

E. Wheal — Firm, edematous plaque resulting from infiltration of the dermis with fluid. Wheals are transient and usually a response to an allergen. Sizes usually range from 3 mm to 12 cm. An allergic response to an insect bite or hives are examples of small and large wheals.

F. Vesicle — A round, raised lesion containing clear or purulent fluid that is less than 0.5 cm. They are either sparsely scattered or specifically grouped. Some examples are impetigo, herpes zoster, and chicken pox lesions.

G. Bulla — This is simply a vesicle that is larger than 0.5 cm. Mostly superficial in nature, it ruptures easily. A bulla may be seen in many blistering diseases.

H. Pustule — Whitish or yellowish elevations of the skin filled with purulent exudate. These, for example, are seen in acne vulgaris or folliculitis.

I. Cyst — A closed sac or pouch within the epidermal, dermal, or subcutaneous layers containing either liquid or semi-solid material. Soft or firm, and usually movable, cysts remain stationary but vary in size. Examples include cystic acne and epidermal inclusion cysts.

J. Comedo — A plug of sebum and keratin at the pilosebaceous opening that occurs when the material can not escape through the follicular opening. Comedo is seen commonly in acne, and described as either open or closed. An open comedo known as a "blackhead" contains keratin and bacteria. The follicular neck is open and has a ballooned-out appearance. The closed comedo, or "whitehead," contains keratin and the neck of the follicle is narrow.

K. Burrow — A linear trail or tunnel in the skin produced by parasites. Burrows may be seen in scabies infestation.

V. SECONDARY LESIONS (see Table 7)

This is the patient's response to a disease process. Types of secondarily produced lesions include:

A. Scale — Accumulated dry or greasy laminated keratin that range from fine and delicate as in pityriasis rosea, to coarse and sheet-like as that found in exfoliative dermatitis. Psoriatic scale appears silvery when air is trapped between the layers.

B. Crust — A scab made of dried masses of serum, bacteria, and possibly blood, mixed with epithelial debris that is covering damaged skin. They vary in size, thickness, and color depending upon the cause and location.

C. Fissures — Linear cracks in the epidermis, caused mainly by injury or disease. Excessive dryness of the skin may also cause this lesion. They vary in size from a tiny crack to a cleft several centimeters in length. The hands, toes, and angles of the mouth are most commonly affected.

D. Lichenification — A condition of epidermal thickening caused by long-term rubbing or scratching. Underlying inflammation often gives a dark red appearance to the skin. Patient's with neurodermatitis will have lichenified areas.

E. Erosion — A temporary loss or break in the epidermis, that unless secondarily infected will heal without a scar. Appearing as a slightly depressed, moist lesion it extends only as deep as the basal layer. Examples of erosions are a

scraped knee or elbow.
F. **Ulcer** — A deep erosion that extends through the epidermis down into the dermis. This type of lesion is likely to scar. The cause and location of the ulcer influence the size and type of discharge produced.
G. **Excoriation** — A superficial linear erosion caused by excessive scratching. Usually self-induced and seen in pruritic conditions, such as patients with eczema, neurodermatitis, and scabies. Fingernails are most commonly used to relieve the itch, so infection is common.
H. **Scar** — A normal result of skin regeneration when the corium or deeper skin elements have been interrupted due to injury or disease. Scars are usually smooth, firm, and appear white over time. Over-production of collagen during the healing process produces a red, raised thickened scar known as a keloid. Burn scars frequently keloid. The opposite can occur when sclerosing of the skin causes an indented atrophic scar seen in severe inflamed cystic acne.
I. **Atrophy** — A thinning of the superficial skin layers or deeper dermal layers most commonly after injury or inflammation. The skin develops a transparent localized indentation. Some examples are post pregnancy stretch marks or healed lesions in patients with chronic discoid lupus.
Note: Refer to Figure 1 for evaluation of a primary lesion into a secondary lesion.

VI. LESION DETAILS THAT HELP DIAGNOSE

Evaluate the distribution, shape, arrangement, and color of the lesion(s). The earliest lesion and the arrangement of the lesions in relation to each other are valuable diagnostic clues.
A. Consider the number of lesions. Are they few or numerous? Are they localized in one spot or one region? The lesions may be generalized or universal involving the hair and nails as well.
 1. Some lesions affect only one side of the body and follow nerve tracts.
 2. Sometimes a lesion has a ringed, crescent, or linear-shaped pattern.
 3. Lesion location is important because some diseases only affect specific areas of the skin. For example, acne most often occurs on the face, chest, and back because of the sebaceous glands; whereas eczema is usually found in the antecubital fossa and posterior knees.
    a. Lesions under a watchband, necklace, or ring might signify a nickel sensitivity.
    b. An eruption isolated where skin is exposed to direct sunlight could likely indicate a polymorphic light eruption.
    c. A rash on the "blush" areas of the face

might indicate rosacea, if the history coincides.
    d. Lesions at the openings of hair follicles on the backs of upper arms would likely signify keratosis pilaris.
B. The shape and the word used to describe the shape of the lesion sometimes coincide with the diagnosis. The first four below are all words for round lesions.
 1. Circinate — circular lesions seen in the herald patch of pityriasis rosea.
 2. Annular — ring shaped with active elevated margins that spread peripherally and regress centrally, seen in granuloma annulare.
 3. Discoid — disk shaped seen in discoid lupus erythematosus.
 4. Nummular — coin shaped, found in nummular eczema.
 5. Linear — in a line as seen in Rhus dermatitis.
 6. Arciform — arc shape with an incomplete circle as found in mycosis fungoides.
 7. Guttate — resembling a drop.
 8. Iris lesion or "bull's eye" lesion which has an erythematous annular macule or papule with a purplish papular or vesicular center.
 9. Herpetiform — in a grouping.
 10. Reticulated — having a net-like appearance.
 11. Confluent — blending together with adjacent lesions.
C. Lesion color is a helpful diagnostic aid, but may be confusing also since everyone's perception of color is different. A few basic shades are listed below:
 1. Brown — seen with increased epidermal melanin pigmentation.
 2. Yellow — lipid skin lesions such as xanthomas.
 3. Orange — accumulated carotene in the dermis.
 4. Purplish-red — extravasation of blood in the dermis.
 5. Blue-black — seen in cellular blue nevi.
D. The condition of lesions can be determined by using a scoring system called the **Overall Lesion Severity (OLS) scale (see Table 8).**
 1. The score selected is one that best describes the overall appearance of the lesion
 2. Scores range from 0 (clear) to 5 (very severe).
 3. Criteria for scoring are plaque elevation, erythema, and scale.
 4. Not all lesions will have all three characteristics, so use plaque elevation as the main evaluating factor.

VII. HAIR AND NAILS AS DIAGNOSTIC INDICATORS

Changes in a person's hair and nails are not necessarily indicative of a disease process. Limited to the skin, changes may be important diagnostic indicators of overall health.

Figure 1.
Evolution of Primary Lesion into Secondary Lesion

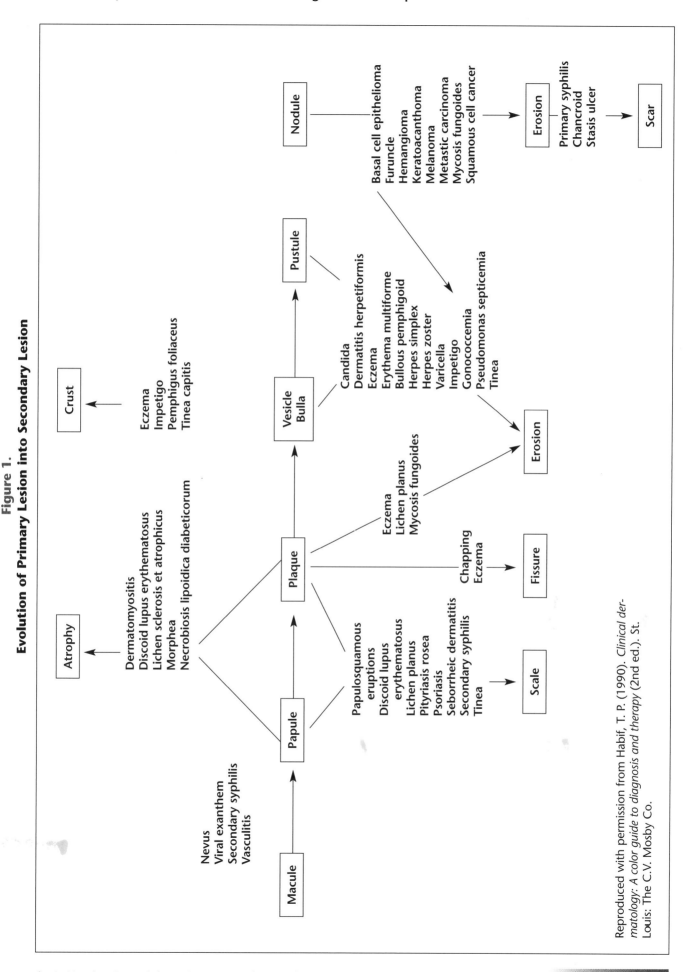

Reproduced with permission from Habif, T. P. (1990). *Clinical dermatology: A color guide to diagnosis and therapy* (2nd ed.). St. Louis: The C.V. Mosby Co.

Table 8.
Overall Lesion Severity (OLS) Scale

The degree of overall lesion severity will be evaluated using the following categories:

Score	Category	Category Description
0	Clear	Plaque elevation = 0 (no elevation over normal skin) Scaling = 0 (no scale) Erythema = ± (hyperpigmentation, pigmented macules, diffuse faint pink or red coloration)
1	Minimal	Plaque elevation = ± (possible but difficult to ascertain whether there is a slight elevation above normal skin) Scaling = ± (surface dryness with some white coloration) Erythema = up to moderate (up to definite red coloration)
2	Mild	Plaque elevation = slight (slight but definite elevation, typically adges are indistinct or sloped) Scaling = fine (find scale partially or mostly covering lesions) Erythema = up to moderate (up to definite red coloration)
3	Moderate	Plaque elevation = moderate (moderate elevation with rough or sloped edges) Scaling = coarser (coarse scale covering most of all of the lesions) Erythema = moderate (definite red coloration)
4	Severe	Plaque elevation = marked (marked elevation typically with hard or sharp edges) Scaling = coarse (coarse, non-tenacious scale predominates, covering most or all of the lesions) Erythema = severe (very bright red coloration)
5	Very Severe	Plaque elevation = very marked (very marked elevation typically with hard, sharp edges) Scaling = very coarse (coarse, thick tenacious scale over most of all of the lesions; rough surface) Erythema = very severe (extreme red coloration; dusky to deep red coloration)

A. **Excessive hair (hypertrichosis) or too little hair (hypotrichosis) are findings worth noting.**
   1. Hypertrichosis is usually associated with malignancy. The excess hair is very fine, light textured, and occurs mainly in females.
   2. Hypotrichosis is seen in Marie Unna syndrome. At birth there is sparse or no hair growth. Then, until puberty is reached there is hair growth that changes to progressive hair loss afterwards.
B. **Generalized thinning or lost patches of scalp hair, or generalized hair loss in multiple body locations may be important symptoms of infections (bacterial and fungal), systemic illness, lupus erythematosus, chemicals/drugs, scarring, and many other less-common conditions.**
C. **Fingernails and toenails protect the digits, and changes in their appearance or color must be considered.**
   1. Pitting — seen in psoriasis and alopecia areata.
   2. Discoloration — found in psoriasis, fungal infections, and when taking certain medications.

3. Telangiectatic nailfolds — may be seen in lupus erythematosus.
4. Half-and-half nails (half white, half normal) — seen in patients with renal failure.
Note: See Chapter 18, Hair and Nails, for more detail.

VIII. PRURITUS

A. **Primary symptom found in many pathologic disease processes from simple dry skin to the early symptoms of Hodgkin's disease.**
B. **The itch threshold is lower at night.**
C. **It is the prominent symptom in many dermatologic disorders (see Table 9), and in some cases there is no apparent skin eruption.**
D. **To help break the itch-scratch cycle, hydration, moisturizers, antihistamines, antipruritic lotions, topical and injectable steroids may be used. Or simply, cool compresses applied to the trigger point, if discernable, may help decrease symptoms.**

E. Labwork such as CBC, sed rate, urinalysis, serum glucose, and/or liver/thyroid/renal function tests may be ordered. A chest x-ray, pap smear, or stool tests for ova and parasites and occult blood might also be useful.

F. Psychologic stress and emotional well-being are considered a contributing factor in pruritus, but not solely the causing influence.

G. Fear, tension, anxiety, stress, boredom, and depression may intensify the itch sensation.

IX. PSORIASIS AREA AND SEVERITY INDEX (PASI)

A. A method used to evaluate the percentage of body involvement and plaque severity evident on the day of exam.
   1. The amount of erythema, scaling, and thickness of an "average" plaque is used to figure overall condition.
   2. Head, trunk, upper extremities, and lower extremities are the four body areas assessed.
      a. Scores range from 0 to 72.
      b. Body areas are assigned a numerical value depending upon the degree of involvement.

B. Evaluator is a dermatologist or experienced physician specially trained to determine PASI.

C. Each body area involved is assessed according to severity (see Table 10).

Table 9.
Disorders for Which Pruritus May Be A Major Complaint

Scabies
Dermatitis herpetiformis
Atopic dermatitis
Lichen simplex chronicus
Pruritus vulvae
Pruritus ani
Miliaria
Insect (flea or bedbug) bites
Pediculosis
Contact dermatitis
Psoriasis (especially on scalp and genitalia)
Lichen planus
Urticaria
Lymphoma

Adapted from Fitzpatrick, T.B. (1979). Fundamentals of dermatologic diagnosis. In T. Fitzpatrick, A. Eisen, K. Wolff, I. Freedberg, & K. Austen (Eds.), *Dermatology in general medicine* (5th ed.) (pp. 10-36). New York: McGraw-Hill Company.

Table 10.
Psoratic Lesion Signs

In addition, the severity of the psoriatic lesions in three main signs — erythema (E), thickness (T), and scaling (S) — will be assessed for each body area according to a scale (0-4) in which 0 represents a complete lack of cutaneous involvement and 4 represents the most severe possible involvement.

	Erythema[a]	Scaling	Thickness
0 = none	No redness	No scaling	No elevation over normal skin
1 = slight	Faint redness	Fine scale partially covering lesions	Slight but definite elevation, typically edges indistinct or sloped
2 = moderate	Red coloration	Fine to coarse scale covering most of all of the lesions	Moderate elevation with rough or sloped edges
3 = severe	Very or bright red coloration	Coarse, non-tenacious scale predominates covering most or all of the lesions	Marked elevation typically with hard or sharp edges
4 = very severe	Extreme red coloration; dusky to deep red coloration	Coarse, thick, tenacious scale over most or all lesions; rough surface	Very marked elevation typically with hard sharp edges

[a] Do not include residual hyperpigmentation, hypopigmentation, pigmented macules, or diffuse slight pink coloration as erythema.

Table 11.
Calculating PASI

To calculate the PASI, the sum of the severity rating for the three main signs will be multiplied with the numerical value of the area affected and with the various percentages of the four body areas. These values will then be added to complete the formula as follows:

PASI = 0.1 (Eh + Th + Sh) Ah + 0.3 (Et + Tt + St) At + 0.2 (Eu + Tu + Su) Au + 0.4 (El + Tl + Sl) Al

Row		Head	Trunk	Upper Limbs	Lower Limbs
1	Erythema[a]				
2	Thickness[a]				
3	Scaling[a]				
4	Total each column				
5	Degree of involvement[b]				
6	Multiply Row 4 by Row 5				
7		x 0.10	x 0.30	x 0.20	x 0.40
8	Multiply Row 6 by Row 7				
9	Total PASI (add together each column from Row 8)				

[a] Rank severity of psoriatic lesions: 0=none, 1=slight, 2=moderate, 3=severe, 4=very severe.
[b] Rank area of psoriatic involvement: 0=none, 1=<10%, 2=10% to <30%, 3=30% to <50%, 4=50% to <70%, 5=70% to <90%, 6=90% to 100%.

1. A "0" score indicates no erythema, scaling, or plaque elevation.
2. A score of "4" means severe erythema, coarse thick scale, and marked plaque elevation.

D. Calculating the PASI is done using the sum of the three main symptoms and the various percentages of the four body areas inserted into a formula (see Table 11).

X. DIAGNOSTIC OPTIONS

As adjuncts to what is seen with the eyes or palpated with the hands, numerous diagnostic tools offer key information in making a diagnosis.

A. An alcohol wipe swept across a lesion is a method used to lucidate the small, delicate telangiectasia and translucence of a basal cell carcinoma.

B. Mineral oil applied to a glass slide, before using magnification helps visualize the scabies mite.

C. The Tzanck test using Wright's or Giemsa's stain and a microscope looks for epithelial giant cells when a vesicle is thought to be viral.

D. In many microscopic examinations the microbe is stained for visibility, but in dark-field examination the slide background is darkened to visualize the causative spirochete for syphilis.

E. Scrapings from a dry patch of skin, nail plate, or under the nail can be introduced onto a dermatophyte culture medium and aerobically incubated for a minimum of 7 to 10 days.

F. Quicker visualization of fungal hyphae and spores is possible using the KOH (potassium hydroxide) mount (see Figure 2-1, page 221).

1. A #15 blade, glass slide, cover slip, and dry scale scrapings are used.
2. One or two drops of 20% KOH are placed on the slide.
3. The slide is gently heated to dissolve the keratin, then examined under the microscope.

G. Another simple, but lesser used diagnostic tool is the Wood's lamp (see Figure 2-2, page 221). This hand-held lamp has ultraviolet bulbs that cause certain microorganisms to appear colorful when illuminated with ultraviolet light.

1. Certain ringworms glow blue-green.
2. Gold indicates tinea versicolor.
3. Urine screen for porphyrins fluoresce orange-red.

H. Direct immunofluorescence of tissue is an option when trying to diagnose immunologic abnormalities in the skin. Bullous diseases and connective tissue disorders are two examples. Special tissue preparations and stains are done at a lab to microscopically visualize immunoglobulins, complement (a natural property of blood), and fibrin found in the skin or circulation.

I. Gram stain — Allows for identification of gram-negative or positive organisms. Exudate from the site is smeared onto a glass slide, then stained, dried, and examined under oil immersion.

J. Diascopy — Examination of the skin by gentle pressure utilizing a translucent object to observe the effect upon the color (erythema) of the skin.

1. Pressure producing a reduction in erythema or

pigmentation means blood vessel dilation.

2. Pressure that does not produce a change in erythema or pigment indicates increased extravasation of blood, or simply an increased amount of pigment.

K. **Hair pull (pluck) — Most accurate technique to evaluate the anagen/telogen ratio; extract approximately 50 hairs of the same length using a rubber-tipped needleholder and pluck with a quick motion. Hairs are floated on a wet microscope slide or petri dish for examination. Dyes will be applied to determine phase of growth — anagen reacts with citrulline, telogen hairs do not stain.**

XI. CRYOSURGERY, SHAVE, PUNCH, AND ELLIPSE

Four common methods used to treat lesions are cryosurgery, shave, punch, and ellipse. Being familiar with each procedure, when each is used, and the scarring potential helps nurses teach and care for their patients more effectively.

A. **The simplest and least invasive method of lesion destruction, but one that yields no tissue for pathology, is cryosurgery. It is the process of applying extreme cold to a localized site.**

1. No anesthesia is necessary.
2. Liquid nitrogen at -195.6 C is the standard agent now used due to its availability, low cost, and noncombustible nature (see Figure 2-3, page 221).
3. Invokes rapid cooling and slow thawing.
4. Damages tissue by causing ice formation at the cellular level, thermal shock to the cell, and vascular stasis, resulting in necrosis.
5. Treatment causes intense stinging and burning that generally peaks 2 minutes later.
6. The lesion develops a wheal, then blisters, dries, crusts, and falls off in the course of 10 to 14 days. Complications include a possible white spot at the treatment site and infection should the blister break.

B. **The shave biopsy/excision is a tangential specimen of tissue for pathology, resulting in minimal to no scarring.**

1. Indicated for dome-shaped intradermal nevi, fibromas, warts, seborrheic keratoses, and actinic keratoses.
2. Involves mainly a portion of the epidermis and underlying papillary dermis.
3. The procedure can be both an excisional and incisional biopsy depending on whether part or all of the lesion is removed.
4. Very little equipment is needed — local anesthesia, gentian marker, a single-edged blade (see Figure 2-4, page 221), curette (optional), hemostatic agent, and pathology bottle.

5. Special wound care or dressings are optional depending upon the shave location and patient compliance.
6. Hypopigmenting at the shave site and localized infection are two complications.

C. **The punch biopsy has multiple uses depending on whether diagnosing a disease, an eruption, or simply to excise a lesion. The punch instrument can be either circular or elliptical with a razor sharp cutting edge (see Figure 2-4, page 221).**

1. An early lesion is selected when an eruption needs diagnosing. If a vesicle is to be studied, a fully intact one is preferred.
2. An older lesion is needed if suspecting discoid lupus erythematosus.
3. Sometimes a punch tool is advantageous in the removal of small nevi because the scar will be smaller than one by the larger elliptical method.
4. Used in diagnosing basal and squamous cell carcinomas, granuloma annulare, and other diseases that involve the deeper dermis.
5. Punch diameters range in size from 1.0 mm to 1.2 cm.
6. Depth extends from the stratum corneum (outermost skin layer) to the underlying fat, providing the entire dermis for evaluation. If nonabsorbable suture is used, the patient returns for suture removal.
7. Complications to consider are infection, scarring, and nerve damage.

D. **The elliptical excision/wedge biopsy is used when both normal skin and lesional skin junctions are needed for study, such as evaluating basal and squamous cell malignancies and nevi.**

1. Offers greater tissue depth down to and, if necessary, into the subcutaneous fat.
2. The incision length is normally 2.5 to 3 times the width of the incision.
3. Repairs require suturing, and frequently layered closures are necessary.
4. With so many different types of absorbable suture material available, patients often don't need to return for suture removal making skin surgery more convenient for their schedules. Nonabsorbable suture must be removed.
5. Flaps and grafts are additional options for closing large and/or inelastic skin surgery sites.
6. Scarring, possible nerve damage, and infection are the most common complications.

XII. HEMOSTASIS DURING AND AFTER SURGERY

Three methods frequently used to achieve hemostasis during, or at the end of a surgical procedure are:

Table 12.
The SOAP Charting Format

S: Statements (the patient's) regarding the problem; symptoms; what worsens or improves the problem.

O: Observations and exam that support the subjective data.

A: Assessment; impression or interpretation.

P: Plan of treatment; therapy; teaching; instructions to attendants.

Adapted from Perry, A.G. & Potter, P.A. (2002). Documenting nurses' progress notes. In A.G., Perry & P.A. Potter (Eds.), *Clinical nursing skills and techniques* (5th ed.) (p. 53). St. Louis, MO: Mosby, Inc.

A. Simple direct pressure, which is the easiest and least traumatizing to tissue.

B. Hemostatic agents such as aluminum chloride or ferric subsulfate, used after shave or curettage procedures.

C. Electrocautery uses high-frequency radio current during surgical procedures. The lowest current needed to achieve hemostasis is used to reduce tissue destruction.

XIII. DOCUMENTATION

Numerous methods and formats for documenting are available to the dermatology specialty. Variations of the S-O-A-P method, freehand illustrations, body stickers, and photography are all popular.

A. The S-O-A-P format, used by both doctors and nurses, has further evolved in the last few years (see Table 12). By standardizing a charting format, important patient information and details are less likely to be neglected or forgotten.

B. Stickers of body areas applied to the chart (purchased from an office supply store), and/or freehand drawings help indicate lesion and surgery locations. These methods work when mapping moles, too.

C. Charting a patient's progress with photos is reassuring to the patient and more reliable than one's memory. A change in an acne condition, scar development, mole mapping, and hair loss or regrowth are examples of when a 35 mm camera or Polaroid-type camera are valuable.

D. Dermatologic photography is also used when teaching medical/nursing students, special courses, or relaying information to other medical associates. Written consent from the patient is necessary.

E. Photo documentation of skin surgery before, during, and after the repair is useful for the referring physician, insurance company, and dermatologist for medico-legal reasons.

Bibliography

Arndt, K.A. (2002). Operative procedures. In K. Arndt (Ed.), *Manual of dermatologic therapeutics* (6th ed.) (pp. 255-263). Philadelphia: Lippincott Williams & Wilkins.

Bertolino, A.P., & Freedberg, I.M. (1993). Disorders of epidermal appendages and related disorders. In T. Fitzpatrick, A. Eisen, K. Wolff, I. Freedberg, & K. Austen (Eds.), *Dermatology in general medicine* (4th ed.) (pp 672-696). New York: McGraw-Hill Company.

Carpenito, L.J. (Ed.). (1995). *Nursing diagnosis application to clinical practice* (6th ed.) (p. 23). Philadelphia: J.B. Lippincott Company.

Edwards, L. (1997). Definitions & principles of diagnostic procedures. In L. Edwards (Ed.), *Dermatology in emergency care* (pp. 1-15). New York: Churchill Livingstone, Inc.

Elder, D., Elenitsas, R., Jaworsky, C., & Johnson, B., Jr. (1997). Introduction. In D. Elder, R. Elenitsas, C. Jaworsky, & B. Johnson, Jr. (Eds.), *Lever's histopathology of the skin* (8th ed.) (pp. 1-2). Philadelphia: Lippincott-Raven Publishers.

Elenitsas, R., & Halpern, A. C. (1997). Biopsy techniques. In D. Elder, R. Elenitsas, C. Jaworsky, & B. Johnson, Jr. (Eds.), *Lever's histopathology of the skin* (8th ed.) (pp. 3-4). Philadelphia: Lippincott-Raven Publishers.

Fitzpatrick, T.B., Bernhard, J.D., & Cropley, T.G. (1999). The structure of skin lesions & fundamentals of diagnosis. In I. Freedberg, A. Eisen, K. Wolff, K. Austen, L. Goldsmith, S. Katz, & T. Fitzpatrick (Eds.), *Dermatology in general medicine* (5th ed.) (pp. 13-38). New York: McGraw-Hill.

Fleischer, A.B. (1998). Pruritis & health-related quality of life. In R. Rajagopalan, E. F. Sherertz, & R.T. Anderson (Eds.), *Care & management of skin diseases* (pp. 223-229). New York: Marcel Dekker, Inc.

Goldsmith, L.A., Lazarus, G.S., & Tharp, M.D. (1997). Examination of the skin. In L.A. Goldsmith, G.S. Lazarus, & M.D. Tharp (Eds.), *Adult & pediatric dermatology: A color guide to diagnosis & treatment* (pp. 11-20). Philadelphia: F.A. Davis Company.

Haake, A.R., & Holbrook, K. (1999). The structure & development of skin. In I. Freedberg, A. Eisen, K. Wolff, K. Austen, L. Goldsmith, S. Katz, & T. Fitzpatrick (Eds.), *Dermatology in general medicine* (5th ed.) (pp. 70-89). New York: McGraw-Hill.

Helm, T.N., Wirth, P.B., & Helm, K.F. (2000). Inexpensive digital photography in clinical dermatology & dermatologic surgery. *Cutis, 65*(2), 103-106.

Larimore, W.L., & Jordan, E.V. (1995). SOAP to SNOCAMP: Improving the medical record format. *Journal of Family Practice, 41*(4), 393-398.

Olsen, E.A. (1999). Disorders of epidermal appendages & related disorders. In I. Freedberg, A. Eisen, K. Wolff, K. Austen, L. Goldsmith, S. Katz, & T. Fitzpatrick (Eds.), *Dermatology in general medicine* (5th ed.) (pp. 729-748). New York: McGraw-Hill.

Perry, A.G., & Potter, P.A. (2002). Documenting nurses' progress notes. In A.G. Perry & P.A. Potter (Eds.), *Clinical nursing skills & techniques* (5th ed.) (pp. 53). St. Louis, MO: Mosby, Inc.

Rapini, R.P. (1994). Obtaining a skin biopsy specimen and interpreting the results. *Dermatologic Clinics, 12*(1), 83-85.

White, G. (1997). Morphology. In G. White (Ed.), *Levene's color atlas of dermatology* (2nd ed.) (pp. 2-8). London: Times Mirror International Publishers Limited.

Wolff, K., Kibbi, A., & Mihm, M.C. (1999). Basic pathologic reactions of the skin. In I. Freedberg, A. Eisen, K. Wolff, K. Austen, L. Goldsmith, S. Katz, & T. Fitzpatrick (Eds.), *Dermatology in general medicine* (5th ed.) (pp. 41-55). St. Louis, MO: Mosby, Inc.

1. Which of the following skin conditions are not passed down along family lines?
   a. Psoriasis.
   b. Lichen planus.
   c. Eczema.
   d. Keratosis pilaris.

2. A sac within the skin containing liquid or semi-solid material is known as a:
   a. Furuncle.
   b. Abscess.
   c. Comedo.
   d. Cyst.

3. The pattern, distribution, and texture of _____ on the body is an indicator of a person's general state of health.
   a. Seborrheic keratosis.
   b. Moles.
   c. Hair.
   d. Warts.

4. A circumscribed, flat discoloration that could be brown, blue, red, or hypopigmented is a:
   a. Macule.
   b. Bulla.
   c. Nodule.
   d. Plaque.

5. Lichenification is not the accumulation of dried masses of serum, bacteria, and possible blood mixed with epithelial debris that covers damaged epidermis.
   a. True.
   b. False.

6. Which of these primary lesions is directly caused by the disease process?
   a. Scales.
   b. Erosion.
   c. Pustule.
   d. Ulcer.

7. A lesion that is a response to a disease process is a secondary lesion. An example would be:
   a. Wheal.
   b. Crust.
   c. Vesicle.
   d. Plaque.

8. Pruritis is a major symptom of:
   a. Rosacea.
   b. Keratosis pilaris.
   c. Herpes zoster.
   d. Atopic dermatitis.

9. A tool used to evaluate the severity and amount of body involvement in patients with psoriasis is:
   a. DIF.
   b. PASI.
   c. Gram stain.
   d. Tzanck test.

10. Which method of lesion destruction involves mainly the epidermis and papillary dermis?
    a. Shave.
    b. Ellipse.
    c. Cryosurgery.
    d. Punch.

11. Two surgical techniques that provide a full-thickness sampling of the dermis for study are:
    a. Shave and punch biopsy.
    b. Ellipse and shave excision.
    c. Punch biopsy and ellipse excision.
    d. Punch excision and cryosurgery.

12. The overall lesion severity (OLA) is scored based on the lesion's:
    a. Scaling, blister formation, erythema.
    b. Erythema, plaque elevation, bleeding.
    c. Plaque elevation, scaling, pruritus.
    d. Erythema, plaque elevation, scaling.

Answers to Study Questions

1. b	5. a	9. b
2. d	6. c	10. a
3. c	7. b	11. c
4. a	8. d	12. d

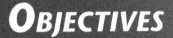

OBJECTIVES

At the end of this chapter, the reader will be able to:
- Describe the two available techniques for patch testing.
- Discuss the presentation of patients with allergic contact dermatitis.
- List general considerations (do's and don'ts) during patch testing.
- Differentiate between allergic and irritant reactions.
- Describe morphology codes for evaluating patches.

KEY POINTS

- Patch testing is an essential tool used in diagnosing allergic contact dermatitis.
- Accurate interpretation of test results is vital to the effective use of patch testing.
- It is critical that test sites are read twice, preferably by the same clinician.
- Patient compliance is vital to effective patch testing and patient education is vital to compliance.
- Patch testing requires patient education at every stage.

Skin Assessment and Diagnostic Techniques
Part II. Patch Testing

Anne Marie Ruszkowski, BSN, RN, DNC

I. OVERVIEW

Patch testing is an essential diagnostic tool used to differentiate irritant versus allergic contact dermatitis. Patients who present with dermatitis or eczema are potential candidates for patch testing.

A. History.
1. The first scientifically derived connection between a sensitizing substance and a dermatologic hypersensitivity reaction was made by Jadassohn in 1895.

B. Available techniques.
1. Finn chamber/Scanpore tape method to test the standard 20 allergens. Consists of shallow aluminum cups or chambers 8 mm in diameter that are affixed to a strip of Scanpore tape. Allergens, chambers, and tape are supplied separately.
2. Al-test filament paper discs affixed to a strip of plastic-coated aluminum may also be used to test the standard 20 allergens.
3. T.R.U.E Test® (thin-layer rapid use epicutaneous test) the first standardized, ready-to-use patch test system. This system delivers 24 of the most common allergens and allergen mixes which are incorporated into hydrophilic gels, printed on a water impermeable sheet of polyester, and mounted on nonwoven cellulose tape.

II. PATIENT SELECTION

All patients selected for patch testing should be tested to the standard allergens (see Tables 1 & 2).

A. Morphology of disease warranting patch testing.
1. Dermatitis or eczema.
2. Erythroderma.
3. Urticaria.
4. Photosensitivity.
5. Dermal inflammatory reaction.
6. Burning and itching skin with no visible pathology.

B. Presentation of patients with allergic contact dermatitis.
1. Highly suggestive history or distribution.
2. Suspected specific antigen or substance.
3. Other dermatitides that flare or do not respond to treatment.
   a. Atopic eczema.
   b. Stasis dermatitis.
   c. Hand dermatitis.
      (1) Irritant contact dermatitis.

Table 1.
Standard Patch Test Screening Tray

1. Benzocaine 5%
2. Mercaptobenzothiazole 1%
3. Colophony 20%
4. p-Phenylenediamine 1%
5. Imidazolidinyl urea 2%
6. Cinnamic aldehyde 1%
7. Lanolin alcohol 30%
8. Carba mix 3%
9. Neomycin sulfate 20%
10. Thiuram mix 1%
11. Formaldehyde 1%
12. Ethylenediamine dihydrochloride 1%
13. Epoxy resin 1%
14. Quaternium-15 2%
15. P-tert-Butylphenol formaldehyde resin 1%
16. Mercapto mix 1%
17. Black rubber mix 0.6%
18. Potassium dichromate 0.25%
19. Balsam of Peru 25%
20. Nickel sulfate 2.5%

From Ruszkowski, A.M, Nicol, N.H., & Moore, J.A. (1995, February). Patch testing basics: Patient selection, application techniques, and guidelines for interpretation. *Dermatology Nursing* (Suppl.). Reprinted with permission.

      (2) Dyshidrotic eczema.
      (3) Psoriasis of the palms and soles.
   d. Seborrheic dermatitis.
   e. Chronic tinea of the hands and/or feet.
   f. Nummular eczema.
4. Occupationally related dermatitis.

III. PATCH TESTING APPLICATION TECHNIQUES

A. General considerations (Do's and Don'ts).
1. Patches should be applied to clean skin that is free of dermatitis.
2. Preferable testing site is upper back, avoiding midline.
3. Avoid applying patches on hairy areas.
4. Patients should not have phototherapy or sun exposure to testing areas for 1 to 2 weeks before testing.
5. Patients should not apply topical corticosteroids to test areas for 1 to 2 weeks before testing.

Table 2.
T.R.U.E. Test® Allergen Series

Panel 1		Panel 2	
Patch	Allergen	Patch	Allergen
1.	Nickel sulfate	13.	p-tert-Butylphenol formaldehyde resin
2.	Wool alcohols	14.	Epoxy resin
3.	Neomycin sulfate	15.	Carba mix
4.	Potassium dichromate		Diphenylguanidine
5.	Caine mix		Zincdiethyldithiocarbamate
	Benzocaine		Zincdibutyldithiocarbamate
	Dibucaine	16.	Black rubber mix
	Tetracaine		N-isopropyl-N'phenyl
6.	Fragrance mix		paraphenylenediamine
	Cinnamyl alcohol		N-cyclohyxyl-N' phenyl
	Cinnamaldehyde		Paraphenylenediamine
	-Amyl-cinnamaldehyde		N, N'-diphenyl paraphenylenediamine
	Eugenol	17.	Cl+ Me- Isothiazolinone
	Isoeugenol	18.	Quaternium-15
	Hydroxycitronellal	19.	Mercaptobenzothiazole
	Geraniol	20.	p-Phenylenediamine
	Oak moss	21.	Formaldehyde
7.	Colophony	22.	Mercapto mix
8.	Parabin mix		Morpholinylmercaptobenzothiazole
	Methyl parahydroxybenzoate		N-cyclohexylbenzothiazylsulfenamide
	Ethyl parahydroxybenzoate		Dibenzothiazyl disulfide
	Propyl parahydroxybenzoate	23.	Thimerosal
	Butyl parahydroxybenzoate	24.	Thiuram mix
	Benzyl parahydroxybenzoate		Tetramethylthiuram monosulfide
9.	Negative control		Tetramethylthiuram disulfide
10.	Balsam of Peru		Dipentamethylenethiuram disufide
11.	Ethylenediamine dihydrochloride		Disulfiram
12.	Cobalt dichloride		

From Ruszkowski, A.M, Nicol, N.H., & Moore, J.A. (1995, February). Patch testing basics: Patient selection, application techniques, and guidelines for interpretation. *Dermatology Nursing* (Suppl.). Reprinted with permission.

6. Patients should not be taking oral steroids or have recent intramuscular injection of corticosteroid before testing.
7. Never test patients to unknown substances.
8. All patients should have two readings of patches.
   a. First reading 48 hours after initial application.
   b. Second reading 24 to 72 hours after removal of patches.
9. Patients should keep patch testing area dry during testing.
10. Patients are instructed to remove patches if "unbearable" to wear for 48 hours. This may include severe burning, stinging, or pruritus at testing areas.
B. **Finn chamber/Scanpore tape method/standard allergens.**

1. Preparing patches for application.
   a. Allergens are kept refrigerated before use.
   b. Anchor strips of Scanpore tape to a hard surface and then apply Finn chambers directly to tape.
   c. Clinician applies a 5 mm ribbon of each petroleum-base allergen directly into individual Finn chambers.
   d. For aqueous allergens, a filter paper disk is placed into the chamber and one drop of solution is placed on the disk immediately before application.
2. Applying patches.
   a. Twenty standard allergen patches are placed on patient's upper back.
   b. Patches are smoothed into place.
   c. Additional Scanpore tape may be necessary to keep patches secure.

Table 3.
Characteristics of Positive Patch Test Reactions

Allergic Reaction	Irritant Reaction
Spreading erythema	Glazed, scaled
Edema	Follicular
Vesicles	Pustular
Persists and/or worsens after patch removal or appears later	Bullous Fades rapidly after patch test removal

From Ruszkowski, A.M, Nicol, N.H., & Moore, J.A. (1995, February). Patch testing basics: Patient selection, application techniques, and guidelines for interpretation. *Dermatology Nursing* (Suppl.). Reprinted with permission.

Table 4.
Morphology Codes for Patch Test Interpretation

1	=	Weak reaction: Nonvesicular, but with erythema, infiltration, possibly papules (+)
2	=	Strong reaction: Edematous and vesicular, with erythema, edema, papules, and vesicles (++)
3	=	Extreme reaction: Spreading, bullous, ulcerative (+++)
4	=	Doubtful reaction: Macular erythema only (+/?)
5	=	Irritant reaction (IR)
6	=	Negative reaction (-)
7	=	Excited skin
8	=	Not tested

From Ruszkowski, A.M, Nicol, N.H., & Moore, J.A. (1995, February). Patch testing basics: Patient selection, application techniques, and guidelines for interpretation. *Dermatology Nursing* (Suppl.). Reprinted with permission.

C. T.R.U.E. test (see Table 2).
 1. Preparing patches for application.
  a. Standardized, ready-to-use system consists of two panels of patches with 12 allergens per test strip.
  b. Allergens should be stored in refrigerator before application.
  c. Remove test strip from the foil outersleeve and take off the protective plastic cover.
  d. Position test panel #1 on the upper part of the patient's back so that allergen #1 is in the upper left corner.
  e. Smooth the panel from the center outward toward the edges.
  f. Indicate the location on the skin by using a medical marking pen to make marks on the two notches found on the panel.
  g. Repeat the same procedure with panel #2 on the opposite side of the upper back so allergen #13 is in the upper left corner.

Table 5.
Patch Testing Do's and Don'ts for Patients

- **Do** keep the patch test area dry for the entire testing period. **Do not** take a bath or shower until the testing period is over. You may *sponge bathe* all areas except the patch test site.
- **Do not** engage in any strenuous activity while the test is in progress. Any activity in which considerable sweating occurs should be avoided, as sweating will cause loosening of the tape.
- **Do** wear loose clothing throughout the day. Wear a T-shirt to bed to avoid catching the edges of the tape on the bedsheets.
- **Do** call the patch testing office immediately if any of the patches appear loose.
- **Do** contact the office immediately if a patch itches or burns severely. You will be given instructions in removing the patch.

From Ruszkowski, A.M, Nicol, N.H., & Moore, J.A. (1995, February). Patch testing basics: Patient selection, application techniques, and guidelines for interpretation. *Dermatology Nursing* (Suppl.). Reprinted with permission.

IV. REMOVING THE PATCHES

All patches should be removed after 48 hours.
A. Supplies needed.
 1. Recording tool.
 2. Surgical marking pen or permanent marker.
 3. Adhesive remover.
 4. Template.
B. Finn chamber method.
 1. Remove test strips so that top portion of each strip remains in place (when using template) or;
 2. Remove test strips and individually mark each individual patch area.
 3. Wait 20 to 30 minutes before reading patches.
C. T.R.U.E. test method.
 1. Check that notches on test strip are marked before removing testing panels.
 2. Position notches on template to correlate with the notch marks on the skin during application.

V. INTERPRETING PATCH TEST RESULTS

A. Timing.
 1. All patches should be read initially at removal time (48 hours).
 2. A second reading is critical 72 to 96 hours after patch application.
B. Irritant vs. allergic reaction (see Table 3).
C. Morphology codes for patch test interpretation (see Table 4).

VI. PATIENT EDUCATION

A. **Pre-patch testing.**
1. Explain procedure, timing of visits, and need for testing.
2. Describe the testing materials.
3. Explain the requirements of testing.
4. Inform patient about patch testing safety.

B. **During patch testing.**
1. Review patch testing do's and don'ts for patient (see Table 5).

C. **After patch testing.**
1. Counsel for negative results.
2. Counsel for positive results.
   a. Discuss avoidance of allergens.
   b. Distribute written info regarding allergens to be avoided.
   c. Be available for phone followup.

Bibliography

Fisher, A.A. (1986). *Contact dermatitis.* Philadelphia: Lea & Febiger.

Marks, J.G., & DeLeo, V.A. (1997). *Contact & occupational dermatology.* St. Louis: Mosby-Year Book, Inc.

Nicol, N.H., Ruszkowski, A.M., & Moore, J.A. (1995, February). Update on patch testing: A roundtable discussion. *Dermatology Nursing* (Suppl.).

Dermatologic Nursing Essentials: A Core Curriculum 2nd Edition © DNA 2003

1. Patch testing should be recommended for patients presenting with:
   a. Atopic dermatitis.
   b. Dyshidrotic eczema.
   c. Vitiligo.
   d. All of the above.
   e. A and b only.

2. Mr. Smith is scheduled for patch testing. The nurse explains to him that the patches will be placed on his upper back for:
   a. 24 hours.
   b. 48 hours.
   c. 72 hours.
   d. 96 hours.

3. Mr. Smith is instructed that during patch testing he should:
   a. Keep patch area dry.
   b. Avoid strenuous activity.
   c. Wear loose clothing.
   d. All of the above.

4. All of the following statements are TRUE except:
   a. Patches should be applied to clean skin that is free of dermatitis.
   b. Patches should not be applied to the midline of the back.
   c. Patients may apply topical corticosteroid cream to the testing area during patch testing.
   d. Patches should not be applied on hairy areas.

5. After the patch tests are removed the patient must return for a second reading of the patches.
   a. True.
   b. False.

6. All patients selected for patch testing should be tested to the standard allergens.
   a. True.
   b. False.

7. Patients can be patch tested to unknown substances.
   a. True.
   b. False.

8. Irritant reactions will usually fade rapidly after patch test removal.
   a. True.
   b. False.

9. The presentation of an extreme reaction (+3) can be characterized by:
   a. Macular erythema only.
   b. Nonvesicular with erythema.
   c. Spreading and bullous.
   d. Edema and papules.

Answers to Study Questions

1. e	5. a	9. c
2. b	6. a	
3. d	7. b	
4. c	8. a	

CE Answer/Evaluation Form

Chapter 2.
Skin Assessment and Diagnostic Techniques

Please photocopy this test page and return.

COMPLETE THE FOLLOWING:

Name: _____

Address: _____

City: _____ State: _____ Zip: _____

Preferred telephone: (Home)_____ (Work) _____

State where licensed and license number: _____

CE application fee: DNA member $10.00
                       Nonmember $13.00

POSTTEST INSTRUCTIONS
1. To receive continuing education credit for individual study after reading the article, complete the answer/evaluation form below.
2. Photocopy and send the answer/evaluation form along with a check or money order payable to **Dermatology Nurses' Association** to: *DNA*, East Holly Avenue Box 56, Pitman, NJ 08071-0056.
3. Test returns must be postmarked by December 31, 2008. Upon completion of the answer/evaluation form, a certificate for 3.0 contact hour(s) will be awarded and sent to you.

This chapter was reviewed and formatted for contact hour credit by Marcia J. Hill, MSN, RN, Core Curriculum Editor; and Sally Russell, MN, RN,C, DNA Education Director.

ANSWER FORM

1. Name one new detail (item, issue, or phenomenon) that you learned by completing this activity.

   _____

   _____

   _____

   _____

2. How will you apply the information from this learning activity to your practice?
   a. Patient education.
   b. Staff education.
   c. Improve my patient care.
   d. In my education course work.
   e. Other: Please describe _____

   _____

   _____

Evaluation

	Strongly disagree				Strongly agree
3. The offering met the stated objectives.					
a. Identify what subjective and objective data are necessary for a diagnosis.	1	2	3	4	5
b. Recognize the apropriate terminology used for primary and secondary lesions.	1	2	3	4	5
c. Determine how lesion location and distribution help indicate specific diagnosis.	1	2	3	4	5
d. Identify various diagnostic methods available for use during assessments.	1	2	3	4	5
e. Recognize which surgical treatment option is optimal and choose a favorable method of documentation.	1	2	3	4	5
f. Describe the two available techniques for patch testing.	1	2	3	4	5
g. Discuss the presentation of patients with allergic contact dermatitis.	1	2	3	4	5
h. List general considerations (do's and don'ts) during patch testing.	1	2	3	4	5
i. Describe the difference between allergic and irritant reactions.	1	2	3	4	5
j. Describe morphology codes for evaluating patches.	1	2	3	4	5
4. The content was current and relevant.	1	2	3	4	5
5. The content was presented clearly.	1	2	3	4	5
6. The content was covered adequately.	1	2	3	4	5

7. I am more confident of my abilities since completing this material.
8. The material was (check one) ☐ new, ☐ review for me

Comments _____

_____

9. Time required to complete reading assignment: _____ minutes.

This independent study is provided by the Dermatology Nurses' Association (DNA) for 3.0 contact hours. DNA is accredited as a provider of continuing education in nursing by the American Nurses Credentialing Center's Commission on Accreditation. DNA is approved as a provider of continuing education by the California Board of Registered Nursing Provider #CEP5708.

Dermatologic Nursing Essentials: A Core Curriculum 2nd Edition © DNA 2003

Therapeutic/Treatment Modalities

Robin Weber, MN, RN, FNP-C

OBJECTIVES

At the end of this chapter, the reader will be able to:

- Identify the advantages and disadvantages of topical treatment vs. systemic treatment.
- Understand the steps to applying an Unna's boot correctly.
- Define the systemic antibiotics related to clinical use, absorption, metabolism, adverse reaction, and dosage.
- Identify the pros and cons of vitamin A therapy.
- Understand the keys to phototherapy treatment.
- Describe the indication for photopheresis treatment.
- Identify the drug used for photopheresis.
- Define the response to photopheresis as documented in the literature.
- List the nursing concerns to follow in patients receiving photopheresis.

KEY POINTS

- Percutaneous absorption in intact skin may be unpredictable; but increased when the skin is compromised.
- Patient education regarding importance of compliance to treatment regimen, benefits, and risks is paramount to successful treatment.
- The proper application of venous compression therapy such as Unna's boot is important to positive outcomes.
- Topical modalities should be used with caution on open wounds; choice of topical medication should consider rate of absorption, healing, presence of infection, and possible sensitivities.
- Assist in evaluating the patient to confirm that photopheresis is the appropriate treatment and that it can be performed safely.
- Educate patients and their significant others to the procedure and its effect.
- Patient education about the drug methoxsalen is necessary for compliance and positive outcome.
- Photopheresis must be performed under controlled and safe circumstances.
- Patient must be provided with appropriate discharge instructions.

CHAPTER 3

Therapeutic/Treatment Modalities

Robin Weber, MN, RN, FNP-C

I. OVERVIEW

The skin is the largest organ of the body. When the skin is intact it regulates percutaneous absorption. The removal of lipids, water, or protein from the epidermis can severely compromise this protective function. This function must be maintained even when the skin is compromised. Topical preparations are used to provide this barrier function when the skin is compromised. For example, alkaline soaps affect the stratum corneum by changing the normal acidity of the skin (normal skin pH is 5.5). Alteration of the acid mantle can decrease bacterial resistance. Most drugs that pass through the stratum corneum into the epidermis are metabolized there; this action may decrease the drug's pharmacologic or toxicologic activity. Drugs not metabolized in the epidermis pass unchanged into the systemic circulation.

II. TOPICAL AGENTS

A. Vehicles.
Choice of the appropriate vehicle is paramount to successful treatment. Vehicles affect the absorption of medicaments. Fat soluble vehicles, especially natural emollients, are more rapidly absorbed than water soluble vehicles.
   1. Ointment: water-in-oil emulsions; water content 40% or less; desirable for dryer lesions/conditions.
      a. Increases lubrication.
      b. Occlusive which increases percutaneous absorption thus enhancing potency of medications.
      c. Usually are preservative free.
      d. Should not be used in extremely eczematous inflammation or in intertriginous area due to occlusive properties.
      e. May cause folliculitis when used in hairy areas.
   2. Creams: oil-in-water emulsion; water content 60% or less; may have preservatives.
      a. Used for lubrication; easily applied.
      b. Highly versatile due to ability to use on almost any area of the body.
      c. Do not increase percutaneous absorption.
      d. Are more cosmetically acceptable.
      e. Some may cause dryness due to the content of alcohol, propylene glycol, and water.
   3. Lotions: powder suspended in liquid (usually water, alcohol, or oil); delivers medication as uniform residual film; has a cooling effect.
      a. Suitable for hairy areas; frequently used for scalp due to ease of penetration.
      b. Have greater content of alcohol and water.
      c. May over dry the skin; wears off easily.
      d. Absorbs moisture, promoting drying.
      e. May cause stinging and drying in intertriginous areas.
   4. Solutions: composition similar to lotions.
   5. Gel: semisolid mixture (usually propylene glycol and water); use in acute exudative inflammation.
      a. Easily applied.
      b. Drying and cooling — good for pruritic eruptions like poison ivy.
      c. Aggravates dry, cracked lesions if it contains alcohol.
      d. May cause burning on eroded skin.
   6. Powder: finely ground solid particles.
      a. Absorptive; promotes drying.
      b. Decreases skin friction.
      c. Good vehicle to deliver medication to intertiginous areas.
   7. Aerosols: medications suspended in a base and delivered under pressure.
      a. Similar to a lotion but more drying.
      b. Useful for applying medication to hairy areas.
      c. Useful on wet lesions.
   8. Paste: powder in ointment; 50% or greater powder content.
      a. Provides protection.
      b. Decreases rate of percutaneous absorption.
      c. Messy.
B. Application of topicals (see Tables 1 & 2): the objective of topical treatment is to lubricate or medicate, or both. Proper application technique should always be used. Hydrating the skin before application will increase percutaneous absorption. Frequency of application will be dictated by severity of dermatosis and the medication chosen.
   1. Remove any "caked" topical before applying additional topical.
      a. Remove creams with water.
      b. Mineral or cottonseed oil may be used to remove ointments or pastes.
      c. Always use gentle motions when removing topical medications.
   2. Applying creams, ointments.
      a. Use approximately one-half inch of medication.
      b. Rub briskly in your hands to ease application.

Table 1.
Amount of Topical Medication Needed for Single or Multiple Application(s)

Area Treated	One Application (gm)	BID for 1 Week (gm)	TID for 2 Weeks (gm)	BID for 1 Month (gm)	TID for 6 Weeks (gm)
Hands, Head, Face, Anogenital Area	2	28	90 (3 oz)	120 (4 oz)	270 (9 oz)
One Arm, Anterior or Posterior Trunk	3	42	120 (4 oz)	180 (6 oz)	360 (12 oz)
One Leg	4	56	180 (6 oz)	240 (8 oz)	540 (18 oz)
Entire Body	30-60	420-840 14-28 oz	1.26-2.52 kg 42-82 oz 2.5-5 lb	1.8-3.6 kg 60-120 oz 3.75-7.5 lb	3.8-7.5 kg 126-252 oz 7.5-15 lb

From *Dermatology Nurses' Association Dermatology Nursing Basics Course.* (2003). Pitman, NJ: Dermatology Nurses' Association.

Table 2.
Guidelines for Patient Education Regarding the Application of Topical Medications

Successful topical therapy depends as much on the patient's understanding of how to apply the topical agent as what product they have been prescribed. Using your knowledge of the drug and the product, teaching your patients the following guidelines to will aid in accomplishing your goal.

- Review any preapplication instructions.
- How often to apply.
- Where to apply.
- How much to apply.
- Which topical to apply to which location.
- The sequence of application for multiple products.
- Assess the patient's ability to comply.
- Review the importance of compliance.
- The expected results.
- Who and when to call with questions.

From *Dermatology Nurses' Association Dermatology Nursing Basics Course.* (2003). Pitman, NJ: Dermatology Nurses' Association.

  c. Apply in long downward (direction of hair growth) strokes using the palm of the hand.
  d. Only a thin film of medication is necessary.
3. Applying pastes.
  a. Use tongue depressor if available.
  b. May warm container of medication in warm water to soften thus facilitating application.

4. Applying lotions/solutions.
  a. Shake well.
  b. Pour small amount in the palm of the hand.
  c. Pat onto the skin.
  d. A brush or gauze may be used for application; avoid use of cotton, it filters out medication and may stick to skin.
5. Applying sprays and aerosols.
  a. Shake well.
  b. Direct spray to affected area (distance as determined by package insert).
  c. Use short bursts when applying.
6. Applying powders.
  a. Dry affected area thoroughly.
  b. "Dust" affected area leaving only a thin layer of powder.
  c. Gauze or powder puff facilitates application.
  d. Use caution around patients with tracheostomies or respiratory problems.
7. Applying gels.
  a. Cleanse affected areas.
  b. If acne medication, wait a minimum of 30 minutes after cleansing before application to reduce incidence of irritation.
C. **Occlusion: this produces an airtight barrier usually by use of plastic film. It enhances absorption by preventing medication evaporation and increases rehydration of stratum corneum by moisture retention.**
  1. Cleanse skin of debris and other medications.
  2. Apply prescribed topical thinly while skin is damp.
  3. Snugly fit plastics; compress air out; seal borders with paper tape.

Table 3.
Potency Ranking of Some Commonly Used Topical Steroids

Group	Generic Name	Brand Name
I	Clobetasol propionate Halobetasol propionate Betamethasone diprionate (optimized vehicle) Diflorasone diacetate	Temovate® 0.05% Ultravate® 0.05% Diprolene® 0.05% Psorcon® 0.05%
II	Amcinonide Betamethasone dipropionate Mometasone furoate Halcinonide	Cyclocort® 0.1% Diprosone® 0.05% Elcon® 0.1% Halog® 0.1%
III	Fluticasone propionate Flucinonide Bethamethasone valerate	Cutivate® 0.0005% Lidex® 0.05% Valisone® 0.1%
IV	Triamcinolone acetonide Fluocinolone acetonide	Kenalog® 0.1% Synalar® 0.02%
V	Hydrocortisone butyrate Hydrocortisone valerate	Locoid® 0.1% Westcort® 0.2%
VI	Alclometasone dipropionate Desonide	Aclovate® 0.05% DesOwen® 0.05%
VII	Hydrocortisone acetate	Hytone® 2.5% Hytone® 1.0%

Adapted from Bogunieqicz, M., Nicol, N.H., & Leung, D.Y.M. (1997). Atopic disease and the skin. In *Cutaneous allergy for the clinician* (p. 220). Boston: Blackwell Scientific Publications.

4. Leave dressing intact for prescribed time.
5. Remove gently and cleanse skin.
6. Problems associated with occlusion.
   a. Sweat retention.
   b. Maceration.
   c. Folliculitis.
   d. Atrophy.
   e. Striae.
   f. May increase risk for bacterial/fungal overgrowth.
7. Long-term occlusion with even a low-potency topical steroid may result in temporary suppression of the hypothalamic pituitary adrenal (HPA) axis; this function returns after occlusion is discontinued.

III. TOPICAL MEDICATIONS

Numerous topical medications are available for treating skin disorders — corticosteroids, antifungals, antibacterials, antivirals, scabicides and pediculicides, keratolytics and caustics, and antineoplastics.

A. Topical steroids.
   1. Used extensively in treating skin disorders.
   2. Reduce inflammation.
   3. Relieve pruritus.
   4. Induce remission of many cutaneous disorders.
   5. Potency ranking — groups from 1 to 7 with 1 being the most potent; most dermatoses may be managed with low to moderately potent topical steroids (see Table 3).
   6. Possible side effects.
      a. Atrophy — older skin, inguinal, genital, and perianal areas most predisposed to atrophy; may be irreversible depending on potency of steroid used.
      b. Striae — irreversible.
      c. Telangiectasia — may disappear after up to 6 months without steroid application.
      d. Acneiform eruptions — develop after months of use; reversible.
      e. Interfere with epithelialization and collagen synthesis in wound healing.
      f. Burning/dryness — usually due to the vehicle.
      g. Hypo/hyperpigmentation — reversible on discontinuation of steroid.
      h. Bruising — reversible.
      i. Hypothalamic pituitary adrenal axis

suppression — results from application of potent (fluorinated) steroids in excess of 50 to 100 gm/week in adults, 10 to 20 gm in children, for 2 or more weeks; reversible.

7. Nursing considerations.
   a. Assess efficacy of medication regularly.
   b. Assess patient for development of side effects; length of therapy increases risk of developing side effects.
   c. Assess for tachyphylaxis. — *write sudden decrease in response*
   d. Assess for signs of superimposed infections.
   e. Assess response related to vehicle — ointment-based preparations are generally more potent than chemically equivalent cream-based agents.
   f. Avoid use of topical steroids on the face, perineal area, or axillae unless otherwise indicated; if required monitor closely.
   g. Hydration increases percutaneous absorption; application after soaking the skin in lukewarm water will increase absorption; in steroid-responsive generalized dermatoses application following a bath or shower is most efficacious.
   h. Compromised skin has increased percutaneous absorption.
   i. Frequency of application depends on steroid potency and severity of dermatoses.

8. Patient education.
   a. Review any preapplication instructions.
   b. Instruct patient on appropriate technique for application; when multiple products are to be applied, instruct patient regarding which topical should be applied first.
   c. Review frequency of applications.
   d. Emphasize that medication is only to be applied to areas for which it is prescribed; self-medication can have disastrous complications.
   e. Stress that overuse or misuse can result in serious cutaneous and systemic complications.
   f. Review expected results from therapy.
   g. Caution patient against lending medication to friends/relatives.
   h. Emphasize importance of using full course of medication unless side effects occur.
   i. Inform patient about who to call if any problems occur.

B. **Topical antifungals (antimycotic agents).**
   1. Used to treat fungal or dermatophyte infections (superficial infections of the skin, hair, and nails); also called tineas.
      a. Tinea pedis.
      b. Tinea cruris. — *groin*
      c. Tinea corporis. — *superficial plaque; light or dark = Tan*
      d. Tinea versicolor. — *like rash; more noticeable. yeast*

2. Antifungal-corticosteroid combinations.
   a. Used to alleviate the symptoms of inflammation and pruritus secondary to fungal infection.
   b. Produce more rapid response/alleviation of symptoms.
   c. May mask superimposed bacterial infections.
   d. Use in chronic dermatophyte-induced infections may make evaluation of response or titration of therapy difficult secondary to the topical steroid.

3. Antifungal chosen based on:
   a. Species of dermatophyte.
   b. Body site involved.
   c. Severity of infection.
   d. Duration of infection (days, weeks, years, recurrent).
   e. Patient's age.
   f. Concurrent medical conditions/drug therapy.

4. Possible side effects.
   a. Skin irritation.
   b. Overgrowth of fungus when occlusion is used.

5. Nursing considerations.
   a. Assess patient's history for pre-existing condition that might preclude use of topical antifungal.
   b. Assess for any evidence of skin irritation secondary to medication.
   c. Assess patient/significant other's knowledge of medication and appropriate application.
   d. Moist areas of the body (intertriginous and perineal areas) are particularly prone to fungal infections.
   e. Ointment-based antifungal products are not desirable due to their occlusive properties.

6. Patient education.
   a. Review any pre-application instructions.
   b. Instruct patient on appropriate technique for application.
   c. Review frequency of applications.
   d. Emphasize that medication is only to be used on areas for which it is prescribed; self-medication can have disastrous results.
   e. Emphasize need to use full course of medication unless side effects occur.
   f. Review expected results from therapy.
   g. Caution patient against lending medication to friends/relatives.
   h. Instruct patient to keep affected areas dry; use nonocclusive footwear and cotton undergarments to minimize moisture buildup.

C. **Topical antipruritics.**
   1. Usually contain camphor, menthol, phenol, or a

topical anesthetic; have anesthetic and counterirritant properties which induce cooling; indicated for the temporary relief of pruritus.

2. Examples.
   a. PrameGel®.
   b. Sarna® lotion.
   c. Calamine lotion.
   d. Aveeno® anti-itch lotion/cream.
   e. Pramosone®. _i hydrocortisone_
3. Nursing considerations.
   a. May be applied liberally 3 to 4 times/day.
   b. Underlining etiology of pruritus must be pursued and corrected.
   c. Monitor for skin irritation especially with topical antipruritics.
4. Patient education.
   a. Explain the objective of an antipruritic agent.
   b. Explain appropriate use.
   c. Emphasize need to report effectiveness of therapy.

D. **Topical antibacterials.**
1. May be used in combination with other topical modalities.
2. Suitable in treating inflammatory acne vulgaris.
3. Suitable for use in open wounds; may facilitate granulation.
4. Preparations chosen based on organism cultured and skin problem.
5. Examples.
   a. Bacitracin — used for gram-positive infections and prophylaxis in minor cuts, burns, and abrasions.
   b. Garamycin — used for aerobic gram-negative and some gram-positive infections.
   c. Meclocycline sulfosalicylate — used for acne vulgaris.
   d. Neomycin sulfate — used for aerobic gram-negative and some aerobic gram-positive infections.
   e. Nitrofurazone — used as adjunct therapy in second and third-degree burns and in skin grafts/donor sites to prevent rejection due to bacterial contamination.
   f. Silver sulfadiazine — used for gram-negative and gram-positive infections.
   g. Erythromycin — indicated for acne vulgaris.
   h. Chloramphenicol — used for prophylaxis and treating superficial bacterial infections.
   i. Tetracycline hydrochloride — used for prophylaxis and treatment of superficial infections.
   j. _Bactroban_ Mupirocin — antistreptococcal and antistaphlococcal action; good for treating impetigo.
6. Nursing considerations.
   a. Use contraindicated in patients with a history of prior sensitization.
   b. Unless otherwise indicated cleanse affected area before application.
   c. Observe for any signs of allergic reaction — burning, swelling, redness, or worsening of condition.
   d. ✳With prolonged use monitor for superinfections and overgrowth of nonsusceptible organisms, especially fungus.
   e. Alcohol-based antibacterial solutions may cause burning upon application.
7. Patient education.
   a. Educate patient/significant other regarding treatment objectives.
   b. Instruct patient/significant other on correct application including pre-application process.
   c. Emphasize need to use full course of medication.
   d. Emphasize importance of using medication only on affected areas.
   e. Instruct patient/significant other regarding what to do in case side effects develop.

E. **Antivirals.**
 Valtrex Above
1. Acyclovir (Famvir®) — used to prevent or treat herpetic viral infections; mode of action is interference with viral replication.
2. Contraindicated with hypersensitivity to any components.
3. Use cautiously during lactation.
4. Possible side effects: burning/stinging, pruritus, or rash.
5. Nursing considerations.
   a. Ointment must thoroughly cover all lesions.
   b. Initiate treatment as soon as possible after onset of symptoms.
   c. Monitor for side effects and process.
6. Patient education.
   a. Educate patient/significant other about treatment objectives.
   b. Instruct patient/significant other on the appropriate application of topical.
   c. Instruct patient on importance of compliance to therapy.
   d. Inform patient/significant other about possible side effects and what to do should they occur.

F. **Scabicides and pediculicides.**
(See Chapter 16 for further detail on infestations and the treatments indicated.)

G. **Keratolytics/Caustics.**
1. Keratolytics dissolve and separate the stratum corneum in diseases where hyperkeratosis is a manifestation; caustics have an antimitotic action.
2. Examples.
   a. Coal tar (cream, shampoo, ointment, gel,

lotion, soap, bath solution).

   b. Salicylic acid (cream, gel, ointment, patch, shampoo, solution).

   c. Anthralin.

   d. Cantharidin.

   e. Podophyllum resin.

   f. Resorcinol.

   g. Silver nitrate.

   h. Sulfur.

3. Possible side effects.

   a. Irritation.

   b. Burning.

   c. Pain.

   d. Inflammation.

   e. Increased dryness.

   g. Erosions.

   h. Hearing loss, tinnitus, dizziness, confusion, headache, hyperventilation with salicylic acid if salicylism develops.

   i. Bleeding, dizziness, hematuria, vomiting may be seen as a side effect of podophyllum resin.

4. Nursing considerations.

   a. Use with caution in pregnant or lactating women.

   b. Do not apply to face, groin, axillae, mucous membranes, broken or inflamed skin.

   c. Do not apply caustics to intertriginous areas.

   d. Do not use occlusion with caustics.

   e. Salicylic acid is contraindicated for use in children under 2 years of age, diabetics, or individuals with impaired circulation.

   f. Do not apply salicylic acid to moles, birthmarks, unusual warts with hair, genital warts or warts on mucous membranes.

   g. Prolonged use of salicylic acid can lead to salicylate toxicity.

   h. When applying caustics, protect uninvolved skin by applying petrolatum.

   i. Apply caustics only to affected areas.

5. Patient education.

   a. Inform patient/significant other of treatment objectives.

   b. Instruct patient/significant other on correct application of topical.

   c. Inform patient/significant other of possible side effects of treatment.

   d. Reinforce importance of compliance with therapy.

   e. Reinforce importance of applying topicals only to affected areas.

   f. Inform patient that topical is not to be applied to broken skin, wounds, or cuts.

   g. Inform patient not use occlusion unless directed to do so.

H. Antineoplastics.

1. Used for treating reactive and proliferative cutaneous malignancies.

2. Exert action through different mechanisms.

   a. Cycle-specific are more effective against proliferating cells.

   b. Phase-specific are more effective against a specific phase of the cell cycle.

   c. Interfere with the synthesis of DNA through different mechanisms.

3. Categories of antineoplastics.

   a. Alkylating agents — nitrogen mustard.

     (1) Disrupt the structure of DNA through nonspecific cell-cycle manner.

     (2) Interfere with normal cell division in rapidly proliferating tissue.

     (3) Used in treating T-cell lymphoma (mycosis fungoides).

   b. Antimetabolites — 5-fluorouracil.

     (1) Interfere with the synthesis of nucleic acids and proteins.

     (2) Phase-specific; primarily affect the cells that actively synthesize DNA.

     (3) Used in treating superficial basal cell carcinomas; multiple actinic or solar keratoses.

   c. Retinoid X receptors bexarotene gel (Tagretin®) gel 1% for the topical treatment of resistant T-cell lymphoma.

     (1) Bexarotine gel inhibits the growth of some tumor cell lines of hematopoietic and squamous cell origin.

     (2) The exact mechanism of action in the treatment of T-cell lymphoma is unknown.

4. Possible side effects.

   a. Pain.

   b. Pruritus.

   c. Hyperpigmentation.

   d. Irritation.

   e. Inflammation.

   f. Burning.

   g. Scarring.

   h. Swelling.

   i. Alopecia.

   j. Photosensitivity.

   k. Scaling.

   l. Contact dermatitis.

5. Nursing considerations.

   a. Apply with care near eyes, nose, and mouth.

   b. Always wear gloves when applying.

   c. Can cause photosensitivity.

   d. Avoid occlusion.

   e. Erythema and crusting are a result of topical treatment with 5-fluorouracil.

   f. Nitrogen mustard is applied total body with exception of eyelids, lips, and genitals.

   g. Nitrogen mustard may be applied in liquid form or compounded in a petrolatum base.

6. Patient education.
   a. Inform patient/significant other regarding the treatment objectives.
   b. Emphasize the importance of compliance to therapy.
   c. Instruct patient/significant other on the correct application of topical.
   d. Inform patient/significant other of possible side effects of treatment.
   e. Inform patient of increased photosensitivity; advise to use a sunscreen of at least SPF 15 daily.
   f. Inform patients on 5-fluorouracil about the various stages of inflammation that will occur.
   g. Remind patient that this is a potent prescription medication which should not be shared with others or used for other skin conditions than the one that it has been prescribed to treat.

I. **Vitamin A/Retinoids.**
   1. Used in treating noninflammatory acne, photoaging, flat warts, molluscum contagiosum, senile comedones, and actinic keratoses.
   2. Mechanism of action.
      a. Initiates increased cell turnover in both normal follicles and comedones.
      b. Reduces cohesion between keratinized cells.
      c. Causes skin peeling and extrusion of comedones.
      d. Improves skin turgor; reduces fine wrinkling.
      e. Improves circulation which improves skin color.
   3. Possible side effects.
      a. Erythema.
      b. Peeling.
      c. Thinning of stratum corneum increasing risk of sunburn/sun damage.
      d. Increased susceptibility to irritation from wind/cold.
      e. Dryness.
      f. Edema.
      g. Blisters.
      h. Stinging.
   4. Nursing considerations.
      a. Use with caution in pregnant or lactating women.
      b. Avoid applying around eyes, mouth, angles of the nose, and mucous membranes.
      c. Increases risk of sunburn.
      d. Astringents, alcohol-based lotions, and acne soaps may not be tolerated while using retinoids.
   5. Patient education.
      a. Educate patient/significant other regarding treatment objectives.

   b. Instruct patient/significant other on correct application.
   c. Advise patient to avoid using keratolytics, alcohol-based products, abrasive cleansers, astringents, and topical products containing spice or lime.
   d. Inform patient that a topical moisturizer can be used if skin becomes too dry.
   e. Inform patient to apply topical after thoroughly cleaning and drying the skin.
   f. Inform patient of increased sensitivity to sun; advise using a sunscreen of at least SPF 15.
   h. Stress importance of compliance to prescribed regimen.
6. Topical immune modulators: tacrolimus 0.03% to 0.1% (Protopic®) pimecrolimus (Elidel®).
   a. Used for treating intermittent flares of atopic dermatitis.
   b. Topical form of anti-rejection medication FK506 (cyclosporine).
   c. Can safely be used on the face and for eyelid dermatitis without the atrophy of topical steroids.
   d. Side effects:
      (1) Burning and stinging with initial use.
      (2) Possible increased risk of secondary infection from bacterial, viral, and fungal infections.
      (3) Theoretical increased risk of skin cancer, remind patient to use daily sunscreen.
      (4) Possible systemic absorption of FK506 if used for long periods on large areas of effected skin.
   e. Use: Apply sparingly to effected areas bid for approximately 4 to 5 days. If no improvement noted, contact health care provider.

IV. INTRALESIONAL THERAPY

A. **Intralesional steroids.**
   1. Injected directly into or just beneath the lesion.
   2. Provides a reservoir of medication that lasts for several weeks to months.
   3. Used to supplement other treatment modalities.
   4. Conditions treated.
      a. Psoriasis.
      b. Alopecia areata.
      c. Cystic acne.
      d. Hypertrophic scars/keloids.
      e. Chronic eczematous inflammation.
      f. Herpes zoster to attenuate/eliminate pain in eruptive stage and in postherpetic neuralgia (mixture of lidocaine and triamcinolone acetonide; dilute 10 mg/5 ml

of steroid with equal parts of 1% lidocaine).
g. Discoid lupus (use lidocaine/steroid solution as for herpes zoster).

5. Most commonly used mixture: 2.5 to 10 mg/ml suspension of triamcinolone acetonide.

6. Other mixtures.
a. 10 mg/ml — effective for chronic eczematous inflammation; acne; hypertrophic scars/keloids.
b. 10 mg/ml diluted with 1% Xylocaine® or physiologic saline — effective for acne; herpes zoster; discoid lupus.
c. 2.5 to 5.0 mg/ml — effective in suppressing inflammation.

7. Possible side effects.
a. Prolonged, continuous use may lead to adrenal suppression.
b. Atrophy may result after multiple injections in same site.

8. Nursing considerations.
a. Injections may be painful.
b. Atrophy can result from multiple treatments.
c. Multiple treatments may be necessary in some conditions such as keloids.
d. Vial of steroid solution must be shaken thoroughly before drawing up solution.
e. If syringe of medication is not used immediately, syringe should be shaken immediately prior to injection.

B. Intralesional antineoplastic agents.
1. Bleomycin sulfate.
a. Useful in treating recalcitrant periungual or plantar warts.
b. Solution: 1 U/ml in physiologic saline (dissolve 15 U vial of bleomycin in 15 ml of sterile physiologic saline).
c. Inject 0.1 to 1.0 ml until wart blanches.
2. Vinblastine.
a. Useful in treating Kaposi's sarcoma.
b. Solution: 0.2 mg/ml.
c. Maximum total dose to be used is 2 mg.
3. Interferon alfa-2b recombinant.
a. Treatment indications.
(1) Genital warts that are unresponsive to all forms of conventional treatment; imposing significant social or physical limitations.
(2) Kaposi's sarcoma.
(3) Basal/squamous cell cancers.
b. Possible side effects.
(1) Injection site reactions — redness, pain, swelling, discoloration.
(2) Flu-like symptoms.
4. Nursing considerations.
a. A thorough history to determine presence of underlying medical problems (cardiac, liver, or renal).

b. Medication must be refrigerated.
c. Initial treatment for warts will be 3 times/week for 3 weeks.
d. Flu-like symptoms can be managed with acetaminophen.

5. Patient education.
a. Inform patient/significant other of the treatment objective.
b. Inform patient/significant other of possible side effects and how to handle.
c. Emphasize the importance of compliance to prescribed treatment regimen.

V. SYSTEMIC MEDICATIONS

A. Antibiotics: act to prevent or treat infection from pathogenic microorganisms.
1. Erythromycin — highly effective; one of the safest antibiotics; drug of choice in treating folliculitis.
a. Member of macrolid group.
b. Bacteriostatic — inhibits protein synthesis.
c. Bacteriocidal in high concentrations.
d. Pharmacokinetics.
(1) Inactivated rapidly by gastric acid.
(2) Dissolves poorly in water.
(3) Distributed well to most tissues with the exception of cerebrospinal fluid (CSF).
(4) Transported across the placenta and excreted in breast milk.
(5) Metabolized in the liver and excreted in the bile; small amount excreted in urine.
(6) Peak serum concentration level occurs 2 to 4 hours after a single 250 mg dose in a fasting patient.
e. Pharmacotherapeutics.
(1) Broad spectrum of antimicrobial activity, effective against:
(a) *Pneumococci.*
(b) Group A *Streptococci.*
(c) *Staphylococci aureus.*
(d) Gram-negative and gram-positive bacteria.
(e) May be used in patients with penicillin allergy who have Group A beta-hemolytic *streptococci* or *S. pneumoniae* infection.
(2) Dosage/Indications.
(a) Adults: 250 mg qid x 10 days; pediatric dose: 30 to 50 mg/Kg/d in divided doses q 6 hrs.
(b) Skin and soft tissue infections.
 i. Chlamydia trichomatis urethritis.
 ii. Erythrasma. *oxilla, groin : Corynebacter*
 iii. Syphilis or gonorrhea.
(c) *Strep pyogenes* infections.
 i. Erysipelas. *B hemolytic strep.*
 ii. Cellulitis. *inflammation SQ, loose connective*

Facial Nasopharynx rapid invasion of lymph system

iii. Lymphangitis.
iv. Impetigo. *Staph. or GrpA strep*
v. Ecthyma. *B-henolytic strep : LE, diabets*
(d) *S. aureus* infections.
i. Folliculitis.
ii. Furunculosis.
iii. Infected dermatitis.
(3) Adverse reactions.
(a) Commonly causes nausea and vomiting when take on an empty stomach.
(b) Diarrhea.
(c) Chloestatic hepatitis with fever, abdominal pain, nausea, vomiting, eosinophilia, elevated serum bilirubin.
(4) Drug interactions.
(a) Theophylline.
(b) Cyclosporine.
(c) Carbamazepine. *Tegretol : Seizure Trigeminal neoralgia*
(d) Warfarin.
(e) Digitalis.
(f) Ergotamine. *~ migrans*
(g) Methyl prednisolone.

2. Penicillins.
a. Derived from strains of *Penicillium motatum* and *Penicillium chrysogenum* which are common molds seen on bread or fruit.
b. First generation.
(1) Penicillin G.
(2) Newer semisynthetic penicillinase — resistant.
(a) Oxacillin.
(b) Cloxacillin.
(c) Dicloxacillin.
c. Second generation.
(1) Aminopenicillin.
(2) Ampicillin.
(3) Amoxicillin.
d. Pharmacokinetics.
(1) Kills bacteria by destroying the cell walls.
(2) Natural penicillins (penicillin G) effective against:
(a) Gram-positive organisms.
(b) Gram-negative organisms.
(c) Anaerobic organisms.
(3) Penicillinase-resistant penicillins (cloxacillin, dicloxacillin, methicillin, nafcilin, oxacillin).
(a) *S. aureus.*
(b) *S. epidermidis.*
(c) Some streptococci infections.
(4) Absorption.
(a) Oral absorption varies; limited by gastric acidity and binding with food.
(b) Completely and rapidly absorbed throughout the body after parental

administration.
(c) Distributed widely in fluids/tissue including liver, kidneys, bones, muscle, placenta.
(d) Does not readily enter CSF.
(e) Limited metabolization in the liver.
(f) Excreted primarily through the kidneys.
(5) Peak serum concentrations vary from one-half hour to 2 hours depending on route of administration.
e. Pharmacotherapeutics.
(1) Broad spectrum of antimicrobial activity.
(a) Procaine penicillin used for susceptible strains of gonorrhea.
(b) Benzathine penicillin G preferred for syphilis.
(c) Dicloxacillin: treatment of suspected or proven staphylococcal infections and most streptococci and *S. aureus* infections.
(d) Aminopenicillins (ampicillin and amoxicillin): broad spectrum; active against gram-negative bacteria; better absorbed with less GI distress.
(2) Dosage/Indications.
(a) Dependent on type of penicillin and route of administration.
(b) Used to treat common infections: syphilis, staph infections.
(3) Adverse reactions.
(a) Hypersensitivity reactions (the major adverse reaction).
(b) Neurotoxicity.
(c) Nephrotoxicity.
(d) Electrolyte imbalances.
(e) Hematologic reactions.
(4) Drug interactions.
(a) Probenecid. *gout : penicillin adjunct*
(b) Methotrexate.
(c) Tetracyclines.
(d) Chloramphenicol. *infection*
(e) Aminoglycosides (penicillin G, azlocillin, carbenicillin, mezlocillin, piperacillin, ticarcillin).
(f) Neomycin (penicillin V).
(g) Oral contraceptives (penicillin V, ampicillin).

3. Cephalosporins.
a. Pharmacokinetics.
(1) Properties and mechanisms of action resemble penicillins.
(2) Semisynthetic derivation of cephalosporin C (produced by fungus *cephalosporin auremonium*); classified by generation which is determined by spectra of activity.
(3) Rapidly absorbed by the GI tract.

(4) Food will delay but not diminish total absorption.

(5) Distributed widely through soft tissue and bodily fluids except CSF.

(6) Excreted essentially unchanged by the kidneys except for cefoperazone and ceftriaxone which are excreted in the feces.

(7) Oral cephalosporins reach a peak serum concentration level within 1 to 2 hours after administration; IV administration levels achieved within 30 minutes; IM administration delays peak serum levels and are 50% of those achieved by IV administration.

b. First generation.
  (1) Parenteral.
    (a) Cefazolin.
    (b) Cephalothin.
    (c) Cephapirin.
    (d) Cephradine.
  (2) Oral.
    (a) Cephalexin.
    (b) Cephradene.
    (c) Cefadroxil.
  (3) Treatment of gram-positive and gram-negative organisms (most staphylococci, Groups A&B hemolytic streptococci, most streptococci).

c. Second generation.
  (1) Parenteral.
    (a) Cefoxitin.
    (b) Cefamandole.
    (c) Ceforamide.
    (d) Cefonicid.
    (e) Cefuroxime.
  (2) Oral.
    (a) Cefaclor. *ceclor*
  (3) Treatment of gram-negative, gram-positive, and anaerobic organisms (same as first generation as well as, *Neisseria gonorroheae, Neisseria meningitidis, Enterobacter, Citrobacter, Clostridium, Bacteroides*).

d. Third generation.
  (1) Parenteral.
    (a) Cefalaxime.
    (b) Ceftriaxone. *Rocephine*
    (c) Cefoperazane.
    (d) Cefoperazone.
  (2) Oral.
    (a) Cefixime.
  (3) Treatment of gram-negative, gram-positive, and anaerobic organisms (same as first and second generation as well as, *Pseudomonas aeruginosa, Acinetobacter*).

e. Pharmacotherapeutics — ineffective against enterococci (*Streptococcus faecalis*),

methicillin-resistant staphylococci, and beta hemolytic streptococci.

f. Dosage/Indications.
  (1) Based on drug and condition being treated and route of administration.
  (2) Treatment of skin infections due to *S. aureus* and Group A&B beta-hemolytic strep.
  (3) Cellulitis due to *H. influenzae*.

g. Adverse reactions (relatively safe).
  (1) Hypersensitivity reactions (most common).
  (2) Cross-reactivity in patients that are sensitive to penicillins (approximately 10% to 20% of patients).
  (3) Pain, induration, and tenderness at site of injection.
  (4) In patients with impaired renal function, confusion, seizures.
  (5) In orally administered drug: nausea, vomiting, diarrhea.
  (6) Cephalosporins may produce nephrotoxicity.
  (7) Possibility of superinfection.

h. Drug interactions.
  (1) Acute alcohol intolerance with cefamandole, cefoperazone.
    (a) Headache.
    (b) Flushing.
    (c) Dizziness.
    (d) Nausea, vomiting, abdominal cramping.
  (2) Concomitant use of cephalosporins and imipenem/cilastatin.
    (a) Antagonizes antibacterial activity of betalactam cephalosporins.

4. Tetracyclines.
  a. Pharmacokinetics.
    (1) Absorbed from the duodenum.
    (2) Distributed widely into the body tissues, fluids.
    (3) Excreted primarily by the kidneys (except for doxycycline and minocycline).
    (4) Onset, peak, and duration of action vary among tetracyclines.

  b. Pharmacotherapeutics.
    (1) Provide broad-spectrum coverage against gram-positive, gram-negative, aerobic, and anaerobic bacteria; spirochetes, mycoplasmas, rickettsieae, chlamydiae, and some protozoa.
    (2) Doxycycline and minocycline provide more action against various organisms.

  c. Dosage/Indications.
    (1) Minocycline hydrochloride (Minocin®).
      (a) Treatment of severe acne: 50 mg qid or 100 mg bid.

(b) Not recommended in children under 8.
(2) Tetracycline hydrochloride (Achromycin®, Sumycin®).
  (a) Treatment of acne, Lyme disease, and syphilis in penicillin-allergic patients.
    i. 250 to 500 mg PO q 6 hr for gram-positive and gram-negative organisms.
    ii. 500 mg PO qid for 10 to 30 days for Lyme disease.
    iii. 250 to 500 mg qid for acne.
  (b) Pediatric dose: 25 to 50 mg/Kg/day PO in divided doses every 6 hours.
d. Adverse reactions.
(1) GI disturbances — nausea, vomiting, diarrhea. (Tetracycline must be taken on an empty stomach with either juice or water for proper absorption).
(2) Risk of superinfection.
(3) Significantly affects tooth enamel, therefore not recommended in children under age of 8, or pregnant patients.
(4) Photosensitivity reactions.
(5) Nephrotoxicity in patients with renal failure.
(6) Hepatotoxic reactions in patients with an excessive serum concentration due to renal failure.
(7) Light-headedness, loss of balance, dizziness, tinnitus (most common with minocycline).
(8) Yeast infections.
(9) Hypersensitivity reactions, though uncommon.
e. Drug interactions.
(1) Antacids with calcium, aluminum and magnesium — chlortetracycline, doxycycline, minocycline, tetracycline.
(2) Iron salts, bismuth, subsalicylate, zinc sulfate — tetracycline, doxycycline.
(3) Barbiturates, carbamazepin, phenytoin — doxycycline.
(4) Oral contraceptives — tetracycline.
(5) Penicillin — all tetracyclines.

B. **Antifungals (antimycotics): used to treat superficial (topical) and systemic infections.**
1. Nystatin.
  a. Pharmokinetics.
    (1) Little or no absorption, distribution or metabolism.
    (2) Excreted unchanged in feces.
  b. Pharmacotherapeutics.
    (1) Primarily treat superficial skin infections.
    (2) Effective against *C. albicans, C. guilliermondii,* and other Candida species.

(3) Oral nystatin is used to prevent fungal infection in neutropenic patients.
c. Dosage.
(1) For oral candidiasis: 500,000 units swish and swallow tid or qid, or 500,000 units oral tablets dissolved in the mouth tid or qid for 10 days.
d. Adverse reactions.
(1) Uncommon.
(2) Bitter taste.
(3) High doses may cause diarrhea, nausea, vomiting, and abdominal pain.
e. Drug interactions.
(1) None.
2. Amphotericin B (IV).
  a. Pharmokinetics.
    (1) Distributed throughout the body.
    (2) Excreted by the kidneys.
  b. Pharmacotherapeutics.
    (1) Indicated for treating severe systemic fungal infections.
    (2) Extremely toxic, therefore risk/benefit must be weighed carefully.
    (3) Used to treat aspergillosis, coccidiomycosis, cryptococcus, candidiasis, and phycomycosis infections.
  c. Dosage.
    (1) Test dose: 1 mg in 250 ml of dextrose 5% over 2 to 4 hours; increase to 5, 10, 20 mg over consecutive days.
    (2) Systemic fungal infections: 0.25 mg to 1.5 mg/kg/day based on organism present, patient's tolerance; infused over 4 to 6 hours.
  d. Adverse reactions.
    (1) Nephrotoxicity.
    (2) Hypokalemia.
    (3) Chills, fever.
    (4) Nausea, vomiting, anorexia.
    (5) Muscle and joint pain.
    (6) Headache.
    (7) Abdominal pain.
    (8) Normochromic or normocytic anemia.
    (9) Phlebitis/thrombophlebitis.
    (10) Hypotension/hypertension.
    (11) Flushing.
  e. Drug interactions.
    (1) Aminoglycosides.
    (2) Cyclosporine.
    (3) Acyclovir.
    (4) Corticosteroids.
    (5) Extended-spectrum penicillins.
    (6) Pancuronium bromide.
    (7) Electrolyte solutions.
3. Fluconazole (Diflucan®).
  a. Pharmokinetics.
    (1) Synthetic, broad-spectrum agent.

(2) 90% absorbed after oral administration.
(3) Distributed in all body fluids.
(4) Excreted unchanged in the urine.
(5) Peak plasma concentration 1 to 2 hours after administration.
b. Pharmacotherapeutics: indicated for treating candidal and cyryptococcal infections.
c. Dosage.
(1) Oropharyngeal candidiasis: 200 mg PO first day, then 100 mg PO daily for 2 weeks.
d. Adverse reactions: all reactions are more common in HIV patients.
(1) Transient elevations in SGOT/SGPT, alkaline phosphatase, and bilirubin.
(2) Dizziness.
(3) Nausea, vomiting, diarrhea, abdominal pain.
(4) Skin rash.
(5) Headache.
e. Drug interactions.
(1) Warfarin.
(2) Levels of phenytoin and cyclosporine may increase with fluconazole.
(3) Patients taking rifampin may require higher doses of fluconazole to get therapeutic results.
4. Terbinafine (Lamisil®).
a. Pharmokinetics.
(1) Disrupts the cell wall of fungal hyphe (fungacidal). Metabolized in the liver and excreted in the feces.
b. Pharmotheraputics.
(1) Indicated for treating widespread tinea infections of the skin and onychmycosis.
c. Dosage: 250 mg po qd X 4 weeks for tinea corporis, 6 weeks for fingernail involvement, and 12 weeks for toenails.
d. Adverse reactions.
(1) Elevated liver enzymes (rare).
(2) Leucocytopenia (rare).
(3) Stevens-Johnson type reaction (rare).
(4) Taste dysruption.
(5) Indigestion.
(6) Headache.
(7) Fatigue.
e. Drug interactions.
(1) Rifampin.
(2) Cyclosporine.
(3) Tagamet (oral antacid may decrease absorption).
5. Ketoconazole (Nizoral®). Oral ketaconazole is less often prescribed now than in the past years because newer azole drugs such as itraconazole and fluconazole are less likely to cause liver dysfunction.
a. Pharmacokinetics.

(1) Varied absorption and distribution.
(2) Metabolized in the liver and excreted through bile and feces.
(3) Peak plasma concentration reached in 1 to 4 hours.
b. Pharmacotherapeutics.
(1) Treatment of superficial and systemic infections with susceptible fungal organisms.
(a) Active against dermatophytes (tinea infections).
(b) Yeasts such as candida and malassezia.
(3) Response to treatment.
(a) Mucosal infections — respond in days.
(b) Skin infections — respond in weeks.
(c) Nail infections — respond in months.
c. Dosage.
(1) 200 mg PO daily; may increase to 400 mg if unresponsive.
(2) Duration varies with organism/site.
(a) 1 to 4 weeks for oral candidiasis.
(b) 1 to 2 months for dermatophyte infections.
(c) 6 to 12 months for chronic mucocuta neous candidiasis and tinea unguium.
d. Adverse reactions.
(1) Nausea/vomiting, diarrhea.
(2) Pruritus, skin rash, dermatitis, urticaria.
(3) Headache.
(4) Insomnia, lethargy.
(5) Dizziness.
(6) Interference with adrenal and corticosteroid synthesis leading to decreased circulatory testosterone.
e. Drug interactions.
(1) Warfarin.
(2) Methylprednisolone.
(3) Cyclosporine.
(4) Some hypoglyclic medications.
(5) Seldane®.
6. Itraconazole (Sporanox®).
a. Pharmacokinetics.
(1) Bioavailability maximal when taken with food.
(2) Metabolized in the liver and excreted in feces.
b. Pharmacotherapeutics: indicated in treating onychomycosis of the nails; deep fungal infections (blastomycosis and histoplasmosis).
c. Dosage.
(1) Toenails with or without fingernail involvement: 200 mg qd for 12 consecutive weeks.

(2) Fingernails only: two treatment pulses of 200 mg bid for 1 week; separate pulses by a 3 week period.
  d. Adverse reactions.
    (1) Elevated liver enzymes.
    (2) GI disorders.
    (3) Rash/pruritus.
    (4) Hypertension/orthostatic hypotension.
    (5) Headache.
    (6) Malaise.
    (7) Myalgia.
    (8) Vasculitis.
    (9) Vertigo.
    (10) Hypertriglyceridemia (with dosing for fingernail involvement).
    (11) Arrhythmias.
  e. Drug interactions.
    (1) Warfarin.
    (2) Antihistamines: terfenadine; astemizole.
    (3) Ritonavir, indinavir.
    (4) Benzodiazepines: midazolam, triazolam, diazepam.
    (5) Calcium channel blockers.
    (6) Cyclosporine.
    (7) Methylprednisolone.
    (8) Digoxin, quinidine.
    (9) Phenobarbital, carbamazepine.
    (10) Isoniazid, rifampin, rifabutin.
Note: Sporanox increases plasma concentrations of drugs 1 through 8; decreases plasma concentrations of drugs 9 through 10.
7. Griseofulvin.
  a. Pharmacokinetics: disrupts mitosis of fungal cells.
  b. Pharmacotherapeutics.
    (1) Indicated for treating fungal infections of the skin; less effective for nails.
    (2) Duration of therapy varies with site of infection.
  c. Dosage.
    (1) Gris-PEG®: 250 mg tid; qid for 12 to 18 months.
    (2) Fulvicin®: 250 mg tid; qid for 12 to 18 months.
    (3) Pediatric: Grifulvin® V 125 mg/5 cc suspension; 10 to 20 mg/Kg/d.
  d. Adverse reactions.
    (1) Nausea, vomiting, diarrhea.
    (2) Fatigue.
    (4) Confusion.
    (5) Headaches.
    (6) Rare: proteinuria, urticaria, rash, serum sickness, photosensitivity, hearing loss, paresthesia, dizziness, insomnia, leukopenia, oral candidiasis.
  e. Drug interactions.
    (1) Alcohol.

(2) Barbiturates.
(3) Warfarin.
(4) Oral contraceptives.
C. Antivirals.
1. Acyclovir.
  a. Pharmacokinetics.
    (1) Absorbed in the GI tract.
    (2) Distributed throughout the body.
    (3) Crosses the placenta.
    (4) Metabolized in the liver.
    (5) Excreted in the urine.
    (6) Peak concentration levels reached within 1.5 to 2.5 hours after oral administration; immediately after IV administration.
  b. Pharmacotherapeutics.
    (1) Effectiveness limited to herpes viruses (HSV 1 & 2; varicella-zoster virus).
    (2) Initial and recurrent genital herpes treated with oral acyclovir.
    (3) Recurrences may be reduced with long-term use.
    (4) Severe initial and recurrent mucocutaneous HSV infections and varicella-zoster, particularly in immunocompromised patients, requires parenteral administration.
    (5) Decreases severity, pain, and viral shedding.
    (6) Decreases duration of lesions.
  c. Dosage (must be adjusted in patients with renal dysfunction).
    (1) Acyclovir: 800 mg 5/day for 7 days.
    (2) Famvir: 500 mg q 8 hrs for 7 days.
    (3) Either medication must be started within 72 hours for optimal reduction in shedding.
    (4) Both medications are indicated to help prevent post-herpetic neuralgia.
  d. Adverse reactions.
    (1) Headache.
    (2) Nausea, vomiting, diarrhea.
    (3) Pruritus.
    (4) Fatigue.
    (5) Insomnia.
    (6) Irritability.
    (7) Depression.
    (8) Hypotension.
    (9) Rare: thrombocytosis, thrombocytopenia, transient lymphopenia, transient leukopenia, and bone marrow hypoplasia.
  e. Drug interactions.
    (1) Probenecid (and other drugs that inhibit tubular secretion or absorption).
    (2) Cimetidine.
    (3) Allopurinol.
    (4) Theophylline.

(5) Digoxin.

D. Antineoplastics.
1. Methotrexate.
   a. Pharmacokinetics.
      (1) Well absorbed and distributed throughout the body.
      (2) Undergoes minimal metabolism.
      (3) Peak plasma concentration reached 1 hour after oral dosing.
   b. Pharmacotherapeutics.
      (1) Used for treating recalcitrant, severe psoriasis, mycosis fungoides, psoriatic/rheumatoid arthritis.
      (2) May be used as steroid-sparing drug in immunobullous diseases.
         (a) A folic acid antagonist; inhibits cell division.
         (b) Has some activity as an immunosuppressive agent.
   c. Dosage: varies from 5 to 30 mg/week.
   d. Adverse reactions.
      (1) Hepatic fibrosis and cirrhosis with long-term use.
         (a) Liver function may be abnormal despite frequently normal blood tests.
         (b) Liver biopsy after first 1.5 gms and repeated after each increase of 1 to 1.5 gms.
      (2) Bone marrow suppression is usually dose dependent; WBC must be monitored carefully.
      (3) Nausea.
      (4) Malaise.
      (5) Headaches.
      (6) Teratogenic in females; harmful to male sperm; birth control indicated during course of medication.
   e. Drug interactions.
      (1) Probenecid.
      (2) Salicylates and NSAIDS.
      (3) Alcohol.
      (4) Cholestyramine.
      (5) Live vaccines.
      (6) Co-trimoxazole.
      (7) Penicillins.
2. Cyclophosphamide (Cytoxan®).
   a. Pharmacokinetics.
      (1) Synthesized derivation of nitrogen mustard.
      (2) Alkylating agent — disrupt the structure of DNA.
      (3) Absorbed well.
      (4) Peak plasma concentration reached 1 hour after oral dosing.
      (5) Hepatic metabolism.
      (6) Excreted in the urine.
   b. Pharmacotherapeutics.
      (1) Used for steroid-sparing therapy of immunobullous diseases and leukocytoclastic vasculitis.
      (2) Used in advanced mycosis fungoides and in connective tissue diseases.
      (3) Activity and effectiveness depend on type of cancer, the extent of disease, and patient's overall condition.
   c. Dosage.
      (1) 2 to 3 mg/kg up to 100 mg/kg PO.
      (2) Dosage must be adjusted in patient with impaired liver or renal function.
   d. Adverse reactions.
      (1) Bone marrow suppression.
      (2) Late lymphoreticular malignancies.
      (3) Hemorrhagic cystitis.
   e. Drug interactions.
      (1) Succinylcholine.
      (2) Chloramphenicol.
E. Retinoid (vitamin A).
1. Isotretinoin (Accutane®).
   a. Pharmacokinetics.
      (1) Isomer of retinoic acid, a metabolite of vitamin A.
      (2) Appears to reduce secretion of sebum; decreases the size of sebaceous glands.
      (3) May prevent abnormal keratinization.
      (4) Peak plasma concentrations reached 2.9 to 3.2 hours after dosing.
      (5) Metabolized in the liver and excreted in urine and feces.
   b. Pharmacotherapeutics.
      (1) Indicated in treating recalcitrant cystic acne.
      (2) May be used in ichthyosis, pityriasis rubra pilaris, Darier's disease.
      (3) May affect BCC, SCC, CTCL, keratoacanthoma, verruca vulgaris, DLE, pustular/erythrodermic psoriasis.
      (4) Females must have a negative pregnancy test before initiation of treatment and must use birth control for the duration of treatment and avoid pregnancy for 3 years after stopping medication.
   c. Dosage.
      (1) 0.5 to 2 mg/kg PO daily in two divided doses for 15 to 20 weeks.
      (2) Contraindicated if patient is sensitive to any ingredients or sensitivity to parabens.
      (3) Use with caution in diabetics and patients with hepatic disease.
   d. Adverse reactions.
      (1) Cheilitis.
      (2) Conjunctivitis.
      (3) Skin fragility.
      (4) Dry skin and mucous membranes.

(5) Epistaxis.
(6) Pseudotumor cerebri.
(7) Corneal opacities.
(8) Inflammatory bowel disease.
(9) Hypertriglyceridemia.
(10) Arthralgia.
(11) Hepatotoxicity.
(12) Photosensitivity.
e. Drug interactions.
(1) Vitamin A or vitamin A supplements.
(2) Minocycline.
(3) Tetracycline.
(4) Abrasives, medicated soaps, and cleansers.
(5) Alcohol-containing acne preparations or cosmetics.
(6) Alcohol.

2. Etretinate.
a. Pharmacokinetics — mechanism of action unknown.
b. Pharmacotherapeutics.
(1) Treatment of severe recalcitrant psoriasis, keratoacanthoma, lichen scleroses atrophicus, pityriasis rubra pilaris, psoriatic arthiritis, seborrheic dermatitis.
(2) Contraindicated in pregnant patients.
(3) CBC, baseline liver function, pregnancy test, cholesterol/triglycerides must be checked before beginning treatment and 1 to 2 week intervals for the first 1 to 2 months decreasing to 1 to 3 months if values within normal limits.
c. Dosage.
(1) 0.75 mg to 1 mg/kg PO initially in daily divided doses.
(2) Maximum initial dose not to exceed 1.5 mg/kg/d.
(3) Maintenance dose 0.5 to 0.75 mg/kg/d.
d. Adverse reactions.
(1) Blood dyscrasias.
(2) Pseudotumor cerebri.
(3) Headache.
(4) Dizziness.
(5) Lethargy.
(6) Dryness of skin and mucous membranes.
(7) Elevated liver enzymes.
(8) Hypo or hyperkalemia; hyperlipidemia.
(9) Bone pain.
(10) Photosensitivity.
e. Drug interactions.
(1) Alcohol.
(2) Hepatotoxic medications.
(3) Milk, high-fat diet.
(4) Tetracyclines.
(5) Vitamin A/vitamin A supplements.

F. Corticosteroids.
1. Pharmacokinetics.
a. Absorbed well through the GI tract; IM absorption varies.
b. Metabolized in the liver.
c. Excreted by the kidneys.
d. Cross the placenta and are distributed in breast milk.
e. Rapid onset of action, usually within 1 hour after oral dosing.
2. Pharmacotherapeutics.
a. Anti-inflammatory.
b. Immunosuppressive.
3. Dosage: based on disease process and severity.
4. Adverse reactions: usually seen with long-term treatment.
a. Adrenocortical insufficiency.
b. Muscle weakness.
c. Cataracts.
d. Cushingoid signs and symptoms.
e. Skin atrophy; striae; hirsutism.
f. Petechiae; ecchymoses.
g. Polycythemia; enhanced coagulability.
h. Fluid/electrolyte imbalance.
i. Weight gain.
j. Immunosuppression.
k. Mood changes.
l. Psychosis.
m. Osteoporosis.
n. Hypertension.
5. Drug interactions.
a. Barbiturates.
b. Phenytoin.
c. Rifampin.
d. Amphotericin B.
e. Furosemide.
f. Thiazide diuretics.
g. Erythromycin.
h. Salicylates.
i. NSAIDS.
j. Vaccines, toxoids.
k. Estrogen, oral contraceptives that contain estrogen.
l. Hypoglycemic agents.
m. Isoniazid.
n. Antihypertensive agents.

G. Psoralens (methoxsalen, oxsoralen, oxsoralen-ultra, 8-MOP).
1. Pharmacokinetics.
a. Increase melanization of the epidermis; thickening of the stratum corneum.
b. Photosensitizer.
c. Bonds with cellular DNA, causes cell damage when exposed to UVA light, decreasing cell turnover rate.
d. 95% absorbed from the GI tract.
e. Peak serum concentration increased when taken with food.

(1) Oxsoralen-ultra reaches peak serum concentration 30 minutes to 1 hour after ingestion.

(2) Oxsoralen reaches peak level in 1.5 to 6 hours after ingestion, with half-life being 2 hours.

 f. Metabolized in the liver, excreted in urine.

2. Pharmacotherapeutics.

 a. Used in treating psoriasis and vitiligo.

 b. Contraindicated if patient has increased risk for developing melanoma, SCC.

 c. Contraindicated if patient is aphakic, has disorder associated with photosensitivity, is an albino, or has documented cataracts.

3. Dosage.

 a. Psoriasis: individualized according to weight.

 b. Vitiligo: 20 mg with food or milk 2 hours prior to treatment.

4. Adverse reactions.

 a. Severe burns (must avoid sun exposure for 24 hours post ingestion).

 b. Rash; pruritus.

 c. Erythema; peeling.

 d. Nausea.

 e. Nervousness.

 f. Insomnia.

 g. Dizziness.

 h. Headache.

 i. Depression.

 j. Malaise.

5. Drug interactions.

 a. Photosensitizing drugs.

  (1) Phenothiazines.

  (2) Thiazides.

  (3) Sulfonamides.

  (4) Tetracyclines.

  (5) Griseofulvin.

  (6) Coal tar derivatives.

  (7) Nalidixic acid.

  (8) Halogenated salicylamides.

H. Immunosuppressants.

1. Cyclosporine A.

 a. Pharmacokinetics.

  (1) Distributed widely throughout the body; skin shows high concentrations.

  (2) Crosses the placenta.

  (3) Metabolized in the liver.

  (4) Excreted primarily in bile.

  (5) Peak serum concentration reached within 1 to 8 hours after oral dosing.

  (6) Variable absorption through GI tract.

 b. Pharmacotherapeutics.

  (1) Prevention of graft rejection without destruction of bone marrow.

  (2) Used for treating psoriasis, alopecia areata, pyoderma gangrenosum, Behcet's disease, atopic dermatitis, and

lichen planus.

  (3) Limited to treating moderately severe to severe recalcitrant psoriasis.

  (4) Contraindicated in patients with renal impairment, uncontrolled hypertension, migraine headaches, other infections, or if prone to infection or malignancy.

 c. Dosage.

  (1) Determined on body weight.

  (2) Psoriasis: 3 to 5mg/kg/d.

  (3) Initial dosing may be at maximum level (5 mg/kg/d) for rapid response with adjustment downward in 0.5 mg/kg/d increments for 2 weeks.

 d. Adverse reactions.

 e. Drug interactions.

2. Azathioprine (Imuran®).

 a. Pharmacokinetics — see cyclosporine.

 b. Pharmacotherapeutics.

  (1) Immunosuppressive effect, steroid sparing.

  (2) Used in immunobullous diseases, leukoplastic vasculitis, recalcitrant eczema, and connective tissue disease.

 c. Dosage.

  (1) 1 to 3 mg/day PO; based on severity of disease.

  (2) If no response after 6 to 8 weeks dose may be increased by 0.5 mg/kg/d.

 d. Adverse reactions.

  (1) Leukopenia, anemia, pancytopenia, thrombocytopenia.

  (2) Bone marrow suppression.

  (3) Nausea, vomiting, anorexia.

  (4) Pancreatitis.

  (5) Mouth ulcerations.

  (6) Hepatotoxicity.

  (7) Rash.

  (8) Alopecia.

  (9) Increased risk of SCC.

 e. Drug Interactions.

  (1) Allopurinol.

  (2) Nondepolarizing neuromuscular blocking agents.

I. Antihistamines.

1. Nonsedating (Claritin®, Zyrtec®, Allegra®).

 a. Pharmacokinetics.

  (1) Peak plasma levels reached in 1 hour.

  (2) Metabolized in the liver; excreted in feces.

  (3) H1-receptor antagonist.

 b. Pharmacotherapeutics.

  (1) Relief of allergic rhinitis.

  (2) Chronic idiopathic urticaria (Zyrtec and Allegra).

 c. Dosage.

  (1) Loratidine (Claritin): one 10 mg tablet daily.

(2) Cetirizine HCL (Zyrtec): Adults and children over 6 years old 5 mg to 10 mg po qd.

(3) Fexofidnine (Allegra): Adults and children 12 or older 60 mg po bid or 180 mg qd.

d. Adverse reactions.
(1) Hypotension.
(2) Syncope.
(3) Headache.
(4) Increased appetite.
(5) Nausea.
(6) Nervousness.
(7) Dry mouth.
(8) Elevated liver enzymes.
(9) Photosensitivity.
(10) Rash.
(11) Urinary retention (with BPH).

e. Drug interactions.
(1) CNS depressants.
(2) Antimuscarinics.
(3) Tricyclic antidepressants.
(4) Monoamine oxidase inhibitors (MAO).
(5) Phenothiazines.
(6) Norepinephrine/phenylephrine.
(7) Aminogylcosides.

2. Benadryl®, Atarax®, Tavist®, Tacaryl®, Temaril®, Periactin®: H1-antagonists have the same pharmacokinetics/pharmacotherapeutics as the nonsedating drugs except they cause drowsiness.

VI. LOCAL ANESTHETICS

A. Local anesthetics are drugs that slow or stop nerve conduction when applied close to nerve tissue. Both temporary sensory and motor nerve paralysis occur in the affected nerve distribution with complete recovery in the normal course of events.

B. Injectable anesthetics.
1. Ester linked — cocaine, procaine (Novocain®), tetracaine.
a. Metabolized in plasma or local tissue by the enzyme pseudocholinesterase.
b. Metabolized to PABA among other metabolites to which patients may already have been sensitized and may lead to severe allergic reactions.
c. Excreted through the kidneys.
2. Amide linked.
a. Metabolized in liver and excreted by the kidneys.
b. Rarely sensitizes.
c. Common amide anesthetics include:
(1) Lidocaine (Xylocaine®) — rapid onset, low toxicity and allergic potential, water soluble, and compatible with

vasoconstrictors and tissue fluid.
(2) Mepivacaine (Carbocaine®) — less toxic than lidocaine or procaine but slower onset of action.
(3) Bupivacaine (Marcaine®) — more potent and toxic than lidocaine and mepivacaine. Longer duration of action, onset of action delayed.
(4) Etidocaine (Duranest®) — four times more potent than lidocaine and lasts two times longer; useful for nerve blocks.

3. Other agents.
a. Antihistamines (Phenergan®, pyribenzamine, Benadryl).
(1) May be combined with epinephrine.
(2) Benadryl produces sedative effect if over 50 mg given. One suggested formula: 2 cc Benadryl (25 mg/cc), 8 cc normal saline, 0.1 cc epinephrine (1:1,000).
(3) Normal saline (to be effective must be injected to produce wheal; is inadequate for large procedures).

C. Vasoconstrictors (epinephrine 1:100,000 to 1: 500,000).
1. Shortens time of onset, prolongs durations, and increases the depth of anesthesia.
2. Reduces systemic toxicity by reducing rate of clearance, gaining more effective anesthesia with less drug volume.
3. Reduces bleeding during procedure (plain lidocaine is a vasodilator).
4. Useful with shorter-acting anesthetics; of little benefit with Marcaine or Duranest.

D. Untoward effects of systemic absorption of epinephrine.
1. Normal reaction to epinephrine includes restlessness, increased heart rate, palpitations, pounding in the head, chest pain. These symptoms alert physician of pending CNS toxicity with further absorption.
2. Avoid vasoconstrictors.
a. Digits.
b. When patient is taking phenothiazines, MAO inhibitors, and tricyclic antidepressants (raises blood pressure).
3. Dilute concentration of epinephrine.
a. Hypertensive patients or those with cardiovascular disease.
b. Anxious or nervous patients.
c. When patients are on beta blockers.

E. Adverse reactions to local anesthesia.
1. Usually related to vasoconstrictors; may result in anxiety, tremor, tachycardia, and diaphoresis when absorbed.
2. Vasovagal reactions include hyperventilation, apprehension, syncope.
3. Local reactions such as swelling, erythema, and

abscess formation usually caused by vasoconstrictors or hydrostatic pressure of large amounts of local anesthetic in confined spaces resulting in vascular occlusion.

4. True allergic reaction includes pruritus, urticaria, and angioedema with bronchospasm manifested by wheezing and coughing.

F. **System toxicity depends on concentration of local anesthesia in blood.**
   1. Maximum safe doses:
      a. Adult: repeated doses at 2-hour intervals.
         (1) 1% lidocaine with epinephrine 50 cc.
         (2) 1% lidocaine without epinephrine 30 cc.
         (3) Suggest 0.5% lidocaine when large amounts required.
         (4) Mepivacaine with/without epinephrine 35 cc.
         (5) Tetracaine without epinephrine 10 cc.
         (6) Bupivacaine with epinephrine 15 cc.
         (7) Etidocaine with epinephrine 30 cc.
         (8) Etidocaine without epinephrine 40 cc.
      b. Children: one-half to one-third adult dose.
   2. Plasma concentration is the result of a balance between the rate of absorption and its rate of elimination dependent upon:
      a. Inadvertent intravascular injection (into an artery or vein).
         (1) May occur with nerve blocks.
         (2) Inadvertent injection into scalp artery may more easily reach cerebral circulation and produce CNS response.
      b. Total dosage (see above).
      c. Speed on injection.
      d. Vascularity of injection site.
      e. Presence of vasoconstrictors in solution.
      f. Physiologic characteristics of local anesthetics.
      g. Decreased metabolism of local anesthesia.
      h. Health status of patient (be cautious in elderly, sick, and patient with renal or hepatic disease).

G. **Systemic toxicity mainly involves CNS and cardiovascular system.**
   1. Toxic blood levels of 1% lidocaine.
      a. Concentrations of 1% lidocaine — 10 mg/ml.
      b. Depending on site, peak blood level of between 0.5 to 2.0 µg/ml is reached for every 100 mg lidocaine given.
      c. 50 mg IV results in blood level of about 1 µg/ml.
   2. Central nervous system toxicity (mirrors blood concentration of local anesthetic).
      a. 1 to 5 µg/ml:
         (1) Ringing in ears.
         (2) Perioral numbness and tingling.
         (3) Metallic taste in mouth.
         (4) Lightheadedness, talkativeness.

         (5) Nausea and vomiting.
         (6) Double vision.
      b. 5 to 8 µg/ml may precede seizure activity:
         (1) Nystagmus.
         (2) Slurred speech.
         (3) Hallucinations.
         (4) Localized muscle twitching.
         (5) Fine tremors of face and hands.
      c. 8 to 12 µg/ml: focal seizure activity may increase to culminate in grand mal seizures (may be life threatening).
         (1) Usually self-limiting.
             (a) Protect from injury; lie patient flat and maintain open airway.
             (b) Oxygen delivery with mask.
             (c) IV diazepam if necessary.
      d. 20 to 25 µg/ml: cardiac toxicity, hypertension, arrhythmias, CNS depression, CV collapse.
   3. Cardiovascular effects (heart and peripheral arteries).
      a. All anesthetics except cocaine are vasodilators and can result in hypotension; patient may become pale, nauseated, with cold sweating.
      b. Inject with patient lying flat.
      c. Trendelenburg position if reactions appear. Apply cool wet washcloth to forehead, monitor vital signs, physician may order oxygen.

H. **Preventing CNS and cardiovascular reactions.**
   1. Use minimum effective dose, especially on head and neck.
   2. Aspirate before injection.
   3. Use nerve block whenever possible.
   4. Allow sufficient time for anesthesia before reinjecting.
   5. Avoid injection of inflamed tissue which results in unsatisfactory anesthesia due to lower tissue pH.
   6. Use vasoconstrictors when indicated.
   7. Some physicians consider preoperative diazepam when large amounts of local anesthetics must be used; this raises seizure threshold but may induce respiratory depression.
   8. Consider pre-existing renal, hepatic, cardiac failure that may decrease clearance and increase risk of toxic dose.
   9. Reduce dose in elderly.

I. **Allergy.**
   1. More common in patients with underlying atopic or immunologic problems, multiple drug allergies (especially procaine penicillin).
   2. Ester groups primarily responsible for allergic reactions.
   3. Allergy to amides very rare — may be allergic to preservative (paraben) in mixture, which is

also present in ester mixtures.

4. Topical sensitization to lidocaine has been substantiated leading to anaphylaxis.
5. Allergy symptoms.
   a. Skin: pruritus, urticaria, erythema, facial swelling.
   b. GI: nausea, vomiting, abdominal cramps, diarrhea.
   c. Respiratory: cough, sneezing, dyspnea, cyanosis, laryngeal edema.
6. Treatment of allergy to local anesthetic.
   a. SQ epinephrine (may need IV epinephrine).
   b. Maintain airway.
   c. Oxygen.
   d. Transport to acute care facility (needs observation for 6 hours).

J. **Effects on fetus/newborns.**
   1. Avoid during first trimester while organogenesis has begun.
   2. Postpone large procedures if possible until after delivery (hepatic system of fetus is immature).
   3. Small procedures require minimal anesthetic and may be performed if necessary. Dilute epinephrine 1:300,000.
   4. All local anesthetics are excreted into breastmilk and toxicity to infant is possible.

K. **Topical anesthetics: the epidermis offers an effective barrier to diffusion of anesthetic agents while absorption through mucous membranes occurs quickly.**
   1. Cocaine (4% solution): a vasoconstrictor useful for anesthesia of nasal mucosa.
      a. Maximum safe dose: 5 cc (200 mg) in adult.
      b. Soak cotton ball in solution and apply topically to nasal mucosa with forceps.
      c. Peak effect is 2 to 5 minutes lasting 30 to 40 minutes.
      d. Absorption in mucosa is slow; increased cocaine blood level may occur 4 to 6 hours after nasal application.
      e. Renders superficial (not deep) anesthesia only.
   2. Benzocaine available as 20% gel or aerosol or 2.5% to 20% solution.
      a. Useful in oral mucosa.
      b. Associated with increased risk of contact allergy.
      c. Cetacaine®, used by otolaryngologists, is:
         (1) 14% benzocaine.
         (2) 2% tetracaine.
         (3) 2% bulylaminobenzoate.
         (4) Spray of 1 second with 0.1 cc solution produces 30 seconds mucosal anesthesia.
   3. 2% lidocaine jelly.
      a. Contains parabens.
      b. Maximum dose: 30 cc (600 mg) in 12-hour

period.

4. EMLA cream (lidocaine 2.5% and prilocaine 2.5%) is an emulsion in which the oil phase is an eutectic mixture of lidocaine and prilocaine in a ratio of 1:1 by weight.
   a. Applied to intact skin under occlusive dressing at least 1 to 2 hours before procedure.
   b. May cause a transient local blanching followed by temporary local erythema.
   c. Application of EMLA cream to larger areas or for longer times than those recommended could result in overabsorption of anesthetic resulting in serious side effects.
5. 0.5% Ophthaine® — 1 to 2 gtt on conjunctival surface prior to administering local anesthesia will prevent sting of lidocaine in eye and help eliminate blink reflex.
6. Viscous lidocaine for oral mucosa.

L. **Injection technique: patient comfort and safety.**
   1. Discuss procedure, goals, and expectations with patient.
   2. Consider need for preoperative sedation.
   3. Comfort measures.
      a. Positioning, distraction (conversation, music), ice prior to injection.
      b. Eliminate preservatives that are acidic and contribute to the "sting" of local anesthesia infiltration by:
         (1) Mix fresh solution of 0.1 cc epinephrine (1:1,000) to each 10 cc plain lidocaine. pH 6.5 to 6.8. Tissue fluid pH is 7.3 to 7.4.
         (2) Buffer stock lidocaine with epinephrine 1:100,000 with 1 cc sodium bicarb (8.4% solution) to every 10 cc lidocaine. Results in pH of 7.0 to 7.3.
            (a) Decreased duration may be due to more rapid absorption of less-charged buffered agents.
            (b) Epinephrine concentration reduced to 1:200,000.
            (c) Do not buffer Marcaine — may result in prolonged numbness of injection site.
            (d) Some physicians keep buffered solution up to 1 week. Loss of 25% epinephrine effect occurs by that time.
   4. Infiltration of anesthesia.
      a. Equipment includes gloves, goggles, 30 gauge 1" needles, Luer-lock syringes, alcohol prep.
      b. Pain is caused by inevitable expansion of tissue on injection and the speed with which it occurs.
         (1) SQ injection is less painful since tissue is

more distensible but onset is delayed (and duration of reaction is longer).

    (2) Intradermal injection produces immediate anesthesia with prolonged effect due to placement but is more painful.

    (3) Whenever dermis is bound tightly to underlying tissue and there is little fat (for example, nose), there is more resistance to instillation of local anesthetic and increased pain.

    (4) Use careful approach to bone.

  c. Proper technique includes:

    (1) Rapid needle penetration into tense skin.

    (2) SLOW INJECTION to lessen burning sensation.

    (3) Limit number of punctures by trailing the needle, inject proximal to distal.

    (4) Proper placement of anesthesia (not too deep).

    (5) Allow time for vasoconstrictors to take effect, at least 5 minutes.

    (6) Carefully test injected areas by "light" touch with needle — not dart-like jabs. Make sure patients are well anesthetized prior to procedure.

M. Field block: circumferential injections in superficial and deep planes.

  1. Avoids distortion of surgical field.

  2. Prevents possible implantation of cancer cells beyond surgical margins.

  3. Limits amount of anesthesia required to anesthetize area.

  4. Paralysis due to anesthesia of motor nerves; prepare patient in advance.

N. Nerve block.

  1. Requires less anesthetic volume, higher concentration such as 2% lidocaine useful.

    a. Duration of action may be prolonged with use of long-acting agent such as Duranest.

    b. Use of vasoconstrictors in blocks do not decrease bleeding at operative site, but does increase duration of anesthetic.

  2. Requires greater skill and knowledge of anatomy.

  3. Allow time for block to take effect — 10 minutes minimum.

  4. Complications of nerve blocks.

    a. Laceration of nerve — long-term or permanent anesthesia in area supplied by nerve.

    b. Intravascular injection may lead to acute toxicity.

    c. Nurse should maintain observation of patient following nerve blocks.

    d. Hematoma formation — apply firm pressure for 5 minutes to injection site to avoid hematoma formation resulting from vessel laceration.

    e. Needle breakage usually resulting from attempt to change needle position while in contact with bone.

    f. Infection — nerve blocks are considered an invasive procedure, maintain sterile technique.

VII. TOPICAL TREATMENTS

A. Balneotherapy.

  1. Objectives.

    a. Cleansing.

    b. Hydration.

    c. Enhance delivery of medication.

  2. Types of baths.

    a. Antibacterial: Potassium permanganate (1:32,000; 1:64,000).

      (1) Used for infected eczema, dirty ulcerations, furunculosis.

      (2) Lowers bacterial load.

    b. Colloidal: Starch/baking soda; Aveeno® colloidal or oilated colloidal.

      (1) Used for red, pruritic, or oozing conditions.

      (2) Soothing; helps relieve pruritus.

    c. Emollient: bath oils.

      (1) Dry skin conditions.

      (2) Cleanse and hydrate.

    d. Tar: oils with tar; coal tar concentrate (liquor carbonic detergens).

      (1) Scaly dermatoses (psoriasis).

      (2) Relieve pruritus.

      (3) Loosen scale.

      (4) Potentiate UVB/UVA.

  3. Nursing considerations.

    a. Average home tub holds 150 to 200 L of water.

    b. Hot water and soap are drying, increasing pruritus; use tepid water and limit soap use.

    c. Pat dry leaving some moisture on the skin.

    d. Apply medication or emollient immediately after patting skin dry.

  4. Patient education.

    a. Inform patient of appropriate bath preparation.

    b. Educate patient to use tepid water to decrease pruritus.

    c. Re-emphasize that bath additives can cause slippery conditions; use rubber mats.

B. Soaks.

  1. Objectives.

    a. Loosen eschar/crusts.

    b. Decrease/prevent infection.

    c. Relieve pruritus.

    d. Promote drying in moist dermatoses.

    e. Enhance re-epithelialization.

    f. Decrease pain.

Table 4.
Examples of Wet Dressings

Agent	Strength	Preparation	Germicidal Activity	Astringent Activity	Comments
Normal saline	0.9%	1 tsp to a pint of water	-	-	Inexpensive, easy to prepare.
Aluminum acetate Burow's solution Domeboro packets/tablets	5% -	Dilute to 1:10 - 1:40 One packet/table to a pint of water yields a 1:40 solution; two yields a 1:20 solution.	Mild Mild	+ +	
Potassium permanganate	65 mg and 330 mg tablets	Dilute to 1:40,000-1:16,000; 65 mg tablet to 250-1,000 cc; 330 mg tablet to 1,500-5,000 cc.	Moderate	-	Stains skin, clothing.
Silver nitrate	0.1%-0.5%	1 tsp or a 50% stock solution to 1,000 cc yields a 0.25% solution.	Good	+	Stains, can cause pain.
Acetic acid	1%	Dilute 1:5 with standard 5% household vinegar.	Good	+	Smells, can be irritating.

From *Dermatology Nurses' Association Dermatology Nursing Basics Course.* (2003). Pitman, NJ: Dermatology Nurses' Association.

2. Types of soaks (see Table 4 Wet Dressings).
   a. Tap water.
      (1) Cooling.
      (2) Relieve pruritus.
      (3) Loosen eschar/crust.
   b. Aluminum acetate (Domeboro®, Aluwets®, Burow's® solution); one tablet in one quart of water.
      (1) Cooling.
      (2) Relieve pruritus.
      (3) Loosen eschar/crust.
      (4) Promote drying in moist dermatoses.
      (5) Provides mild antiseptic effect (mix 1 tablet with 1 pint water).
   c. Potassium permanganate (KMnO4): 0.25% to 0.5%.
      (1) Cooling.
      (2) Relieve pruritus.
      (3) Loosen eschar/crust.
      (4) Provide astringent effect.
      (5) Provide antimicrobial effect (especially Pseudomonas aeruginosa).
   d. Normal saline: 0.9%.
      (1) Cooling.
      (2) Relieve pruritus.
      (3) Loosen eschar/crust.
   e. Silver nitrate (AgNO3): 1:1,000 to 1:10,000.
      (1) Astringent.
      (2) Antibacterial.
3. Nursing considerations.
   a. Soaks must be kept wet.
   b. Gauze pads with fillers should not be used for soaks (retain too much solution/fibers

   may be left in wounds).
4. Patient education.
   a. Instruct patient on objective of soak.
   b. Demonstrate mixing of solution (if applicable) and appropriate application technique.
C. **Therapeutic shampoos.**
1. Objective.
   a. Cleansing.
   b. Remove accumulated scales, crusts, or medications.
   c. Deliver medication.
2. Types of shampoos.
   a. Salicylic acid/sulfur.
   b. Zinc pyrithione.
   c. Surfactants.
   d. Tar.
   e. Selenium sulfide.
   f. Nizoral®.
3. Nursing considerations.
   a. Avoid scrubbing scalp with fingernails to remove scale.
   b. Allow shampoo to stay on scalp to enhance penetration.
   c. Dryers may increase scaling and pruritus.
   d. Rinsing with a solution of two tablespoons of white vinegar in one gallon of water will help prevent hair from becoming dry.
4. Patient education.
   a. Inform patient regarding the objective of therapy.
   b. Demonstrate appropriate technique for therapeutic shampoo.

VIII. CRYOSURGERY

A. Definition: the destruction of tissue through freezing, most commonly with liquid nitrogen; less scarring due to ability to control depth of tissue destruction.
B. Indications.
   1. Actinic keratoses.
   2. Seborrheic keratoses.
   3. Leukoplakia.
   4. Molluscum contagiosum.
   5. Condyloma acuminatum.
   6. Superfical BCC and SCC in situ (rarely).
C. Nursing considerations.
   1. Good cosmetic results with little anesthesia.
   2. Most painful when used to treat lesions on nose, lips, ears, or eyelids.
   3. Few side effects but can damage vital vessels and tear ducts.
   4. Application with cotton-tipped applicator allows for more control of tissue depth.
   5. Blisters form in 3 to 6 hours after application; flattens in 2 to 3 days and peels off in approximately 2 to 3 weeks.
   6. If site is kept clean infection is rare.
D. Patient education.
   1. Explain the objective of treatment.
   2. Inform patient that there will be some discomfort associated with the treatment.
   3. Explain the sequence of skin changes associated with treatment.

IX. LASER

A. Definition: laser is an acronym for Light Amplification by Stimulated Emission of Radiation. The energy from the laser is directed at the skin and the majority will be absorbed by chromophores. Lasers produce measurable, repeatable, consistent zones of tissue damage. They can cut, coagulate, and vaporize tissue to some degree.
B. Types: see Tables 5 & 7 for types and indications for use.
C. Nursing considerations.
   1. Must have thorough knowledge of laser safety for both patient and health care providers.
   2. Written policy and procedures addressing laser safety should be in place.
   3. Pre and post-treatment education is essential.
   4. Photosensitivity may occur after photodynamic therapy, lasting 4 to 6 weeks.
D. Patient education.
   1. Inform patient about objective of treatment.
   2. Educate patient regarding pre and post-treatment interventions.
   3. Inform patient regarding increased vulnerability of skin and need to avoid environmental stresses including UV radiation.

   4. Inform patient regarding need for multiple treatments when indicated.

X. DERMATOLOGIC SURGERY

A. Shave biopsy: see Diagnostic Options, Chapter 2.
B. Punch biopsy: see Diagnostic Options, Chapter 2.
C. Excisional biopsy: see Diagnostic Options, Chapter 2.
D. Wedge biopsy: see Diagnostic Options, Chapter 2.
E. Mohs: see Chapter 6.
F. Dermabrasion.
   1. Definition: the process of planing the superficial layer of epidermis and dermis. The area to be treated may be anesthetized by injecting local anesthesia or freezing the area with fluoroethyl spray.
   2. Indications.
      a. Removal of superficial scars.
      b. Removal of hyperplastic tissue.
      c. Tattoo removal.
      d. To smooth out rhinophyma.
      e. Sun-damaged skin.
   3. Nursing considerations.
      a. Patient expectations may be unrealistic.
      b. Results are seen slowly.
      c. Discomfort may increase as lesions dry and heal.
      d. Risk of infection due to loss of protective barrier.
      e. Photosensitivity post-procedure.
      f. Edema is common post-procedure, keep head elevated at least 45 degrees during first 24 to 48 hours.
      g. Analgesics may be indicated for post-procedure discomfort.
   4. Patient education.
      a. Educate patient regarding the procedure.
      b. Explain what outcomes may be expected; patient may be unrealistic in expectations.
      c. Inform patient of post-procedure care.
         (1) Petrolatum to relieve tightness.
         (2) Keep head elevated for 24 to 48 hours post-procedure to reduce edema.
         (3) Use saline solution for wound cleansing and to help reduce edema.
         (4) Signs of infection.
         (5) Need for sun protection.
         (6) Take analgesics as directed for discomfort.
      d. Inform patient to expect oozing for at least 24 hours.
      e. Inform patient that crust will form and will last approximately 1 week.
      f. Inform patient that skin will remain red for approximately 2 to 3 months.

Table 5.
Lasers Used to Treat Cutaneous Lesions

Laser Type	Wavelength (nm)	Mode of Output	Clinical Use
Argon	488	Continuous	Vascular and pigmented lesions
Argon	514	Continuous	Vascular and pigmented lesions
Flashlamp-pumped pigmented lesion dye	510	Short-pulsed	Pigmented lesions; tattoos
Copper vapor	511	Pseudo-continuous	Pigmented lesions
Krypton	521; 530	Continuous	Pigmented lesions
KTP	532	Pseudo-continuous	Vascular and pigmented lesions
Frequency-doubled Q-switched Nd:YAG	532	Pulsed-continuous	Vascular and pigmented lesions; tattoos
Krypton	568	Continuous	Vascular lesions
Cooper vapor	578	Pseudo-continuous	Vascular lesions
Flashlamp-pumped dye	585	Long-pulsed	Vascular lesions
Argon-pumped tunable dye	585-690	Continuous	Vascular lesions; photodynamic therapy
Q-switched ruby	694	Pulsed	Pigmented lesions; tattoos
Q-switched alexandrite	755	Pulsed	Pigmented lesions; tattoos
Q-switched Nd:YAG	1,064	Pulsed	Pigmented lesions; tattoos
Nd:YAG	1,064	Continuous	Deep coagulation of tissue
Carbon dioxide	10,600	Continuous	Tissue cutting; coagulation; vaporization

From Marcus, J., & Goldberg, D.J. (1996). Lasers in dermatology: A nursing perspective. *Dermatology Nursing, 8*(3), 181-195.

Table 6.
Vascular Lesions Treated with Lasers

Laser Type	Clinical Use	Other Considerations
Argon	Telangiectases; thick PWS in adults	Increased risk of scarring.
KTP	Telangiectases; thick PWS in adults	Increased risk of scarring.
Frequency-doubled Q-switched Nd:YAG	Telangiectases; cherry angioma; capillary hemangioma	Temporary unsightly purpura.
Krypton	Telangiectases; thick PWS in adults	Better for large caliber vascular lesions; increased risk of scarring.
Copper vapor	Telangiectases; thick PWS in adults	Better for large caliber vascular lesions; increased risk of scarring.
Flashlamp-pumped dye	Flat PWS and PWS in children; telangiectases	Least risk of scarring; temporary unsightly purpura.
Argon-pumped tunable dye	Telangiectases; thick PWS in adults.	
Nd:YAG	Deep coagulation of tissue; cavernous hemangioma	Better for deep, large caliber vascular lesions; increased risk of scarring.

Port-wine stain (PWS)
Capillary (cutaneous) hemangioma
Cavernous (subcutaneous) hemangioma
Cherry angioma
Nevus araneus
Venous lake
Glomus tumor
Kaposi's sarcoma
Pyogenic granuloma

Angiokeratoma
Adenoma sebaceum
Angiolymphoid hyperplasia
Rosacea
Poikiloderma of Civatte
Telangiectases
Verrucae
Hypertrophic scars

From Marcus, J., & Goldberg, D.J. (1996). Lasers in dermatology: A nursing perspective. *Dermatology Nursing, 8*(3), 181-195.

Table 7.
Pigmented Lesions Treated with Lasers

Laser Type	Clinical Use	Other Considerations
Argon	Epidermal pigmented lesions	Scarring
Argon	Epidermal pigmented lesions	Scarring
Flashlamp-pumped pigmented lesion dye	Epidermal pigmented lesions; tattoos (red, orange, purple, yellow, tan)	
Copper vapor	Epidermal pigmented lesions	
Krypton	Epidermal pigmented lesions	
KTP	Epidermal pigmented lesions	
Frequency-doubled Q-switched Nd:YAG	Epidermal pigmented lesions; tattoos (red, orange, purple, tan)	
Q-switched ruby	Dermal and epidermal pigmented lesions; tattoos (black, blue, green)	
Q-switched alexandrite	Dermal and epidermal pigmented lesions; tattoos (black, blue, green)	
Q-switched Nd:YAG	Dermal pigmented lesions; tattoos (black, blue)	
Nd:YAG	Dermal pigmented lesions; tattoos (black, blue).	

TATTOOS

Dermal Pigmented Lesions — Nevus of Ota, Nevus of Ito, Becker's nevus, Melasma

Epidermal Pigmented Lesions — Solar lentigo, Ephelides, Epidermal nevus, Melasma, Café au lait, Becker's nevus

From Marcus, J., & Goldberg, D.J. (1996). Lasers in dermatology: A nursing perspective. *Dermatology Nursing, 8*(3), 181-195.

XI. PHOTOTHERAPY

A. Definition: the exposure of nonionizing radiation for therapeutic benefit; ultraviolet light is not visible and is classified by wavelength — UVC, UVB, UVA; UVB and UVA are used in treating dermatologic diseases.
B. Types of phototherapy.
  1. UVB.
    a. Wavelength of 290 to 320 nm.
    b. Sunburning spectrum of light, therefore the most damaging.
    c. Potential carcinogenesis following long-term exposure.
    d. Indications.

(1) Treatment of photosensitive dermatoses.
(2) Pregnant women and children may be treated since there are no drugs needed for UVB to be effective.
(3) Used for patients with UVA; contraindications such as previous arsenic or x-ray therapy.
  e. Contraindications.
(1) Can exacerbate photodermatoses.
(2) Previous nonmelanoma skin cancers or family history of melanoma.
(3) Inability of patient to stand due to physical limitations.
(4) Noncompliance with regular treatment schedule.

Dermatologic Nursing Essentials: A Core Curriculum 2nd Edition © DNA 2003

Table 8.
Skin Typing by Pigmentation, Erythema, and Genetic History

Skin Type I	
Pigmentation & Erythema History	Has very poor ability to tan; burns easily and severely, and then peels.
Genetic History	Very fair skin, freckling evident; blue green, grey eye color, blonde, red, or light brown hair; unexposed skin is white; Celtic, Northern European heritage.
Skin Type II	
Pigmentation & Erythema History	Tans minimally or lightly following exposure, usually burns easily resulting in a painful burn.
Genetic History	Fair skin, unexposed skin is white; blue, green, grey, or brown eye color; blonde, red, or brown hair; German, European heritage.
Skin Type III	
Pigmentation & Erythema History	Tans gradually following exposure, burns moderately.
Genetic History	Unexposed skin is white; hair and eye color usually brown; Southern European heritage.
Skin Type IV	
Pigmentation & Erythema History	Burns minimally, tans well with initial exposure.
Genetic History	White or light brown skin color; unexposed skin is white or light brown; dark hair and eye color; Mediterranean, Oriental, or Hispanic heritage.
Skin Type V	
Pigmentation & Erythema History	Tans easily and profusely, rarely burns.
Genetic History	Brown skin, unexposed skin is brown; African, American Indian, East Indian, Hispanic heritage.
Skin Type VI	
Pigmentation & Erythema History	Deeply pigmented, never burns.
Genetic History	Black skin, unexposed skin is black; African, American Indian, East Indian, Hispanic heritage.

From Leach, E.L., McClelland, P.B., Morgan, P., & Shelk, J. (1996). Basic principles of photobiology and photochemistry for nurse phototherapists and phototechnicians. *Dermatology Nursing, 8*(4), 235-258.

f. Dosing.
　(1) Skin type — estimate of patient's ability to tolerate ultraviolet light (see Table 8 for skin types).
　(2) Minimal erythema dose — the smallest amount of ultraviolet light needed to produce mild erythema.
　　(a) Small sections of the patient's skin are exposed to increasing doses of UVB.
　　(b) Results are read within 18 to 24 hours.
g. Schedule for treating psoriasis.
　(1) Initially three or more treatments/week.
　(2) Treatments should be scheduled with 1 day of "rest" in between (erythema from UVB should show up 6 to 8 hours after exposure).
h. Nursing considerations.
　(1) Always evaluate extent of erythema before retreating a patient.
　(2) Arms and legs may require extra dosing; all other areas must be shielded.
　(3) Always question the patient regarding medications that may be photosensitizers.
　(4) Protective goggles must be worn during treatment.
　(5) Do not increase treatment if a treatment has been missed.
i. Patient education.
　(1) Explain objective of treatment.
　(2) Explain possible side effects of treatment.
　(3) Emphasize the importance of patient reporting any new medications, prescription or OTC, to avoid photosensitization.
　(4) Reinforce the importance of compliance with treatment regimen.
　(5) Instruct patient to use emollients after treatment to prevent dryness and pruritus.
　(6) Instruct patient on interventions for UVB burns.
2. UVA (Photochemotherapy, PUVA).
　a. Wavelength of 320 to 400 nm.
　b. 1,000 times less effective in producing erythema than UVB.
　c. May enhance the photobiologic effects of UVB.
　d. Can produce skin damage in the presence of photosensitizers.
　e. Requires a photosensitizing drug, psoralen either topically or systemically, to be effective.
　　(1) Topical psoralen (paint PUVA).

Table 9.
MED Approach

The second method of establishing a starting dose is called MED testing. MED stands for minimal erythema dose. This is the smallest amount of ultraviolet light needed to product a slight sunburn. With this method, several small sections of the patient's skin are exposed to increasing doses of UVB. This test is read 18 to 24 hours later. Remember not to do MEDs on Fridays unless the center is open on Saturdays.

When doing MEDs, it is important to test an area of the body that is not normally exposed to the sun, such as the buttocks or abdomen. Sun-exposed areas such as forearms, produce higher readings than unexposed areas. Always calculate the light dose for the unexposed areas.

SUGGESTED MED DOSE GUIDELINE

Skin Type					Dose Range in mj				
I	5	10	15	20					
II		10	20	30	40				
III			20	30	40	50	60		
IV				30	40	50	60	70	80
V					40	50	60	70	80	90	100

A rule-of-thumb is to double the expected MED for each skin type. For example, the expected MED for a skin Type III is 30 mj. Multiply 30 times 2 equals 60 mj.

Six test sites are chosen and the rest of the body is completely protected from UVB light. All sites are open at the beginning of the test and closed individually after each dose of light is given.

Outline the test sites with a skin marker. This provides clear identification of the test sites.

From *Dermatology Nurses' Association Phototherapy Administration Symposium*. (2003). Pitman, NJ: Dermatology Nurses' Association.

(a) Useful for localized lesions and is very potent.
(b) Higher risk of burning or blistering than with systemic psoralen.
(c) Application must be done meticulously 30 minutes prior to exposure to UVA.
(d) Post treatment with topical psoralen, site must be washed with soapless cleanser; moisturizing sun block and/or appropriate clothing must be worn over site 8 hours.
 f. Dosage.
(1) MED or skin type dosing (see Table 9).
(2) Intensity and dosage length are increased as tolerated.
 g. Treatment schedule.
(1) Three times/week on alternate days until clearing.
(2) Maintenance program is individualized based on response.
 h. Indications.
(1) Failure of topical steroid, tar, anthralin, and UVB.
(2) Extensive skin involvement.
(3) Nail disease.
(4) Geographic, social, or occupational factors that necessitate keeping treatments to a minimum.

Table 10.
Assessment Prior to Initiating PUVA Photochemotherapy

Subjective Data
1. Motivation to adhere to regimen.
2. Ability to alter work and personal schedule to adhere to therapy schedule.
3. Financial needs/concerns regarding prescribed drug and treatment, physicians' fees, and transportation.

Objective Data
1. Determine skin type.
2. Perform thorough assessment of skin area to be treated.
3. Obtain results of patient's initial ophthalmology exam.
4. Obtain complete history of other medications patient is taking — prescription and over-the-counter. Pay particular attention to any that may cause photosensitivity.
5. Obtain complete health history — particularly in regards to liver problems, skin cancer, heart problems, hypertension, and lupus erythematosus.

The nurse will notify physician of inability to initiate therapy if a problem exists with the patient's ability to begin PUVA therapy.

From Galloway, G.A., & Lawson, G.B. (1995). Photochemotherapy (PUVA) protocol. *Dermatology Nursing, 7*(6), 348-351.

Table 11.
PUVA Treatment Outcomes

The patient will:
1. Verbalize understanding of PUVA therapy.
2. Verbalize understanding of action and side effects of oral methoxsalen.
3. Demonstrate adherence to correct regimen for PUVA therapy.
   a. Take methoxsalen as directed — 1.5 to 2 hours prior to scheduled PUVA treatment.
   b. Wear protective glasses and protective clothing immediately after taking the methoxsalen and for 24 hours following PUVA treatment.
4. Demonstrate physical signs of therapeutic response to PUVA without side effects as evidenced by:
   a. Light-to-medium pink erythemal response 24 to 48 hours following each treatment.
   b. Tolerance of methoxsalen by no complaints of nausea and vomiting.
   c. Lab values maintained within normal limits.
   d. Ophthalmologic exams saw no evidence of cataract formation.

The nurse will:
1. Assess patient's understanding, ability, and motivation to adhere to PUVA regimen.
2. Monitor patient's response to PUVA therapy for:
   a. Adverse side effects of oral medication and light treatment.
   b. Inability to cope with altered body image and stress of managing therapy regimen.

From Galloway, G.A., & Lawson, G.B. (1995). Photochemotherapy (PUVA) protocol. *Dermatology Nursing, 7*(6), 348-351.

Table 12.
Monitoring During PUVA Therapy

1. Assess patient's response to psoralen for adverse side effects once treatment is begun.
2. Assess patient's skin before each treatment for adverse erythemal response from previous treatment.

From Galloway, G.A., & Lawson, G.B. (1995). Photochemotherapy (PUVA) protocol. *Dermatology Nursing, 7*(6), 348-351.

Table 13.
Actions if Adverse Side Effects Are Suspected

1. If patient's skin is extremely red or blistered, suspect hypersensitivity to ultraviolet light. Contact physician before proceeding with treatment.
2. If patient is exhibiting side effects of the psoralen such as depression, dizziness, headache, swelling, rash, or leg cramps for more than 24 to 48 hours, contact physician.

Table 14.
Patient Instructions Prior to Initiating PUVA

1. Instruct patient on what PUVA therapy is and how it works.
2. Instruct patient on action and side effects of medication.
3. Instruct patient on PUVA therapy regimen and necessary precautions while taking photosensitizing medication. Patient should protect his/her skin and eyes from sunlight and artificial UVA light sources (fluorescent lights) for 24 hours following ingestion of psoralens and the light treatment.
4. Instruct patient on what to expect from PUVA therapy.
5. Caution patient against taking any medications or using anything topical without approval of physician since some medications cause photosensitivity.

From Galloway, G.A., & Lawson, G.B. (1995). Photochemotherapy (PUVA) protocol. *Dermatology Nursing, 7*(6), 348-351.

      (5) Photosensitivity to UVB.
   i. Absolute contraindications.
      (1) Xeroderma pigmentosum.
      (2) LE.
      (3) Lactation.
      (4) Porphyria cutanea tarda, erythropoietic porphyria, variegate porphyria.
      (5) Albinism.
      (6) Pregnancy.
   j. Relative contraindications.
      (1) Age, infirmity.
      (2) Pemphigus and pemphigoid exacerbated by UVA/UVB.
      (3) Uremia or severe hepatic failure.
      (4) History or family history of melanoma.
      (5) Past history of nonmelanoma skin cancer.
      (6) Extensive solar damage.
      (7) Previous treatment with ionizing radiation or arsenic.
      (8) Patients with cataracts or who are aphakic.
      (9) Dysplastic nevus syndrome.
      (10) Photosensitizing medications.
      (11) Severe cardiac disease.
      (12) Noncompliant patient.
      (13) Immunosuppression.
   k. Nursing considerations (see Tables 10-13).
   l. Patient education (see Table 14).

XII. UNNA'S BOOT

A. Definition: a dressing for varicose ulcers formed by applying a layer of a gelatin-glycerin-zinc oxide paste to the leg and then a spiral bandage

Figures 1-14.
Stages of Wrapping

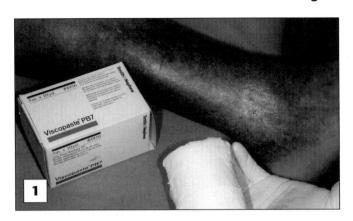

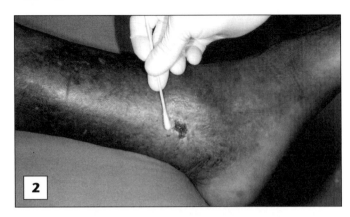

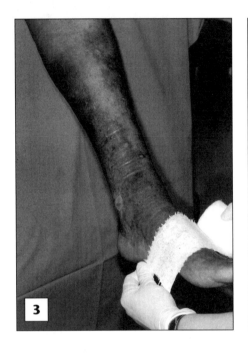

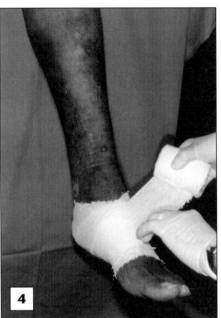

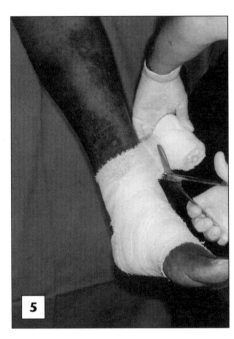

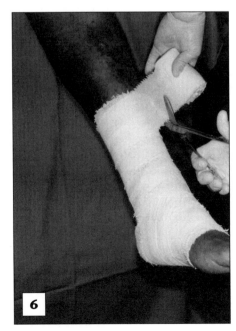

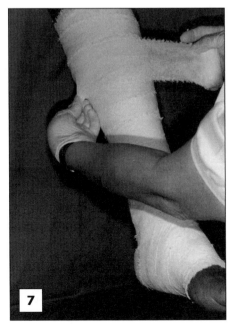

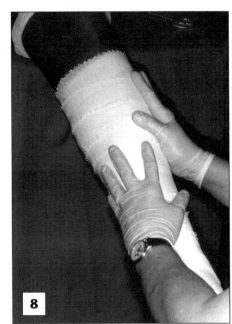

Dermatologic Nursing Essentials: A Core Curriculum 2nd Edition © DNA 2003

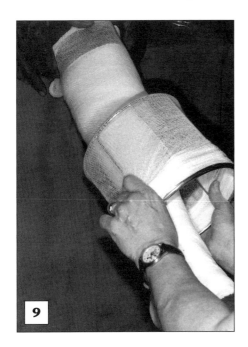

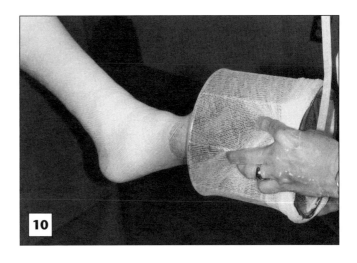

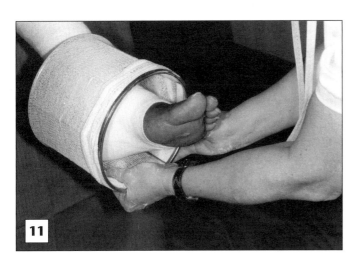

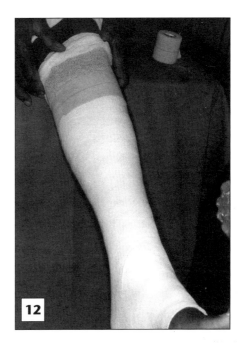

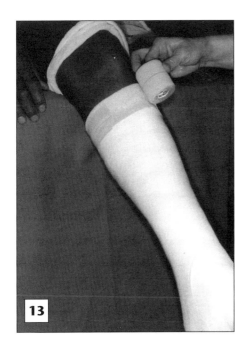

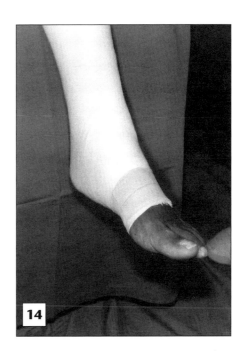

that is covered with successive coats of paste to produce a rigid boot.

B. Indications.
1. To reduce edema.
2. Decrease healing time in stasis ulcers.
3. Give support to surgical wounds.
4. Protect lesions from manipulation.
5. Excellent alternative to elastic wraps particularly for patients who are not self-sufficient.

C. Application.
1. Should be applied to legs before arising in the morning to prevent edema.
2. Applied with graduated pressure with greatest pressure at ankle and gradually lessening as wrapped up the leg.
3. Specialized dressing of 3 inch x 10 yard of gauze impregnated with zinc oxide (see Figure 1).
4. Wash leg with warm water and dry thoroughly.
5. Apply a thin layer of topical medication, when indicated (bacitracin zinc/polymyxin B sulfate ointment) (see Figure 2).
6. Apply hydrocolloid or hydrogel dressing over ulcer (see Figure 3).
7. Begin wrap behind first metatarsal prominence (see Figure 4).
8. Wrap, enclosing the heel and being certain there are no wrinkles to cause discomfort (see Figure 5).
9. Use only one layer of gauze over the foot to minimize thickness of dressing in patient's shoe.
10. When passing over the ulcer DO NOT allow edge of gauze to lie directly on ulcer, this will cause pain.
11. Continue wrapping, overlapping about half the gauze with each wrap (see Figures 6 & 7).
12. Be sure that pressure of wrap is greater at ankle, decreasing to knee.
13. Stop wrap just below popliteal space.
14. Begin wrap down the leg in continuous fashion tucking small pleats on the side to conform to shape of the leg (see Figure 8).
15. Wrap should end just at the top of the ankle.
16. Gently mold the wrap by gently rubbing (see Figure 9).
17. Place about 2.5 yards of tube gauze over the form (see Figure 10).
18. Have patient secure the gauze at the knee and then begin stretching while rotating the tube gauze form.
19. Relax tension when at the foot (see Figure 11), rotating the form once.
20. Push back over the foot rotating toward the knee (see Figure 12).
21. Pull tension on loose ends of tube gauze and secure with 2 inch elastoplast (see Figure 13).
22. Fold down and trim loose edges and secure with tape (see Figure 14).

23. Unna's boot should remain comfortably in place for 1 to 2 weeks.

Note: It may be helpful to apply a bland emollient to the unaffected areas of the legs to decrease dryness and pruritus during time boot is in place.

PHOTOPHERESIS

I. INDICATIONS

Photopheresis is indicated for the palliative treatment of the skin manifestations of cutaneous T-cell lymphoma.

II. OVERVIEW

Photopheresis, or extracorporeal photochemotherapy (ECP), is an FDA-approved therapy for cutaneous T-cell lymphoma (see Chapter 6). Cutaneous T-cell lymphoma is a malignancy of human t-lymphocytes (helper T-cells). These malignant lymphocytes often target the skin and spend part of their life cycle residing there. This infiltration of malignant cells into the skin can be seen in several variations and ranges. From a patch-plaque type disease to a universal erythrodermic scaly version that may cover the entire skin surface.

The photopheresis UVAR® XTS instrument integrates three main subsystems designed to collect and separate a portion of the patient's blood and to photoactivate the collected white blood cells (WBCs). In photopheresis, the injectible drug, methoxsalen (UVADEX®) is given directly into the reservoir collection bag (collected WBCs) just prior to the photoactivation phase. UVADEX® is delivered at a dose of 0.017 times the total treatment volume in milliliters (ml). For example, if the total treatment volume of collected WBCs is 260 ml, the calculation would be 0.017 X 260 ml treatment volume for a total dose of 4.4 ml of UVADEX®.

Using a 16 to 17 gauge butterfly needle inserted in the antecubital vein, a portion of blood is removed (300 to 400 cc), then processed through a centrifuge where the individual components of the blood are separated. Some of the plasma and as many of the white blood cells as can be collected are stored in a reservoir bag. The red blood cells are returned to the patient immediately. The plasma and the white blood cells are then circulated through an ultraviolet light field where the UV light activates the methoxsalen that is now attached to the lymphocytes (see Figure 15).

How the UVA-activated methoxsalen affects the white blood cells and primarily the malignant T-cells found in CTCL is still not completely understood. We

Figure 15.
Photopheresis Procedure

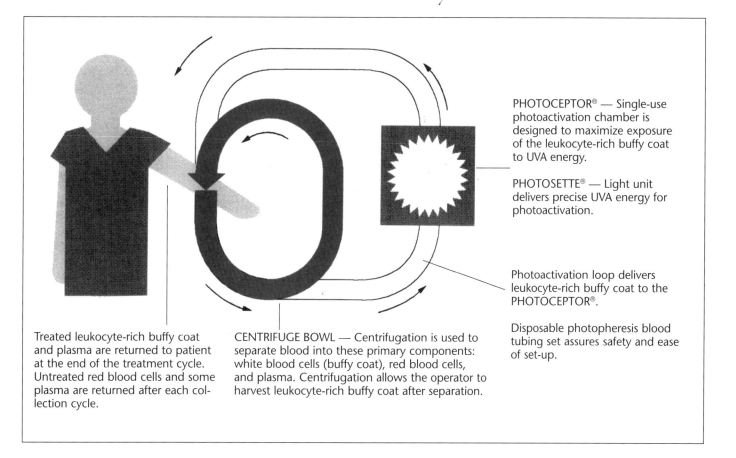

PHOTOCEPTOR® — Single-use photoactivation chamber is designed to maximize exposure of the leukocyte-rich buffy coat to UVA energy.

PHOTOSETTE® — Light unit delivers precise UVA energy for photoactivation.

Photoactivation loop delivers leukocyte-rich buffy coat to the PHOTOCEPTOR®.

Disposable photopheresis blood tubing set assures safety and ease of set-up.

Treated leukocyte-rich buffy coat and plasma are returned to patient at the end of the treatment cycle. Untreated red blood cells and some plasma are returned after each collection cycle.

CENTRIFUGE BOWL — Centrifugation is used to separate blood into these primary components: white blood cells (buffy coat), red blood cells, and plasma. Centrifugation allows the operator to harvest leukocyte-rich buffy coat after separation.

do know that the UVA light activates the methoxsalen inside the cell. This leads to cross linking of the DNA and the death of the cell. Ongoing research also suggests that the methoxsalen combined with UVA may somehow affect the presentation of endogenous antigens on the cell surface. When these treated white blood cells are returned to the patient, it appears that they are now capable of stimulating the patient's previously unresponsive immune system, thereby fighting the disease. The total understanding of how these processes take place is unknown.

III. PRE-TREATMENT WORKUP

A. Prior to the patient being referred for treatment, a skin biopsy, lymph node biopsy, flow cytometry, or monoclonal antibody test must be performed to confirm the diagnosis. In addition, results from the following tests should be evaluated prior to starting photopheresis.
   1. CBC with differential.
   2. Chemistries.
   3. Hepatitis screening.

   4. Chest x-ray and electrocardiogram.
B. It is important that the patient is screened for any underlying renal, hepatic, cardiovascular, or infectious disease prior to starting the photopheresis procedure. The removal of close to a unit of blood during the procedure can put the patient at risk for a hypotensive/hypovolemic episode. Therefore, the above tests should be performed and the results evaluated very carefully by the medical staff to ensure that the patient can tolerate the procedure.

IV. ORIENTATION TO THERAPY

A. Prior to starting the actual treatment, the patient should be introduced to the photopheresis nursing staff and undergo an orientation to the unit and its procedures.
B. Any interested relatives should be invited to participate with the patient to establish as much support as possible.
C. Written material regarding the disease and the procedure should be offered to the patient and copies given to relatives.

D. Additional written instructions regarding policies and unit procedures should be provided for the patient.

E. Written information regarding the ultraviolet light should be presented; precautions should be discussed and provided.

F. The patient should be instructed in how to contact the medical/nursing staff in case of potential emergency situations (fever, pain, bleeding, or other acute symptoms).

G. The primary nurse in charge should also arrange for the patient to meet with the office staff to review health insurance coverage for the procedure.

V. PROCEDURE INFORMATION

A. After a thorough explanation by a member of the medical staff, a consent form is obtained by the physician in charge.

B. The patient is given an appointment for the procedure.

C. The patient is reminded about the most common precautions that must be taken (use sunscreen, UV-protective glasses). These instructions should be provided to the patient in writing.

D. A followup telephone call prior to starting therapy to review all instructions and to evaluate the patient's level of understanding is beneficial.

E. Prior to the actual procedure the patient is examined by the medical staff and an assessment is performed by the primary nurse. This assessment includes:
   1. Recent medical history.
   2. Review of allergies.
   3. Review of medications currently being used.
   4. Vital signs.
   5. Physical exam.
   6. A brief review of the recent social history.

F. If the patient is cleared, the procedure is performed. After the procedure, the patient may be discharged if:
   1. Vital signs are normal.
   2. He/she has no new complaints.
   3. He/she has a secured pressure dressing on the needle site.
   4. He/she uses appropriate sun protection.
   5. He/she is cleared for discharge by the medical staff.

G. The photopheresis procedure in most institutions is a 3 to 4 hour outpatient procedure.
   1. After the patient has been cleared for treatment, venous access is obtained using a 16 to 17 gauge intravenous needle.
   2. The preferred access site is one of the large antecubital veins.
   3. In some patients it can be very difficult to obtain a sufficient access. It might be necessary to insert some type of a central line, similar to those used for chemotherapy or hyperalimentation. This increases the risk for infections in this high-risk group of patients and should be avoided if possible.
   4. The photopheresis UVAR XTS system automatically sets the photoactivation time (light exposure time) based upon the total treatment volume, hematocrit of the treatment volume, and remaining UVA lamp life. Approximately 1.5 joules/cm^2 of UVA dose is delivered to the treatment volume. Photoactivation times vary, but generally average 30 to 40 minutes. The total treatment time, including cell collection, separation, and photoactivation generally averages between 2.5 and 3.5 hours.
   5. During the procedure the patient will also receive between 500 to 650 cc of 0.9% saline, some mixed with heparin to prevent the blood from clotting as it goes through the instrument. It is also given to maintain the patient's blood volume and to prevent any hypovolemia.

VI. POST-TREATMENT PRECAUTIONS

A. Prior to leaving, the patient is instructed as to the following precautions.
   1. Bleeding tendency.
      a. Due to the use of heparin as an anticoagulant during the procedure the patient should be instructed to watch for bleeding immediately after the treatment primarily from the needle site. The amount of heparin used during the treatment is fairly low (between 6,000 to 10,000 units of heparin) and will rarely cause such complications.
      b. The pressure dressing that is applied to the needle insertion site should remain in place for at least 4 hours. When it is removed, the patient may place an adhesive bandage over the site.
      c. If any bleeding occurs from the needle site, the patient should be instructed to apply pressure to the site. If the bleeding does not stop within a reasonable period of time, the patient should be instructed to seek help either from his/her local physician, emergency room, or call 911 and request help.
   2. Methoxsalen.
      a. When using methoxsalen, a drug that causes sensitivity when activated by ultraviolet light, the patient should be instructed in specific precautions (as

Table 15.
Sample Nursing Care Plan for Patient Undergoing Photopheresis

NURSING DIAGNOSES AND THE PLAN OF CARE		
Nursing Diagnoses Anxiety related to: 1. Knowledge deficit regarding photopheresis.	**Outcomes** Reduced level of anxiety.	**Interventions** 1. Explain to patient what photopheresis is. 2. Provide written information about photopheresis. 3. Have patient and significant other visit unit and meet staff and other patients if desired.
Photosensitivity as related use of methoxsalen.	No photosensitivity.	1. Encourage patient to wear UV-resistant glasses. to 2. Encourage patient to wear protective clothing. 3. Encourage minimal sun exposure even on cloudy days. 4. Encourage use of a sunscreen of SPF 15. 5. Provide patient with a list of drugs that are photosensitizing.
Potential imbalance of fluids as related to volume.	Maintain normal fluid balance in patient.	1. Assess patient frequently for signs of fluid imbalance. 2. Elevate legs above heart. 3. Replace fluids as needed. 4. Check vital signs frequently. 5. Observe color and temperature of skin. 6. Observe for mental status change (confusion or agitation of patient).

recommended by the manufacturer). (See *Physician's Desk reference* for additional information.)

(1) A sunscreen should be applied to the skin areas that may be exposed to sunlight.

(2) Protective UV wrap-around sunglasses should be worn during daylight for the next 24 hours.

(3) It is recommended by the drug manufacturer that all patients should have an annual eye exam to monitor the effects of the methoxsalen.

3. Additional information.

a. Patient should be instructed that a small fever spike may occur 4 to 6 hours after the treatment. This is a common reaction and there is no cause for alarm. This usually will subside without any need for treatment. If it does persist for longer than 24 hours, patient should notify the unit staff.

b. Patient should be instructed how to avoid potential light-sensitive medications that might interfere with the photopheresis treatment. A list of light-sensitive drugs should be provided and reviewed with the patient and/or significant other.

c. Patient and significant others should be informed how to contact the unit staff for any emergencies or concerns.

VII. SCHEDULING

A. **The photopheresis treatments are always given on 2 consecutive days 2 to 4 weeks apart. The physician in charge determines the actual treatment schedule depending on the severity of the patient's condition. As the patient's condition improves the interval between the treatments may be extended.**

VIII. ADJUNCTIVE THERAPY

A. **Patients with a partial response to photopheresis can often gain additional improvement if an adjunctive therapy is selected. The physician, together with the patient, will determine when and if any additional therapy is needed. Some of the adjunctive therapies used are:**

1. Electron beam radiation treatment given to selected skin areas or to the total skin surface.

2. Chemotherapeutic agents such as methotrexate, nitrogen mustard, and carmustine.

3. The different interferons can also be used.
4. PUVA.
5. Targretin (oral or topical).

IX. COMPLICATIONS

A. **Photopheresis has been used worldwide since 1987. Presently no major side effects have been identified. The photopheresis treatment does not appear to suppress the immune system or expose the patient to an increased risk of opportunistic infections or other malignant diseases.**
   1. Minor side effects that can occasionally occur:
      a. Hematoma and bleeding from needle site that can be easily treated with pressure dressings and ice packs.
      b. Slight fever spike 4 to 8 hours after re-infusion of the treated cells that usually does not require treatment.
      c. Increased erythema and itching immediately after the treatment. This will most often respond to oral antihistamines.
      d. Hypovolemia/hypotension during treatment. This is primarily seen in patients with low body weight or patients with a low Hgb/Hct and can in most situations be corrected by infusion of intravenous fluids and positioning the patient in a Trendelenburg position.

X. RESPONSE

A. **During the initial clinical trials that led to the FDA approval of photopheresis (1984 to 1987), the data showed that approximately 30% of patients treated with photopheresis had an excellent response to the therapy. Thirty percent had some response but might benefit from adjunctive treatments and 30% showed no response. Recent clinical publications have described similar results.**

XI. NURSING CONSIDERATIONS (see Table 15)

A. **Evaluation and teaching.**
   1. It is very important that the patient receives a general medical evaluation prior to starting therapy to exclude any significant medical problems that might be a contraindication to photopheresis (cardiac, renal, hepatic disease, or any infectious disease).
   2. Both the patient and significant others should receive a detailed orientation to the procedure, the unit, and its policies.
      a. The unit coordinator or the primary nurse should meet with the patient and significant others and provide additional verbal information as needed. Make sure

that the patient has plenty of opportunities to ask questions.
      b. If possible, have the patient observe an actual treatment and meet other patients who are receiving therapy.
   3. Allow the patient time to absorb the information given. Do not start treatment on the same day patient is being oriented to the procedure.
   4. Give the patient detailed instructions regarding possible side effects, expectations, and information regarding other forms of therapy that may be needed.
   5. Communicate all test data and results to the patient directly, if the patient has requested this information.
   6. Provide a multidisciplinary approach using all disciplines within the system (medical, nursing, social work, psychiatry, dietary, and other resources from within the institution as they are needed).
   7. In addition to the nursing diagnosis related to primary disease (CTCL) of the patient, the following additional issues may be covered:
      a. Increased risk of bleeding due to anticoagulation with heparin.
      b. Increased risk of fever from the re-infusion of the treated cells.
      c. Increased risk of potential infection from venous line.
      d. Increased risk of alterations in mental status due to long-term chronic illness.
      e. Issues related to the patient's loss of control during the time he/she is connected to the UVAR instrument.

Bibliography

Arndt, K.A., Burton, C., & Noe, J.M. (1983). Minimizing the pain of local anesthesia. *Plastic and Reconstructive Surgery, 72,* 676-679.

Auletta, M.J., & Grekin, R.C. (1990). *Local anesthetics for dermatologic surgery.* New York: Churchill Livingstone.

Baer, C.L., & Williams, B.R. (1992). *Clinical pharmacology and nursing.* Springhouse, PA: Springhouse Corporation.

Bennett, R.G. (1988). *Fundamentals of cutaneous surgery* (pp. 100-135, 194-239). St. Louis: C.V. Mosby.

Bielan, B., & Rudy, S.J. (1996). *Dermatology in primary care, for nurse practitioners and physician assistants.* Pitman, NJ: Dermatology Nurses' Association.

Brown, C.D. (1992). Drug interactions in dermatologic surgery. *Journal of Dermatologic and Surgical Oncology, 18,* 512-516.

Carpenito, L.J. (1991). *Nursing care plans and documentation.* Philadelphia: J.B. Lippincott.

Dean, F.A. (1990). Caring for CTCL patients undergoing photopheresis. *Dermatology Nursing, 2*(1), 26- 28.

Duvic, M., Hester J., & Lemak, N. (1996). Photopheresis therapy for cutaneous T-cell lymphoma. *Journal of the American Academy of Dermatology, 35*(4), 573-579.

Edelson, R.L., Heald, P., Perez, M., & Berger, C. (1994). Extracorporeal photochemotherapy. *Biologic Therapy of Cancer Update, 4*(5), 1-12.

Edelson, R.L., Berger, C., Gasparro, F., Jegasothy, B., Heald, P., Wintroub, B., Vonderheid, E., Knobler, R., Wolf, K., Plewig, G., McKiernan, G., Christensen, I., Oster, M., Honigsmann, H., Wilford, H., Kokoschka, E., Rehle, T., Perez, M., Stingl, G., & Laroche, L. (1987). Treatment of cutaneous T-cell lymphoma by extracorporeal photochemotherapy. *New England Journal of Medicine, 316*(6), 297-303.

Eriksson, E. (Ed.). (1979). *Illustrated handbook in local anesthesia.* London: Lloyd-Luke Medical Books, Ltd.

Galloway, G.A., & Lawson, G.B. (1995). Photochemotherapy (PUVA) protocol. *Dermatology Nursing, 7*(6), 348-351.

Gasparro, F.P. (1994). Mechanistic events underlying the response of CTCL patients to photopheresis. In Extracorporeal photochemotherapy: *Clinical aspects and the molecular basis for efficacy* (pp. 101-120). Austin, TX: RG Landes Co.

Grekin, R.C., & Auletta, M.J. (1988). Local anesthesia in dermatologic surgery. *Journal of the American Academy of Dermatology, 19,* 599-614.

Habif, T.P. (1990). *Clinical dermatology.* St. Louis: Mosby.

Heald, P.W., Rook, A., Perez, M., Wintrougb, B., Knobler, R., Meschig, R., Jegasothy, B., Gasparro, F., Berger, C., & Edelson, R. (1992). Treatment of erythrodermic cutaneous T-cell lymphoma with extracorporeal photochemotherapy. *Journal of the American Academy of Dermatology, 27*(3), 427-433.

Hill, M.J. (1994). *Skin disorders.* St. Louis: Mosby-Year Book Inc.

STUDY QUESTIONS

1. Intralesional steroids can be appropriate in all of the following *except:*
   a. Neurodermatitis.
   b. Inflamed epidermal cyst.
   c. Hypertrophic scars.
   d. Inflamed stasis ulcer.
   e. Keloids.

2. Local cytotoxic agents include all of the following *except:*
   a. Bleomycin.
   b. Warfarin.
   c. Nitrogen mustard.
   d. Vinblastine.

3. Careful monitoring of a patient undergoing topical psoralen therapy include all of the following *except:*
   a. Eye exams for cataracts.
   b. Skin biopsy for direct immunofluorescence.
   c. Birth control.
   d. Lab values (CBC, SMAC, ANA).

4. 5-Fluorouracil occasionally can be used on superficial basal cell carcinoma when:
   a. Conventional surgical intervention is not feasible.
   b. Difficult location.
   c. Produce disfigurement.
   d. On multiple recurrent tumors.
   e. a, b, and c.

5. Side effects of retinoid therapy include all *except:*
   a. Erythema and dryness of skin.
   b. Dryness of mucous membranes producing cheilitis and nosebleeds.
   c. Peeling of palms and soles.
   d. All of the above.
   e. None of the above.
   f. a and c.

6. Side effects of steroid therapy include:
   a. Mood changes.
   b. Muscle wasting.
   c. Hypotension.
   d. All of the above.
   e. a and b.

7. Local anesthetics act to slow or stop nerve conduction.
   a. True.
   b. False.

8. Epinephrine:
   a. Is a vasoconstrictor.
   b. May cause restlessness.
   c. Is okay to use in a patient with atrial fibrillation.
   d. All the above.
   e. a, b only.
   f. a, b, c.

9. To prevent CNS and cardiovascular reactions with local anesthetics:
   a. Use minimum effective dose.
   b. Avoid injection of inflamed tissue.
   c. Inject quickly.
   d. a, b, c.
   e. a and b.
   f. None of the above.

10. Aluminum acetate soaks are not used for antiseptic effect.
    a. True.
    b. False.

11. Cryosurgery is indicated in all the following *except:*
    a. Actinic keratoses.
    b. Molluscum contagiosum.
    c. Psoriasis.
    d. Leukoplakia.

12. Intralesional bleomycin is useful in treat recalcitrant periungual or plantar warts.
    a. True.
    b. False.

13. The anticipated complications from photopheresis therapy include which of the following?
    a. Low-grade fever.
    b. Hair loss.
    c. Transient rise in liver function tests.
    d. Abdominal pain.

14. Photopheresis is FDA-approved for which of the following disorders?
    a. Kaposi's sarcoma
    b. Cutaneous T-cell lymphoma.
    c. Herpes zoster.
    d. Metastatic melanoma.

15. Patient education related to photopheresis therapy should include which of the following?
    a. Ultraviolet light precautions.
    b. Possible increased itching and redness post-treatment.
    c. Potential light-sensitizing medications.
    d. Expected response rate based upon early clinical trials.
    e. All of the above.

Answers to Study Questions

1.	d	6.	d	11.	c
2.	b	7.	a	12.	a
3.	b	8.	e	13.	a
4.	e	9.	e	14.	b
5.	e	10.	b	15.	e

Dermatologic Nursing Essentials: A Core Curriculum 2nd Edition © DNA 2003

DNAP303

CE Answer/Evaluation Form

Chapter 3.
Therapeutic/Treatment Modalities

Please photocopy this test page and return.

COMPLETE THE FOLLOWING:

Name: _____

Address: _____

City: _____ State: _____ Zip: _____

Preferred telephone: (Home)_____ (Work) _____

State where licensed and license number: _____

CE application fee: DNA member $15.00
                        Nonmember $20.00

POSTTEST INSTRUCTIONS

1. To receive continuing education credit for individual study after reading the article, complete the answer/evaluation form below.
2. Photocopy and send the answer/evaluation form along with a check or money order payable to **Dermatology Nurses' Association** to: *DNA*, East Holly Avenue Box 56, Pitman, NJ 08071-0056.
3. Test returns must be postmarked by December 31, 2008. Upon completion of the answer/evaluation form, a certificate for 6.6 contact hour(s) will be awarded and sent to you.

This chapter was reviewed and formatted for contact hour credit by Marcia J. Hill, MSN, RN, Core Curriculum Editor; and Sally Russell, MN, RN,C, DNA Education Director.

ANSWER FORM

1. Name one new detail (item, issue, or phenomenon) that you learned by completing this activity.

_____
_____
_____
_____

2. How will you apply the information from this learning activity to your practice?
   a. Patient education.
   b. Staff education.
   c. Improve my patient care.
   d. In my education course work.
   e. Other: Please describe _____

_____
_____

Evaluation

	Strongly disagree				Strongly agree
3. The offering met the stated objectives.					
a. Identify the advantages and disadvantages of topical treatment vs. systemic treatment.	1	2	3	4	5
b. Understand the steps to applying an Unna's boot correctly.	1	2	3	4	5
c. Define the systemic antibiotics related to clinical use, absorption, metabolism, adverse reaction, and dosage.	1	2	3	4	5
d. Identify the pros and cons of vitamin A therapy.	1	2	3	4	5
e. Understand the keys to treating the phototherapy patient.	1	2	3	4	5
f. Identify the drug used for photopheresis.	1	2	3	4	5
g. Define the response to photopheresis as documented in the literature.	1	2	3	4	5
h. List the nursing concerns to follow in patients receiving photopheresis.	1	2	3	4	5
4. The content was current and relevant.	1	2	3	4	5
5. The content was presented clearly.	1	2	3	4	5
6. The content was covered adequately.	1	2	3	4	5
7. I am more confident of my abilities since completing this material.	1	2	3	4	5

8. The material was (check one) ☐ new, ☐ review for me.

Comments _____

9. Time required to complete reading assignment: _____ minutes

This independent study is provided by the Dermatology Nurses' Association (DNA) for 6.6 contact hours. DNA is accredited as a provider of continuing education in nursing by the American Nurses Credentialing Center's Commission on Accreditation. DNA is approved as a provider of continuing education by the California Board of Registered Nursing Provider #CEP5708.

Diseases of the Epidermis

Melissa Cooper, RN, CWOCN, DNC

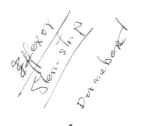

OBJECTIVES

At the end of this chapter, the reader will be able to:

- Understand T-cell mediated inflammation as it relates to psoriasis.
- Define etiology, immunopathogenesis, and therapy for each disease state.
- Make a nursing diagnosis and establish proper intervention.

KEY POINTS

- Understanding of T-cell mediated inflammation as a multiple-step activation cascade is essential to understand the new immune biologic therapeutics.
- Proper medical intervention is essential to proper and appropriate outcomes.
- Patient education and support can alter the course of the disease or the patient's response.

Diseases of the Epidermis

Melissa Cooper, RN, CWOCN, DNC

These are exciting times in the area of increased knowledge of the immune system of the skin. New areas of biologic therapeutic interventions are here or on the horizon for diseases of the epidermis. Many biological therapeutic targets in the immunologic cascade of events leading to diseases of the epidermis have been identified. Rapid growth of epidermal cells and scaling disorders have been called papulosquamous (squamous means scaly) diseases; this is a reactive characteristic that distinguishes these diseases from other skin disorders. Patients who suffer with psoriasis, pityriasis rosea, lichen planus, and keratosis pilaris may soon benefit from new biologic therapeutic agents.

The psychological affects of visual alterations of the skin are far reaching and should not be taken lightly. The reader is referred to Chapter 22 for further details of these effects.

PSORIASIS

I. OVERVIEW

Epidermal hyperplasia is a reaction to the activation of the immune system in focal skin regions, which, in turn, is mediated by CD8+ and CD4+ T lymphocytes that accumulate in diseased skin. Within psoriatic lesions, the keratinocyte cell cycle time is reduced approximately 8-fold (36 versus 311 hours in normal skin) and the number of dividing cells is doubled, resulting in a hyperplastic epithelium. Infiltration of T lymphocytes in skin lesions has been recognized to be an integral feature of psoriasis, current evidence suggests that epidermal changes in psoriasis are caused by actions of T lymphocytes in these skin lesions.

A. **Definition: psoriasis is a T-cell mediated inflammatory disease. Sometimes genetically determined and characterized by exacerbation and remission. Although there are many types of psoriasis, the common forms are psoriasis vulgaris, guttate, and pustular. Psoriatic lesions may be present on any skin surface. The most common areas are the elbows, knees, scalp, gluteal cleft, fingernails, and toenails. It affects extensor surfaces more than flexural surfaces. The face and lips are commonly not involved in adults and oral lesions in the form of whitish areas on the mucosa are quite rare.**

B. **Etiology.**

1. There is evidence for a potential "psoriasis gene" on chromosome 17q. Attention has been focused on chromosome 1q21; genes clustered in this region are responsible for epidermal proliferation.

Table 1.
Abbreviations

APCs:	antigen-presenting cells
CLA:	cutaneous lymphocyte-associated antigen
CTLs:	cytotoxic T lymphocytes
DC-LAMP:	dendritic cell lysosome-associated membrane protein
UDB-γ	interferon gamma
GM-CSF:	granulocyte-macrophage colony-stimulating factor
HEV:	high endothelial venules
HLA:	human leukocyte antigen
ICAM:	intercelleular adhesion molecule
IL:	interleukin
IL-12R:	IL-12 receptor
IL-2R:	IL-2 receptor
LFA:	lymphocyte function associated antigen
MHC:	major histocompatibility complex
NK:	natural killer
NK-T:	natural killer (T) cell
PNAd:	peripheral lymph node addressin
PUVA:	psoralens and ultraviolet A
RANTES:	regulated upon expression, normal T-cell expressed and secreted
Tc1:	type 1 cytotoxic T cell
Tc2:	type 2 cytotoxic T cell
TCR:	T-cell receptor
T_H1:	type 1 helper T cell
T_H2:	type 2 helper T cell
TNF-α:	tumor necrosis factor α
TRANCE:	tumor necrosis factor-related activation-induced cytokine ultraviolet B
UVB:	ultraviolet B
VCAM:	vascular cell adhesion molecule
VEGF:	vascular endothelial growth factor
VLA-4:	very late antigen 4

2. The major histocompatibility complex is located on chromosome 6. Psoriasis is associated with an increased frequency of certain human leukocyte antigens (HLA) found here, specifically HLA-CW6, HLA-1113, and HLA-B17 which are all associated with plaque psoriasis. HLA-B17 is usually associated with a mild form of psoriatic arthritis. HLA-B27 is associated with the pustular form of psoriasis. 60% to 70% of arthritis patients who also have psoriasis are also positive for HLA-B27. Epidermal keratinocytes in psoriatic lesions synthesize HLA-DR molecules; the specific product of activated T cells is interferon gamma (IFN-Y), which induces synthesis of HLA-DR keratinocytes.

Figure 1.
Epidermal Hyperplasia with Elongated Ridges

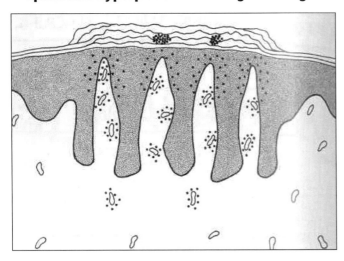

3. Environment and stress are believed to affect the course of the disease. Our immune system is also affected by the environment and stress. The skin is an active player on the immunologic field of action, as it is involved with normal homeostasis and host defense. Physical trauma, scratching, sunburn, and surgery are known to initiate psoriatic lesions; this is known as Koebner's phenomenon (see Figure 4-1, page 222).

C. **Immunology and pathophysiology.**
   1. A psoriasiform reaction pattern is defined morphologically as the presence of epidermal hyperplasia with elongation of the rete ridges in a regular manner (see Figure 1). The increased mitotic activity is presumed to be secondary to the release of various mediators from the dilated vessels in the papillary dermis in psoriasis. Rapid cell growth at the epidermal layer of the skin manifests as lesions on the skin. These lesions can present as scaling papules, plaques, or patches with white or silver scale. Pustules may also be seen (see Figure 4-2, page 222).
   2. T cells orchestrate pathogenic inflammation in psoriasis vulgaris (see Figures 4-3 & 4-4, pages 222 & 223). Monoclonal antibodies have permitted extensive characterization of T cell subsets and other leukocytes found in psoriatic lesions. Identified infiltrates include accumulations of both CD4+ and CD8+ T lymphocytes (mainly cytotoxic or "killer" lymphocytes), increased dermal Langerhans' cells, and scattered dermal monocytes (macrophages).
   3. Both CD4+ and CD8+ T cells have markers of persistent activation such as increased interleukin IR-2 receptor (IR-2R) and HLA-DR surface molecules. Infiltrating T cells in psoriasis are mainly activated type 1 helper T cells (T_H1) (CD4+) and type 1 cytotoxic T cells (T_C1) (CD8+).
   4. T_H1 and T_C1 lymphocytes have the inflammatory cytokines IFN-γ and tumor necrosis factor alpha (TNF-α) upon activation, and both of these cell types are considered to be effector cell populations (as opposed to regulation T cells). Clonal expansion of T cells in psoriasis vulgaris lesions has been observed only in CD8+ T cells, which suggests that the Tc1 subset is the major antigen-reactive population in this type of psoriasis (see Figures 4-5, 4-6, & 4-7, pages 224-226).
   5. In guttate psoriasis, a precise characterization of CD4+ versus CD8+ T-cell differentiation needs to be established. It has been suggested that T cells are initially reactivated with streptococcal antigens.
   6. Skin capillaries enlarge and there is a tendency to bleed. When the scale is removed punctate bleeding may be seen; this is called the Auspitz's sign.

D. **Incidence.**
   1. About 2% of the population is affected by psoriasis and involves all racial groups. The estimate of incidence among African Americans is about 0.1% and is rare in South American Indians. There is equal distribution between males and females.
   2. The prevalence of arthritis with psoriasis is higher than that found in the general population. It occurs in about 5% to 42% of patients with psoriasis.
   3. Nonpustular psoriasis usually develops under the age of 16 and is known as early onset or type 1 psoriasis. Psoriasis, which develops after the age of 16 until the age of 60, is called late onset psoriasis or type 2.
   4. Psoriasis vulgaris or classic plaque psoriasis is most common. Guttate and pustular psoriasis are usually seen in older populations. Other forms of psoriasis: erythrodermic, light-sensitive, HIV-induced, and keratoderma blenorrhagicum or Reiter's syndrome are seen less frequent.

E. **Considerations across the life span.**
   1. The disease is chronic with periods of exacerbation and remission; it can last a lifetime and can occur at any age.
   2. Scratching and rubbing may stimulate the proliferation process and areas of physical trauma have an increased tendency to develop psoriasis. Perturbation of the immune system by infection (for example, streptococcal and

HIV) may also trigger exacerbation of psoriasis.

3. Medications such as lithium, beta-blockers, systemic cortico steroids, antimalarial drugs, systemic interferon, and class I topical corticosteroids may cause an exacerbation of the disease known as psoriasiform drug eruption.

II. ASSESSMENT

A. History and physical exam.

1. Common forms of psoriasis:
   a. Psoriasis vulgaris — chronic plaque psoriasis.
      (1) Clinical appearance is well-defined plaques that have elevated sharply demarcated boundries and are easily palpable. Plaques appear whitish to silvery in color, on a salmon-colored, blue or violaccous or purplish bed, and may be round, oval, polycyclic, annular, or linear base. Lesions may be localized or generalized. The smaller papules and plaques may coalesce to form large plaques (see Figures 4-8 to 4-10, pages 226-227). Occasionally plaques appear to be immediately encircled by a paler peripheral zone referred to as the halo or ring of Woronoff. Fissuring of plaques can occur.
      (2) The predominate areas affected are the scalp (see Figure 4-11, page 227), elbows, knees, and sacral-lumbar areas. Lesions usually present in a symmetrical fashion.
      (3) Temporary white, red, or purplish macules and patches may remain after the elevated plaque has resolved.
   b. Guttate psoriasis.
      (1) Relatively uncommon, occurring in less than 2% of the psoriatic population. Usually proceeded by a history of upper respiratory infection secondary to group A B-hemolytic *Streptococcus* (*S. pyogenes*) pharyngitis or viral URI, which may precede the eruption of lesions 2 to 3 weeks prior.
      (2) Over 30% of patients have first episode before age 20.
      (3) A distinctive, acute clinical presentation of scattered 1 to 10 mm drop-like papules that usually spare the palms and soles. The lesions are spot-like and salmon pink or purplish in color.
      (4) Pruritus is variable.
      (5) May resolve spontaneously in weeks or months or develop into chronic plaque-type psoriasis.

      (6) Good response to therapy.
   c. Pustular type.
      (1) An uncommon variant, presents as either generalized or palm plantar, which is localized to palms and soles. Pustule lesions evolve into dusky-red crusts, which are studding more typical plaques.
      (2) Generalized pustule psoriasis, Von Combust, is the most common variant. It is has an explosive onset characterized by burning erythema and within hours develops into pinpoint pustules that appear in clusters. The pustules form lakes filled with purulent fluid, which is sterile. The distribution of erythema can be generalized. Areas of increased involvement are the flexural, anal region, and genitalia. Individuals with pustular psoriasis may present with high fever, leukocytosis, rapid pulse, and breathing. Without adequate treatment this form of psoriasis carries a mortality as high as 30%. Onset in pregnancy is usually in the third trimester, although it develops earlier in subsequent pregnancies. It usually remits postpartum, but may flare with use of oral contraceptives. Fetal mortality is high as a consequence of placental insufficiency.
   d. Nail psoriasis.
      (1) Common in plaque psoriasis, as much as 10% to 55%, it only occurs in less than 5% of patients with no other cutaneous findings of psoriasis.
      (2) Nails may exhibit pitting and small ice-pick like depressions in the nail plate from loss of parakeratotic cells from the surface of the nail plate (see Figures 4-12a & 4-12b, page 227).
      (3) Onycholysis/nail bed and nail hyponychium is a white area of the nail plate due to a functional separation of the nail plate from its underlying attachment to the nail bed. It usually starts distally and progresses proximally, causing a traumatic uplifting of the distal nail plate. Secondary microbial colonization may occur.
      (4) Subungual hyperkeratosis/hyponychium is a subungual hyperkeratosis that affects the nail bed and hyponychium. Excessive proliferation of the nail bed can lead to onycholysis.
      (5) The oil-drop sign or salmon patch/nail bed is a translucent yellow-red discoloration in the nail bed resembling

a drop of oil beneath the nail plate that is diagnostic of nail psoriasis.

    (6) Splinter hemorrhage/dilated tortuous capillaries in the dermal papillae are longitudinal black lines due to minute foci of capillary hemorrhage between the nail bed and the nail plate. This is analogous to the Auspitz sign of cutaneous psoriasis.

  e. Psoriasis in children.

    (1) Plaques are not as thick and are less scaly.

    (2) Appears in diaper region and flexural areas.

    (3) More commonly affects the face.

2. Family history is as high as 35%; many generations may have had some form of the disease. However, the disease may skip generations making familial history hard to discern. Studies of twin siblings have shown concordant disease in 73% of monozygotic twins compared with 20% in dizygotic twins. While this certainly points to a genetic mechanism, the absence of 100% concordance among monozygotes suggests that environmental factors must play a role in the pathophysiology of this disease.

3. Lesions are usually present for months in psoriasis vulgaris. Acute guttate and generalized pustular onset may be sudden. If an individual has no history of psoriasis and has a sudden onset consideration must be given to psoriasis induced by HIV or other infections.

4. Pruritus is common in most psoriatic patients.

5. Joint pain may be an indication that psoriatic arthritis is present.

6. Complete skin examination should include scalp, soles of feet, anal, and genitalia areas.

B. **Diagnostic tests.**

1. Lesions of vulgaris, guttate, and pustular psoriasis are distinctive; therefore a biopsy is usually not necessary. Psoriasis is a dynamic process and consequently the histopathological changes vary during the evolution and subsequent resolution of individual lesions. However, if a biopsy was performed it would show increased mitosis of keratinocytes, fibroblasts, and endothelial cells. Early lesions show few neutrophils collecting in the stratum corneum, some psoriasiform acanthosis, and dilated vessels in dermal papilla. More mature plaques will show psoriasiform hyperplasia of the epidermis, neutrophils present in the upper layers of the overlying parakeratotic scale, and Munro's abscesses.

2. Serum in patients with generalized pustular psoriasis or erythroderma may show electrolyte imbalance and low protein.

III. COMMON THERAPEUTIC MODALITIES

The goal of therapy is to decrease the epidermal hyperplasia and inflammation. Serendipity has played a major role in drug discovery for psoriasis. Prior and many current therapeutics come with toxicities with long term use. The need to rotate therapies every 1 to 2 years to minimize cumulative toxicity is the norm. Understanding the role of T cells in the pathogenesis of psoriasis has lead to a re-examination of the therapeutic mechanism of many standard agents.

In psoriasis the primary strategies are for reducing or eliminating the role of T cells in inducing psoriasis. Biologic therapeutics are mainly proteins that are produced in vitro and made through recombinant DNA techniques. In psoriasis treatment they are designed to bind to extracellular targets, usually with the intent of blocking molecular activation in one of many cellular pathways.

Current targets in the immune pathways of cutaneous inflammation have focused mainly on extracellular adhesion proteins, receptors, cytokines, and chemokines because these molecules are the main pharmacologic targets of new biologic therapeutics. New biologic treatment options offer potentially highly selective therapeutics that can minimize side effects on cells outside the immune system. Consequently, it may be possible to improve the therapeutic index for long-term treatment of patients with psoriasis.

A. **Medical interventions.**

1. Vulgaris and guttate psoriasis.

  a. Biologic therapies for psoriasis are very new and efficacy and safety information from clinical trials is just becoming available. Protein-based therapeutics fall into three classes of agents: antibodies, fusion proteins, and recumbrant cytokines.

    (1) LFA-3/TIP is an immunoglobulin/receptor fusion protein made by Biogen. Proposed mechanism is to bind to CD2 to block co-stimulation. It may also eliminate memory in activated T cells. In clinical trials the mean decrease in Psoriasis Activity and Severity Index (PASI) scores were 53%. Patients who cleared, remained clear for a mean period of almost 8 months.

    (2) IL-2/DAB is a cytokine/toxin fusion protein made by Ligand Pharmaceuticals. Proposed mechanism is to introduce B-subunit of diphtheria toxin into activated T cells and eliminate activated T cells.

(3) Anti-CD3a (HuM291) is a humanized monoclonal antibody made by Protein Design Labs. Proposed mechanism of action is to bind to activated T cells and induce apoptosis.

(4) Anti-CD11a is an humanized monoclonal antibody made by Genentech/Xoma. Proposed mechanism of action is to block LFA-1/VCAM-1 interactions, inhibiting co-stimulation and T-cell migration into skin. Clinical trials have shown approximately 60% reduction of PASI scores. There seems to be no increase in infections. Headache and flu-like symptoms lessen with continued use.

(5) Anti-B7-1 is an humanized monoclonal antibody made by IDEC Pharmaceuticals. Proposed mechanism of action is to block B7/CD28 interaction and inhibit co-stimulation.

(6) Anti-CD25 (daclizumab®) is a humanized monoclonal antibody made by Protein Design Labs. Proposed mechanism is to block IL-2 receptor and potential T-cell growth.

(7) CTLA-4/Ig is an immunoglobulin/receptor fusion protein made by Bristol-Myers/Squibb. Proposed mechanism is to bind to B7 and block co-stimulation.

(8) rIL-11 (oprelvekin) is a recombinant cytokine made by Genetics Institute. Proposed mechanism is to induce T_H2 type differentiation in activated T cells.

(9) Anti-IL-8 is an human monoclonal antibody made by Abgenix. Proposed mechanism is to block activity of IL-8, inhibiting immune cell migration into the skin and angiogenesis.

(10) Anti-TNF-alpha (infliximab) is a humanized monoclonal antibody made by Centocor. Proposed mechanism is to bind to and block activity of TNF-alpha, decreasing immune activity.

(11) Anti-TNF-alpha (etanercept) is an immunoglobulin/receptor fusion protein made by Immunex. Proposed mechanism is to bind and block activity of TNF-alpha, decreasing immune activity.

b. Topical corticosteroids (TCS) are both antimitotic and anti-inflammatory. TCS are most useful for localized psoriasis or psoriasis of the scalp. High-potency TCS are used for usually 2 to 3 weeks then either switched to weekly, lower-potency TCS or combined with other therapies. Long-term use of topical steroids have a potential to cause atrophy, rebound effect, tachyphylaxis (loss of effect with continued use of a drug) and steroid-induced acne. If topical steroids are used with occlusion for prolonged periods, systemic effects of steroids may be seen.

c. Broad-band ultraviolet B (UVB) (wave length range 290 to 320 nanometers) has been used for decades. Ultraviolet B radiation reduces the adhesive interactions, expression and adhesion molecules, possibly explaining its mode of action in treating psoriasis. Ultraviolet A (UVA) (wavelength range 320 to 400 nanometers) therapy has been used in a psoralen plus (PUVA) program since the mid 1970s. PUVA therapy depleted lymphocytes in concert with disease improvement. Both therapies have been successful but limited. UVB rays are most energetic, and therefore, produce the most erythema (sunburn). UVA rays are the least energetic and are noted for their tanning effect (melanogenesis) rather than burning. The recent advent of narrow-band UVB lamps (wave length 311 to 313 nanometers), hence the term narrow-band, derive their most theraputic effects from these three wavelengths. Wavelengths in the lower nanometer range of 290 to 310, which have been eliminated in narrow-band lamps, are associated with nontherapeutic responses such as burning, premature aging, and skin cancer.

d. Topical tars and anthralin are hydrocarbons with antimitotic activity; tars can also be anti-inflammatory. Estar® 5% coal tar gel, Sebutone Cream Shampoo® (0.5% coal tar/2% salicylic acid/2% sulfur), and Balnetar Bath Oil® (2.5% coal tar) are no longer available for purchase in California because of the Safe Drinking Water and Toxic Enforcement Act. Alternative agents are available. These products tend to stain the skin (temporary) and fabrics (permanently), and are slow to produce a response but the response lasts longer. Tachyphylaxis is less likely to develop than with topical steroids. The tar bath oils will stain plastic but not porcelain bathtubs. Skin irritation and staining are the main disadvantages of anthralin therapy.

e. Goeckerman regimen is the application of a tar-based topical preparation followed by exposure UVB light. This has been shown to induce disease remission in less than 80% of patients.

f. Ingram method is based on anthralin

application following a tar bath and UVB. Time commitment and unfavorable odor are main complaints of patients on this regimen.

g. With thin-plaque psoriasis the use of emollients and UVB light is effective. This regimen often takes place in day care psoriasis treatment centers.

h. Calcipitrene is a vitamin D derivative with antimiotic activity and has suppressive effects on IFN-γ elaboration from activated T lymphocytes.

i. More resistant disease is treated with systemic retinoids, methotrexate, or cyclosporine.

   (1) Topical retinoids are available in gels and creams. Systemic retinoids are approved for severe recalcitrant psoriasis. They are given by mouth and are based on body weight. A complete blood cell count and lipid levels should be monitored. Pregnancy prevention program should be activated with initiation of retinoids because of the teratogenic effects.

   (2) Methotrexate is given by mouth on a weekly basis. A complete blood cell count, liver function test, and liver biopsy must be completed and continuously monitored with this medication. Reserved for more severe forms.

   (3) Cyclosporine is given by mouth daily. Monitoring of serum for creatinine, BUN, liver function, and cyclosporine levels is necessary. Cyclosporine has a major inhibitory effect on T-cell activation and strong antiproliferative effects on epidermal keratinocytes. Reserved for more severe form.

   (4) Most treatments are rotated, starting with the one that is the least harmful.

2. Pustular psoriasis.

a. Treatment options for generalized pustular and palmoplantar psoriasis are PUVA therapy, systemic retinoids, or parenteral methotrexate once a week. Analysis of 385 cases of generalized pustular psoriasis revealed that retinoid treatment was effective in 84% of patients, methotrexate in 76% of patients, cyclosporine in 71% of patients, and psoralen plus ultraviolet A (PUVA) in 46% of patients.

b. Topical corticosteroids and/or tar products are not known to be effective for this type of psoriasis.

3. Difficult psoriasis sites.

a. Scalp psoriasis: treatment is focused on removing the scale. Removing the scale usually requires salicylic acid in mineral oil under a shower cap overnight; alternatively tar or ketoconazole shampoos may be used. Both should be followed by betamethasone valerate 0.1% lotion or a vitamin D analogue applied to the scalp. Newer topical foam formulations have proven effective and with increased patient compliance.

b. Nails: PUVA using topical or oral methoxsalen for 3 to 6 months can improve nail psoriasis. Systemic treatments (retinoids, vitamin D derivatives, methotrexate, or cyclosporine) are also effective. Short-term therapy with high-potency topical cortical steroid solution or ointment under occlusion with cellophane wrap at bedtime can improve psoriasis. Intradermal injection with triamcinolone acetonide is also used. Avulsion therapy, or topical 5-fluorouracil 1% solution or 5% cream bid to the matrix area for 6 months without occlusion improves the subungual hyperkeratosis.

c. Perianal and genital regions: the use of low-potency steroids or vitamin D preparations is advised.

d. Rotation of treatments is often used to keep psoriasis under control due to the disease becoming recalcitrant to long-term therapy with one modality.

e. Other treatment for localized disease includes the vitamin D analogue capcipotriene (Dovonex®) ointment, cream, or solution applied twice daily; and the topical retinoid tazarotene (Tazorac®) gel or cream applied at bedtime.

IV. COMMON NURSING DIAGNOSES, OUTCOMES, AND INTERVENTIONS

A. Nursing diagnosis: altered comfort — pruritus related to presence of skin lesions as manifested by itching, areas of excoriated skin, agitation, and anxiety due to pruritus.

1. Outcome: patient will express satisfactory control of pruritus.

2. Interventions.

a. Decrease environmental irritants (for example, heat, scratchy coverings) to reduce vasodilatation and sensory stimulation.

b. Use topical and systemic anti-inflammatory medications to reduce inflammation and cause vasoconstriction.

c. Provide a cool environment. Use cool, wet dressings, soaks, bland emollients, and lubricating baths.

d. Administer antihistamines as necessary.

e. Patient should be advised to keep nails trimmed short.

f. Provide diversion activities (for example, music).

B. **Nursing diagnosis: risk for infection related to open lesion, presence of environmental pathogens and exudate.**

1. Outcome: patient will show no evidence of secondary infection such as redness, edema, or exudate.

2. Interventions.

a. Monitor for open, draining lesions; redness, swelling, and pain at lesion sites; lymphadenopathy and fever; indications of scratching.

b. Teach patient measures to prevent scratching, such as tepid baths and cool environment. Use of patting versus scratching as a behavior modification.

c. Practice and teach careful handwashing and proper disposal of dressing and contaminated linens. Have patient carry and use personal size hand sanitizer.

d. Advise patient of dangers of scratching — Koebner's phenomenon.

C. **Nursing diagnosis: altered comfort — dry skin related to inadequate fluid intake, too frequent cleansing, dryness from treatments as manifested by dry, flaking skin.**

1. Outcome: patient will have moist, well-lubricated skin.

2. Interventions.

a. Use nonirritating moisturizing agents.

b. Avoid moisturizers with alcohol content.

c. Provide adequate fluid intake (2,000-3,000 ml/day).

d. Avoid frequent bathing.

e. Encourage use of superfatted soap.

f. Suggest patient apply skin lotion or cream immediately after bathing.

D. **Nursing diagnosis: self-esteem disturbance related to presence of unsightly lesions as manifested by verbalization of self-disgust and despair over appearance of lesions, isolation, reluctance to look at lesions, or participate in self-care.**

1. Outcome: patient will express realistic hope for resolution of open lesions; maintain normal social relationships.

2. Interventions.

a. Discuss situation with patient in open, accepting manner.

b. Do not show shock or disgust at the sight of lesions.

c. Touch the patient, if appropriate to the situation.

d. Point out and show patient progress of skin lesions in clinic room mirror.

e. Provide counseling, or self-help groups if indicated.

f. Encourage patient's family and friends to participate in patient's care.

E. **Nursing diagnosis: altered health maintenance related to lack of knowledge of disease process, management plan, prevention of scarring, care of lesions, possible cosmetic solutions, and use of OTC medications as manifested by questions on self-care activities and possibilities for improved appearance, lack of understanding of chronic disease process, or management plan.**

1. Outcome — patient will:

a. Verbalize confidence in ability to care for self and explore options.

b. Describe disease process and management plans.

c. Determine when to seek medical help if self-medication is ineffective or condition worsens.

2. Interventions.

a. Answer questions completely.

b. Teach patient about disease process, management plan, care of lesions.

c. Advise patient to carefully follow guidelines for OTC medications.

d. Inform patient of signs that indicate a worsening of condition, such as increase in number of lesions, increase in erythema, pain, swelling, and fever.

F. **Nursing diagnosis: anxiety related to chronic nature of problem and personal appearance as manifested by verbalization of anxiety and frustration over appearance of skin scarring and lichenification. Request for information on suitable cover-up techniques.**

1. Outcome: patient will express hope regarding cessation of new lesions, and improved appearance with use of cover ups.

2. Interventions.

a. Encourage patient to continue medical regime.

b. Counsel patient regarding healthy life practice.

c. Advise patient on skilled use of cover ups, refer to cosmetic experts.

d. Involve family members for support.

G. **Nursing diagnosis: social isolation related to decreased activities secondary to poor self-image, fear of rejection, and lack of knowledge related to cover-up techniques as manifested by lack of social activities and verbalization of dissatisfaction with social life.**

1. Outcome: patient will express satisfaction with social life.

2. Intervention.

a. Encourage socialization in patient's interest areas.

b. Arrange counseling referral, if indicated.
c. Refer patient to organizations that allow a forum for discussion such as the National Psoriasis Foundation.
H. **Nursing diagnosis: alteration in self-esteem related to diseases manifested by verbalization of physical or psychological discomfort related to psoriatic arthritis.**
1. Outcome: patient will accurately describe discomfort and verbalize options for managing discomfort.
2. Interventions.
a. Suggest use of OTC medications for joint pain of arthritis or ask their doctor about some of the new biological therapies available.
b. Encourage moderate exercise of low-impact activities such as walking, yoga, or swimming for arthritis.
c. Suggest alternative treatments for relaxation and healing such as massage or music therapy.
d. Refer patient to appropriate organizations for further information and assistance on how to cope and actively participate in healing process.

PSORIATIC ARTHRITIS

I. OVERVIEW

Psoriatic arthritis (PA) is a progressive, chronic, inflammatory form of arthritis associated with psoriasis. Five types of PA have been described. Because the different patterns of PA may change in time in individuals, or patients may have overlapping features or more than one type, prevalence of each type is difficult to establish. Estimations of the frequency of PA ranges from at least 10% to 30% of the 3 million people with psoriasis in the United States. Affecting men and women equally, PA is usually seen between the ages of 30 and 50, but can begin in childhood. PA occurs at higher frequencies when skin involvement is severe (for example, pustular psoriasis). It may precede the diagnosis of psoriasis in up to 15% of patients.

A. Definition: psoriatic arthritis is a form of inflammatory arthritis associated with psoriasis. PA affects the ligaments, tendons, fascia, and joints. It may be characterized by severe inflammation and joint destruction but more often it is milder than rheumatoid arthritis. Although the cause of PA is unknown it is believed that genetic factors are involved and, with the new information on psoriasis as a T-cell mediated disease, it is believed that PA appears to also be an autoimmune disease. There are five types of psoriatic arthritis (see Table 2). Onset of symptoms may vary; either gradual and subtle or sudden and dramatic.

Table 2.
Types of Psoriatic Arthritis

Asymmetric peripheral joint involvement
Symmetric peripheral joint involvement
Distal interphalangeal predominant (DIP)
Spondylitis
Arthritis mutilans

B. Etiology.
1. Exact cause is not known, but believed to be a combination of genetic, immune, and environmental factors. It is classified as one of the seronegative spondyloarthropathies (which include ankylosing spondylitis, enteropathic arthritis, and Reiter's syndrome).
C. Immunology and pathophysiology.
1. Studies have shown that certain MHC class I allele associations govern susceptibility to psoriasis and psoriatic arthritis. This, in conjunction with T-cell infiltration, lead to the conclusion that PA, like psoriasis, is an autoimmune disease.
2. It is believed that CD8 T-cells are the major players in the immunopathogenesis of PA.
3. Development (like psoriasis) occurs in stages, beginning with a genetically defined predisposition and ending with a overt disease.
D. Incidence.
1. Estimations of 10% to 30% of patients with psoriasis have a form of PA.
2. Affects both sexes equally.
3. Generally seen between ages 30 to 50 (may be seen in children).
4. Prevalence of each form is difficult to establish.
E. Considerations across the life span.
1. Disease is chronic.
2. Onset generally between 30 to 50; if it occurs earlier it is associated with a poorer prognosis.
3. It has remissions and exacerbations that may follow the remissions and exacerbations of cutaneous disease.
4. PA may precede the onset of cutaneous disease in up to 15% of patients.
5. A considerable amount of damage and disability tends to occur early in the disease process.
6. May cause permanent deformities of the involved joints.
7. No cure for the disease, but new treatments are available.

II. ASSESSMENT

A. **History and physical exam.**
1. Forms of psoriatic arthritis (see Table 2).
   a. Symmetric arthritis (resembles rheumatoid arthritis) — affects the same joints (typically joints in the fingers and toes), usually in matching pairs; less severe than rheumatoid arthritis; can be disabling, with development of varying degrees of progressive, destructive disease.
   b. Asymmetric arthritis — typically involves one to three joints (large or small).
   c. Distal interphalangeal predominant (DIP) — involves primarily the distal joints (small peripheral joints in fingers and toes); may be confused with oseoarthritis.
   d. Spondylitis — affects the spinal column; may cause inflammation and stiffness in the neck, lower back, spinal vertebrae, or sacroiliac region; may restrict motion; may also attack connective tissue; may involve joints of the arms, legs, hips, or feet.
   e. Arthritis mutilans — severe, deforming, and destructive; primarily affects the distal joints of the hands and feet; may be associated with lower back and neck pain.
2. Family history: patients with PA may have close relatives with the disease or with psoriasis only.
3. Clinical characteristics.
   a. Characteristic psoriatic skin and nail changes must be present to make a diagnosis of psoriatic arthritis.
   b. Elevated erythrocyte sedimentation rate.
   c. Mild anemia.✷
   d. Elevated levels of blood uric acid may be seen in some patients (rule out gout).
   e. Symptoms (vary from gradual/subtle to severe/dramatic) — discomfort, stiffness, pain, throbbing, swelling, or tenderness in one or more joints; reduced ROM in joints; morning stiffness and fatigue; inflammation or stiffness in lower back, wrists, knees or ankles, or swelling in the distal joints (sausage-like appearance); tenderness, pain, or swelling where tendons and ligaments attach to bone; conjunctivitis.
   f. Constitutional symptoms — fever and malaise (rare); elevated ESR and serum complement (due to activation of acute phase reactants by cytokines).
   g. NOTE: pediatric PA resembles the disease in adults, with monoarticular disease more prevalent (especially during early stages); most common presentation in children at onset is monoarticular, often acute, arthritis of the knee.

B. **Diagnostic tests (none are considered diagnostic on their own).**
1. ESR, CBC, rheumatoid factor (to rule out rheumatoid arthritis), serum complement.
2. X-ray of joints.

III. COMMON THERAPEUTIC MODALITIES

A. **Overview: the goal of therapy is to control the inflammation of arthritis, restore function, and to help minimize deformity. For years treatment choices were limited to nonsteroidal anti-inflammatory drugs (NSAIDS), gold salts, and sulfasalazine, which had minimal to no effect on the cutaneous disease; etretinate, methotrexate, and cyclosporine which benefit both joint and cutaneous disease; PUVA may benefit both joint and cutaneous disease. Choice of treatment modality is based on type and severity of involvement.**
B. **Mild to moderate joint involvement.**
1. Goal — control inflammation.
2. First-line treatments.
   a. Use NSAIDS (for example, naproxen, indomethacin).
   b. Adverse reactions: gastric and renal toxicity, hypersensitivity reactions, CNS symptoms (for example, tinnitus and headache), and coagulation abnormalities.
   c. May see idiosyncratic flare of psoriasis (prior to initiating drug ask patient whether ASA causes psoriasis to flare).
   d. If no response to NSAIDS or progression of disease may change therapy to sulfasalazine, gold salts, or vitamin D.
   e. Gold injections may cause leukopenia, thrombocytopenia, and nephropathy.
3. Intra-articular steroid injections — may relieve isolated episode of severe synovitis.
4. Maintain joint ROM and function.
5. Avoid potentially injurious joint stress.
C. **Severe destructive arthritis (multiple joint involvement).**
1. Add potent anti-inflammatory agent to NSAIDS.
2. Methotrexate or cyclosporine (both oral and parenteral).
3. Most common side effects if methotrexate — ✷ stomatitis (use folic acid to minimize stomatitis) and GI pain.
4. Serious side effects of methotrexate — ✗ pulmonary and hepatic toxicity.
5. Patients with diabetes mellitus and antecedent liver disease are at greater risk for developing overt hepatic complications.
6. Most common side effects of cyclosporine — ✗ renal toxicity and potential development of B cell lymphoma.

D. **Immunotherapies.**
1. Infliximab (Remicade®).
   a. Approved for the treatment of rheumatoid arthritis and Crohn's disease.
   b. Chimeric monoclonal antibody.
   c. Specifically targets and irreversibly binds to TNF-alpha.
   d. Administered intravenously.
   e. Good to excellent or clear rating at week 10 of treatment.
   f. Warnings.
      (1) Increased risk of infection/sepsis.
      (2) Hyper and hypotension.
      (3) Lupus-like syndrome; rheumatoid nodules.
      (4) Pancreatitis.
      (5) Cardiac failure; myocardial ischemia.
      (6) Anemia, thrombocytopenia, leukopenia.
      (7) Pulmonary embolism.
   g. Required monitoring.
      (1) TB skin testing/chest x-ray (before initiation of drug).
      (2) Serum pregnancy testing (category C rating).
      (3) CBC with differential.
      (4) Chemistries.
2. Etanercept (Embrel®).
   a. Approved for treating early-stage rheumatoid arthritis; treatment of children with polyarticular juvenile rheumatoid arthritis and psoriatic arthritis.
   b. Significant improvement and reduction in joint pain and swelling after 3 months of treatment.
   c. Can be used with or without methotrexate.
   d. Warnings.
      (1) Increased risk of infection.
      (2) Neurologic events — rare cases of new onset or exacerbation of CNS demyelinating disorders; mental status changes; transverse myelitis, optic neuritis, multiple sclerosis.
      (3) Hematologic events — aplastic anemia (rare).
      (4) May worsen CHF.
      (5) Do not vaccinate with live vaccines.
3. Subcutaneous administration.
E. **Surgery and related techniques.**
1. Arthroscopic synovectomy.
2. Intra-articular injection of short-lived radioactive isotopes (experimental).
3. Joint replacement and some reconstructive therapy occasionally necessary.
F. **Supportive interventions.**
1. Exercise — moderate, regular exercise may relieve joint stiffness and pain (ROM, strengthening exercises combined with low-impact aerobics).
2. Hydrotherapy or aquatherapy — easier on painful joints, proceed with ROM, strength and aerobic exercise to reduce chance of injury.
3. Heat and cold therapy — alternating application of moist heat and cold to affected joints to provide temporary relief of pain and swelling.
4. Joint protection and energy conservation — perform daily activities in a way that reduces excess stress and fatigue on joints.

IV. **COMMON NURSING DIAGNOSIS, OUTCOMES AND INTERVENTIONS**

A. **Nursing diagnosis: altered comfort — joint pain related to arthritis.**
1. Outcome — patient will express satisfactiory control of arthritic symptoms.
2. Interventions.
   a. Decrease stress and fatigue on joints.
   b. Use prescribed medications.
   c. Use supportive interventions as appropriate.
B. **Nursing diagnosis: increase risk for infection — immunotherapy decreases immune response.**
1. Outcome — patient will show no evidence of secondary infection due to therapy.
2. Interventions.
   a. Educate patient regarding possibility of infection.
   b. Monitor blood work.
   c. Instruct patient on signs of generalized infection.
C. **Nursing diagnosis: altered comfort — swollen painful joints secondary to arthritic involvement.**
1. Outcome — patient will experience level of comfort.
2. Interventions.
   a. Medication.
   b. Exercise.
   c. Hot/cold therapy.
   d. Splinting (as necessary).
D. **Nursing diagnosis: restricted mobility.**
1. Outcome — patient will achieve maximum mobility.
2. Interventions.
   a. Medication.
   b. Exercise regimen.
   c. Hot/cold therapy.
   d. Splinting (as necessary).
   e. Physical therapy as indicated.

PITYRIASIS ROSEA

I. **OVERVIEW**

Pityriasis rosea (PR) is an acute, self-limiting, inflammatory dermatosis with a characteristic course. Its diagnosis is important, as it may resemble secondary syphilis.

A. **Definition:** pityriasis rosea is a pruritic condition characterized by rose-colored bran-like scaly lesions, which are scattered. The condition is most common in the spring and fall months.

B. **Etiology.**
   1. Considered to be a viral exanthem. Its clinical presentation supports this concept. It has been linked to upper-respiratory infections, can cluster within families and close contacts, and has increased incidence in the immunocompromised. There are increased CD4 T cells and Langerhans' cells in the dermis. Also, anti-IgM keratinocytes has been found in patients with pityriasis rosea. Recent work demonstrated HHV-7 viral DNA in both lesions and plasma in patients with PR. Also, a separate study found HHV-7 DNA in lymphocytes in 75% of patients with PR compared to 9% of controls. A single outbreak tends to elicit lifelong immunity.
   2. Twenty percent of patients have a recent history of acute infection with fatigue, headache, sore throat, lymphedema, and fever.

C. **Pathophysiology.**
   1. The "herald patch" is a plaque 2 to 10 cm, bright red, oval to round in shape, often has a flesh-colored center and raised, pink borders, with a fine scale. It occurs 1 to 2 weeks prior to an eruptive rash.
   2. The patches typically appear on the trunk and extremities and have a tendency to arise in lines of cleavage. The lesions can grow to become I to 2 cm plaques; typically salmon colored in light-skinned individuals and hyperpigmented in people with darker-skinned people (see Figures 4-13a & 4-13b, page 227). Lesions often show a narrow rim of scale, called a "collarette scale" that overhangs the well-circumscribed edge. The lesions are bilateral and symmetrically distributed; lesions on the back typically resemble a "Christmas tree" pattern.
   3. The disease is self-limiting and usually subsides in about 6 weeks.

D. **Incidence.**
   1. Estimates of about 2% of outpatient dermatology patients worldwide are affected. It has been reported in patients of all ages, from infants to elderly, but 75% of cases occur in people between the ages of 10 to 35, with a mean age of 23 years.
   2. Two percent of patients have a recurrence.
   3. Slightly more common in women more than men (1.5:1).

E. **Consideration across the life span.**
   1. Patient may be symptomatic or may complain of mild itching.
   2. Disease may result in post-inflammatory hyper pigmentation, especially in patients with dark skin. African Americans tend to have more widespread disease.

II. ASSESSMENT

A. **History and physical exam.**
   1. The herald patch is typically seen on the trunk.
   2. History of infection within the last month, especially viral.
   3. Complete examination of skin, asking patient if any pruritus is associated with patch.
   4. If lesions present on face, suspect atypical pityriasis rosea.
   5. Other conditions that can mimic pityriasis rosea include tinea versicolor, drug eruption, nummular eczema, or guttate psoriasis.
   6. Medication history is important. PR-like drug eruptions may be difficult to distinguish. Medication-induced eruptions have been reported with captopril, metronidazole, isotretinoin, penicillamine, levamisole, bismuth, gold, barbiturates, ketotifen, clonidine, and omeprazole. A single case has been reported with terbinafine. Certain vaccinations such as BCG and diphtheria have been reported to cause similar eruptions. Lesions also are thought to be increased in highly stressed individuals.

B. **Diagnostic tests.**
   1. Rapid plasma reagin (RPR) or VDRL to rule out syphilis if herald patch is absent and there is history of high-risk sexual contact, a previous genital ulcer, or significant involvement of the palms and soles.
   2. Biopsy in atypical cases. Biopsy results show erythrocytes within dermal papillae and dyskeratotic cells within the dermis.

III. COMMON THERAPEUTIC MODALITIES

A. **Medical interventions.**
   1. The disease is self-limiting, therefore treatment is usually not needed or aimed at controlling pruritus.
   2. Low-dose UVB phototherapy starting at 80% of the minimum erythrogenic dose may relieve pruritus rapidly in resistant cases. If itching is not controlled, the UVB dose should be increased by 20% until symptoms decrease. However, a recent study failed to bring improvement in the pruritus, but did note decreased lesion severity with UVB therapy.
   3. Suggest exposing skin to natural sunlight when appropriate.
   4. Relief of pruritus is helpful and can be accomplished by topical steroids, oral antihistamines, topical menthol-phenol lotions, and oatmeal baths. Systemic steroids are not recommended, as they suppress pruritus but do

not shorten the overall disease. They may prolong or exacerbate the disease. For vesicular PR, a single case was considerably improved with 20 mg of dapsone twice a day.

5. Prognosis is excellent. Patients may return to work or school, as they are not considered contagious. If rash persists more than 3 months it is better classified as pityriasis lichenoides chronica.

IV. COMMON NURSING DIAGNOSES, OUTCOMES, AND INTERVENTIONS

A. **Nursing diagnosis: potential for skin injury related to itchiness or scratching.**
   1. Outcome: patient's skin will remain intact and without injury.
   2. Interventions.
      a. Request patient use topical corticosteroids as directed.
      b. Teach patient to take cool baths and keep skin well-moisturized.

B. **Nursing diagnosis: potential self-image reduction related to unsightly patches.**
   1. Outcome: patient will maintain positive self-image.
   2. Interventions.
      a. Reassure patient that patches will subside 2 to 8 weeks with or without therapy.
      b. Instruct patient that the disease is not contagious and to reassure family and friends.

LICHEN PLANUS

I. OVERVIEW

Lichen planus is an idiopathic inflammatory dermatosis, which could be chronic or acute. The disease can affect the skin and/or mucous membranes of the mouth. The papules on the skin are usually flat (planus) and surrounded by subtle, fine white dots and lines that with imagination, resemble the appearance of lichen (see Figures 4-14a & 4-14b, page 228).

A. **Definition: lichen planus means flat, which describes the typical papule seen in lichen planus.**

B. **Etiology.**
   1. The cause of the disease is unknown.
   2. An eruption may occur as a response to medication.

C. **Pathophysiology.**
   1. Lichen planus is usually very pruritic.
   2. The lesions appear as purple, polygonal, and flat-topped papules. The surface has a fine reticulate pattern of white dots and lines. The lesions are the result of the inflammatory process.

D. **Incidence.**

1. Uncommon but not rare. Prevalence in the United States is estimated at 4.4 per 1,000. Usually occurs in women between the ages of 30 to 70 years of age.
2. Hypertrophic lichen planus is more common in darkly pigmented skin.
3. There is a oropharyngeal involvement in about 40% to 60% of patients. Mucous membrane involvement sometimes results in painful erosions.
4. The cellular immune mechanisms involved are as follows; activated helper T cells are present in early lesions and appear to target the basal cells that may have been antigenically altered. Cytokines and macrophages also play a role. In older lesions, suppressor T cells have been shown to predominate.

E. **Considerations across the life span.**
   1. The mucous membrane may be involved.
   2. Streaks may occur as a result of scratching or trauma.
   3. Hyperpigmented lesions occur from the post-inflammatory process.
   4. The soles of feet, palms of hands, nails, and scalp and genitalia may also be affected. Nail and hair follicles are occasional involved with dystrophic changes and even scarring.

II. ASSESSMENT

A. **History and physical exam.**
   1. Obtain a list of medications patient is currently taking. Thiazide, phenothiazine, gold, quinidine, quinacrine, and chloroquine have been associated with eruptions of lichen planus.
   2. The lesion usually presents as a flat-topped papule about 1 to 10 mm. Plaque-type lichen planus appears with a reticulate pattern of white dots and lines called Wickham's striae — a whitish cross-hatching on lesions. Reticular lichen planus may also appear in a netlike pattern of lacy white hyperkeratosis on the buccal mucosa, lips, tongue, and gums.
   3. The lesions are grouped, linear, annular, or disseminated and can occur on the wrists, lumbar region, eyelids, shins, scalp, and glans penis.
   4. When palms and soles are involved serology tests to rule out syphilis should be performed.
   5. Complete skin examination including scalp and mouth is indicated.

B. **Diagnostic tests.**
   1. Diagnosis is confirmed by biopsy.
   2. A biopsy finds increased granular layer, irregular acanthosis, liquefaction degeneration of basal cell layer, and band-like mononuclear infiltrate. Lymphocytes are CD4+ helper-inducer cells. Degenerate keratinocytes are found in the dermal-epidermal junction.

concave nula.

3. Wickham's striae is best seen by pressing the lesions with a microscopic lens plate following the application of mineral oil to the lesions.

III. COMMON THERAPEUTIC MODALITIES

A. Medical interventions.
1. Systemic or topical corticosteroids used for a short duration for relief of pruritus. Antihistamines are used with varying success for pruritis.
2. Topical immunotherapy, tacrolimus 0.1% in hydrophilic ointment.
3. Oral cyclosporine may be used as a last resort, 5 mg/kg per day, for very resistant cases.
4. PUVA may be used for patients resistant to topical therapy.
5. Systemic retinoids have been used successfully in some patients with mucous membrane lesions.
6. The course may be chronic, ranging from months to years. Almost two-thirds of patients experience spontaneous resolution within 1 year. Patients with mucous membrane involvement usually have a more prolonged course.

IV. COMMON NURSING DIAGNOSES, OUTCOMES, AND INTERVENTIONS

A. Nursing diagnosis: potential for skin injury related to scratching.
1. Outcome: patient will not experience any breakage of skin.
2. Interventions.
   a. Instruct patient on importance of not scratching pruritic areas.
   b. Teach patient how to apply topical antipruritic medications.
   c. Suggest patient take cool baths using oatmeal to assist in relieving pruritus.
   d. Keep nails manicured, teach patting pruritic area versus scratching.
   e. Use distractions such as music, reading, walking.

KERATOSIS PILARIS

I. OVERVIEW

A common, benign finding on the posterolateral aspects of the upper arms and anterior thighs.
A. Definition: a group of small, pinpoint, folliculocentric keratotic papules (see Figure 4-15, page 228). Seen in the same anatomical area for years; seen more commonly in association with ichthyosis vulgaris and less commonly with atopic dermatitis.
B. Etiology: unknown but common in an isolated condition or in association with hereditary

koilonychia as well as other diseases including ichthyosis, xerosis, atopy, monilethrix, trichothiodystrophy, Noonan's syndrome, Down syndrome, uremia, and some forms of alopecia such as atrophoderma vermiculata, keratosis pilaris atrophicans, and keratosis pilaris decalvans.
C. Pathophysiology.
1. Considered a disorder of keratinization. Apparent because of lack of desquamation of keratinocytes, follicular keratinous plugs of 1 to 2 mm in size develop.
D. Incidence.
1. Present in a up 40% of the general population.
2. Seen more commonly in association with ichthyosis vulgaris and less commonly with atopic dermatitis.
3. Likely a genetically inherited disorder.
E. Considerations across the life span.
1. Any age group may be affected; onset most frequent in 2nd decade.
2. Common in young children. About 30% to 50% of patients have a positive family history.
3. Peaks during adolescence and in women with hyperandrogenism. No racial predilection. Females may be more frequently affected.

II. ASSESSMENT

A. History and physical exam.
1. Ichthyosis or atopic dermatitis.
2. Age at onset.
3. Small 1 to 2 mm rough follicular papules.
4. Predilection for posterolateral aspects of the upper arms and anterior thighs.
5. Any area can be involved except palms and soles.
6. Lesions on the face may be misdiagnosed as acne.
7. Associated with dry skin and chapping.
8. May resemble heat rash or milaria.
9. Most often asymptomatic, but lesions may become red, inflamed, and pustular (resembles bacterial folliculitis).
10. In adults lesion may present with a red halo.
11. Systemic steroids may accentuate lesions and distribution.
B. Diagnostic tests: no specific studies.

III. COMMON THERAPEUTIC MODALITIES

A. Medical interventions.
1. Tretinoin — may give temporary improvement in roughness, but only increases irritation.
2. Short course of mid-potency topical steroids to reduce inflammation for 7 days, emollient-based topical steroid once or twice a day.
3. Application of lactic acid (12%), alpha and beta hydroxy acid (3%) lotions may be most

effective treatment. Mild cases may improve with emollients. Administer antihistamines as indicated to control pruritus.

B. **Nonmedical treatment.**
   1. Avoid scratching lesions — implement measures to reduce pruritus.
   2. Avoid tight clothing.
   3. Do not use abrasives for treatment.

IV. COMMON NURSING DIAGNOSIS, OUTCOMES, AND INTERVENTIONS

A. **Nursing diagnosis: body image alteration secondary to clinical presentation.**
   1. Outcome: patient will have positive body image.
   2. Interventions.
      a. Assess patient's feelings regarding skin appearance.
      b. Assess patient's coping process.

B. **Nursing diagnosis: increased risk for infection secondary to scratching.**
   1. Outcome: patient will remain free of secondary infection.
   2. Intervention: instruct patient on the use of antihistamines; bland emollients to reduce pruritus.
   3. Use and carry instant hand sanitizer.
   4. Keep fingernails manicured.

C. **Nursing diagnosis: knowledge deficit related to skin disorder.**
   1. Outcome: patient/significant other will understand disorder and appropriate interventions.
   2. Interventions.
      a. Educate patient/significant other about keratosis pilaris.
      b. Instruct patient on appropriate use of topical medications.
      c. Instruct patient/significant other to avoid tight-fitting clothing, scratching, and use of abrasives.

WEB SITES OF INTEREST:

National Psoriasis Foundation: www.psoriasis.org
American Skin Association: www.skinassn.org
American Academy of Dermatology: www.aad.org

Bibliography

Allan, R.A. (2002). Pityriasis rosea. *eMedicine Journal. 3*(4), 1-11.

American College of Rheumatology (2000). *Psoriatic arthritis.* Retrieved March 9, 2003, www.rheumatology.org/patients/factsheet/psoriati.html.

Arffa, R., (2001). Psoriasis, *eMedicine Journal, 2*(3), 1-10.

Eisen, D. (2002). The clinical features, malignant potential, and systemic associations of oral lichen planus: A study of 723 patients. *Journal American Academy of Dermatology, 46,* 207-214.

The Cleveland Clinic (2001). *What you need to know about psoriatic arthritis.* Retrieved March 9, 2003, www.clevelandclinic.org/arthritis/treat/facts/psoriatic.htm.

Doctor's Guide. (2001). Retrieved February 26, 2003, www.pslgroup.com/dg/1FED7E.htm.

Ellis, C.N., & Krcuger, G.G. (2001). Treatment of chronic plaques psoriasis by selective targeting of memory effector T lymphocytes. *The New England Journal of Medicine, 345*(4), 248-255.

Gottlieb, A.B., & Krueger, J.G. (2002). Psoriasis as a model for T-Cell mediated disease. *Archives of Dermatology, 138,* 591-600.

Hall, J.C. (2000). *Sauder's manual of skin diseases* (8th ed.). Philadelphia: Lippincott Williams & Wilkins.

Jones, G., Crotty, M., & Brooks, P. (2002). *Interventions for treating psoriatic arthritis.* Retrieved December 31, 2002, www.medscape.com/viewarticle/434754.

Kahn, C.E. (2003). *Psoriatic arthritis.* Retrieved March 9, 2003, www.chorus.rad.mcw.edu/doc/01047.html.

Kaliakatsou, F., & Hodgson, T.A. (2002). Management of recalcitrant ulcerative oral lichen planus with topical tacrolimus. *Journal of the American Academy of Dermatology, 46,* 35-41.

Kim, J.H., & Krivda, S.J. (2002). Lichen planus confined to a radiation therapy site. *Journal American Academy of Dermatology, 46,* 604-605.

Krueger, J.G. (2002). The immunologic basis for the treatment of psoriasis with new biologic agents. *Journal of American Academy of Dermatology, 46,* 1-23.

Lebwohl, M.G. (2002). *The role of TNFF Inhibition in the treatment of psoriasis.* A supplement to skin and allergy news, produced in affiliation with the 26th annual Hawaii dermatology seminar January 25 - February 2, 2002.

Lookingbill, D.P., & Marks, J.G. (2000). *Principles of dermatology* (3rd ed.). Philadelphia: W.B. Saunders Company.

Lorenzo, A.L.D. (2001). HLA-B27 Syndromes. *eMedicine Journal, 2*(9),1-10.

Lui, H., & Mamelak, A. (2002). Psoriasis, plaque. *eMedicine Journal, 3*(2), 1-11.

Lyer, S, Yamauchi, P., & Lowe, N.J. (2002). Etanercept for severe psoriasis and psoriatic arthritis: Observations on combination therapy. *British Journal of Dermatology, 146*(1),118-121.

Mason, J., Mason, A.R., & Cork, M.J. (2002). Topical preparations for the treatment of psoriasis: A systematic review. *British Journal of Dermatology, 146,* 351-364.

O'Quinn, R.P., & Miller, J.L., (2002). The effectiveness of tumor necrosis factor alpha antibody (infliximab) in treating recalcitrant psoriasis. *Archives of Dermatology, 138,* 644-648.

Rozycki, T.W., & Rogers, R.S. (2002). Topical tacrolimus in the treatment of symptomatic oral lichen planus: A series of 13 patients. *Journal of American Academy of Dermatology, 46,* 27-34.

Sege-Peterson, K., & Winchester, R. (1999). *Psoriatic arthritis.* In Freedberg, I.M., et al (Eds.), Fitzpatrick's dermatology in general medicine (5th ed.). (CD-ROM). Philadelphia: McGraw Hill.

Shelk, J., & Morgan, P., (2000). Narrow-band UVB: A practical approach. *Dermatology Nursing, 12*(6), 407-411.

Singri, P., & West, D.P. (2002). Biologic therapy for psoriasis. *Archives of Dermatology, 138*, 657-663.

Taylor, C.R., & Baron, E. (2001). Psoriasis, pustular. e*Medicine Journal, 2*(10),1-10.

Taylor, C.R., & Baron, E. (2002). Psoriasis, guttate. *eMedicine Journal, 3*(5),1-10.

Thai, K., & Sinclair, R.D. (2001). Keratosis pilaris and hereditary koilonychia. *Journal American Academy of Dermatology, 45*, 627-629.

Tosti, A., & Piraceini, B.M. (2001). Nail lichen planus in children. *Archives of Dermatology, 137*, 1027-1032.

Weedeon, D. (1997). *Skin pathology.* London: Churchill Livingstone.

Wolverton, S.E. (2001). *Comprehensive dermatologic drug therapy.* Philadelphia: W.B. Saunders Company.

Youngquest, S. (2001). It's beginning to look a lot like Christmas. *Western Journal of Medicine, 175*, 227-228.

Richard is a 23-year-old man and a junior in college. He presents with a history of small, well-defined, salmon-colored plaques with silvery scales for a few years. Recently he has been under a lot of stress and the plaques have enlarged and coalesced to form even larger plaques. His father has had psoriasis for years.

1. What type of psoriasis does Richard have?
   a. Plaque
   b. Guttate
   c. Pustular
   d. Type 11

2. Can stress cause an exacerbation of psoriasis?
   a. Yes
   b. No

3. Are there heredity factors related to psoriasis?
   a. Yes
   b. No

4. Richard's nail plate is pitted, what is happening?
   a. He needs a manicure.
   b. He has nail psoriasis.
   c. He bites his nails.
   d. He has a fungal infection.

5. Narrow-band UVB has the most therapeutic wavelength?
   a. True
   b. False

6. Topical corticosteroids are both antimiotic and anti-inflammatory?
   a. True
   b. False

7. Richard picked one of his plaques off and it began to bleed. This is called Auspitz's sign.
   a. True
   b. False

8. Fissures have been a problem as a port of entry for infections. What can Richard do?
   a. Wear bandages over all his plaques.
   b. Carry and use instant hand sanitizers often.
   c. Use antibiotic ointment prn.
   d. b & c.

9. Richard's father has lower back and joint pain. What are his chances of developing psoriatic arthritis?
   a. 5% to 42%
   b. 75%
   c. 100%
   d. 15%

10. Recent understanding of the immune system has created a new way of treating at psoriasis. Protein-based therapeutics fall into three classes of agents: antibodies, fusion proteins, and recombinant cytokines.
    a. True
    b. False

11. Are T cells part of the immune system of the skin?
    a. Yes
    b. No

12. Psoriasis is a T-cell mediated inflammatory disease.
    a. True
    b. False

13. Pityriasis rosea is a self-limiting inflammatory disease?
    a. True
    b. False

14. A herald patch is the first lesion seen in pityriasis rosea?
    a. True
    b. False

15. What does your patient, who has a flat, pruritic patch with fine white lines and dots likely have?
    a. Lichen planus
    b. Psoriasis
    c. Pityriasis rosea
    d. Keratosis pilaris

16. Your patient is complaining of papules over both arms; says her mother had it too. What is your diagnosis?
    a. Acne
    b. Keratosis pilaris
    c. Skin cancer
    d. Herald patch

Answers to Study Questions

1. a	7. a	13. a
2. a	8. d	14. a
3. a	9. a	15. a
4. b	10. a	16. b
5. a	11. a	
6. a	12. a	

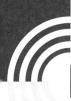

CE Answer/Evaluation Form

Chapter 4.
Diseases of the Epidermis

Please photocopy this test page and return.

COMPLETE THE FOLLOWING:

Name: _____

Address: _____

City: _____ State: _____ Zip: _____

Preferred telephone: (Home)_____ (Work) _____

State where licensed and license number: _____

CE application fee: DNA member $13.00
                      Nonmember $16.00

POSTTEST INSTRUCTIONS
1. To receive continuing education credit for individual study after reading the article, complete the answer/evaluation form below.
2. Photocopy and send the answer/evaluation form along with a check or money order payable to **Dermatology Nurses' Association** to: *DNA*, East Holly Avenue Box 56, Pitman, NJ 08071-0056.
3. Test returns must be postmarked by December 31, 2008. Upon completion of the answer/evaluation form, a certificate for 3.5 contact hour(s) will be awarded and sent to you.

This chapter was reviewed and formatted for contact hour credit by Marcia J. Hill, MSN, RN, Core Curriculum Editor; and Sally Russell, MN, RN,C, DNA Education Director.

ANSWER FORM

1. Name one new detail (item, issue, or phenomenon) that you learned by completing this activity.

_____
_____
_____
_____

2. How will you apply the information from this learning activity to your practice?
   a. Patient education.
   b. Staff education.
   c. Improve my patient care.
   d. In my education course work.
   e. Other: Please describe _____

_____
_____

Evaluation

	Strongly disagree				Strongly agree
3. The offering met the stated objectives.					
a. Understand T-cell mediated inflammation as it relates to psoriasis.	1	2	3	4	5
b. Define etiology, immunopathogenesis, and therapy for each disease state.	1	2	3	4	5
c. Make a nursing diagnosis and establish proper intervention.	1	2	3	4	5
4. The content was current and relevant.					
5. The content was presented clearly.	1	2	3	4	5
6. The content was covered adequately.	1	2	3	4	5
7. I am more confident of my abilities since completing this material.	1	2	3	4	5

8. The material was (check one) ☐ new, ☐ review for me

Comments _____
_____

9. Time required to complete reading assignment: _____ minutes

This independent study is provided by the Dermatology Nurses' Association (DNA) for 3.5 contact hours. DNA is accredited as a provider of continuing education in nursing by the American Nurses Credentialing Center's Commission on Accreditation. DNA is approved as a provider of continuing education by the California Board of Registered Nursing Provider #CEP5708.

Dermatitis/Eczemas

Noreen Heer Nicol, MS, RN, FNP

OBJECTIVES

At the end of this chapter, the reader will be able to:

- Understand that eczema and dermatitis are terms that describe the same response in the skin.
- Recognize several types of eczemas and their various clinical presentations.
- Discuss the therapeutic interventions frequently used to treat various eczemas.
- Identify important patient teaching issues for managing various eczemas.

KEY POINTS

- Eczema and dermatitis are terms that can be used interchangeably to describe a type of inflammatory disease characterized by pruritus and lesions with indistinct borders.
- Eczema or dermatitis can present in multiple phases including acute, subacute, and chronic.
- Many types of eczema or dermatitis exist including atopic dermatitis, contact dermatitis (allergic or irritant), seborrheic dermatitis, and nummular eczema.

Dermatitis/Eczemas

Noreen Heer Nicol, MS, RN, FNP

DERMATITIS/ECZEMAS

Eczema and dermatitis are both general terms that describe a particular type of inflammatory response in the skin. Diseases that are considered eczematous disorders are generally characterized by pruritus, lesions with indistinct borders, and epidermal changes. These lesions can appear as either erythema, papules, or lichenification of the skin; they can present in an acute, subacute, or chronic phase. In this category of disease, the inflammation process takes place at the level of the epidermis. Atopic dermatitis, contact dermatitis, whether nonallergic (irritant) or allergic, lichen simplex chronicus, nummular eczema, and seborrheic dermatitis are all examples of specific types of eczema or dermatitis.

I. ATOPIC DERMATITIS

A. Definition.
1. A chronic hereditary disorder associated with inflammation of the skin leading to pruritus and disruption of the skin surface. Usually associated with a personal or family history of asthma, allergic rhinitis, or eczema.
2. Fifty percent of patients with atopic dermatitis (AD) go on to develop respiratory manifestations of asthma or allergic rhinitis.
3. Commonly seen in children.
   a. Onset before 5 years of age in almost 90% of cases.
   b. Almost 75% of all cases clear by adolescence, but can reoccur in adults.
B. Etiology.
1. The exact pathogenesis is unknown.
2. Commonly there is a family history of atopic dermatitis, asthma, and/or allergic rhinitis.
C. Immunopathogensis.
1. T-cell activation.
2. Antigen presenting/dendritic cells.
3. Th1/Th2 cytokine imbalance.
4. IgE prodution.
5. *Staphylococcal aureus* and staphylococcal toxins trigger several processes.
D. Assessment.
1. Clinical manifestations.
   a. Characterized by basic diagnostic criteria: patient must have three or more basic features.
      (1) Pruritus.
      (2) Typical morphology and distribution:
         (a) Facial and extensor involvement in patients.
         (b) Flexural lichenification or linearity in

adults.
      (3) Chronic or chronically relapsing dermatitis.
      (4) Personal or family history of atopy (asthma, allergic rhinitis, atopic dermatitis).
   b. Severity ranges from mild to severe; tends to wax and wain with seasonal variation, often worsening in the winter.
   c. Precipitating factors.
      (1) Extremes in temperature and humidity: hot/humid or cold/dry.
      (2) Sweating.
      (3) Course or irritating clothing such as wool and some synthetic fabrics.
      (4) Drying cleansers or cosmetics.
      (5) Emotional stress.
      (6) Environmental allergens (for example, dust mite, cat).
      (7) Food allergens (for example, milk, soy, egg, wheat, fish, and nuts).
   d. Primary lesions.
      (1) Some believe no primary lesion can be identified and that all visible skin lesions in AD are secondary to scratching.
      (2) Erythematous papules that may coalesce or dry scaly patches.
   e. Secondary lesions.
      (1) Scale.
      (2) Excoriations.
      (3) Lichenification.
      (4) White dermatographism.
   f. Distribution.
      (1) Tends to be symmetrical.
      (2) Is more pronounced in areas not covered by clothing.
      (3) The extensor surfaces and face tend to have greater involvement in infants. Diaper area is generally clear.
      (4) The flexor surfaces tend to have greater involvement in older patients.
      (5) The hands and feet frequently are involved in adults.
   g. Complications.
      (1) Secondary bacterial infection usually caused by *S. aureus*.
      (2) Eczema herpeticum as well as other viral and fungal infections including molluscum and tinea.
2. Diagnostic tests.
   a. Serum IgE tests are frequently elevated but are not helpful diagnostically.
   b. Allergy testing if allergies are suspected

(prick skin testing and patch testing can be useful in assessing triggers). Clinical correlation necessary prior to any restrictions.

   c. Skin cultures and sensitivities in cases of suspected secondary infection.

E. Nursing considerations.

   1. Interventions.

      a. Relief of xerosis.

         (1) Bathe or shower at least once per day. Use warm, not hot, water for at least 15 to 20 minutes. Avoid scrubbing skin with a washcloth.

         (2) Use a gentle cleansing bar or wash such as Dove®, Oil of Olay®, Eucerin®, Basis®, Cetaphil®, Aveeno®, or Oilatum®. During a severe flare, limit the use of cleansers to avoid possible irritation. Gentle cleansers are generally perfume free and dye free.

         (3) After the bath or shower, gently pat away excess water and immediately apply the moisturizer or the special skin medications prescribed onto damp skin. This will seal in the water and make the skin less dry and itchy. Moisturizers should not be applied over the medications. Vaseline® is a good occlusive preparation to seal in the water; however, it contains no water so it only works effectively after a soaking bath. Recommended moisturizers include Aquaphor® Ointment, Eucerin® Creme, Vanicream®, Cetaphil® Cream, or Lubrex® Cream.

         (4) Wet dressing with occlusion twice a day when severe, or overnight to treat individuals with multiple excoriations, crusting, and weeping lesions.

           (a) Wet one pair of cotton sleepers, pajamas, or long underwear in warm water, wring out until damp, and put on immediately after applying topical medications.

           (b) Place a dry layer on top of the damp ones.

           (c) Keep the room warm to avoid chilling.

      b. Decrease inflammation.

         (1) Mild-to-moderate strength topical corticosteroids or topical immunomodulators twice a day as needed.

         (2) Cream or ointment vehicle may be used on face and body; solution or lotion vehicle to scalp. Some patients with AD are sensitive to the ingredients of topical preparations.

         (3) Topical corticosteroids and topical immunomodulators may be used in combination with wet dressings in severe cases.

         (4) Systemic corticosteroids are rarely used in the chronic condition of atopic dermatitis.

         (5) The two immunomodulatory drugs, tacrolimus (Protopic®) ointment and Elidel® cream, are effective in both adults and children without the side effects of topical steroids.

      c. Relief of pruritus.

         (1) Sedating antihistamines such as diphenhydramine (3 to 5 mg/kg/day) or ✱hydroxyzine (1 to 2 mg/kg/day) may help to relieve pruritus.

         (2) Use sedating antihistamines at bedtime to decrease itching and to promote more restful sleep.

         (3) The relatively low-sedating antihistamine cetirizine may be used to provide relief from pruritus in children as young as 6 months of age during the daytime.

         (4) Cool soaks to limited areas of the body followed by emollients, topical corticosteroids, or topical immunomodulators may help to relieve pruritus.

      d. Treatment of infections.

         (1) Topical antibiotic — mupirocin 2% ointment may be applied 3 times a day to small areas of impetigo. Use 3 times per day for at least 3 to 5 days or until clearing; never use PRN.

         (2) For more widespread infection, use an antistaphylococcal oral antibiotic (for example, cephalexin 25 to 50 mg/kg/day).

      e. Environmental control.

         (1) Decrease exposure to predisposing factors.

         (2) Avoid exposure to anyone with active herpes lesions.

   2. Patient education.

      a. Methods of skin hydration.

      b. Proper methods of application of medications.

      c. Signs of skin infection.

      d. Ways to incorporate treatments into daily routines.

      e. Sources of psychosocial support such as the National Eczema Association for Science and Education.

   3. Followup.

      a. First followup visit in 7 to 14 days to assess treatment effectiveness.

      b. Monthly visits (if insurance allows) until

patient is using moisturizers.

   c. When skin condition is stable visits every 6 months for re-evaluation.

   d. As needed for flairs and failure to respond to treatment.

II. SEBORRHEIC DERMATITIS

A. Definition.
1. Common chronic dermatitis occurring primarily in areas of increased sebaceous gland concentration resulting in an overproduction of sebum.
2. Occurs in multiple age groups — the neonate, the adolescent, and the adult.

B. Etiology and pathology.
1. Pathology has been attributed to excessive sebum accumulation on skin surface but the mechanism for this remains unclear.
2. Occurrence in the neonate is believed to be related to intrauterine exposure to maternal hormones.
3. The role of the overgrowth of Malassezia furfur (Pityrosporum ovale) remains controversial.
4. Occasionally, may be associated with serious illness and failure to thrive. It may be an early sign of HIV or other immunodeficiency diseases.

C. Incidence.
1. The incidence in the general population is 2% to 5%.
2. In infants, tends to regress by 5 to 6 months of age.
3. In adolescents and adults, may improve with age, tends to wax and wain.

D. Assessment.
1. Clinical manifestations.
   a. Minimal to no pruritus in infancy. Adolescents or adults may complain of pruritus.
   b. Lesions are symmetric and typically red with greasy yellow to salmon-colored scale.
   c. Areas of involvement are primarily the scalp, medial eyebrows, central face, retroauricular area, presternal area, or perineum.
   d. Varies from minimal to widespread involvement.
   e. Primary lesions — erythematous papules/patches, poorly marginated.
   f. Secondary lesions — greasy scale, excoriations if pruritic.
2. Diagnostic tests.
   a. Not helpful unless another severe systemic disease is suspected.

E. Nursing considerations.
1. Interventions.
   a. Low-potency topical corticosteroid creams or topical immunomodulators applied twice

daily for several days will usually clear the dermatitis and then used occasionally will control recurrences.

   b. Frequently in infants, tear-free shampoos are adequate to loosen the scales when allowed to remain on the scalp for several minutes and lightly scrubbed with a soft brush to remove the scale. In more difficult cases, scale may be loosened with mineral oil prior to shampooing.

   c. Keratolytic/antiseborrheic shampoos may be helpful for adolescents and adults to control scalp scaling. For more stubborn cases, use ketoconazole (Nizoral®) shampoo.

2. Patient teaching.
   a. Review the expected course of the disorder.
   b. Encourage gentle therapy in removal of the scales.
   c. Instruct on proper use of the medication.
3. Followup.
   a. One week visit to evaluate response.
   b. Thereafter, the patient is seen only if the dermatitis does not resolve.

III. CONTACT DERMATITIS

A. Definition.
1. Irritant contact dermatitis from a local irritant is the most common form of contact dermatitis. The intensity of the inflammation is related to the concentration of the irritant and the exposure time.
2. Allergic contact dermatitis triggers an immunologic event which is the result of a Type IV delayed hypersensitivity reaction to an allergen.

B. Etiology.
1. Irritant nonallergic contact dermatitis results from direct contact with an irritating substance. Possible irritants are numerous; for example, oil products such as fuels and lubricants, corrosives, detergents, bleaches, ammonia, oven cleaners, and ingredients in common skin products.
2. Allergic contact dermatitis affects a limited number of susceptible individuals and is a manifestation of a sensitivity to a substance to which the patient has had previous contact. Possible allergens are many; common examples include fragrances, dyes, nickel, antibiotic ointments or creams, rubber-containing products, formaldehyde, and poison ivy/oak.

C. Presentation.
1. Irritant contact dermatitis.
   a. Can be either acute or chronic. In the acute stage erythema, blister formation, erosion, crusting, shedding, and scaling are seen.

The distribution is usually isolated or localized; pruritus is always present.

b. In chronic contact dermatitis thickening of skin, scaling, fissures, and crusting are present. Distribution is usually isolated or localized.

2. Allergic contact dermatitis.
   a. Can be either acute or chronic. In acute allergic dermatitis erythema, papules, vesicles, erosion, crusts, and scaling are seen. The dermatosis is usually confined to the area of exposure but can spread to peripheral areas.
   b. In allergic contact dermatitis the patient has been previously exposed to the allergen. This exposure creates a sensitization phase which results in antigen formation. The resulting sensitized T cells remain in the body. Re-exposure to the antigen in the elicitation phase results in a cutaneous eczematous inflammation. Although these reactions are usually localized, patients who are sensitized to topical medications may develop generalized eczematous reactions.

D. Incidence.
   1. Anyone at any time could acquire irritant contact dermatitis. Suspect patients working with cleaning agents such as ammonia or bleach, and health care workers who work with various lotions and alcohol solutions. Repeated higher concentrates of chemicals can cause a contact dermatitis. Approximately eighty percent of contact dermatitis is irritant in nature.
   2. Individuals must be sensitized to a chemical to acquire contact allergic dermatitis. Patients initially come in contact with a sensitizing agent and have a reaction upon subsequent exposure to the agent. Approximately 20% percent of contact dermatitis is allergic in nature.

E. Assessment
   1. History and physical exam.
      a. History of sensitivity to chemicals or substances.
      b. Occupation and history of exposure to, for example, neomycin, procaine, benzocaine, sulfonamides, turpentine, balsam of Peru, formalin, mercury, chromate, nickel sulfate, cobalt sulfate, p-phenylenediamine, and parahydroxybenzoic acid ester.
      c. In an acute exposure erythema, papules, vesicles, and edema are present and are usually confined to area of exposure.
      d. In chronic exposure plaques of lichenification with small, firm, round, or flat-topped papules with mild erythema are present.

   2. Diagnostic tests.
      a. Patch testing can help determine the responsible allergen in allergic contact dermatitis. The goal of patch testing is to reproduce the eczema in a controlled process. Small amounts of suspected chemical are applied to the skin and subsequent examination will reveal reaction. This process must be done in a standardized format to be realible. The product True Test® offers standardized easy-to-use patch testing. Patient counseling of results is key in management.
      b. Biopsy may not be helpful; complete history of clinical findings and patch testing are the most important diagnostic tools.

F. Common therapeutic modalities.
   1. Medical interventions.
      a. Eliminate the irritant or allergen when possible.
      b. In severe cases a short course of systemic corticosteroids may be required.
      c. Topical corticosteroids are used but only in chronic cases; they should be used carefully to avoid side effects.

G. Common nursing diagnoses, outcomes, and interventions.
   1. Nursing diagnosis: potential alteration in skin integrity related to acute or chronic condition.
      a. Outcome: patient will not experience any skin changes.
      b. Interventions.
         (1) Remove causative agent. If not possible suggest patient avoidance strategies such as to wear gloves, mask, and goggles when working with agent.
         (2) Teach patient proper way to apply topical medications.
   2. Nursing diagnosis: anxiety related to need for occupation change where required.
      a. Outcome: patient will experience minimal anxiety and verbalize ways to control anxiety.
      b. Interventions.
         (1) Suggest patient pursue patch testing to determine cause of dermatitis.
         (2) Give patient information on caustic agents.
         (3) Suggest career counseling if applicable.

IV. DIAPER DERMATITIS

A. Definition.
   1. A cutaneous eruption in the diaper area and the majority of cases represent the most common form of primary irritant contact dermatitis seen in pediatrics.

B. Etiology and pathology.
1. Is caused by an interaction between several factors.
   a. Frequent and prolonged skin wetness from occlusion and urine and feces trapping close to the skin.
   b. Friction by movement of the skin against skin, the diaper, plastic leg gathers, or fastening tape.
   c. Fecal enzymes causing cutaneous irritation.
2. Administration of oral antibiotic medication may predispose a child to develop diaper dermatitis.

C. Incidence.
1. Diaper dermatitis is one of the most frequent skin disorders of infancy, with peak incidence between 9 and 12 months of age.
2. May occur in any child or adult who is incontinent of urine or stool.

D. Assessment.
1. Clinical manifestations.
   a. Erythema with or without papules, erosions, scale, and/or maceration on the lower abdomen, groin, perineum, buttocks, labia majora, scrotum, penis, or upper thigh that initially spares skin creases.
   b. If diaper dermatitis is present for longer than 3 days there is likely to be a secondary *C. albicans* infection. This presents as confluent erythema with satellite papules and often involves skin creases.
   c. Fragile bulla or erosions with a collarette of scale may indicate bullous impetigo.
2. Diagnostic tests.
   a. KOH preparation to identify *C. albicans* infection.
   b. Bacterial culture may be needed to rule out secondary bacterial infection.
   c. Skin biopsy may be required in dermatitis that is unresponsive to therapy to rule out other associated problems.

E. Nursing considerations.
1. Interventions.
   a. Prevention is the single most important intervention. Most irritant diaper dermatitis is self-limited and may resolve, or be prevented quickly with the following steps.
      (1) Airing of the diaper area.
      (2) Applying barrier creams and ointments (such as petrolatum or zinc oxide).
      (3) Frequent diaper changes. If dermatitis is present, change at least every 2 hours during the day and once at night.
   b. *C. albicans* diaper dermatitis is treated with a topical antiyeast cream such as nystatin applied TID or with each diaper change.
   c. In severe dermatitis, hydrocortisone 1% cream twice daily for 1 or 2 days may help

to decrease discomfort in between use of other topicals
2. Patient education.
   a. Diaper dermatitis is less prevalent in those whose diapers are changed at least 8 times a day.
   b. Use of barrier ointments.
   c. Signs of *C. albicans* infection.
3. Followup.
   a. Routine visits for care is sufficient followup.
   b. In severe diaper dermatitis, a return visit in 2 days to assess response is recommended.

V. NUMMULAR ECZEMA

An inflammatory skin disorder with coin-shaped lesions usually affecting lower extremities.
A. Etiology.
1. Unknown although secondary infection is common.
B. Pathophysiology.
1. Lesions are 2 to 10 cm or more, circular, and often distributed symmetrically on the legs.
2. Usually subacute with erythema, edema, and in some cases vesiculation.
3. Pruritus may be present; color is usually pink to dull red; plaque may be present.
C. Incidence.
1. Peaks and usually occurs in old age.
2. Occurs mainly in the winter season.
3. Affects males more than females.
D. Considerations across life span.
1. The condition is chronic.
2. Plaques may be lichenified.
E. Assessment.
1. History and physical exam.
   a. History of psoriasis, atopic dermatitis, and contact dermatitis associated with subsequent nummular eczema.
   b. Lesions may be present for months to weeks.
   c. Change in seasons or excessive cold may initiate nummular eczema.
   d. Coin-shaped, small vesicles and papules with regional clusters of lesions seen on lower legs.
2. Diagnostic tests.
   a. Bacterial culture to rule out *S. aureus* infection.
   b. Biopsy reveals inflammation with acanthosis and spongiosis.
F. Common therapeutic modalities.
1. Medical interventions.
   a. Hydration of skin with moisturizing lotions.
   b. Applications of topical steroids.
   c. Use of topical tar preparations.
   d. Use of systemic antibiotics if secondary bacterial infection.

e. PUVA may be used in very difficult cases.

G. **Common nursing diagnoses, outcomes, and interventions.**
1. Nursing diagnosis: impaired skin integrity related to possible lichenification process.
   a. Outcome — patient's skin will not appear lichenified.
   b. Intervention — teach patient how to apply moisturizers and topical medications if applicable.

VI. LICHEN SIMPLEX CHRONICUS

The disease is a secondary result of inflammatory eczematous diseases. Pruritus is always present. Rubbing and scratching becomes an unconscious activity which precipitates the problem.

A. **Etiology.**
1. Proliferation of cells of the epidermal layer and hyperplasia in response to repeated scratching and itching.
2. Emotional stress has been linked to occurrence of the disease.

B. **Pathophysiology.**
1. Hyperplasia occurs and lesions may appear as lichenificated plaques with small papules. The skin is thickened.

C. **Incidence.**
1. Usually occurs in individuals over 20 years.
2. There is higher incidence in females, Asians, and Native Americans.

D. **Consideration across the life span.**
1. Patients with atopic dermatitis are at risk for developing skin lichenification.
2. Diseases such as psoriasis and contact dermatitis must be ruled out in order to deliver appropriate treatments.
3. Dark-skinned individuals present with lichenificated papules rather than plaques.

E. **Assessment**
1. History and physical exam.
   a. Familial history of psoriasis, contact dermatitis, atopic dermatitis, or seasonal rhinitis.
   b. History of localized pruritus which the patient often scratches.
   c. Most lesions occur on the scalp, ankles, lower legs, upper thighs, and exterior forearms.
   d. Lesions are always pruritic.
   e. Areas of excoriation are common and usually dull red. The shape of the lesion varies; it may be round, oval, or linear.
2. Diagnostic tests.
   a. Potassium hydroxide — KOH preparation to rule out dermatophytosis.
   b. Biopsy shows hyperplasia of the components of epidermis. In the dermis

there is a chronic inflammatory infiltrate.

F. **Common therapeutic modalities.**
1. Medical interventions.
   a. Rehydration therapy followed by emollients and/or topical steroids.
   b. Sedating oral antihistamines such as hydroxyzine and diphenhydramine to relieve itching.
   c. Tranquilizers and antidepressants may be helpful to alleviate emotional stress.

G. **Common nursing diagnoses, outcomes, and interventions.**
1. Nursing diagnosis: potential for depression related to chronic condition.
   a. Outcome — patient will be aware of what control he/she has over the disease process.
   b. Interventions.
      (1) Give patient educational information on the disease.
      (2) Teach patient relaxation techniques.
      (3) Refer patient to counseling to talk about feelings.

VII. ICHTHYOSIS

A. **Definition.**
1. Excessive scaling of the skin. The scale may be "fish scale-like."
2. Four major hereditary types have been described.
   a. Lamellar ichthyosis and congenital nonbullous ichthyosiform erythroderma.
   b. Bullous ichthyosis (also called congenital bullous ichthyosiform erythroderma or epidermolytic hyperkeratosis).
   c. Ichthyosis vulgaris.
   d. X-linked ichthyosis.

B. **Etiology and pathology.**
1. Ichthyosis vulgaris (IV) is inherited as an autosomal dominant disease
2. X-linked ichthyosis (XLI) is inherited as a X-linked recessive trait that is due to a deficiency of the enzyme, steroid sulfatase. Female carriers are asymptomatic.
3. Lamellar ichthyosis (LI) and congenital nonbullous ichthyosiform erythroderma (CNIE) are inherited in an autosomal recessive trait pattern.
4. Bullous ichthyosis (BI) is inherited as an autosomal dominant disorder.
5. Increased epidermal turnover with excessive production of stratum corneum cells has been demonstrated in LI and BI.
6. In XLI and IV there appears to be normal epidermal turnover, and the accumulated scale is thought to be due to faulty shedding of the stratum corneum.

C. **Incidence.**

1. IV is extremely common with 1:250 children having some variant of this disorder from mild to severe.
2. XLI is estimated to occur in 1 in 60,000 males.
3. LI and CNIE appear to occur in approximately 1 per 100,000 live births.
4. Incidence of BI is unknown.

D. Assessment.
1. Clinical manifestations.
   a. Ichthyosis vulgaris.
      (1) The skin of the newborn with IV usually remains normal throughout the newborn period.
      (2) Manifestations are limited to the skin with fine scales predominately over the legs and buttocks that may be evident by 6 months to 2 years of age.
      (3) Dry, follicular, horny plugs (keratosis pilaris) are present on the extensor surface of extremities and may become widespread.
      (4) The entire surface of the skin is dry and may be associated with atopic dermatitis.
   b. X-linked ichthyosis.
      (1) Presents in infancy with scales over the posterior neck, upper trunk, and extensor surfaces of the extremities.
      (2) Scaling is usually mild during the first 30 days of life and the skin is a normal color.
      (3) As the child ages, the scales become thicker and dirty-yellow/brown in color. Antecubital and popliteal areas are often spared as well as the palms and soles.
      (4) Corneal opacities are a clinical marker in XLI, but are usually not present until adulthood.
      (5) Cryptorchidism may occur in as many as one-fourth of males with XLI.
   c. Lamellar ichthyosis and congenital nonbullous ichthyosiform erythroderma.
      (1) Large, plate-like, dark scales with or without erythematous skin are present in LI.
      (2) In CNIE, generalized fine scales on erythematous skin are present. The erythema may fade as the child ages.
      (3) With either condition, the affected infant may be born with a collodion membrane.
      (4) Facial tautness commonly produces ectropion and eclabium that appears shortly after birth in children with LI.
      (5) The skin of the palms and soles are generally thickened.
      (6) Cicatricial alopecia may develop as well as thickening of the nails and inflammation of the nail folds.
      (7) Heat intolerance is common and due to obstruction of the eccrine glands.
   d. Bullous ichthyosis.
      (1) Presents at birth with extensive scaling, erythroderma, and recurrent episodes of bullous formation.
      (2) The bullae frequently become infected with *S. aureus* causing problems in the neonatal and infant periods.
      (3) With age, the involvement is more limited in extent and by school age, thick, warty, malodorous, dirty-yellow/brown scales will develop on the palms, soles, elbows, and knees.
      (4) Flexure areas tend to have greater involvement and frequently become macerated and secondarily colonized with bacteria producing a foul body odor.
      (5) After the neonatal period the mechano-bullous component becomes less prominent; however, focal blistering continues.
      (6) Facial involvement is common, but ectropion does not occur. Nails may become dystrophic due to nail fold inflammation.
2. Diagnostic tests.
   a. Skin biopsy helps to demonstrate the histologic changes in the epidermis and hyperkeratosis.
   b. Measurement of steroid sulfatase activity in red blood cells may be useful in diagnosing X-linked ichthyosis.
   c. Molecular genetic diagnosis is useful to distinguish the various forms of ichthyosis.

E. Nursing considerations.
1. Interventions.
   a. Daily use of emollients.
      (1) Bland emollients such as petrolatum or Aquaphor. For example, Vaseline, Eucerin, or Johnson's Ultra Sensitive product line.
      (2) Alpha-hydroxy acid (lactic acid, urea, glycolic acid 5% to 10%) in petrolatum.
      (3) Propylene glycol 40% to 60% in water applied at bedtime with occlusion.
   b. Oral synthetic retinoids to alleviate the hyperkeratosis. Due to their toxicity their use is warranted only in patients with severe physical or emotional complications.
   c. Adequate provision of calories in diet, especially protein, and monitoring of child's iron status due to the metabolic drain of erythroderma on a growing child and substantial iron loss in hyperproliferative states.

d. Infants with widespread blistering are cared for in the NICU with precautions to avoid further trauma to the skin and prevent infection.

e. Psychosocial support to deal with issues related to body image, social relationships, and demanding complex therapy.

2. Patient education.

a. Prevent heat prostration particularly during strenuous physical activity and/or warm temperatures.

b. Bath with antibacterial soaps to decrease bacterial colonization of scales.

c. Consideration of choice of clothing and shoewear for children with mechanically induced blisters.

d. Blistering after infancy often signifies a bacterial infection requiring treatment with an oral antibiotic effective against *S. aureus*.

e. Referral to the Ichthyosis Foundation for family support.

3. Followup.

a. One week after discharge from the newborn nursery.

b. Routine visits for pediatric care and additional visits may be necessary, depending on the severity of the ichthyosis.

VIII. KERATOSIS PILARIS

A group of small, pinpoint, follicular papules or pustules that are seen in the same anatomic area for years; seen more commonly inpatients with atopic dermatitis.

B. Etiology: unknown.

C. Pathophysiology.

1. Follicular keratinous plugs of 1 to 2 mm in size.

D. Incidence.

1. Present in a large portion of the normal population.

2. More common in patients with atopic dermatitis.

E. Considerations across the life span.

1. Any age group may be affected; onset most frequent in 2nd decade.

2. Common in young children.

3. Peaks during adolescence.

F. Assessment.

1. History and physical exam.

a. Atopic dermatitis.

b. Age at onset.

c. Small 1 to 2 mm rough follicular papules or pustules.

d. Predilection for posterolateral aspects of the upper arms and anterior thighs.

e. Any area can be involved except palms and soles.

f. Lesions on the face may be misdiagnosed as acne.

g. Associated with dry skin and chapping.

h. May resemble heat rash or milaria.

i. Most often asymptomatic, but lesions may become red, inflamed, and pustular (resembles bacterial folliculitis).

j. In adults lesion may present with a red halo.

2. Diagnostic tests — no specific studies.

G. Common therapeutic modalities.

1. Medical interventions.

a. Tretinoin — may provide temporary improvement in roughness, but may increase irritation.

b. Short course of low-potency topical steroids to reduce inflammation, when present.

c. Application of urea or lactic acid-based cream.

2. Nonmedical treatment.

a. Avoid scratching lesions — implement measures to reduce pruritus.

b. Avoid tight-fitting clothing.

c. Do not use abrasives for treatment.

H. Common nursing diagnosis, outcomes, and interventions.

1. Nursing diagnosis: body image alteration secondary to clinical presentation.

a. Outcome — patient will have positive body image.

b. Interventions.

(1) Assess patient's feelings regarding skin appearance.

(2) Assess patient's coping process.

2. Nursing diagnosis: increased risk for infection secondary to scratching.

a. Outcome — patient will remain free of secondary infection.

b. Intervention — instruct patient on the use of antihistamines; bland emollients to reduce pruritus.

3. Nursing diagnosis: knowledge deficit related to skin disorder.

a. Outcome — patient/significant other will understand disorder and appropriate interventions.

b. Interventions.

(1) Educate patient/significant other about keratosis pilaris.

(2) Instruct patient on appropriate use of topical medications.

(3) Instruct patient/significant other to avoid tight-fitting clothing, scratching, and use of abrasives.

Bibliography

Berger, T.G., James, W.D., & Odom, R.B. (2000). *Andrews' diseases of the skin: Clinical dermatology* (9th ed.). Philadelphia: W.B. Saunders Co.

Boguniewicz, M., & Nicol, N.H. (2002). Conventional therapy for atopic dermatitis. *Immunology and Allergy Clinics of North America, 22,* 107-124.

Callen, J.P. (2000). *Color atlas of dermatology.* (2nd ed.). Philadelphia: W.B. Saunders Co.

Deleo, V.A., Elsner, P. , & Marks, J.G. Jr. (2000). *Contact & occupational dermatology* (3rd ed.). St. Louis: Mosby.

Fitzpatrick, T.B., Johnson, R.A., & Wolff, K. (2001). *Color atlas and synopsis of clinical dermatology: Common and serious diseases* (4th ed.). New York: McGraw-Hill.

Freeberg, I.M. (Ed.) (1999). *Fitzpatrick's dermatology in general medicine* (5th ed.). New York: McGraw-Hill, Health Professions Division.

Gilchrest, B.A. (Ed.). (2002). *Geriatric dermatology part II.* Philadelphia: W.B. Saunders.

Greaves, M.W., & Leung, D.Y.M. (Eds.). (2000). *Allergic skin disease: A multidisciplinary approach.* New York: Marcel Dekker, Inc.

Lane, A.T., Morelli, J.G., & Weston, W.L. (1996). *Color textbook of pediatric dermatology* (3rd ed.). St. Louis: Mosby.

Lookingbill, D.P., & Marks, J.G. Jr. (2000). *Principles of dermatology* (3rd ed.). Philadelphia: W.B. Saunders Co.

Moore, J.A., Nicol, N.H., & Ruszkowski, A.M. (1995). What patients need to know about patch testing. *Dermatology Nursing, 20*(1), 20-26.

STUDY QUESTIONS

1. The most common form of ichthyosis seen in children is:
   a. Bullous ichthyosis.
   b. Congenital nonbullous ichthyosiform erythroderma.
   c. Ichthyosis vulgaris.
   d. Lamellar ichthyosis.

2. The cutaneous manifestations of atopic dermatitis are the same at any age.
   a. True
   b. False

3. The infant with seborrheic dermatitis generally presents with all of the following signs and symptoms *except:*
   a. Erythematous papules.
   b. Greasy yellow scale.
   c. Intense pruritus.
   d. Rash on scalp and forehead.

4. A parent can best prevent irritant diaper dermatitis in a healthy 6-month-old infant by:
   a. Changing diapers frequently.
   b. Increasing dietary vitamin C intake.
   c. Using cloth diapers only.
   d. Using commercial diaper wipes regularly.

5. Nummular eczema is an inflammatory skin disorder usually affecting:
   a. Scalp.
   b. Torso.
   c. Upper extremities.
   d. Lower extremities.

6. Lichen simplex chronicus is always accompanied by:
   a. Coin-shaped lesions.
   b. Pruritus.
   c. Fish scale-like lesions.
   d. Facial tautness.

7. The clinical manifestations of ichthyosis include:
   a. Fine scales predominantly over the legs and buttocks.
   b. Dry, follicular, horny plugs.
   c. Dry skin associated with atopic dermatitis.
   d. All of the above.

8. Interventions for ichthyosis include:
   a. Daily use of emollients.
   b. Exercise.
   c. Antihistamines.
   d. Steroids.

9. Keratosis pilaris comprises follicular keratinous plugs of what size?
   a. 4 to 5 mm.
   b. 2 to 3 mm.
   c. 1 to 2 mm.
   d. 0.5 to 1 mm.

10. Nonmedical treatment of keratosis pilaris includes:
    a. Scratching lesions to reduce pruritus.
    b. Avoid tight-fitting clothing.
    c. Using abrasives for treatment.
    d. a & c.

Answers to Study Questions

1.	c	5.	d	9.	c
2.	b	6.	b	10.	b
3.	c	7.	d		
4.	a	8.	a		

Dermatologic Nursing Essentials: A Core Curriculum 2nd Edition © DNA 2003

Chapter 5.
Dermatitis/Eczemas

Please photocopy this test page and return.

COMPLETE THE FOLLOWING:

Name: _____

Address: _____

City: _____ State: _____ Zip: _____

Preferred telephone: (Home)_____ (Work) _____

State where licensed and license number: _____

CE application fee: DNA member $10.00
                     Nonmember $13.00

POSTTEST INSTRUCTIONS
1. To receive continuing education credit for individual study after reading the article, complete the answer/evaluation form below.
2. Photocopy and send the answer/evaluation form along with a check or money order payable to **Dermatology Nurses' Association** to: **DNA**, East Holly Avenue Box 56, Pitman, NJ 08071-0056.
3. Test returns must be postmarked by December 31, 2008. Upon completion of the answer/evaluation form, a certificate for 2.2 contact hour(s) will be awarded and sent to you.

This chapter was reviewed and formatted for contact hour credit by Marcia J. Hill, MSN, RN, Core Curriculum Editor; and Sally Russell, MN, RN,C, DNA Education Director.

ANSWER FORM

1. Name one new detail (item, issue, or phenomenon) that you learned by completing this activity.

_____

_____

_____

_____

2. How will you apply the information from this learning activity to your practice?
   a. Patient education.
   b. Staff education.
   c. Improve my patient care.
   d. In my education course work.
   e. Other: Please describe _____

   _____

   _____

Evaluation	Strongly disagree				Strongly agree
3. The offering met the stated objectives.					
a. Understand that eczema and dermatitis are terms that describe the same response in the skin.	1	2	3	4	5
b. Recognize several types of eczemas and their various clinical presentations.	1	2	3	4	5
c. Discuss the therapeutic interventions frequently used to treat various eczemas.	1	2	3	4	5
d. Identify important patient teaching issues for managing various eczemas.	1	2	3	4	5
4. The content was current and relevant.	1	2	3	4	5
5. The content was presented clearly.	1	2	3	4	5
6. The content was covered adequately.	1	2	3	4	5
7. I am more confident of my abilities since completing this material.	1	2	3	4	5

8. The material was (check one) ☐ new, ☐ review for me.

Comments _____

_____

9. Time required to complete reading assignment: _____ minutes

This independent study is provided by the Dermatology Nurses' Association (DNA) for 2.2 contact hours. DNA is accredited as a provider of continuing education in nursing by the American Nurses Credentialing Center's Commission on Accreditation. DNA is approved as a provider of continuing education by the California Board of Registered Nursing Provider #CEP5708.

Cutaneous Malignancies

Nancy Vargo, RN, DNC

OBJECTIVES

At the end of this chapter, the reader will be able to:
- Identify and differentiate the growth patterns of common skin malignancies.
- Describe the risk factors and incidence of skin cancers.
- Identify the relationship of UV irradiation and genetic mutations.
- Describe the clinical appearance of skin cancers and certain precursors.
- Discuss the various treatment options available for patients diagnosed with skin cancer based on clinical and histologic assessment.

KEY POINTS

- Tumors of the skin may be benign, premalignant, or malignant.
- Early and accurate diagnosis of tumors is paramount for correct intervention.
- Malignant melanoma has the potential for metastasis and may be life threatening.
- Skin cancer is the most common malignancy found in humans.
- Visibility on the skin surface and the relative slow growth of most skin cancers contributes to early detection and treatment resulting in high cure rates for adequately treated lesions.

Cutaneous Malignancies

Nancy Vargo, RN, DNC

BASAL CELL CARCINOMA

I. OVERVIEW

A tumor of the epidermis that demonstrates its malignant nature by its expansive growth and invasion of local structures. Basal cell carcinoma (BCC) rarely metastasizes beyond the skin.

A. Definition: an epidermal tumor predominantly found on exposed surfaces of the skin. BCC arises from the single layer of spherical-shaped basal cells that line the basement membrane, separating the epidermis from the dermis.

B. Etiology.
1. Ultraviolet radiation.
   a. Cumulative exposure to ultraviolet light is the most important environmental carcinogen causing nonmelanoma skin cancer.
   b. Depletion of earth's protective ozone layer allows dangerous UV rays to penetrate the atmosphere.
   c. UV radiation results in mutations in cellular DNA leading to unrestricted growth and tumor formation.
   d. Mutation of the *p53* tumor suppressor gene is an early event in UV carcinogenesis resulting in unchecked mitoses of keratinocytes.
   e. Langerhans' cells, found in the basal layer of the epidermis is functionally impaired by UVB and PUVA treatment leading to morphologic changes within the cell.
2. Ionizing radiation exposure through occupation or as a treatment of disorders such as acne, tinea, eczema, or skin cancer.
3. Exposure to chemical carcinogens such as arsenic found in some well water, in household or agricultural insecticides, or pharmacological mixtures (Fowler's solution).
4. Genetic determinations.
   a. Inherited skin type.
   b. Basal cell nevoid syndrome — a complex group of disorders that affects the skin, endocrine, central nervous, and skeletal systems characterized by skin cancers that develop at an early age.
      (1) *PTCH* gene mutation (as a result of UV irradiation) causes an inherited mutated gene contributing to nevoid basal cell syndrome.
5. BCC may arise in nevus sebaceous.

C. Pathophysiology.
1. Basal cells fail to mature into keratinocytes resulting in tumor cells that retain the capability of mitotic division beyond the basal layer of the epidermis.
2. Growth results in a bulky tumor that fills the epidermis, dermis, and eventually projecting finger-like strands of tumor along tissue planes, fascia, cartilage, or bone.
3. Growth occurs in a continuous cellular structure that may invade surrounding healthy skin, nerves, lymphatic and blood vessels as well as cartilage or bone.
4. BCC has a nonmetastasizing nature due to its dependence on the integumental system for viability.
   a. Metastasis via lymphatic or hematogenous spread is rare, reported at 0.0028% to 0.1%.
   b. Very rare distant metastases to lungs, lymph nodes, bone, liver, and other viscera.
   c. Predisposing factors for metastasis include large primary tumors and resistance of tumor to surgery and radiotherapy.
   d. Basosquamous BCC (containing typical basal cells as well as squamoid-appearing cells) has a metastatic potential of 9.7% due to its aggressive behavior.

D. Incidence.
1. Nonmelanoma skin cancer (BCC and squamous cell carcinoma [SCC]) compose the most common cancers in the country.
2. Over one million new cases of skin cancer will occur in 2002, 70% of which are nonmelanoma skin cancers.
3. Risk factors include.
   a. Chronic UV exposure.
   b. Race.
   c. Fair complexion.
   d. Gender.
   e. Occupational exposure to carcinogens.
   f. Genetics.
   g. DNA repair capability.
   h. PUVA treatment for psoriasis.

II. CLASSIFICATION OF BCC

A. Nodular (see Figure 6-1, page 229).
1. Most common classification composing 40% to 54% of all BCCs.
2. A bulky nodular growth on exposed skin that fails to heal.
3. Epidermis thins as tumor slowly grows, stretching intact skin and producing a shiny,

translucent bump with a pearly hue.

4. Tiny blood vessels rupture causing telangiectasias to course within the lesion.
5. Steady growth results in raised borders and central ulceration and necrosis.
6. Bleeds easily from mild injury, doubles in size every 6 to 12 months at a rate of 5 mm/yr.

B. **Superficial (see Figure 6-2, page 229).**
1. Appears most frequently on the trunk and in actinically damaged skin.
2. Well-demarcated, erythematous scaly patch that may grow up to 15 cm on the skin surface.
3. May develop in multiple sites growing peripherally across skin surface forming pearly, raised borders.
4. Small ulcerations will appear signifying invasive growth.
5. Associated with arsenic ingestion/exposure.

C. **Morpheaform or Sclerotic (see Figure 6-3, page 229).**
1. Appears as pale yellow or white flat or depressed scar-like plaque.
2. Indistinct margins lacking rolled border.
3. More aggressive variant that often produces fibroepitheliomatous strands of tumor found in the tissue planes of the dermis.
4. May remain undetected due to clinical appearance.

D. **Pigmented (see Figure 6-4, page 229).**
1. Contains melanin appearing as blue, black, or brown lesion.
2. More commonly found in dark-complexioned persons such as Latinos, Japanese. (Not common in blacks).
3. Lesions contain telangiectasias and raised pearly borders.

III. ASSESSMENT

A. **Clinical appearance.**
1. Asymptomatic except possibly pruritic.
2. Lesions mostly occur on exposed surfaces and present as a persistent or recurrent nonhealing sore, scaly spot, or pink/red growth.
3. Variants appear as yellowish-white flat, scar-like patch or plaque-like flat, nonulcerated, flaky erythematous lesion.
4. Some lesions may contain pigment.
5. Deeply invasive tumors may present with paresthesias and/or may be fixed to deep structures such as bone.
6. Recurrent tumors appear as palpable lumps beneath scar or nodular lesions along scar surface.

B. **Diagnosis: by biopsy (either shave, punch, or excisional).**

IV. THERAPEUTIC MODALITIES

A. **Electrosurgery (electrodesiccation and curettage).**
1. Local anesthesia, minimal equipment, quick office procedure.
2. Useful in primary BCCs located on sites over fixed underlying surface such as temple, ear, post-auricular area, chest, and trunk.
3. Site is curetted followed by electrocautery, repeated 2 to 3 times if needed based on physician's clinical judgment.
4. Wounds heal by secondary intention producing flat, depressed scar.
5. Disadvantages include lack of specimen for margin evaluation and possible hypertrophic scar.
6. Advantages include ease of procedure, especially for patients who are poor surgical risk.
7. Contraindicated in patients with demand pacemaker, BCCs 2 cm or larger, recurrent BCC, or an BCC located in high risk location for recurrence. (Discussed later in Mohs' micrographic surgery).
8. Electrodesiccation and curettage offers cure rate of 94.7% to 96.7%.

B. **Carbon dioxide laser (CO_2).**
1. May be used in conjunction with a curette in place of electrocautery.
2. Advantages include minimal nonspecific thermal injury to adjacent cells with more rapid healing and less pain postoperatively.

C. **Surgical excision.**
1. Local anesthesia in office setting.
2. Useful for primary BCC less than 1 cm.
3. Provides specimen for random evaluation of surgical margins.
4. Scars heal quickly as sutured wound resulting in fine-line scar.
5. More time-consuming procedure requiring surgical skill, assistants, and more equipment.
6. Cure rate of 96.8% to 99%.

D. **Cryosurgery.**
1. Local anesthesia in office setting.
2. A noninvasive process by which heat is extracted from tumor cells using liquid nitrogen.
3. Ice crystallization destroys cells potentiated by a rapid freeze and slow thaw cycle.
4. Useful in primary BCC in or around skin with fixed undersurface including areas such as ear, nose, digits.
5. Liquid nitrogen is administered by cone spray apparatus or by use of cryoprobes that conduct cold evenly.

6. Wound requires up to 10 weeks to heal and is edematous, painful, and weepy with blistering and inflammation.
7. Scars may be hypopigmented due to damage to melanocytes.
8. No specimen available for evaluation of margins; skill and judgment of physician of primary importance.
9. Cure rate of 87% to 92.5%.

E. **Radiation therapy.**
   1. Superficial x-ray or high-energy beam; most tumors treated over 5-day period.
   3. Low morbidity, painless with excellent functional result in appropriate lesions.
   2. Useful for BCC on eyelids, periorbital regions, medial triangle of cheek, earlobes, and nose.
   4. Useful for patients who are poor surgical risk.
   5. Contraindicated for lesions on trunk, extremities, dorsum of hands, scalp, or those arising in sweat and sebaceous glands.
   6. Not recommended for morpheaform BCC, large tumors over 8 cm, intra-oral lesions, or those appearing on upper lip/nostril.
   7. May cause radionecrosis over bone.
   8. Radiation therapy is blind method depending on judgment and skill of physician in determining margins of treatment.
   9. Scars become atrophic, erythematous, and irregular over time.
   10. Disadvantages include further aging of skin, radiodermatitis. Recurrences often difficult to detect.
   11. Cure rate of 92.6%.

F. **Mohs' micrographic surgery, named after Frederic Mohs, MD, is defined as excision of skin cancer with histological margin control of deep and peripheral margins.**
   1. Office procedure using local anesthetic.
   2. Indications.
      a. Primary BCC larger than 2 cm.
      b. Morpheaform BCC or tumors with indistinct margins.
      c. Incompletely excised and recurrent BCC.
      d. Certain anatomic areas best treated by the precision of Mohs' surgery include central "H" zone of the face comprising the upper lip, nose, medial canthus, and temple.
   3. Tumor is debulked and a layer of tissue is removed to be processed for margin evaluation in on-site laboratory.
   4. Tissue specimen is marked and color-coded to correspond with a map drawn of the tumor removed.
   5. Specimen pieces are frozen with horizontal processing of the base of the specimen and the epidermal edges.
   6. Surgeon reads slides observing for persistent BCC. If present, another layer or portion of layer is removed from patient.
   7. Reconstruction, if necessary, is performed once margins are free of tumor.
   8. Offers improved cure rates over other methods and conservation of normal tissue due to precise margin control.
   9. Disadvantages include possible lengthy procedures with waiting periods; requires special training of surgeon, assistants, and technicians and specialized equipment.

G. **Other treatment modalities.**
   1. Photodynamic therapy for superficial and nodular BCC, which selectively destroys tumor cells by the administration of a photosensitizing drug that is activated by light creating oxygen products capable of cell destruction.
      a. Beneficial for patients with nevoid basal cell carcinoma syndrome.
   2. Interferon therapy.
      a. Useful for treating primary nodular and superficial BCCs.
      b. Selected tumors are injected with genetically engineered recombinant interferon alfa-2b 3 times a week for 3 weeks resulting in tumor disappearance.

V. **NURSING CONSIDERATIONS/INTERVENTIONS (see Table 1)**

SQUAMOUS CELL CARCINOMA

I. **OVERVIEW**

A tumor of the epidermis that grows by expansion and infiltration of the surrounding skin and structures. Unlike BCC, squamous cell carcinoma (SCC) may metastasize via lymphatic or hematogenous spread.

A. **Definition: a tumor of the keratinizing cells of the epidermis appearing anywhere on the skin and on mucous membranes.**
B. **Etiology.**
   1. Ultraviolet radiation.
   2. Ionizing radiation.
   3. Scar including thermal injury.
   4. Chronic ulcer/sinus and other chronic inflammatory disease such as lupus, hidradenitis, lichen planus, lichen sclerosis, osteomyelitis, etc.
   5. Immunosuppression; prolonged immunosuppression in organ transplant recipients is associated with a dramatically increased risk of SCC.
   6. Genetic determinations (xeroderma pigmentosum, albinism, epidermolysis bullosa).

Table 1.
Nursing Interventions Associated with Tumors of the Skin

Nursing Diagnoses	Outcomes	Interventions
Fear related to diagnosis, treatment and prognosis. Fear of disfigurement, disability, or death.	Patient has up-to-date, adequate information. Patient understands treatment options and recommendations. Recognizes stages of wound healing and measures for optimal scar formation. Patient has opportunity to express fears.	Patient teaching regarding: disease, causes, and interventions. Provide information on disease progression, explanation of tests and procedures to confirm diagnosis and information on treatment recommendations. Talk to patient about "what to expect" regarding surgery and/or treatments. Assist with access to resources regarding disease, treatment, and prevention. Promote family involvement. Participate in multidisciplinary team intervention to provide emotional support, clarification of information, and to identify patient's fears and expectations.
Impaired skin integrity related to presence of lesions. Impaired skin integrity during post-operative healing.	Patient understands principles of skin self-care. Avoidance of infections in surgical wounds, the immunosuppressed, and patients at risk for infections.	Promote barrier function of skin via dressings, topical medications, and emollients. Post-surgical wound management including care of granulating wound, stitches, flaps, and grafts. Identify signs and symptoms of complications including infection.
Psychological impact of disease includes lifestyle changes, time-consuming skin regimens, possibility of incurable disease, fatigue, intensive systemic treatments, and possible financial concerns.	Patient and family receive information and practical interventions for self-care, assistance, and emotional support.	Communicate with and assist in multidisciplinary care including access to nutritionist, social worker, and nurses/physicians in other specialties involved in care of patient. Assist in access to support groups. Teach stress-reduction techniques.

Dermatologic Nursing Essentials: A Core Curriculum 2nd Edition © DNA 2003

Table 1. (continued)
Nursing Interventions Associated with Tumors of the Skin

Nursing Diagnoses	Outcomes	Interventions
Altered body image related to presence of skin lesions and/or post-treatment scars.	Patient will focus on living and quality of life; promote wellness (not necessarily absence of disease) and other positive measures such as adequate nutrition, exercise.	Encouragement, ongoing support and continued teaching on dermatologic interventions for individualized patient needs. Maintain contact and accessibility to patient and family, including surgical patients as they undergo stages of healing that include edema, erythema, scarring, and risk of complications.
Patient is at risk for new, recurrent, or progressive disease.	Patient is empowered to participate in followup care and preventative measures. Patient understands how to identify lesions and/or other symptoms of disease.	Stress importance of followup. Discuss side effects of medications, adequate nutrition, pain, need for on-going lab work (Sezary syndrome). Teach self-skin examination of pigmented and suspicious lesions. Recognize ABCDEs of melanoma identification and other signs of skin cancer. Teach self-lymph node exam. Promote awareness of risk factors of individual diagnosis. Promote activities that lessen risks of UV radiation including use of sunscreens, seeking shade, protective clothing, sun avoidance between 10 am and 4 pm, and avoiding artificial sources of UV light. Target children and parents in teaching photo protection.

a. Mutated *ras* gene is associated with the development of sporadic nonmelanoma skin cancer and the genetic syndrome xeroderma pigmentosum.
7. Human papilloma virus: HPV-16, HPV-18, HPV-31, HPV-5, and HPV-8.
8. Organic hydrocarbons (coal, tar, pitch, crude, paraffin oil, lubricating oil, fuel oil, anthracene oil, and creosote) and inorganic arsenic.
9. PUVA: risk increases with number of treatments, previous exposure of ionizing radiation, and history of prior skin cancers.
10. Precursor lesions include solar keratosis, arsenical keratoses, thermal keratoses, chronic radiation keratoses, tar keratoses, chronic cicatrix keratoses, Bowen's disease, erythroplasia of Queyrat and EV (Lewandowsky-Lutz syndrome).
C. Pathophysiology.

1. Grows by expansion and infiltration as well as by skating and shelving along tissue planes, perichondrium, and/or periosteum.
2. Conduit spread occurs via perineural and perivascular extension.
3. Metastasis is almost exclusively via lymphatics and rarely via blood.
4. Metastasis occurs relatively late and only after the tumor has invaded subcutaneous lymph nodes and lymphatics of the deeper fascial planes and periosteum.
5. Overall metastatic rate is estimated to be 2% to 3% to 10%, depending on tumor location, underlying medical conditions, cell differentiation, and size.
6. The degree of metastatic risk varies according to causative factors, morphologic characteristics, and size and depth of penetration of tumor.
7. Deep SCC, invasive below the dermal sweat glands, large tumors (greater than 3 cm in diameter), anaplastic SCC, and histologically poorly differentiated SCCs have an increased risk of metastases.
8. SCC metastatic rates:
   a. Primary SCC — 0.5%.
   b. Skin with solar keratoses — 2%.
   c. SCC occurring in post-transplant patients — 7%.
   d. Hematogenous to distant organs — 5% to 10%.
   e. Mucocutaneous — 11% to lymph nodes
   f. Within burn scars — 18%.
   g. De novo — 18%.
   h. SCC with previously irradiated site — 20%.
   i. In genital region — 30% to 50% to regional nodes, with distant metastases reported at a rate of 10%.
   j. SCC within lupus — 30%.
   k. Induced by chronic osteomyelitis — 31%.
   l. Verrucous carinoma rarely metastasizes.

D. Incidence
   1. The second most common skin cancer occurs in over 300,000 Americans each year.
   2. Found more frequently in the 6th decade or later, occurs in a male/female ratio of 3:1.

II. VARIANTS

A. **Noninvasive (well-differentiated).**
   1. Arising in sun-damaged skin growing by elevation and diameter of lesions. Margins are often indistinct (see Figure 6-5, page 229).
   2. Verrucous carcinoma (see Figure 6-6, page 229) is a well-differentiated, slow-growing warty lesion appearing in the mouth (oral florid papillomatosis), foot, glans penis as well as arising on the vulva, scrotum, or buttocks.
   3. Bowen's disease (superficial SCC).

   a. Associated with arsenic ingestion.
   b. Exposed and nonexposed sites including mucous membranes of the vulva, vagina, nose, and conjunctiva.
   c. Once Bowen's invades the dermis (5% to 11%) it becomes invasive SCC Bowenoid type.

B. **Invasive (high risk) (poorly differentiated).**
   1. Recurrent tumor.
   2. Tumor invading to a depth at or below reticular dermis.
   3. Greater than 1 to 3 cm in size.
   4. Immunocompromised patient.
   5. Arising in chronic ulcer, sinus, or radiation dermatitis, or burn scar.
   6. Histologically poorly differentiated or anaplastic, spindle cell SCC, or acantholytic.
   7. Arising in certain anatomic sites such as ear, lip, temple, dorsal hand, forehead, preauricular, columella, and nasal vertibule.
   8. Perineural invasion.

III. ASSESSMENT

A. **Expansion of skin at the surface caused by growth of SCC reveals a hyperkeratotic, flesh-colored nodule or plaque, often arising in sun-damaged skin.**
   1. Occurs in sun-exposed and nonexposed skin including mucous membranes of the vulva, vagina, nose, and conjunctiva.
   2. More rapidly growing than BCC, SCCs appear bulkier, often red and raised.
   3. Further invasion reveals a firm, erythematous dome-shaped nodule with a core-like center.

C. **Bowen's disease (superficial SCC).**
   1. Appears as nodular reddish-brown plaque with areas of scales and crusting of varying thickness. Multiple tumors may be present.
   2. Erythroplasia of Querat occurs as a velvety bright red plaque on the penis of uncircumsized males.

D. **Invasive (see Figure 6-7, page 230).**
   1. Ulceration occurs with invasive SCC Bowenoid type (see Figure 6-8, page 230).
   2. Central ulceration that appears early suggests an aggressive variant of SCC.
   3. May be smooth or warty and papillomatous, dull red with telangiectasias.
   4. De novo (occurring on normal skin) appears with slightly raised indurated borders.
   5. Infiltrative lesions may be fixed to undersurfaces or bone.
   6. Paresthesias may be present in tumors with perineural involvement most frequently associated with large tumors.
   7. Lip lesions appear on lower lip 95% of the time as thickened, firm nodular lesions with

destructive ulceration; may appear as small fissure or ulcer within sun-damaged skin.
8. Previously damaged by various hydrocarbons or in chronic ulcers or sinuses caused by burns, syphilis, lupus, etc.; become indurated containing new ulcerations and exhibit increased pain, draining, and bleeding.

E. Laboratory/pathology testing.
1. Diagnosis by biopsy provides diagnosis and histologic staging.
   a. Irregular nests of nonuniform epidermal cells invade the dermis in varying degrees and are termed well, moderately, or poorly differentiated.
   b. Depth of tumor.
   c. Degree of anaplasia (histologically seen as increased numbers of irregularly shaped and sized cells, enlarged nuclei, abnormal mitoses, and loss of intercellular bridges).
2. Sentinel node biopsy when indicated by palpable nodes.
3. MRI, x-ray, and CT scans useful in determining deep invasion.

IV. THERAPEUTIC MODALITIES

A. Local disease.
1. Electrosurgery, cryosurgery, or radiation therapy for small, select primary SCC (cure rate 90% to 95%). Recurrent SCC is best treated by other modalities.
2. Excision of small, noninvasive SCC (90.5% to 95.6% cure rate). Invasive SCC treated with this method has a disappointing cure rate of 50% to 75%.
3. Mohs' micrographic surgery — cure rate for primary non-invasive SCC — 94% to 97%. Cure rate for invasive SCC is 90%, recurrent SCC — 84%.
4. Other treatment modalities and/or research such as:
   a. PDT topical or systemic application of prophyrin derivatives that responds to light irradiation to destroy cancer cells.
   b. Biologic modifiers such as autologous interferon along with applications of imiquimod cream results in eradication of superficial neoplasms.
   c. Investigational trials of liposomal formulation of tyentonuclease for xeroderma pigmentosum patients.
   d. Ongoing research to discover possible human papilloma vaccine.

B. Regional control.
1. Nonpalpable nodes.
   a. Close monitoring for lymphadenopathy.
   b. Sentinel node biopsy for high-risk SCCs, followed by elective lymph node dissection if node is positive, or
   c. Radiation to draining (primary eschalon) nodes for high-risk lesions.
2. Palpable nodes.
   a. Radiation.
   b. Surgery.
   c. Chemotherapy.
   d. Combination of above.

V. NURSING CONSIDERATIONS AND INTERVENTIONS (see Table 1)

MALIGNANT MELANOMA

I. OVERVIEW

An epidermal tumor producing a potentially lethal form of skin cancer that is the leading fatal illness arising in the skin. Melanoma can be successfully cured when detected and adequately treated early. Melanoma may disseminate to any organ, most commonly in skin and subcutaneous tissue, lymph nodes, lungs, liver, brain, bone, and gastrointestinal tract.

A. Definition: a tumor of the melanocytes characterized by uncontrolled growth found on exposed and nonexposed skin surfaces. May arise in pre-existing nevus or de novo (from a new nevus).

B. Etiology.
1. Ultraviolet radiation including history of repeated bursts of sun exposure and blistering sunburn.
   a. Traumatic solar exposure early in life increases risk of melanoma susceptibility.
2. Identification of melanoma susceptibility gene, p16, has clarified the genetics of melanoma.
   a. UV exposure to p16 mutated cells allows uncontrolled proliferation of cells resulting in promotion of cell division of UV damaged melanocytes.
   b. Random mutations at the p16 location are responsible for many sporadic (nonfamilial) cases of melanoma and is present in 40% of familial melanoma patients.
2. Precursor lesions.
   a. Lentigo maligna (occurs most frequently in 5th or 6th decade of life).
   b. Congenital melanocytic nevi.
   c. Dysplastic (atypical) nevi.
   d. Acral and mucosal lentiginous melanocytic proliferation.

C. Pathophysiology: once melanoma breaks through the basement membrane of the epidermis, it has the potential for growth horizontally along the epidermal-dermal junction. This radial growth phase may be followed by a latent phase as the body's immune system restrains the malignant growth.

Table 2.
Risk Factors for Melanoma

Blonde, fair, or red hair with blue eye, light complexion.

Tendency to freckle, sunburn.

Personal history of melanoma.

Family history of melanoma.

Weakened immune system.

Age-risk of melanoma increases with age.

Large numbers of ordinary moles, atypical or congenital nevi; "changing mole."

Ultraviolet radiation, especially intense, intermittent exposure.

Continued growth results in invasion of the dermis, signifying the vertical growth phase. This invasive phase results in thicker lesions often seen clinically as changes in topography of the lesion. The vertical growth phase carries a more guarded prognosis.

D. **Incidence: concurrent with rising incidence, melanoma is being detected earlier resulting in identification of thinner lesions.**
   1. Estimated 53,600 new cases occur annually in United States resulting in approximately 7,800 deaths.
   2. Seventh most common type of cancer (excluding BCC/SCC); most common cancer in women between 25 to 29 years of age.
   3. Projected lifetime risk of 1 in 50 for persons born in year 2010.
   4. Incidence rates are rising more rapidly than any other cancer at 4% per year since 1970.
   5. Affects sexes equally.
      a. Males — back, anterior torso, upper extremity, head and neck
      b. Females — back, lower leg, upper extremity, head, and neck.
   6. Incidence in whites is ten times that of blacks in same geographic locations; less common in Orientals than whites
   7. Incidence varies over 100 fold around the world from a low of 0.2 per 100,000 person-years in parts of Japan to nearly 40 per 100,000 person-years in Queensland, Australia.
   8. A history of BCC/SCCs multiplies risk of melanoma by 17.
   9. Childhood melanoma.
      a. Malignant melanoma is rare in the pediatric population accounting for 13% of all pediatric malignancies and 0.3% to 0.4% of all cases of melanoma.
      b. The prognosis for congenital and infantile melanoma is poor with death occurring in

40% of all cases within 18 months of diagnosis.
      c. A history of severe sunburns in childhood and adolescence doubles the risk for developing melanoma as an adult.

E. **Risk factors (see Table 2).**

II. SUBTYPES

A. **Melanoma in situ (see Figure 6-9, page 230).**
   1. Flat or elevated lesions with histologic features of melanoma but confined to epidermis and adnexal epithelium.
   2. Once totally removed has no impact on patient's longevity.
B. **Lentigo maligna melanoma (see Figure 6-10, page 230) (4% to 15%).**
   1. Occurs on exposed surface of body, often in elderly persons.
   2. Macular lesion may be large (3 to 6 cm or larger) with varied coloration and convoluted borders with prominent notching. Brown lesions may exhibit black flecks.
   3. Regression may appear as blue-grey or white areas.
C. **Superficial spreading (see Figure 6-11, page 230).**
   1. Most common subtype appears on any anatomic surface (70%).
   2. May arise within pre-existing melanocytic nevus.
   3. Slightly raised to elevated lesion usually 2.5 cm or less in size.
   4. Color varies greatly with brown, black, pink, grey, or white areas (possible regression) with irregular borders.
D. **Nodular (15% to 30%) (see Figure 6-12, page 230).**
   1. Elevated throughout, sometimes quite large and polypoid found on any anatomic surface but most commonly on the trunk, head, and neck.
   2. Commonly arises de novo in uninvolved skin, but may arise within a nevus.
   3. Associated with rapid dangerous vertical growth and almost complete lack of radial growth phase.
   4. Lesions may be dark blueberry-like or a uniformly dark, raised lesion. Color may be black, blue, bluish red or amelanotic, often appearing as a polypoid lesion with a stalk.
E. **Acral-Lentigenous (2% to 8%) (see Figure 6-13, page 231).**
   1. Occurs on palms, soles, nailbeds, mucocutaneous or mucosal surfaces most frequently in blacks and Asians (may occur in whites).
   2. Variation of color includes tan, brown to darkly

pigmented lesion, often apparent with papules or nodules.

3. Variant of acral-lentigenous melanoma is subungual melanoma appearing commonly on the great toe or thumb.

   a. Brown to black discoloration beneath the nailbed, usually at proximal location.

F. Amelanotic: commonly nodular in nature, these lack pigment and are often raised and pink.

III. METASTATIC AND RECURRENT MELANOMA

A. Local recurrence is related to tumor thickness and defined as a recurrence in close proximity to the surgical scar or site of primary cutaneous melanoma (3% rate).

B. In-transit metastases/satellites are small cutaneous tumors present in the dermis and subdermal between the primary melanoma site and the draining nodal basin.

1. Lesions occurring within 2 cm of primary tumor are termed satellites whereas in-transit metastases are more than 2 cm from site.

C. Regional lymph mode metastasis.

1. Highly predictive of visceral metastases.
2. Risk varies based on tumor thickness of primary.

D. Distant metastasis is most frequently to nonvisceral sites; skin, subcutaneous tissue and distant lymph nodes (42% to 57%).

1. Lungs — 18% to 36%.
2. Liver — 14% to 20%.
3. Brain — 12% to 20%.
4. Bone — 11% to 17%.
5. Intestines — 1% to 7%.

E. Late recurrences occur 10 or more years after initial diagnosis and treatment (0.93% to 6.7% incidence).

F. Metastatic melanoma in unknown primary occurs in 2% to 6% of all melanoma cases.

   a. Normally, melanoma is detected in lymph nodes in two-thirds of cases.
   b. Five year survival rates in these cases:
      (1) Cutaneous or subcutaneous metastases: 83%.
      (2) In transmit mets: 50%.
      (3) Lymph node metastases: 50%.
      (4) Visceral metastases: median survival 6 months.

IV. ASSESSMENT

Early detection and diagnosis are the most critical factors in overall survival rates.

A. Suspected lesions most commonly include Asymmetry, Border irregularity, Color variation, Diameter greater than 6 mm and Elevation of lesion (change in topography) (ABCDEs of melanoma).

B. The most suspicious sign for melanoma is persistently changing (size, color, elevation, itching) pigmented lesion.

C. Other findings that are suspicious include new pigmented lesions after the age of 30 to 40 and multiple halo nevi in mid to late adult life.

D. Ulceration correlates with tumor thickness and is a significant feature.

E. Physical examination of patient with melanoma should include:

1. History of patient and family, including history of the lesion.
2. Computerized digital imaging to allow retrieval and comparison of previously stored images of new and existing lesions (if available).
3. Meticulous skin examination of entire skin surface including scalp and genitalia.
   a. Suspect pigmented lesions may be evaluated with epiluminescence microscopy (ELM) — a noninvasive test using surface microscope in combination with oil immersion to show patterns that improve clinical diagnosis of melanoma.
   b. Optimal lighting including use of Wood's light.
4. Careful palpation of all lymph nodes with special attention to primary draining nodes.
5. Body systems evaluation especially of brain, bone, gastrointestinal, and constitutional symptoms.

F. Laboratory/histology (AAD guideline of care for primary cutaneous melanoma, 2001).

1. Routine labs and imaging studies are not required in asymptomatic patients with primary melanoma less than 4 mm for initial staging or routine followup. CXR and LDH are optional.
2. Results of routine interval history and exam direct need for laboratory tests and imaging studies.
3. Lymphatic mapping with sentinel lymph node biopsy (SNB) for patients at risk for occult regional lymph node metastases.
   a. Indications for SNB include newly diagnosed primary invasive melanoma with an estimated greater than 5% chance of having identifiable nodal disease with no evidence of existing regional or systemic disease.
   b. Indicated for intermediate thickness or thick melanomas or thin melanomas that have a history of ulceration.
   c. Less morbid procedure to identify occult metastases and is a significant prognostic indicator of risk of recurrence.
4. Biopsy — excisional biopsy with narrow margins is preferred.
   a. Incisional biopsy if necessary.
   b. Repeat biopsy if initial specimen inadequate.

Table 3.
2002 American Joint Committee on Cancer (AJCC)
Melanoma Staging

T Classification	N Classification	M Classification

T1: Tumor 1.0 mm or less
T1a: No ulcer, Clark level II, III
T1b: Ulcer or Clark level IV
 	
T2: Tumor 1.01 to 2.0 mm
T2a: Without ulceration
T2b: With ulceration
 	
T3: Tumor 2.01 to 4.0 mm
T3a: Without ulceration
T3b: With ulceration
 	
T4: Greater than 4 mm
T4a: Without ulceration
T4b: With ulceration
	N1: Metastatic node
	N1a: Micrometastasis
	N1b: Macrometastasis
	
	N2: 2 to 3 metastatic nodes
	N2a: Micrometastasis
	N2b: Macrometastasis
	N2c: In-transit or satellite metastasis
	   with involved nodes
	
	Note: Primary tumor ulceration
	incorporated into State III grouping.
		M1a: Distant skin, subcutaneous or
		   lymph node metastasis
		
		M1b: Lung metastasis
		
		M1c: Metastasis to all other sites or
		   any site with increased LDH.

Balch et al. (2001).

c. Biopsy read by physician experienced in diagnosis of pigmented lesions.
d. Required elements:
   (1) Diagnosis, identifying features.
   (2) Thickness in millimeters (Breslow depth).
   (3) Ulceration.
   (4) Margin involvement.
   (5) Optional, but encouraged include: Clark's level, growth phase, mitotic rate, regression, angiolymphatic invasion, neurotropism, histologic subtype.
5. Immunohistology including S100 protein and HMB-45 used with panel of antibodies against other tumor markers to help diagnose otherwise nonobvious melanoma (if indicated).

IV. STAGING CLASSIFICATION

Summary of American Joint Commission on Cancer (AJCC) staging table: (see Table 3).
A. **2002 AJCC Melanoma Staging Summary.**
1. Clark level is only used for T1 tumors.
2. Thickness cutoffs changed to 1, 2, and 4 mm.
3. Tumors greater than 4 mm staged as Stage II C, previously III A.
4. Ulceration is a modifier on T status.
5. Ulceration of primary tumor is now incorporated into the N positive staging.
6. Satellite and in-transit metastasis is grouped together as N2c or N3.
7. *Number* of involved nodes is primary determinant of N status.

8. Incorporates microscopic LN data from sentinel node biopsy.
9. Metastatic involvement divided based on site and LDH level.
B. **Staging for melanoma.**
1. Stage I and II — localized melanoma.
2. Stage III — regional metastatic melanoma.
3. Stage IV — distant metastatic melanoma.

V. THERAPEUTIC MODALITIES

A. **Melanoma in situ: excision with 0.5 cm margins.**
B. **Melanoma less than 2 mm thick: 1 cm margins.**
C. **Melanoma greater than or equal to 2 mm thick: 2 cm margins.**
D. **Elective regional lymph node dissection (ERLND).**
1. Controversial treatment modality when nodes are not palpable that (some believe) improves survival by removing occult nodal metastases before they spread to distant sites.
2. ERLND is the removal of nodes from the draining site of the primary melanoma when there is no clinical evidence of nodal involvement.
3. Benefit of ERLND is based upon the belief melanoma metastases will most probably spread to the nodes before distant sites.
4. Allows for adequate staging.
5. Randomized prospective trials are ongoing to clarify whether ERLNDs improve survival.
E. **Regional metastasis (regional lymph nodes and in-transit mets.**

1. Therapeutic lymph node dissection.
2. Possible adjuvant therapy.
3. Excision of in-transit mets.
4. Hyperthermic regional limb perfusion.

F. **Adjuvant therapy recommended for post-surgical melanoma patients who are free of disease but at high risk for relapse and to complement surgery in the management of melanoma metastatic to lymph nodes. Randomized trials of adjuvant therapy include:**
    1. Interferon.
    2. Interferon alfa-2b trial and four other interferon trials.
    3. Immunotherapy. The discovery of melanoma-associated antigens as well as antibodies reacting with membrane antigens on melanoma cells spurred the development of several melanoma vaccines.
        a. Immunotherapy with nonspecific agents to potentiate anti-tumor immunity (BCG, Corynebacterium parvum, transfer factor, or immunomodulators (levamisole).
    4. Adjuvant chemotherapy and chemo-immunotherapy.
    5. Isolated limb perfusion.
    6. Adjuvant radiation therapy for postoperative malignant melanoma.
    7. Adjuvant hormonal therapy.
    8. Adjuvant retinoid therapy (vitamin A) has been shown to provide no significant benefit in a recent randominzed trial.

G. **Stage III: therapeutic lymph node dissection is always recommended when clinically suspect nodes are identified (unless uncontrolled distant metastases is apparent).**

H. **Stage IV: promising treatment regimens and ongoing investigational protocols are occurring in multiple centers to identify a cure or to relieve/prevent debilitating symptoms. There is, however, no "cure" for Stage IV melanoma at this time.**
    1. Surgical management of isolated metastases may prolong survival or provide palliative benefit.
    2. Radiation therapy for palliation.
    3. Isolation perfusion and infusion therapy provide maximum effect of chemotherapy in melanoma-involved limb.
        a. For in-transit mets.
        b. Adjuvant therapy for primary melanoma on the limb.
    4. Intralesional injection of Bacillus Calmette-Gueron (BCG) injected in intradermal metastases.
    5. Systemic.
        a. Chemotherapeutic agents as single agent or combination of dacarbazine (DTIC), nitrosureas, temozolomide.

    b. Immunotherapy.
        (1) Trials of interleuken 2 and interferon (highly toxic protocols) ongoing.
        (2) Monoclonal antibodies as direct therapeutic agent for improving host immune response and for diagnostic imaging of metastases.
        (3) Melanoma vaccine to stimulate immune response to melanoma-associated antigens.

VI. FOLLOWUP RECOMMENDATIONS

A. **Follow up 1 to 4 times per year, for 2 years, depending on the thickness of the primary lesion and other risk factors, then 1 to 2 times per year thereafter.**
    1. Considerations on an individual basis include tumor thickness, history of multiple melanomas, presence of atypical nevi, family history of melanoma, patient axiety and patient ability to recognize signs and symptoms of disease.
    2. Patient education regarding self-skin examination including lymph nodes. (Strong evidence suggests the majority of metastases and recurrences are discovered by the patient or a family member.

VII. NURSING CONSIDERATIONS/INTERVENTIONS (see Table 1)

KERATOACANTHOMA (KA)

I. OVERVIEW

A common benign, self-healing lesion with rapid growth and histologic pattern resembling SCC that only rarely progresses into an aggressive SCC.
A. **Defnition: compact tumor comprising well-differentiated squamous epithelium. Unlike SCC, KA show little pleomorphism or anaplasia.**
B. **Etiology (origin of KA is uncertain).**
    1. Ultraviolet light.
    2. Chemical carcinogens.
        a. Contact with pitch and tar in industrial workers.
        b. Higher incidence in smokers than in nonsmokers.
    3. Mechanical trauma in skin rendered susceptible to tumor formation by genetic or actinic/chemical carcinogen factors.
    4. Secondary to other skin lesions such as eczema, seborrheic dermatitis, psoriasis.
    5. Genetic determinations in certain types of multiple keratoacanthomas.
C. **Pathophysiology.**
    1. Probable derivation from hair follicles with

hyperplasia of epithelium causing cystic hair follicles and irregular growth in basal layer.
2. Grows rapidly, usually attaining size of 10 to 25 mm in 6 weeks followed by slow involution over 2 to 6 months (possibly as long as 12 months).
3. Arises from the superficial part of the hair follicle, or more deeply situated KA, arising from the hair germ, or from the hair germ at each hair growth cycle.
   a. Static phase — few or no mitoses are seen and few new epithelial cells are formed.
      (1) Keratinous plug detaches to form saucer or cup-shaped lesion that eventually regresses leaving a puckered scar.
      (2) May form keratinous horn prior to regression.
      (3) Ulceration and exfoliation may produce flat papillomatous lesion.
   b. Regression — lesion shrinks upward and lies close to skin surface.
4. Mucosal KA develops from ectopic sebaceous glands.
D. Incidence.
   1. True accurate information on incidence is not available.
   2. Occurs twice as frequently in men as in women; rare under the age of 20.
   3. Rare in blacks and colored races.
   4. Seen on skin of face and hands more frequently than on unexposed skin.

II. TYPES OF KA

A. Common solitary KA (see Figure 6-14, page 231).
   1. Grows rapidly, up to 2.5 cm in 6 weeks.
   2. Involution occurs over period of 2 to 6 months.
   3. Following regression, a puckered or pitted scar may remain.
B. Multiple KA may be apparent.

III. ASSESSMENT

A. Clinical appearance.
   1. Occurs on exposed hairy site often in actinically damaged skin.
   2. Lesion may also present on mucosal membranes including hard palate, lips, bulbar conjunctiva, nasal mucosa, and genitalia.
   3. Clinical growth phase.
      a. Proliferative phase seen as firm, smooth, enlarging papule; flesh-colored with erythema; may have translucency and telangiectasias.
      b. Mature phase contains central keratinous core, as lesion expands plug is dislodged leaving crater-like nonulcerative center.
B. Laboratory/histology — biopsy to establish diagnosis and rule out SCC.

IV. TREATMENT MODALITIES

Although lesions spontaneously regress, treatment provides hastened cure, prevents rapid enlargement, and improves overall cosmetic results.
A. Conservative excision.
B. Mohs' micrographic surgery for recurrent or aggressive lesions.
C. Electrodesiccation and curettage.
D. Radiotherapy.
E. Cryosurgery for small early KA.
F. Intralesional injection of 5-fluorouracil weekly.
G. Systemic methotrexate for multiple KAs and the larger, more aggressive KAs.

V. NURSING CONSIDERATIONS/INTERVENTIONS (see Table 1)

CUTANEOUS T-CELL LYMPHOMA

I. OVERVIEW

A cutaneous T cell lymphoma (CTCL) also known as mycosis fungoides (MF) consists of malignant cells that resemble mature T cells. The cell of origin is white blood cells (circulating lymphocytes) with a predisposition to the skin and immune surveillance. The disease has a long natural history that, after a variable amount of time, progresses to involve lymph nodes, peripheral blood, visceral organs, and frequently results in death.
A. Definition: a rare malignancy that originates in the reticulo-endothelial cells of the skin characterized by remission and exacerbation of skin diseases. CTCL constitutes a spectrum of diseases which include mycosis fungoides, Sézary syndrome, and other lymphoreticular neoplasms.
B. Etiology.
   1. Viral — human T-cell leukemia/lymphoma virus (HTLV 28), an exogenous RNA retrovirus.
   2. Genetic factor.
      a. Observation of 4% occurrence in first-degree relatives.
      b. Certain histocompatibility antigens are found with increased frequency in CTCL.
   3. Development from other dermatoses as many patients have a preceding eruption of variable duration.
   4. Environmental factors in susceptible host (retrospective studies).
      a. Chemicals (air pollutants, pesticides, solvents and vapors, detergents, disinfectants).
      b. Drugs (tobacco, analgesics, tranquilizers, thiazides).
      c. Occupational exposure (manufacturing

especially in petrochemical, textile, metal, and machinery industries).

C. **Pathophysiology.**
   1. Disruption of T-cell regulation results in T cell cycling and division without the usual "elimination" of immune reactive cells.
   2. Early CTCL malignant cells are small lymphocytes that progress to large tumor cells which are identifiably different from the nonmalignant counterparts.
   3. Initially invades the skin; eventually there is dissemination to lymph nodes, peripheral blood, and/or visceral organs.
   4. Early lesions are often infiltrated with CD8+ cytotoxic T lymphocytes, most likely indicating a mediating anti-tumor response.
      a. Loss of normal immunity with advancing disease compromises antitumor response.

D. **Incidence.**
   1. In United States there are 40,000 to 50,000 individuals affected with CTCL.
   2. 800 to 1,000 new cases occur annually with perhaps 200 deaths per year due to vital organ involvement.
   3. Incidence of CTCL is equal to that of Hodgkin's disease.
   4. Seen in both sexes (more frequently in males) and all races (more commonly in blacks).
   5. Could occur in late teens but more commonly occurs in middle age and later decades of life.

II. CLINICAL STAGES

A. **Patch phase.**
   1. Clinically found in skin initially appearing as single or multiple erythematous scaly macules and patches that are well-defined and vary in size.
   2. Eruption may be asymptomatic although most eruptions are pruritic.
   3. May be transitory, spontaneously disappearing without scarring.
   4. Phase may last months or years; diagnosis at this stage is often difficult.

B. **Plaque phase.**
   1. Plaques may occur from patch-stage lesions or arise de novo.
   2. Lesions may spontaneously regress or may form large plaques.
   3. As cells proliferate, lesions become firm and the plaque varies in surface contour.

C. **Tumor phase.**
   1. May occur in CTCL plaques or de novo.
   2. Tumor cells behave in a more biologically malignant manner with vertical spread into the reticular dermis and subcutaneous tissue.
   3. In addition to cutaneous involvement, disease will invade lymph nodes, liver, and spleen.

There may be involvement of the respiratory system, bone, as well as heart, gastrointestinal tract, kidney (rarely), brain, and peripheral nervous system.

III. ASSESSMENT

A. **Clinical appearance (history and physical exam).**
   1. Patch phase (see Figure 6-15, page 231).
      a. Single or multiple macules or papules that usually present on unexposed sites as erythematous rash.
      b. Size varies, well-defined lesions are orange to dusky violet-red.
      c. May be persistently pruritic.
      d. Classic distribution is buttocks, groin, underneath breasts and axilla.
   2. Plaque phase (see Figure 6-16, page 231).
      a. May present before, simultaneously, or after patch phase and is infiltrative.
      b. Lesions are well-defined, scaly, elevated, and irregularly shaped occurring on any body surface.
      c. Eruptions are dusky red and may appear shiny with wart-like infiltrates; a reddish-blue halo may be observed outside areas of infiltration.
      d. Lesions in this stage may spontaneously disappear or may coalesce and ulcerate.
      e. Scaly scalp and hair loss and thickened, discolored nails are associated symptoms.
      f. May be diagnosed as eczema or psoriasis at this stage.
      g. Erythroderma may be present.
         (1) Patient will be unable to maintain body temperature, suffer weight loss, insomnia, malaise.
         (2) Vasodilation and exfoliations will cause loss of protein, iron, and electrolytes.
         (3) Hyperkeratosis and scaling is present (fissuring of palms and soles).
   3. Tumor phase (T cells lose their affinity for the skin).
      a. Tumors gradually appear in infiltrative lesions often at the border; may shrink and disappear leaving a pigmented atrophic scar.
      b. Lesions appear as dull reddish-brown or purplish red with smooth surface; softly palpable nodular lesions that rapidly grow in size and number.
      c. May be excoriated secondary to pruritus and infection.
      d. Appears on face, back, and body folds.
      e. Absence of pruritus, extremely painful if ulcerated.
   4. Sézary syndrome ("red man disease").
      a. Term relates to generalized exfoliating

erythrodermic CTCL patients with leukocytes and peripheral blood appearance of "monster" cells.

    b. Intensely pruritic with lymphadenopathy starting either de novo, following pre-malignant eruption or after established plaque stage of the disease.

5. Widespread CTCL invasion is evidenced by palpable lymph nodes, bone marrow involvement in advanced stages, pulmonary involvement, and osteolytic lesions in the bone with pathologic fractures.

6. Complications of CTCL and cause of death include viral, fungal, and bacterial infections, immunosuppression and vital organ involvement.

B. **Laboratory/histology.**
1. Skin biopsy.
    a. Diagnosis of CTCL is made on light microscopic examination of hematoxylin and eosin-stained sections.
    b. Multiple punch biopsies at 3-month intervals if diagnosis is nonspecific.
2. CBC with determination of absolute lymphocytes count, serum chemistries (including liver and renal function tests), uric acid, LDH and quantitative immunoglobulins.
3. Most sensitive test is Southern Blot test for T-cell antigen receptor rearrangements in peripheral blood (T-cell receptor gene rearrangement test).
    a. Laborious and expensive.
    b. Tests detect tumor cells down to levels of 1% to 5% of lymphocyte population.
4. Depending on extent of disease, Sézary count, CT scans, lymph node or bone marrow biopsy or as suggested by history or physical examination.
5. In vivo and in vitro response to cell incompetence.

IV. TREATMENT MODALITIES

A. **Skin-directed therapy.**
1. Phototherapy with UVB.
2. Topical nitrogen mustard (HN2).
3. Photochemotherapy (PUVA).
4. Electron-beam therapy (limited penetration of electrons spares mucous membranes, bone marrow, gastrointestinal tract, and other vital internal organs).
    a. Whole body electron beam irradiation results in 85% complete remission rates with medial survival time of 9 years.
5. Surgical removal of solitary nodule or plaque confined to the skin.
6. Topical or intralesional steroids to control symptoms.

B. **Chronic disease (with nodal involvement).**
1. As above.
2. Total skin electron beam therapy followed by topical HN2, PUVA, or photopheresis to maintain remission.
3. If necessary, systemic drug such as interferon-α, retinoids, or chemotherapeutic agent such as methotrexate.

C. **Post remission maintenance includes topical corticosteroids, nitrogen mustard, interferon (alpha), and phototherapy.**

D. **Tumors.**
1. No nodal involvement — as above.
2. Histologic nodal involvement.
    a. Individualized palliative treatment.
    b. Local radiations to local symptomatic disease.
    c. Photopheresis.
    d. Retinoids/experimental protocols.

E. **Visceral involvement/Sezary syndrome.**
1. Individualized palliative treatment.
2. Systemic chemotherapy (fludarabine, 2-CDA, chlorambucil, pentostatin).
3. Extracorporal photopheresis (palliative treatment) whereby leukocytes are selectively removed from peripheral blood by extracorporeal centrifugation technique, exposed to UVA light, and reinfused into the patient.
    a. Causes selective destruction of cancerous cells in the blood.
    b. Has been the only single treatment that has been shown to improve survival in patients with Sezary syndrome.
4. Immune boosters such as interferon, interleukin 2, monoclonal antibodies.
5. Bone marrow transplant, currently limited by graft vs. host disease, offers greatest potential for disease cure.
6. Combinations of skin-directed therapies and biological response modifiers to improve response rates.
7. Recent developments in CTCL therapy include:
    a. Targretin® (bexarotene) — a retinoid X receptor-selective retinoid for all stages CTCL and topical gel formation for the treatment of localized lesions.
    b. Ontak® (denileulkin diftitox) fusion toxin proteins selective for specific T cells, targets malignant T-cell clones.
    c. Systemic chemotherapy development including pegylated liposomal doxrubicin, gencitabine, pentostatin appear to have greatest potential.

V. NURSING CONSIDERATIONS (see Table 1)

KAPOSI'S SARCOMA

I. OVERVIEW

First described by Kaposi as idiopathic multiple pigment sarcoma, this multifocal neoplasm is seen primarily as multiple vascular nodules in the skin and other organs. Kaposi's sarcoma (KS) is associated with other neoplasms or immune disorders that occur before or after the diagnosis. Kaposi's is seen frequently in patients with HIV.

A. Definition: arises in the endothelial cell and produces tumors that appear in a multicentric fashion.

B. Etiology, cause may be multifactorial.
   1. Viral.
      a. New human herpesvirus (HHV-8/KS) and subsequent identification of humoral immune response to this agent in patients with KS may be causally related to KS.
      b. Causative agents of KS associated with disease among young homosexual men with signs of profound immunosuppression include HIV and other specific serologic association between cytomegalovirus (CMV) and classic endemic KS.
      c. Other causative agents of KS may include various micro-organisms such as hepatitis B virus, human papilloma virus (HPV), and *Mycoplasma penetrans* as possible sources of KS.
      d. With the replication of retroviral particles in KS lesions, some hypothesize a non-HIV retrovirus etiological linkage to KS.
   2. Genetic predisposition.
   3. Geographic factors.
   4. Possible hormonal influences.

C. Pathophysiology.
   1. Classic KS develops slowly and runs a benign course although, infrequently, rapid courses with involvement of lung, spleen, heart, and gastrointestinal tract have been reported.
   2. In addition to cutaneous lesions, may develop on mucous membranes of the oral cavity and gastrointestinal tract.

D. Incidence.
   1. Incidence of KS varies according to geography.
      a. Annual incidence in United States of classic KS is 0.02% to 0.06% of all malignant tumors.
      b. Mostly affects people of either Jewish descent and/or of Mediterranean descent.
      c. Male-female ratio is 1:1 or 3:1 in recent literature.
      d. In classic KS, two-thirds of patients develop lesions only after the age of 50.
      e. Disease is strikingly frequent in a region in Africa that includes Kenya, Tanzania, and Zaire with a frequency of 1.3% to 10% depending on region.
      f. In Africa, is more prevalent in males, 3:1 in children, 10:1, 18:1 in adults with a mean time of onset of 48 years for males (36 years for females).
      g. Among people with acquired immunodeficiency syndrome (AIDS), KS predominates in the 3rd and 4th decade with a mean age of 40 years.

II. CLASSIFICATION OF KS

A. Classic KS.
   1. Chronic skin disease affecting predominantly elderly men of Mediterranean, East European, or Jewish heritage with a peak incidence in men after the age of 60. Lesions often appear on the legs.
   2. Affected individuals survive an average of 10 to 15 years from diagnosis and most often die from an unrelated cause.

B. African or endemic KS.
   1. Found in eastern half of African continent near the equator.
   2. Described in two distinct age groups.
      a. Young adults with a mean age of 35 and a male/female ratio of 13:1.
      b. Young children with a mean age of 3 and a male/female ratio of 3:1.

C. Iatrogenic, immunosuppressive, drug-associated KS.
   1. Found in organ transplant patients, particularly renal transplants.
   2. Seen in patients receiving chronic immunosuppressive drug therapy. Spontaneous remission after discontinuation of immunosuppressive therapy usually occurs.

D. AIDS-associated, epidemic KS.
   1. KS is often the primary AIDS-defining illness.
   2. Sexually transmitted co-factor may play a role in the development of AIDS-KS.
   3. Incidence of AIDS-KS continues to rise as more HIV-infected patients progress to AIDS.
   4. Lesions may occur, not only on the skin, but on the mucocutaneous regions, lymph system, and viscera.

III. ASSESSMENT

A. Clinical appearance evolving through stages of macules, papules/plaques and nodules/tumors.
   1. Classic KS (see Figure 6-17, page 231).
      a. Lesions occur most commonly on lower limbs, then upper limbs and may occur on the trunk, head, neck, genitalia, or any skin surface.
      b. Classic KS appears as red or purple multiple dermal plaques, nodules, and tumors in

light-skinned people; a blue hue in dark-skinned individuals.

c. As lesions age, they become brownish in color.

d. Telangiectasias may be evident on or near the tumors, ulceration may occur or the surface may appear verrucous.

e. Lesions may be painful; burning or itching may also be present.

f. Lesions may spontaneously regress as new ones appear; spontaneous remissions have been documented.

g. Early lesions are small papules, as they grow they feel spongy and may grow up to 10 cm or more in diameter.

h. Occurrence may be in the hundreds in a single patient; nodules may cluster along veins.

2. African-endemic KS.

a. Most commonly nodular that may regress spontaneously.

b. Florid variety is rapid growing, ulcerated, and may bleed with tumors extending deep into dermis and may involve underlying bone.

c. Infiltrative type are confined to hand or foot appearing as deeply invasive, fibrotic, indurated tumors with nonpitting edema.

d. Rapidly growing enlarged lymph nodes, often confused clinically with lymphoma, typify lymphadenopathic type of KS occurring in children and young adults.

3. AIDS-KS (see Figure 6-18, page 231).

a. Lesions occur in the oral cavity, nose, post-auricular, trunk, penis, legs, and feet appearing as small pink macules mimicking insect bites, or small brown, tense papules.

b. Examination should include lymph node exam.

c. Macular lesions begin as salmon-colored with a pink halo.

(1) Small, slightly elevated, and round.

(2) Macule becomes purple or brown within a week and halo disappears.

(3) Multiple lesions widely distributed; may demonstrate a mirror-image distribution.

d. Papular and nodular lesions.

(1) May begin as macules.

(2) Facial papules are round and less than 1 cm in size; lesions of trunk, neck, and extremities are 1 to 2 cm and oblong.

e. Plaques and lymphatic disease.

(1) Large purple plaques containing nodules with hyperkeratosis; resemble psoriasis.

(2) Lymphatic involvement may produce numerous firm, red, round papules with local edema in affected nodal sites.

f. Mucocutaneous and ocular lesions.

(1) Oral involvement most commonly seen as lesions on the palate.

(2) Macular lesions of the conjunctiva are relatively benign.

g. Visceral lesions may affect gastrointestinal tract and lungs as well as the pharynx, heart, bone marrow, urogenital tract, brain, kidney, and adrenal glands.

B. Histology.

1. While clinical diagnosis may appear obvious, diagnosis must be histologically confirmed.

2. Biopsy of firm papule or nodule that has been present for several weeks to months is preferred.

IV. THERAPEUTIC MODALITIES

A. At present there is no treatment modality that will cure KS.

B. Local therapy.

1. Excision of cutaneous lesions (often for cosmesis).

2. Radiation therapy.

3. Chemotherapy either single or multi-agent. Most promising results in use of liposomal encapsulated doxorubicin and daunorubicin for both AIDs-associated KS and classic KS.

4. Systemic treatment of interferon alpha, alone or in combination with cytotoxic therapy, or with zidovudine for AIDS-KS.

V. NURSING INTERVENTIONS (see Table 1)

Bibliography

American Cancer Society. (2002). *Cancer facts and figures.* Atlanta, GA: American Cancer Society.

Apisarnthanarax, J., Talpur, R., & Duvic, M. (2002). Treatment of cutaneous T cell lymphoma: Current status and future directions (Review). *American Journal of Clinical Dermatology, 3*(3), 193-215.

Balch, C.M., Ross, M., Buzaid, A.C., Soong, S.J., Atkins, M.B., Cascinelli, N., Coit, D.G., Flemming, D., Gershenwald, J.E., Houghton, A., Kirkwood, J.M., McMasters, K.M., Mihm, M.F., Morton, D.L., Reintgen, D.S., Sober, A., Thompson, J.A., & Thompson, J.F. (2001). Final version of the American joint committee on cancer staging system for cutaneous melanoma. *Journal of Clinical Oncology, 19*(16), 3635-3648.

Berg, D., & Otley, C.C. (2002). Skin cancer in organ transplant recipients: Epidemiology, pathogenesis and management. *Journal of the American Academy of Dermatology, 47*(1), 1-17.

Bouwhuis, S., & Davis, M.D. (2001, June). Sezary syndrome: A summary. *Dermatology Nursing, 13*(3), 205-209.

Ghadially, R., & Ghadially, F.N. (2002). Keratoacanthoma. In T.B. Fitzpatrick, A.Z. Eisen, K. Wolff, I.M. Freedberg, K.F. Austen, L.A. Goldsmith, & S.L. Katz (Eds), *Dermatology in general medicine* (5th ed.) (pp. 865- 871). New York: McGraw-Hill.

Grekin, R.C., Samlaska, C.P., & Van-Christian, K. (2000). Epidermal nevi, neoplasms and cysts. In R.B. Odom, W.D. James, & T.G. Berger (Eds.), *Andrew's diseases of the skin clinical dermatology* (9th ed.) (pp. 820-825, 1082-1087) Philadelphia: WB Saunders Co.

Guill, C.K., & Orengo, I. (2001, June). Cutaneous malignant melanoma. *Dermatology Nursing, 13*(3), 210-213.

Heald, P.W. (2002). Identifying and treating T-cell lymphoma. *Skin Cancer Foundation Journal, Vol XIX,* 39-40.

Heald, P.W., & Edelson, R.L. (1999). Cutaneous T cell lymphomas. In T.B. Fitzpatrick, A.Z. Eisen, K. Wolff, I.M. Freedberg, K.F. Austen, L.A. Goldsmith, & S.L. Katz (Eds), *Dermatology in general medicine* (5th ed.) (pp. 1227-1250) New York: McGraw-Hill.

Lange, J.R. (2000). The current status of sentinel node biopsy in the management of melanoma. *Dermatologic Surgery, 26*(8), 809-810.

Langley, R.C. et al. (1999). Neoplasms: Cutaneous melanoma. In T.B. Fitzpatrick, A.Z. Eisen, K. Wolff, I.M. Freedberg, K.F. Austen, L.A. Goldsmith, & S.L. Katz (Eds), *Dermatology in general medicine* (5th ed.) (pp. 1080-1116) New York: McGraw-Hill.

Liskay, A., & Nicol, N.H. (1998). Anatomy and physiology of the skin. In M.J. Hill (Ed), *Dermatology nursing essentials: A core curriculum* (pp. 3-13), Pitman, NJ: Dermatology Nurses' Association.

Musse, L. (2002, February). Cutaneous T-cell lymphoma. *Dermatology Nursing, 14*(1), 55.

Petter, G., & Haustein, U.F. (2000). Histologic subtyping and malignancy assessment of cutaneous squamous cell carcinoma. *Dermatologic Surgergy, 26*(6), 521-529.

Piepkorn, M. (2001). A new look at genetics breakthrough in melanoma. *Skin Cancer Foundation Journal, Vol. XIX,* 46-47.

Rigel, D.S. (2001). Melanoma update—2001. *Skin Cancer Foundation Journal, Vol XIX,* 13-l4.

Schmid-Wnedtner, M.H., Volkenandt, M., Plewig, G., Berking, C., Baumert, J., Schmidt, M., & Sander, C.A. (2002). Cutaneous melanoma in childhood and adolescence: An analysis of 36 patients. *Journal of the American Academy Dermatology, 46*(6), 874-879.

Schwartz, R.A., & Stoll, H.L. (1999). Squamous cell carcinoma. In T.B. Fitzpatrick, A.Z. Eisen, K. Wolff, I.M. Freedberg, K.F. Austen, L.A. Goldsmith, & S.L. Katz (Eds.), *Dermatology in general medicine* (5th ed.) (pp. 840-850). New York: McGraw-Hill.

Rappersberger, K., Stingl, G., & Wolff, K. (1999). Kaposi's sarcoma. In T.B. Fitzpatrick, A.Z. Eisen, K. Wolff, I.M. Freedberg, K.F. Austen, L.A. Goldsmith, & S.L. Katz (Eds.), *Dermatology in general medicine* (5th ed.) (pp. 1195-1203). New York: McGraw-Hill.

Sober, A.J., Chuang, T.Y., Duvic, M., Farmer, E.R., Grichnik, J.M, Halpern, A.C., Ho, V., Holloway, V., Hood, A.F., Johnson, T.M., & Lowery, B.J. (2001). Guidelines of care for primary cutaneous melanoma. *Journal of the American Academy of Dermatology, 45*(4), 579-586.

Swanson, N.A., & Johnson, T.M. (1998). Management of basal and squamous cell carcinoma. In C.W. Cummings, J.M. Fredrickson, C.J. Krause, L.A. Harker, & D.E. Schuller (Eds.), *Otolaryngology head and neck surgery* (3rd ed.). St. Louis: Mosby.

Vargo, N.L. (2003). Basal cell and squamous cell carcinoma. *Seminars in Oncology Nursing, 19*(1), 12-21.

1. The basement layer between the epidermis and dermis is lined by:
   a. An orderly row of melanocytes.
   b. Basal cells.
   c. A fibrous, protective sheath.
   d. Squamous cells.

2. The most important environmental carcinogen is:
   a. Coal tar.
   b. Arsenic.
   c. Ultraviolet radiation.
   d. Ionizing radiation.

3. Inherited mutated tumor suppressor gene responsible for xeroderma pigmentosum is:
   a. PTCH gene.
   b. Ras gene.
   c. P-16.
   d. P-53.

4. Indentifcation of the "melanoma" susceptibility gene has:
   a. Led to recent advances in a cure for melanoma.
   b. Clarified the genetics of melanoma.
   c. Resulted in identification of increased infantile melanoma.
   d. Been found in 80% familial patients.

5. Melanoma growth and spread includes all *except*:
   a. Blatant growth phase.
   b. Horizontal growth phase.
   c. Vertical growth phase.
   d. Hematogenous spread.

6. American Joint Commission on Cancer (AJCC) staging:
   a. Cuts tumor thickness categories at 1, 2, and 4 mm.
   b. Determines ulceration to be an unremarkable factor.
   c. Recommends full profile liver function studies at regular intevals.
   d. Separates in transit mets from satellite lesions in staging.

7. Elective lymph node dissection refers to
   a. A sentinel node biopsy.
   b. Removal of clinically suspicious lymph nodes.
   c. Removal of nodes with no evidence of clinical evidence of nodal involvement.
   d. Treatment of choice for invasive squamous cell carcinoma.

8. Mohs' micrographic surgery is indicated for:
   a. All primary squamous cell carcinoma.
   b. Initial treatment for Kaposi's sarcoma.
   c. Sclerotic basal cell carcinoma.
   d. Tumor phase CTCL.

9. Keratoacanthoma is a variant of anaplastic squamous cell carcinoma.
   a. True
   b. False

10. Assessment of infiltrative squamous cell carcinoma includes:
    a. Dome-shaped lesion with central ulceration.
    b. Pearly lesion with raised borders with telangiectasias on the surface.
    c. Scaly irregular, raised red patches occurring in actinically-damaged skin.
    d. Vague, yellowish, scar-like plaque with indistinct margins.

11. Melanoma 2.1 cm thick by Breslow level should be excised with a margin of:
    a. 0.5 cm.
    b. 1.0 cm.
    c. 1.5 cm.
    d. 2.0 cm.

Answers to Study Questions

1.	b	5.	a	9.	b
2.	c	6.	a	10.	a
3.	b	7.	c	11.	d
4.	b	8.	c		

CE Answer/Evaluation Form

Chapter 6.
Cutaneous Malignancies

Please photocopy this test page and return.

COMPLETE THE FOLLOWING:

Name: _____

Address: _____

City: _____ State: _____ Zip: _____

Preferred telephone: (Home)_____ (Work) _____

State where licensed and license number: _____

CE application fee: DNA member $15.00
                     Nonmember $20.00

POSTTEST INSTRUCTIONS
1. To receive continuing education credit for individual study after reading the article, complete the answer/evaluation form below.
2. Photocopy and send the answer/evaluation form along with a check or money order payable to **Dermatology Nurses' Association** to: **DNA**, East Holly Avenue Box 56, Pitman, NJ 08071-0056.
3. Test returns must be postmarked by December 31, 2008. Upon completion of the answer/evaluation form, a certificate for 4.3 contact hour(s) will be awarded and sent to you.

This chapter was reviewed and formatted for contact hour credit by Marcia J. Hill, MSN, RN, Core Curriculum Editor; and Sally Russell, MN, RN,C, DNA Education Director.

ANSWER FORM

1. Name one new detail (item, issue, or phenomenon) that you learned by completing this activity.

_____

_____

_____

_____

2. How will you apply the information from this learning activity to your practice?
   a. Patient education.
   b. Staff education.
   c. Improve my patient care.
   d. In my education course work.
   e. Other: Please describe _____

_____

_____

	Strongly disagree				Strongly agree
Evaluation					
3. The offering met the stated objectives.					
a. Identify and differentiate the growth patterns of common skin malignancies.	1	2	3	4	5
b. Describe the risk factors and incidence of skin cancers.	1	2	3	4	5
c. Identify the relationship of UV irradiation and genetic mutations.	1	2	3	4	5
d. Describe the clinical appearance of skin cancers and certain precursors.	1	2	3	4	5
e. Discuss the various treatment options available for patients diagnosed with skin cancer based on clinical and histologic assessment.	1	2	3	4	5
4. The content was current and relevant.	1	2	3	4	5
5. The content was presented clearly.	1	2	3	4	5
6. The content was covered adequately.	1	2	3	4	5
7. I am more confident of my abilities since completing this material.	1	2	3	4	5

8. The material was (check one) ☐ new, ☐ review for me.

Comments _____

_____

9. Time required to complete reading assignment: _____ minutes

This independent study is provided by the Dermatology Nurses' Association (DNA) for 4.3 contact hours. DNA is accredited as a provider of continuing education in nursing by the American Nurses Credentialing Center's Commission on Accreditation. DNA is approved as a provider of continuing education by the California Board of Registered Nursing Provider #CEP5708.

Dermatologic Nursing Essentials: A Core Curriculum 2nd Edition © DNA 2003

Benign Neoplasms/Hyperplasia

Bonita Drones, MSN, RN, C, CS

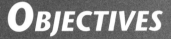

OBJECTIVES

At the end of this chapter, the reader will be able to:
- Define benign neoplasms/hyperplasia.
- Describe the signs and symptoms of benign neoplasms/hyperplasia.
- Understand the various treatment options available to the patient with benign neoplasms/hyperplasia.

KEY POINTS

- Benign neoplasms are noncancerous skin lesions or tumors.
- Benign neoplasms are common skin growths.
- Benign neoplasms have no malignant potential.
- Some benign neoplasms require treatment for cosmetic purposes only.

Benign Neoplasms/Hyperplasia

Bonita Drones, MSN, RN, C, CS

ACROCHORDONS (SKIN TAGS, PAPILLOMAS, CUTANEOUS TAGS, SOFT FIBROMAS)

I. OVERVIEW

Acrochordons are benign neoplasms. Acrochordons are cosmetic disorders (see Figure 7-1, page 232).

A. Definition: acrochordons are soft pedunculate, flesh-colored, tan, brown, or pigmented growths, commonly on the neck, shoulders, axillae, groin, inguinal folds, eyelids, upper chest, and trunk. These lesions are asymptomatic but may become irritated or inflamed if exposed to repeated trauma from jewelry or clothing.

B. Etiology is unknown.

C. Pathophysiology.
   1. Out-pouch at the skin's surface with connective tissue and dilated capillaries covered by normal epidermis.
   2. Varies in size from one to five millimeters.
   3. Single or multiple lesions.

D. Incidence.
   1. Increases during middle age and older adulthood, pregnancy, acromegaly, menopause, and family history.
   2. Equal in males and females.
   3. Associated with obesity and hyperhidroses.
   4. Frequently higher in diabetics.

II. ASSESSMENT

A. History and current health status.

B. Diagnosis by clinical presentation: location, number, size, irritation, tenderness, and inflammation.

C. Biopsy recommended if pigmented or erythematous.

III. COMMON THERAPEUTIC MODALITIES

A. Electrodesiccation.

B. Scalpel or simple scissor excision at the lesion's base.

C. Cryosurgery.

IV. COMMON NURSING DIAGNOSES, OUTCOMES, INTERVENTIONS

A. Common nursing diagnoses.
   1. Body image disturbance related to aesthetics.
   2. Impaired skin integrity related to lesions.
   3. Pain related to trauma and lesions.
   4. Risk of infection related to impaired integument.

B. Outcomes.
   1. Patient exhibits improved positive body image.
   2. Skin integrity improved or maintained.
   3. Pain relieved; need for analgesics decreased.
   4. Free from infection.

C. Interventions.
   1. Patient education.
      a. Potential irritation from jewelry and clothing or friction of body parts.

V. HOME CARE CONSIDERATIONS

A. Wound care (see Table 1).

B. Control bleeding.

C. Watch for signs of infection.

CALLUSES

I. OVERVIEW

A. Definition: a callus is an elevated superficial, hyperkeratotic area. Nontender, but pressure may produce dull pain (see Figures 7-2a to 2c, page 232).

B. Etiology.
   1. Repeated friction or pressure.

C. Pathophysiology.
   1. Reaction of the epidermis to increased cellular division, hyperkeratosis, causing the stratum corneum to thicken.

D. Incidence.
   1. Frequently on palms and weight-bearing surfaces of the foot.

II. ASSESSMENT

A. Physical examination.

B. History of chronic pressure or friction.

III. COMMON THERAPEUTIC MODALITIES

A. Topical keratolytics (40% salicylic acid plaster or ointment).

B. Orthopedic shoes, braces, and support devices to redistribute weight.

IV. COMMON NURSING DIAGNOSES, OUTCOMES, INTERVENTIONS

A. Common nursing diagnoses.
   1. Impaired skin integrity related to pressure and friction.
   2. Potential infection related to improper home interventions such as cutting or paring of calluses.

B. Outcomes.
 1. Relief of pressure sources.
 2. Free of infection.
 3. Reduced callus thickness.
 4. Pain free.
 5. Resolved lesions.
 6. Absence of new lesions.
C. Interventions.
 1. Patient education.
  a. Apply keratolytic plaster, sticky medicated side to skin, making sure plaster covers the affected area. Cover the plaster with adhesive tape for 1 to 7 days. Soak the area in warm water after removing the tape. Rub the soft macerated skin with a rough towel or pumice stone. Reapply the plaster and repeat the process until all hyperkeratotic skin is removed.
  b. Apply keratolytic substance to site (avoid normal skin to prevent tissue damage)
 2. Wound care (see Table 1).

V. HOME CARE CONSIDERATIONS

A. Encourage proper-fitting shoes (for example, wide toe, appropriate length).
B. Avoid socks with seams.
C. Wear gloves when gardening and during activities of repetitive friction.

CORNS (CLAVI)

I. OVERVIEW

Corns are found over bony prominences such as the interphalangeal joints of toes (see Figures 7-3a to 3d, pages 232-233).
A. Definition: hyperkeratotic, painful, flat or slightly elevated with a smooth, firm circumscribed area. "Hard" corns have a sharply defined conical appearance; frequently over the interphalangeal toe joints and pressure site from foot wear. "Hard" corns are usually painful; dull constant pain or sharp pain when pressure is applied. "Soft" corns appear as whitish thickening, usually between the fourth and fifth toes.
B. Etiology.
 1. Repeated external pressure creates localized accumulation of keratin.
C. Pathophysiology.
 1. Localized pinpoint accumulation of keratin forms an elongated, hard plug in the horny layer of the epidermis. The plug presses downward on the dermal structure, causing inflammation and irritation of sensory nerves, resulting in marked tenderness.

Table 1.
Wound Care

- Rest as much as possible for the next 24 hours as ordered.
- Keep surgical dressing dry and in place for 24 to 48 hours as ordered. Then wet dressing in the shower or with a wet towel. Peel off gently.
- Then clean surgical site with soap and water 2 to 3 times a day as ordered. Do not apply alcohol or peroxide. Pat wound dry.
- Apply antibiotic ointment or white petrolatum (petroleum jelly) to keep site moist, 2 times a day and cover with appropriate dressing.
- If bleeding or oozing occurs at the site, gently apply pressure with a clean gauze or wash cloth for 20 minutes. The bleeding/oozing should stop within 25 minutes; if not, call the doctor.
- Watch for signs of infection: redness, swelling, pain, pus, and temp > 101. Take nonaspirin product for pain and discomfort — Tylenol®, if not allergic. Avoid Aleve®, Advil®, Motrin®, ibuprofen, and aspirin products

II. ASSESSMENT

A. Physical examination.

III. COMMON THERAPEUTIC MODALITIES

A. Surgical excision of superficial layer of corn and hard plug in the horny layer.
B. Corticosteroids: triamcinolone injection (Kenalog®, Aristocort®) at corn's base to relieve pain.
C. Topical keratolytics.

IV. COMMON NURSING DIAGNOSES, OUTCOMES, INTERVENTIONS

A. Common nursing diagnoses.
 1. Impaired skin integrity related to pressure and friction.
 2. Potential infection related to improper home interventions such as cutting or paring.
 3. Acute pain related to pressure.
B. Outcomes.
 1. Relief of pressure sources.
 2. Free of infection.
 3. Reduced corn thickness.
 4. Resolved lesions.
 5. Absence of new lesions.
 6. Pain free.
C. Interventions.
 1. Patient education.
  a. Demonstrate proper application of corn pads to relieve pressure.
  b. Avoid cutting and paring.

V. HOME CARE CONSIDERATIONS

A. Encourage proper-fitting shoes.
B. Avoid socks with seams.

> ## CYSTS
> ### (EPIDERMAL, EPIDERMAL INCLUSION CYST, EPIDERMOID CYST, KERATINOUS CYST, PILAR CYST, INFUNDIBULAR CYST, SEBACEOUS CYST, ACNE CYST)

I. OVERVIEW

A cyst is a benign, sac-like growth in the skin layers, which originates from the follicle orifice (see Figures 7-4 & 7-5, page 233).

A. Definition: Asymptomatic noninflammatory dermal cysts lined with epidermis and contain keratin. Frequently occurs after trauma, inflammation, or rupture of closed comedones or acne lesions.
B. Etiology uncertain.
   1. Cyst wall probably formed from occluded pilosebaceous follicles.
   2. Result of cutaneous surface trauma and a portion of the epithelium is forced into the superficial dermis.
C. Pathophysiology: cyst ruptures and keratin is released, causing an inflammatory foreign body response.
D. Incidence.
   1. Higher incidence in young and middle-aged males; increases with a family history.
   2. Multiple lesions (70%).
   3. Solitary (30%).

II. ASSESSMENT

Diagnosis by clinical presentation and examination of expressed material confirmation by biopsy.
A. Location.
B. Number.
C. Size.
D. Firmness.
E. Mobility.
F. Globular.
G. Tenderness.
H. Inflammation.
I. Infection.

III. COMMON THERAPEUTIC MODALITIES

A. Cure by complete excision, including wall to prevent recurrence.
B. Incision and drainage of infected or severely inflamed cysts (optional antibiotics, topical or oral).
C. Intralesional corticosteroid injections (triamcinolone, Aristocort, Kenalog) to decrease lesion size.

D. Extraction: comedome extractor for small cysts or milia.

IV. COMMON NURSING DIAGNOSES, OUTCOMES, INTERVENTIONS

A. Common nursing diagnoses.
   1. Impaired skin integrity related to mechanical factors.
   2. Body image disturbance related to skin appearance.
   3. Pain related to inflammation.
   4. Risk of infection related to disruption of integument.
B. Outcomes.
   1. Healing of site, minimal scarring. Skin intact and smooth.
   2. Increase patient satisfaction.
   3. Absence of pain.
   4. Free of infection (no redness, swelling, tenderness, pus, or fever).
C. Interventions.
   1. Patient education: avoid picking or squeezing to prevent infection. Post-op wound care and dressing changes.

V. HOME CARE CONSIDERATIONS

A. Wound care (see Table 1).

> ## DERMATOFIBROMA (FIBROMA)

I. Overview

A. Definition: a benign tumor of fibrous connective tissue (see Figure 7-6, page 233).
B. Etiology.
   1. The exact cause is unknown.
   2. Localized accumulation of fibroblasts from spontaneous development or as a reaction to trauma (insect bite or splinter).
C. Pathophysiology.
   1. Interwoven histocytes and collagen mesh dermal nodule, with overlying epidermal hyperplasia.
D. Incidence.
   1. Frequently occurs in middle age; dominant in females.
   2. Multiple lesions in 20%.

II. ASSESSMENT

A. Asymptomatic, single or multiple, papule or nodules.
B. Firm, hemispherical disc/dome-shaped.
C. Color: skin-colored, reddish, or tan to brown
D. Surrounding ring of pigmentation; 2 to 3 cm and less.
E. Common on friction areas: neck, axillae, near elbows, lateral trunk, medial thighs, and lower extremities.

Table 2.
Cysts

Type	Common Names	Location
Atheromas Globular, elastic, mobile tumor covered with atrophic thin skin, thick wall, filled with white paste, without external opening. Tender if infected. Baldness over large cyst skin due to follicular pressure damage. No inflammation or proliferation from trauma. No malignant degeneration.	Wen, pilar cyst, trichilemmal cyst	Scalp, hair follicle epithelium
Retention cysts Spheric, mobile, firm under tense skin. Ruptures easily by manipulation. Keratinous material can be pressed into the surrounding tissue; then acts as a foreign body and can cause granuloma abscess formation from bacterial infection	Milia, acne cysts, and traumatic inclusion cysts	Face, trunk, hair follicles areas, scalp, neck, back, and cheeks. One mm to several centimeters in diameter. Cutaneous or subcutaneous — fluctuant, easily movable, tense, swelling. Expanded gland duct and foul-smelling rancid lipids and debris will reoccur if wall remains intact.
Sebocystomatosis Central opening exudes a pasty, cheesy odoriferous material composed of necrotic keratin.	Sebaceous cysts (fat), Wen	Scalp, scrotum, and vulva
Keratinous cysts Firm, movable, globular, and nontender unless infected. Contents are soft and yellow-white, with a rancid odor.	Epidermal and sebaceous, pilar	Face, neck, and upper trunk
Milium Arise in underdeveloped sebaceous glands or within damaged eccrine sweat gland ducts following subepidermal bulla formation (for example, epidermolysis bullosa, porphyria cutanea tarda, bullous pemphigoid) or skin radiotherapy.	Subepidermal cyst	Eyelids and cheeks. Young to middle-aged women and infants. Small (1-2 mm) white papules.
Dermoid cysts Present at birth.		Deep subcutaneous tissue. Walls composed of keratinizing epidermis containing hair follicles, sebaceous glands, and sweat glands.

F. "Dimples" when gently pinched between the thumb and forefinger.

G. Diagnosis by clinical presentation; confirmation biopsy.

III. COMMON THERAPEUTIC MODALITIES

A. Excision for cosmetic reasons only

B. Cryosurgery every 3 to 4 weeks causes gradual involution.

IV. COMMON NURSING DIAGNOSES, OUTCOMES, INTERVENTIONS (see Table 3)

V. HOME CARE CONSIDERATIONS

A. Wound care (see Table 2).

HYPERTROPHIC SCARS

I. OVERVIEW

Hypertrophic scars result from skin trauma in genetically predisposed individuals. Characterized by excess of collagen deposition during wound healing.

II. ASSESSMENT

A. Asymptomatic; pruritic occasionally; and restricted to the area of injury.

Table 3.
Nursing Interventions Associated with Benign Neoplasms/Hyperplasia

Nursing Diagnoses	Outcomes	Interventions
Impaired skin integrity related to presence of lesions.	Skin lesions have been accurately diagnosed and treated; patient understands principles of wound care.	Assess skin lesions, including distribution and signs of progression.
Increased risk of secondary infection related to impaired skin integrity.	Lesions are not infected.	Assess for signs of infection.
Body image disturbance related to presence of skin lesions.	Positive body image is restored.	Assess patient's current preceptions and feelings.

B. Commonly over the sternum, deltoid, mandible, or upper lip.
C. Less exuberant than keloids.
D. Diagnosis by clinical exam and confirmation by skin biopsy.

III. COMMON THERAPEUTIC MODALITIES

A. Involute spontaneously.
B. Resolve without treatment within 6 to 18 months.

IV. COMMON NURSING DIAGNOSES, OUTCOMES, INTERVENTIONS (see Table 3)

KELOIDS

I. OVERVIEW

Keloids are proliferations of connective tissues (collagen) at site of a scar or traumatic injuries (thermal or chemical burns). Keloids may develop spontaneously (see Figure 7-7, page 233).
A. Description: nodular, nonencapsulated, highly hyperplastic mass of scar tissue.
B. Keloids begin as pink to red, firm, rubbery fibrous plaques with telangiectasias; 3 to 5 weeks after trauma. They are smooth, circumscribed, irregularly shaped, and hyperpigmented. May become tender and puritic. Enlargement and extension outside injury area.
C. More prevalent among African Americans and Asians.
D. Not present at birth and rare before puberty.
E. Increased prevalence in patients with severe acne and hidradentitis suppurativa.

F. Frequently affected areas are the earlobes (after piercing), face, neck, abdomen, chest, and upper back.
G. More exuberant than hypertrophic scars.

II. ASSESSMENT

A. Physical exam: location; size, color, tenderness, pain, pruritus, and burning.

III. COMMON THERAPEUTIC MODALITIES

A. Prevention by avoiding accidental and intentional skin trauma if prone to keloid. Apply pressure dressings to skin disruption site over 8 hours daily for 4 to 6 months.
B. Intralesional corticosteroid therapy.
C. Topical retinoic acid.
D. Carbon dioxide laser.
E. Surgical excision: 60% recurrence after surgery.
F. Radiation therapy.
G. Cryosurgery.
H. Topical silicone gel sheeting may minimize scarring extent and promote gradual resolution.

IV. COMMON NURSING DIAGNOSES, OUTCOMES, INTERVENTIONS

A. Common nursing diagnoses.
   1. Impaired skin integrity.
   2. Disturbed body image.
B. Outcomes.
   1. Intact skin integrity.
   2. Improved self-image and increased patient satisfaction.
C. Interventions.
   1. Patient education — wound care (see Table 2).

V. HOME CARE CONSIDERAITONS

A. Avoid scratching and irritation.
B. Avoid injury to keloid.
C. Use protective clothing and equipment.
D. Allow patient to express feelings concerning body appearance and fear of reaction/rejection by others.

LIPOMA

I. OVERVIEW

A. Definition: subcutaneous fatty tissue with fine capsule (see Figures 7-8 & 7-9, page 234).
B. Etiology cause unknown.
C. Incidence.
  1. Solitary or multiple; asymmetric irregular distribution.
  2. Equal sex.

II. ASSESSMENT

A. Soft, without central pore.
B. Freely moveable, slightly compressible.
C. Usually 1 cm or larger.
D. Frequently in areas of subcutaneous fat; trunk and extremities.

III. COMMON THERAPEUTIC MODALITIES

A. No therapy necessary when diagnosis confirmed.
B. Surgical excision.

IV. NURSING DIAGNOSIS, OUTCOMES AND INTERVENTIONS (see Table 3)

SEBACEOUS HYPERPLASIA

I. OVERVIEW

Etiology unknown, related to chronic sun damage. Incidence: seen more often in fair-skinned individuals (see Figure 7-10, page 234).

II. ASSESSMENT

A. Solitary.
  1. Umbilicated cauliflower-like.
B. Muliltiple soft yellowish and erythematous papules 2 to 3 mm in size, on forehead and cheeks.
C. Surface telangiectasis in the valleys between the small, yellow lobules.
D. Asymptomatic; persist unless treated.
E. Diagnosis by physical examination.

III. COMMON THERAPEUTIC MODALITIES

A. No treatment necessary except for patient's request for cosmetic improvement.
B. Isotretinoin (Accutane®).
  1. Normal liver function.
  2. Not currently pregnant or planning pregnancy for at least 1 month after therapy cessation.
C. Light electrodesiccation.
D. Liquid nitrogen cryosurgery.
E. Shave excision.

SEBORRHEIC KERATOSIS (SEBORRHEIC WART, SENILE WART, BASAL CELL PAPILLOMA)

I. OVERVIEW

A. Definition: wart-like, round to oval, superficial, epithelial, pigmented papule or plaque, with sharply circumscribed round to oval; sharply demarcated borders (see Figure 7-11, page 234).
  1. Slow growing.
  2. "Greasy, stuck on the skin."
  3. Hyperkeratotic lesions.
  4. Varied size from millimeters to centimeter.
  5. Color from dark yellow to tan, brown to black.
  6. Common on the face, chest, shoulders, scalp, and back.
B. Etiology is unknown.
C. Pathophysiology: proliferations of immature epidermal kertinocytes; keratinization occurs, causing the lesions to become warty, dry, and fissured. Initially flat, coin size with flesh-brown pigmention. Then develop into papillomatous hemispherical raised tumors with dark brown to black pigmentation. A keratotic, conical protuberance (cutaneous horn) or open comedones may develop.
D. Incidence: common in middle-age and older adults. Onset by age 30. Equal sex. More numerous, smaller, and occur earlier in African Americans and Hispanics. A family history and sunlight exposure history predispose to development. Inherited as a dominant trait. Associated with obesity and acne.

II. ASSESSMENT

A. History and current health status.
B. Physical exam: location, size, number, appearance, color, borders, pruritus, changes, and irritation — erythema, tenderness, increased pruritus.
C. Diagnosis by clinical presentation and confirmation by biopsy.

III. COMMON THERAPEUTIC MODALITIES

A. No treatment necessary if small and asymptomatic.
B. Shave excision.
C. Electrodesiccation and curettage.

Dermatologic Nursing Essentials: A Core Curriculum 2nd Edition © DNA 2003

D. Cryosurgery.

E. Carbon dioxide laser.

IV. COMMON NURSING DIAGNOSES, OUTCOMES, INTERVENTIONS

A. Common nursing diagnoses.
   1. Disturbed body image; perception of appearance related to aesthetics.
   2. Impaired skin integrity related to presence of lesions.
   3. Potential irritation and inflammation related to location.

B. Outcomes.
   1. Patient exhibits improved positive body image.
   2. Skin integrity improved or maintained.
   3. Free from infection.

C. Interventions.
   1. Patient education.
      a. Identify lesions that itch, are irritated, or cosmetically embarrassing.
      b. Patient will identify lesions irritated by clothing or rubbing against other body parts.

V. HOME CARE CONSIDERATIONS

A. Wound care (see Table 2).

B. Control bleeding.

C. Watch for signs of infection.

Bibliography

Bork, K., & Brauninger, W. (1997). *Skin diseases in clinical practice* (2nd ed.). Philadelphia: W.B. Saunders.

Dains, J.E. (2002). Integumentary system. In J.M. Thompson, G.K. McFarland, J.E. Hirsch, & S.M. Tucker, (Eds.), *Mosby's clinical nursing* (5th ed) (pp. 434-454). St. Louis: Mosby.

Hooper, B.J., & Goldman, M.P. (1999). *Primary dermatologic care.* St. Louis: Mosby.

Luckmann, J. (Ed.). (1997). *Saunders manual of nursing care.* Philadelphia: W.B. Saunders.

Nettina, S.M. (2001). *The lippincott manual of nursing practice* (7th ed.). Philadelphia: Lippincott Williams & Wilkins.

Rycroft, R.J., & Robertson, S.J. (1999). *A colour handbook of dermatology.* London, UK: Manson Publishing Ltd.

Stein, A.M., & Miller, J.C. (Eds.). (2000). *National Student Nurses' Association, Inc.: NCLEX-RN™ review* (4th ed.). Albany, NY: Delmar.

1. Acrochordons are benign neoplasms and cosmetic disorders.
   a. True
   b. False

2. Calluses are caused by:
   a. Spontaneous development.
   b. Accompanying cancerous tumors.
   c. Repeated friction or pressure.
   d. Internal pressure.

3. Corns are:
   a. Found over bony prominences.
   b. Hyperkeratotic circumscribed area.
   c. Soft and hard.
   d. a & b.
   e. All of the above.

4. All of the following are common therapeutic modalities for cysts *except:*
   a. Complete excision and wall removal.
   b. Partial excision.
   c. Incision and drainage.
   d. Intralesional corticosteroid injections.

5. Dermatofibroma is caused by spontaneous development of localized accumulation of fibroblasts or a reaction to an insect bite.
   a. True.
   b. False.

6. Hypertrophic scars:
   a. Require excision.
   b. Require incision and drainage.
   c. Require intralesional injections.
   d. Involute spontaneously.

7. Keloid development is common on:
   a. Earlobes after piercing.
   b. Face.
   c. Chest.
   d. All of the above.

8. Lipoma is composed of:
   a. Connective tissue.
   b. Epidermal.
   c. Subcutaneous fatty tissue.
   d. Dermis.

9. Sebaceous hyperplasia is not related to chronic sun damage.
   a. True.
   b. False.

10. Seborrheic keratosis appears as a:
    a. Cyst.
    b. Nodule.
    c. "Greasy, stuck on" papule or plaque.
    d. Bullae.

Answers to the Study Questions

1.	a	5.	a	9.	b
2.	c	6.	d	10.	c
3.	e	7.	d		
4.	b	8.	c		

Dermatologic Nursing Essentials: A Core Curriculum 2nd Edition © DNA 2003

CE Answer/Evaluation Form

Chapter 7.
Benign Neoplasms/Hyperplasia

Please photocopy this test page and return.

COMPLETE THE FOLLOWING:

Name: _____

Address: _____

City: _____ State: _____ Zip: _____

Preferred telephone: (Home)_____ (Work) _____

State where licensed and license number: _____

CE application fee: DNA member $7.00
                        Nonmember $10.00

POSTTEST INSTRUCTIONS
1. To receive continuing education credit for individual study after reading the article, complete the answer/evaluation form below.
2. Photocopy and send the answer/evaluation form along with a check or money order payable to **Dermatology Nurses' Association** to: **DNA**, East Holly Avenue Box 56, Pitman, NJ 08071-0056.
3. Test returns must be postmarked by December 31, 2008. Upon completion of the answer/evaluation form, a certificate for 1.7 contact hour(s) will be awarded and sent to you.

This chapter was reviewed and formatted for contact hour credit by Marcia J. Hill, MSN, RN, Core Curriculum Editor; and Sally Russell, MN, RN,C, DNA Education Director.

ANSWER FORM

1. Name one new detail (item, issue, or phenomenon) that you learned by completing this activity.

   _____

   _____

   _____

   _____

2. How will you apply the information from this learning activity to your practice?
   a. Patient education.
   b. Staff education.
   c. Improve my patient care.
   d. In my education course work.
   e. Other: Please describe _____

   _____

Evaluation

	Strongly disagree				Strongly agree
3. The offering met the stated objectives.					
a. Define benign neoplasms/hyperplasia.	1	2	3	4	5
b. Describe the signs and symptoms of benign neoplasms/hyperplasia.	1	2	3	4	5
c. Understand the various treatment options available to the patient with benign neoplasms/hyperplasia.	1	2	3	4	5
4. The content was current and relevant.	1	2	3	4	5
5. The content was presented clearly.	1	2	3	4	5
6. The content was covered adequately.	1	2	3	4	5
7. I am more confident of my abilities since completing this material.	1	2	3	4	5

8. The material was (check one) ☐ new, ☐ review for me.

Comments _____

_____

9. Time required to complete reading assignment: _____ minutes

This independent study is provided by the Dermatology Nurses' Association (DNA) for 1.7 contact hours. DNA is accredited as a provider of continuing education in nursing by the American Nurses Credentialing Center's Commission on Accreditation. DNA is approved as a provider of continuing education by the California Board of Registered Nursing Provider #CEP5708.

Cutaneous Manifestations of Systemic Disease

Sue Ann McCann, MSN, RN, DNC

OBJECTIVES

At the end of this chapter, the reader will be able to:

- Identify at least five systemic disorders demonstrating significant cutaneous signs and symptoms.
- Describe the cutaneous signs and symptoms common to leukemia/lymphoma.
- Discuss the potential skin alterations in the patient with sarcoidosis, hypothyroidism, Behcet's disease, pyoderma gangrenosum, graft-versus-host disease, and diabetes mellitus.
- List at least five cutaneous signs of possible internal malignancy.
- Discuss nursing care for the patient with body image disturbance.
- Identify common therapeutic modalities for systemic illnesses with cutaneous manifestations.

KEY POINTS

- The skin is fundamentally related and integrated with all body systems and functions.
- Cutaneous signs and symptoms may be the first indication of a systemic illness.
- Dermatology nursing care for patients with systemic illness presents unique challenges requiring a multidisciplinary approach.
- Skin changes may precede, follow, or have a parallel course with suspected internal malignancies.
- Patients with suspected systemic illness and concurrent skin signs and symptoms require a comprehensive multi-system assessment and relevant diagnostic workup.

Cutaneous Manifestations of Systemic Disease

Sue Ann McCann, MSN, RN, DNC

INTERNAL MALIGNANCY: LEUKEMIA/LYMPHOMA

I. OVERVIEW

A. Definition: hematopoietic and lymphoid malignancies with multiple classifications by dominant cell type and duration from onset to death (acute vs. chronic). Some classifications include:
  1. Acute myleomonocytic: monocytosis involving peripheral blood.
  2. Monocytic: large numbers of monocytes and related reticuloendothelial tissue cells "overrun" the blood and reticuloendothelial system.
  3. Aleukemic: leukemic cells are not found in the peripheral blood.
  4. Acute lymphocytic: an uncontrolled proliferation of lymphoblasts and enlargement of lymphoid tissue.
  5. Hairy cell: proliferation of hairy cells in reticuloendothelial organs and blood, usually chronic.
  6. Acute myeloblastic: proliferation of immature myeloblasts in tissues, organs, and blood.
  7. Non-Hodgkin's: represents multiple cytologic classifications, other than Hodgkin's disease, of either nodular or diffuse tumor patterns with low, intermediate, or high-grade malignancy patterns.
B. Etiology is unknown for both leukemias and lymphomas; however, some studies may indicate a possible genetic, environmental, or viral link.
C. Pathophysiology.
  1. Leukemia is characterized by neoplasia of the white blood cells (WBC) in the bone marrow.
    a. Abnormal WBC production suppresses the normal function of the bone marrow.
    b. Characterized by anemia, decreased platelet production, and granulocytopenia.
  2. Non-Hodgkin's lymphoma is characterized by abnormal proliferation of various cell types, categorized as either histiocytic, lymphocytic, or mixed cell type. Malignant cells may spread to lymph nodes, bone marrow, liver, spleen, and GI tract.
  3. Skin lesions as a direct result from invasion of the skin by tumor cells may manifest as papules, macules, infiltrated plaques, nodules, or ulcers.
  4. Skin lesions as an indirect result of the malignancy may, for example, manifest as pallor (anemia), excoriations (pruritus), petechiae (thrombocytopenia), and

opportunistic infections such as severe candidiasis (neutropenia).
D. Incidence.
  1. Leukemia prevalence is reported at 9 per 100,000 yearly.
  2. Non-Hodgkin's is a broad spectrum of lymphomas three times more common than Hodgkin's lymphoma.
E. Considerations across the life span.
  1. Acute leukemia is most common in children while chronic leukemia is more common in adults in the 3rd to 6th decade of life.
  2. Non-Hodgkin's lymphoma is most common in the 5th and 6th decades of life.

II. ASSESSMENT

A. History and physical exam.
  1. A careful review of systems is essential to determine constitutional symptoms such as headaches, fatigue, fever, weight loss, and anorexia.
  2. Skin exam may demonstrate both specific and nonspecific lesions found in leukemias and lymphomas.
B. Specific skin changes.
  1. Most common are rubbery, erythematous/purplish papules, plaques or nodules, randomly distributed. Less common are flesh-colored lesions (see Figure 8-1, page 235).
  2. Less common are lesions similar in appearance to mycosis fungoides (plaques, arciform papules, and ulcerated nodules).
  3. Early skin changes are most common in acute myelomonocytic and monocytic leukemia and include infiltrated, hyperplastic, friable gingiva.
  4. Aleukemic leukemia cutis presents in the skin as erythematous papules or nodules in the absence of malignant cells in the peripheral blood.
C. Nonspecific skin changes.
  1. Skin and mucous membrane findings attributable to cytopenia include pallor, purpura, gingival bleeding, oral ulcerations, and skin infections.
  2. Skin changes in which the pathogenesis is unknown include acute febrile neutrophilic dermatosis (Sweet's syndrome), atypical pyoderma gangrenosum, generalized pruritus, vasculitis, acquired ichthyosis, vesicular disease, and xanthomas.
D. General clinical manifestations.
  1. Leukemia.

a. Hematologic abnormalities.
b. Local/systemic infections (respiratory, skin).
c. Nutritional deficits (anorexia, nausea, vomiting, diarrhea).
d. Hepatomegaly, splenomegaly, lymphadenopathy.
e. Musculoskeletal and neurological related pain.
f. Neurologic-related symptoms such as headaches, visual changes, vertigo, tinnitus.
g. Fatigue, fever, weakness, malaise.
2. Lymphoma.
a. Painless lymphadenopathy.
b. Anorexia, fatigue, fever, weight loss.
c. Hematologic abnormalities (anemia).
d. Hepatosplenomegaly.
e. Local/systemic infections.
f. Neurologic-related symptoms include pain and/or parasthesias/paralysis of affected nerve pathways.
E. **Diagnostic tests.**
1. General diagnostic tests include lymph node and/or bone marrow biopsy, CBC with differential, and x-rays/scans of the chest, abdomen, and bone.
2. Skin biopsy will demonstrate specific type of malignant cell but must be correlated with the history, physical exam, and other diagnostic data.
3. Differential diagnosis for skin lesions.
a. Psuedolymphoma of the skin (infestations or bites, lymphomatoid papulosis, drug-induced pseudolymphoma, actinic reticulosis).
b. Viral, fungal, or bacterial infections.

III. COMMON THERAPEUTIC MODALITIES

A. **Systemic therapy.**
1. Chemotherapy.
2. Radiation therapy.
3. Immunotherapy.
4. Bone marrow transplant.
5. Supportive therapy with antibiotic prophylaxis and blood/platelet transfusions and/or bone marrow growth factors (erythropoetin, GMCSF).
B. **Local therapy.**
1. Radiation therapy to specific skin lesions.
2. Intralesional corticosteroid injection.
3. Supportive management of pruritus, oral ulceration or bleeding, and xerosis.

IV. COMMON NURSING DIAGNOSES, OUTCOMES, AND INTERVENTIONS

A. **Nursing diagnosis: high risk for infection related to increased susceptibility from inadequate primary and secondary defenses.**

1. Patient outcomes.
a. Patient's skin integrity is maintained.
b. Patient's vital signs, temperature, and laboratory tests indicating possible infection are within normal limits. Clinical assessments of pulmonary and genitourinary systems are free of signs of infection.
c. Patient is able to verbalize infection-prevention measures.
2. Interventions.
a. Prevent skin breakdown with frequent skin assessments, positioning, adequate fluid intake and nutrition, and maintaining patient mobility.
b. Assess for opportunistic skin infections such as candidiasis or herpes simplex.
c. Promote and assist with effective overall skin cleansing and hygiene of perianal area.
(1) Avoid over-drying the skin with excessive bathing. Lubricate the skin after bathing with a cream or ointment-based skin care product.
(2) Use a gentle, nondeodorant cleansing agent.
(3) If incontinent, keep skin clean, dry, and protect with barrier ointment to prevent chafing, breakdown, and overgrowth of candida organisms.
d. Monitor vital signs and clinical status.
(1) Administer nonaspirin antipyretics or use a cooling blanket as needed.
(2) Obtain appropriate wound, body fluid, or skin cultures.
(3) Encourage 3 to 4 liters of fluid per day if medical condition permits to maintain hydration.
e. Maintain good pulmonary toilet to prevent respiratory illness.
f. Assist with effective bowel/bladder elimination to prevent constipation or inadequate bladder emptying and bladder infections.
g. If neutropenic or during acute exacerbation, consider reverse isolation to protect patient from infection.
h. Avoid any unnecessary invasive procedures such as venipunctures, injections, or urethral catheterizations.
i. Provide information to patient and family members on importance of avoiding possible infectious agents or persons with obvious communicable illnesses such as the flu, upper respiratory infections/pneumonia, or contact with herpes simplex lesions.
B. **Nursing diagnosis: altered mucous membranes related to disease process and/or treatment.**

1. Patient outcomes.
   a. Patient's mouth and associated mucous membranes are free of ulcerations, edema, and bleeding.
   b. Patient is able to tolerate chewing and swallowing food.
   c. Patient states oral cavity is pain free.
2. Interventions.
   a. Encourage/perform frequent oral hygiene every 2 hours while awake.
      (1) A solution of tepid water and dilute hydrogen peroxide help to soothe and cleanse tissues.
      (2) Oral hygiene should be performed before meals to increase appetite, taste, and enjoyment of foods.
   b. Assess oral cavity TID for lesions, edema, bleeding, infection, or foreign material.
   c. Emollients applied frequently to the lips may decrease chapping, dryness, or pain and improve comfort.
   d. Provide reassurance that lesions will subside as the condition is treated.
   e. Offer mild analgesics if topical measures are ineffective in pain control.
   f. Encourage a bland diet consisting of soft foods. Avoid spicy and acidic foods/beverages.
      (1) Encourage fluid intake of 3 to 4 liters/day if medical condition permits.
      (2) Offer frequent, small feedings.
      (3) Cool or cold foods may be more soothing.

V. HOME CARE CONSIDERATIONS

A. **The home may need to be adapted to the patient's needs for elimination, activity, and safety.**
   1. A one-level bedroom, bathroom, and dining area may be required for patients with significant alterations in mobility and activity.
   2. Assistance with activities of daily living may be required during treatment or recuperation periods.
B. **Home care nurses are beneficial in monitoring patient status and providing ongoing emotional support and physician liaison services.**

CUTANEOUS SIGNS OF SYSTEMIC MALIGNANCY

I. OVERVIEW (see Table 1)

METABOLIC/NUTRITIONAL DISORDERS: HYPOTHYROIDISM

I. OVERVIEW

A. **Definition: metabolic disorder with decreased production of free thyroid hormone involving systemic and cutaneous manifestations.**
B. **Etiology.**
   1. Primary hypothyroidism is related to a defect within the thyroid gland itself.
      a. Chronic thyroiditis (Hashimoto's thyroiditis).
      b. Autoimmune process.
      c. Congenital (cretinism).
      d. Surgical/radiotherapy ablation.
      e. Rare causes include pituitary tumor and pituitary failure (Sheehan's syndrome).
   2. Secondary hypothyroidism may be due to pituitary failure to secrete thyroid-stimulating hormone or hypothalamic failure to secrete thyroid-releasing hormone.
   3. Dietary deficiencies (iodine) or excessive dietary intake of goitrogens (inhibit T4 production) such as cabbage, soybeans, peanuts, peaches, peas, spinach, and strawberries.
C. **Pathophysiology.**
   1. Deficiency of circulating thyroxine and triiodothyronine decrease basal metabolism and oxygen consumption in tissues.
   2. Severe hypothyroidism results in the deposition of hydrophillic mucopolysaccharides in interstitial tissues (myxedema).
   3. Thyroid gland becomes atrophied and fibrotic.
D. **Incidence.**
   1. More common in women than men in 10:1 ratio.
   2. About 95% have primary form of disease and about 5% of cases result from pituitary/hypothalamic dysfunction.
E. **Considerations across the life span.**
   1. Primary hypothyroidism most commonly occurs in 3rd to 6th decade of life.
   2. Fetal or infantile hypothyroidism affecting physical or mental development is termed cretinism. Early detection and treatment are often preventative.
   3. Detection in the elderly is more difficult since the signs and symptoms develop slowly and can be attributed to arteriosclerotic manifestations.

II. ASSESSMENT

A. **History and physical.**
   1. A thorough history is essential to determine presence of nonspecific, early symptoms such as excessive fatigue, somnolence, and lethargy.
   2. Allow extra time for the patient to assimilate questions and formulate a response since

Table 1.
Skin Changes with Potential Suspicion for Systemic Neoplasia (Callen, 1995)

Lesion	Description	Associated Malignancy	Comment
Acanthosis nigricans (AN)	Hyperpigmented velvety thickening of intertriginous skin. Neck, axilla, inguinal area, nipple, umbilicus most common.	Most common are GI/GU tracts. Adenocarcinoma of stomach commonly associated with AN. Usually occurs simultaneously with malignancy.	Must rule out other endo-crinopathies, familial tendency, or obesity related. AN most common in older adults and associated with weight loss.
Bazex's syndrome (Acro-keratosis paraneo-plastica)	Three stage, progressive development from 1) erythematous, violaceous macules with scale over acral areas (fingers, toes, ears, nose) to 2) development of a keratoderma to 3) eruption becomes generalized.	Upper airway and upper GI tract, most commonly squamous cell carcinoma. Course of skin changes often parallels course of malignancy.	
Porphyria cutanea tarda	Hyperpigmentation of sun-exposed areas, hypertrichosis and, less commonly, intact vesicles and bullae.	Hepatic tumors.	Careful liver evaluation is required.
Paraneoplastic pemphigus	Bullous lesions.	Thymomas (benign and malignant). Course of skin disorder does not parallel the malignancy.	Chest x-ray should be carefully reviewed for evidence of a thymoma.
Dermatomyositis	Inflammatory myopathy and associated skin changes.	Gynecologic (ovarian) and nasopharynx carcinomas.	Course is not parallel with skin changes. Debated among authors.
Sudden onset multiple seborrheic keratoses	Raised papules or plaques with "stuck-on" appearance. Lesion surface is usually wart-like.	Intra-abdominal adenocarcinoma.	Known as the sign of Leser-Trélat syndrome. May also occur simultaneously with AN.
Exfoliative erythroderma	Generalized erythema, scaling, and edema.	Lymphoreticular system most common, solid tumor association also reported.	Concurrent course of skin and tumor burden.
Erythema gyratum repens	Erythematous, serpiginous bands across skin form a "wood-grained" appearance.	No specific associated site.	Skin course parallel to neoplasm. Requires extensive evaluation to determine site.
Hypertrichosis lanuginosa (malignant down)	Sudden development of fine, downy, excessive hair growth without signs of virilization.	Varied sites and cell types.	Malignancy often discovered at time of skin change. Must evaluate for neoplastic growth in patients without cause for sudden hair growth (medication or endocrine abnormality).

Table 1. (continued)
Skin Changes with Potential Suspicion for Systemic Neoplasia (Callen, 1995)

Migratory thrombo-phlebitis (Trousseau's syndrome)	Superficial thrombo-phlebitis commonly affecting veins of the neck, chest, abdomen, and lower extremities.	Pancreas or prostate.	Believed related to a chronic, low-grade, intra-vascular coagulopathy. Abdominal CT scan is recommended.
Paget's disease of the breast	Erythematous, eczematous plaque surrounding nipple and areola.	Occurs in conjunction with adeno-carcinoma of the breast.	Believed due to migration of malignant cells and most accurately considered a malignant infiltrate rather than a paraneoplastic sign.
Sweet's syndrome (acute febrile neutrophilic dermatosis)	Tender, erythematous plaques.	Myelogenous leukemia.	Associated with fever and anemia, course parallels that of the leukemia.

mental functioning may be slowed.
3. Assess for weight gain, nonpitting, interstitial edema (found in myxedema), and other associated clinical signs.

B. **Skin, hair, and nail changes.**
1. Skin changes.
   a. Skin texture is coarse, dry, scaly. Excessively dry skin may develop an acquired ichthyosis vulgaris.
   b. Cold intolerant. Skin is cool to touch and pale.
   c. Skin appears puffy, boggy, or swollen (nonpitting) and waxy due to the deposition of hydrophillic mucopolysaccharides, most noted in dependent tissue such as the pretibial area.
   d. Palms and soles are hypohydrotic and hyper-keratotic.
   e. The skin may have an ivory or yellow cast due to improper metabolism of beta-carotene in the liver. Xanthomatosis is common due to hyperlipidemia.
   f. The skin bruises easily due to capillary fragility with resulting ecchymoses and purpura. Telangiectasia is noted on arms and fingertips.
2. Hair changes.
   a. Grows slowly with an increase in telogen (resting) hairs.
   b. Classic pattern of hair loss is lateral 1/3 of eyebrows. Diffuse alopecia is rare, but there is often loss of pubic, axillary, and facial hair.
   c. It appears dull and is coarse and brittle.
3. Nail changes.
   a. Grows slowly.
   b. Characteristically brittle, thin, and striated either longitudinally or transversely.
   c. Onycholysis is rare, but may occur.

C. **Systemic manifestations are multisystem and generally related to decreased metabolic state.**
1. Early symptoms include fatigue, lethargy, somnolence, and cold intolerance.
2. General signs and symptoms include slow heart rate, anemia, impaired wound healing, constipation, decreased appetite, weight gain, parasthesias of hands or feet, slurred speech/hoarseness, myalgias/arthralgias, slowed muscle movement and reflexes, headaches, apathy, and forgetfulness.
3. Reproductive effects include menorrhagia, infertility, and decreased libido in women. Men experience decreased libido and impotence.

D. **Diagnostic tests.**
1. Thyroid function studies, antithyroid antibody titer, and calcitonin level.
   a. TSH is elevated in primary hypothyroidism.
   b. TSH is low or nondetected in pituitary failure.
2. Thyroid scan and radioactive iodine uptake.
3. Skin biopsy to verify myxedema.

III. COMMON THERAPEUTIC MODALITIES

A. **Thyroid hormone replacement such as levothyroxine sodium (Synthroid®) or liothyronine sodium (Cytomel®).**
B. **Dietary management if applicable.**
C. **Surgical excision of large goiters or those nonresponsive to treatment.**
D. **Supportive skin care (see Nursing Interventions).**

IV. COMMON NURSING DIAGNOSES, OUTCOMES, AND INTERVENTIONS

A. **Nursing diagnosis: high risk for impaired skin integrity related to edema, dryness, poor circulation.**

B. **Patient outcome: skin integrity will remain intact.**
C. **Interventions.**
1. Assess routinely for skin breakdown, especially over bony prominences such as elbows, spine, sacrum, coccyx, and any other potential pressure points.
2. Provide for passive range of motion and frequent repositioning (at least every 2 hours) as indicated by patient status. Specialty beds may be indicated for immobile patients.
3. Elevate dependent extremities whenever possible to decrease edema and promote venous return.
4. Promote wound healing and skin repair through adequate nutrition and fluid intake.
5. Apply emollients to dry skin frequently.
6. Avoid excessive bathing and use gentle cleansing agents.
7. Avoid bruising or injuring skin.

V. HOME CARE CONSIDERATIONS

A. **The patient must be monitored for adherence to medication regime and potential side effects of either hypo/hyperthyroidism.**
B. **Periodic thyroid hormone levels must be obtained to ensure adequate response to treatment.**
C. **Ensure proper diet containing iodine and high-fiber foods and avoidance of excessive goitrogenic foods.**

DIABETES MELLITUS

I. OVERVIEW

A. **Definition: system-wide metabolic disorder involving altered insulin utilization or production with resultant abnormalities in metabolism of dietary nutrients.**
B. **Etiology is unknown. Current theories include genetic, autoimmune, or environmental factors (obesity, stress).**
C. **Pathophysiology.**
1. Type I diabetes primarily involves decreased or absent insulin production within the pancreas.
2. Type II diabetes involves one or more factors including too much or too little insulin production, diminished responsiveness of tissues to the available insulin, and abnormal glucose regulation within the liver.
3. The complications related to diabetes mellitus primarily affect the heart, kidneys, and eyes due to micro and macro angiopathy. Neuropathy and skin alterations are also common complications.
D. **Incidence.**
1. The number of existing and new cases are increasing in the United States.
2. Seventeen million people in United States are now affected.

3. About 80% of diabetics are Type II.
4. Trends in incidence demonstrate minority and elderly populations are disproportionately affected.
E. **Considerations across the life span.**
1. Type II more commonly associated with adults older than 40, but may occur at any age.
2. Type I more commonly associated with children and young adults, but may occur at any age.

II. ASSESSMENT

A. **History and physical exam should include a system-wide approach to determine family and patient history, coping and compliance skills, general state of health, and potential/actual complications.**
B. **Potential skin manifestations.**
1. Rubeosis — chronic flushing of face and neck, may also be found on the extremities.
2. Diabetic dermopathy — hyperpigmented, atrophic patches on lower extremities. Initially develops as a cluster of red papules that later coalesce.
3. Bullous diabeticorum — nonscarring, tense bullae more common to the lower extremities (see Figure 8-2, page 235).
4. Necrobiosis lipoidica diabeticorum — yellow-brown, well-circumscribed patches with erythematous borders on lower extremities. Ulceration is common.
5. Acanthosis nigricans — hyperpigmented, velvety thickening in intertriginous areas.
6. Xanthomas — small, yellow-red papules (see Figure 8-3, page 235).
7. Skin infections — Candida, tinea pedis, mucormycosis (acute periorbital swelling and rhinorrhea due to fungal *Phycomycetes* infection, with potential for cerebral involvement and death).
8. Carotenemia — yellowish skin discoloration.
9. Vascular changes — ulcerations, gangrenous digits.
10. Hemochromatosis — bronze skin tones.
11. Sclerotic skin — most common on hands and over joints, limiting mobility.
12. Scleredema — dermal induration of skin on posterior neck and upper back.
13. Perforating folliculitis — keratotic papules and nodules with central plug or excoriation seen in 5% to 10% of patients on renal dialysis.
14. Lipodystrophy — localized at insulin injection sites.
15. Vitiligo — depigmented macular patches.
16. Neurotrophic ulceration and muscle atrophy.
C. **Diagnostic tests.**
1. Type I and Type II diagnostic tests include fasting blood glucose, postprandial blood sugar,

glycosylated hemoglobin, blood urea nitrogen and creatinine, electrolytes, complete urinalysis, complete eye and neurologic exam.

2. Skin biopsy may be required if skin lesion in question is related to diabetic changes or complications.

III. COMMON THERAPEUTIC MODALITIES

A. Diet and exercise management.
B. Pharmacologic management with insulin or oral hypoglycemics.
C. Preventive care and complication management.

IV. COMMON NURSING DIAGNOSES, OUTCOMES, AND INTERVENTIONS

A. Nursing diagnosis: altered tissue perfusion related to degenerative vascular changes.
B. Outcomes.
   1. The patient will maintain skin integrity.
   2. The patient will have decreased extremity edema, with normal capillary refill time of less than 3 seconds.
   3. The patient will have blood pressure, pulse within normal patient range, and palpable peripheral pulses.
   4. The patient will verbalize improved sensation in extremities with decreased parasthesias.
C. Interventions.
   1. Monitor for signs of altered tissue perfusion such as changes in vital signs, delayed capillary refill, and dusky or deep red color to lower extremities.
   2. Educate patient to monitor for changes in circulatory status and to report observed changes or onset of pain, nonhealing ulcer, or parasthesias.
   3. Encourage active range of motion or perform passive range of motion to improve circulation to extremities.
   4. Encourage active exercise with walking and gentle stretching with frequent rest periods as needed.
   5. Assess for loss of skin integrity, especially over bony prominences and the feet.
   6. Maintain vigilant skin care through daily hygiene, avoidance of injuries, scratching, and dryness. Skin should be kept well-lubricated and hydrated.
   7. Instruct patient on means to avoid trauma to skin, especially the feet and lower extremities. Encourage daily practice of skin and foot inspection.
   8. Avoid activities or clothing that impair circulation (girdles, tight shoes, crossing legs, standing or sitting for long periods, constrictive clothing, cold temperatures, and cigarette smoking).

V. HOME CARE CONSIDERATIONS

A. Regular followup is essential to health maintenance and preventing complications.
B. Good personal hygiene is essential with emphasis on foot care.
C. Medical alert cards, bracelets, and necklaces are crucial to identifying diabetics within the home and community.
D. Self-management is ideal, but supervision and continuing education are key to the successful management of diabetes for some patients.

NEUROLOGIC DISORDERS: NEUROFIBROMATOSIS (von RECKLINGHAUSEN'S DISEASE)

I. OVERVIEW

A. Definition: heterogeneous group of disorders (8 subtypes identified) with multiple benign nerve sheath tumors and characteristic skin findings.
B. Etiology.
   1. In 50% of cases, it is related to an inherited, autosomal dominant trait.
   2. Fifty percent of cases are considered new mutations.
C. Pathophysiology.
   1. The cutaneous neurofibromatous lesions originate from Schwann cells of the peripheral nervous system. Proliferation of perineural fibroblasts produce tumor-like growths.
   2. The genetic defect has been localized to chromosome 17 for Type 1 disease and is characterized by at least two of the following:
      a. Six or more café au lait macules.
      b. Axillary or inguinal freckling.
      c. At least two neurofibromas or one plexiform neurofibroma.
      d. Optic glioma.
      e. Lisch's nodules (yellow-brown smooth nodules within the iris).
      f. Thinning of long bone cortex or sphenoid bone dysplasia.
      g. First-degree relative meeting at least two of the above criteria.
   3. Type 2 disease is linked to chromosome 22 and is characterized by bilateral acoustic neuromas and less skin involvement.
   4. Type 3 disease (formerly called mixed type) is characterized by multiple intracranial tumors, paraspinal neurofibromas, neurofibromas primarily of the palms, and café au lait spots.
   5. Type 4 (coined variant neurofibromatosis) includes the range of phenotypes that don't neatly fit elsewhere and are placed in this category.
   6. Type 5, also called segmental type, is typified by café au lait spots or neurofibromas limited to a

single unilateral or dermatomal area.

7. Type 6 is familial, characterized by multiple café au lait spots without neurofibromas (rare).

8. Type 7 includes the presentation of neurofibromas, after the age of 20, without other cutaneous changes (rare).

9. Type 8 is for all other atypical cases of neurofibromatosis not fulfilling any other specified criteria. Type 4 and type 8 cases are often interchanged.

D. **Incidence: Type 1 occurs in 1 out of 3,000 live births; Type 2 occurs in about 1 out of 40,000; and prevalence for Types 3 to 8 is considered uncommon or rare.**

E. **Considerations across the life span.**
   1. Often manifests initially in late childhood.
   2. Lesions become more extensive and cosmetically disfiguring during adulthood.
   3. Malignant tumors (sarcomas) may develop in up to 5% of lesions over time.

II. ASSESSMENT

A. **History and physical exam.**
   1. Cutaneous findings are usually the presenting signs of neurofibromatoses.
   2. The differential diagnosis should include dermal nevi and papillomas.
   3. The clinician should assess for familial history and one or more skin/optic findings.

B. **Skin changes.**
   1. Cafe' au lait spots (hyperpigmented macules) (see Figure 8-4, page 235).
   2. Axillary freckling most common (Crowe's sign) but inguinal or infra-mammary freckling is also seen.
   3. Soft cutaneous and subcutaneous tumors that invaginate when palpated (button-holing sign) (see Figure 8-5, page 235).
      a. Tumors are sessile or pedunculated.
      b. Large drooping masses that develop along a nerve (plexiform neuromas) may develop.
   4. Distribution is generalized but commonly spares the palms and soles.

C. **Systemic manifestations.**
   1. Systemic involvement is variable in incidence, extent, and severity.
   2. Central nervous system.
      a. Optic nerve glioma (most common).
      b. Acoustic neuroma.
      c. Meningiomas.
      d. Intellectual deficiency.
      e. Speech impediments.
      f. Macrocephaly.
   3. Musculoskeletal.
      a. Pseudo arthritis.
      b. Kyphoscoliosis.
   4. Gastrointestinal.

a. Visceral tumors (leiomyomas, neurofibromas).
b. Constipation, obstruction, intussusception, and hemorrhage related to tumor involvement.

   5. Pheochromocytoma.

D. **Diagnostic tests.**
   1. Skin biopsy demonstrates a well-circumscribed dermal tumor.
   2. Multisystem evaluation for diagnosis and disease progression or disease complications is recommended.

III. COMMON THERAPEUTIC MODALITIES

A. **Medical interventions.**
   1. Genetic counseling is advised.
   2. Symptomatic treatment of neurological, gastrointestinal, and musculoskeletal symptoms may be offered.

B. **Surgical interventions.**
   1. Surgical excision of fast growing lesions is recommended, not only for cosmesis, but for threat of malignant degeneration.
   2. Surgical excision is also recommended for lesions with cosmetic or functional concerns.

IV. COMMON NURSING DIAGNOSES, OUTCOMES, AND INTERVENTIONS

A. **Nursing diagnosis: knowledge deficit related to surgical procedure, anesthesia, postsurgical expectations, and postoperative care.**
   1. Patient outcomes.
      a. Patient verbalizes an understanding of pre and postoperative procedures.
      b. Patient demonstrates postsurgical wound care.
   2. Interventions.
      a. Provide rationale for excision of lesions that are fast growing, impair function, or interfere with cosmetic appearance.
      b. Instruct patient on routine preoperative expectations including any presurgical diagnostic studies, time and approximate length of surgery, any food/fluid/drug restrictions prior to surgery, type of anesthesia to be used, and the general sensations (if any) that may be experienced during the procedure.
      c. Discuss postoperative pain control plan and wound care and instruct on signs and symptoms of infection. Review time, date, and purpose of first postoperative visit. Provide with emergency/followup phone numbers.
      d. Review any postoperative activity restrictions such as work, exercise, and bathing/grooming.

Table 2.
Nursing Care Plan for Patients with Body Image Disturbance

NURSING DIAGNOSIS: Body image disturbance related to chronic disease, skin changes, long-term treatment, immobility, and decreased ability to perform routine ADL/job/home functions.		
Outcomes	**Interventions**	**Home Care Considerations**
The patient: Accepts change in physical appearance and abilities. Verbalizes a positive and realistic self-image. Maximizes positive attributes, abilities, and skills. Identifies sources of family, community, and significant other support. Continues participation in family, social, and work activities.	Assess perception of self-image and allow/assist patient to express feelings related to the disease and its impact on self-image and daily life. Determine the extent of problem and assess for exaggerated or unrealistic feelings. Validate patient's express-ions rather than trying to diminish them (avoid statements such as "don't be silly, you don't look THAT bad"). Provide emotional support and guidance to patient and family. Assist in recognition of unreal-istic fears, self-image, or expectations. Deal with behavioral changes that include denial, anger, and dependence. Discuss ways to augment self-image with enhancements such as make-up, hair styles, and clothing. Address potential for sexual dysfunction related to decreased mobility, poor self-esteem, fatigue, dry vaginal mucosa. Refer to appropriate health practitioner. Provide positive reinforcement for actions/statements indicating improved body image. Encourage compliance with routine medical care and followup to maintain state of optimal health. Promote self-care: involve patient and family in planning care, and encourage active participation in all activities. Address any needed lifestyle changes and limitations with accompanying coping strategies.	Consider referral to individual counseling if indicated. Ensure patient and family have available support system within the community. Assure that appropriate followup plan is in place. Ensure adequate understanding of disease process, prescribed medical regimen, and appropriate followup care.

B. Nursing diagnosis: body image disturbance related to chronic, disfiguring illness, decreased mobility, and long-term treatment requirements (see Table 2).

V. HOME CARE CONSIDERATIONS

A. Assess ability to understand and comply with pre and postoperative instructions and care within the patient's cognitive and physical abilities.
B. Enlist family support and visiting nurse services as needed to ensure adequate postsurgical care.
C. Assess need to involve social services in view of chronicity of disease requiring multiple procedures over the life span.

LYMPHORETICULAR DISORDERS: SARCOIDOSIS

I. OVERVIEW

A. Definition: an inflammatory, granulomatous, multisystem disorder primarily affecting the lungs, liver, lymph nodes, spleen, skin, glandular tissues, and eyes.
B. Etiology is unknown but may be related to a variety of infectious agents in genetically predisposed individuals.
C. Pathophysiology.
    1. Lymphoreticular disorder characterized by several abnormal immune-related functions.
        a. Impaired delayed hypersensitivity.
        b. Imbalanced CD4/CD8 ratio.
        c. Hyperreactivity of B cells.
        d. Increased production of circulating immune complexes.
    2. In the presence of a causative antigen, an abnormal immune response among T-lymphocytes and macrophages/monocytes is initiated and sarcoidal granulomas ultimately develop in targeted tissues.
D. Incidence.
    1. Ranges from 11 to 40 per 100,000 people in the United States.
    2. Fourteen times more common in African Americans than Caucasians.
    3. In nonblack populations, the male:female ratio is approximately 1:1.
    4. In black populations, the male:female ratio is approximately 1:2.
E. Considerations across the life span.
    1. Onset is most common during ages 20 to 40.
    2. Sarcoidosis may regress spontaneously.

II. ASSESSMENT

A. History and physical exam.
    1. Up to one-third of patients are asymptomatic;

diagnosis is often incidentally made with chest x-ray demonstrating hilar adenopathy and pulmonary fibrosis.
    2. Patients should be questioned regarding systemic symptoms such as fatigue, weight loss, fever, malaise, and weakness.
B. Systemic involvement.
    1. Respiratory involvement (most common) includes hilar adenopathy and pulmonary parenchymal disease. Symptoms may include dyspnea, dry cough, hemoptysis, or pneumothorax.
    2. Ocular involvement, affecting 25% to 50% of patients, most commonly results in uveitis. Symptoms may include conjunctival injection, photophobia, and tearing.
    3. Lymph node and splenic involvement occurs in about 30% of patients. Lymphadenopathy and splenomegaly are often asymptomatic for the patient.
    4. Bone involvement occurs in 10% to 15% of patients, manifesting with cystic bone lesions. Patients complain of arthralgias and demonstrate arthritic changes. The wrists, knees, and ankles are most commonly affected.
    5. Neurologic involvement occurs in 5% to 15% of patients with systemic involvement. This most commonly manifests as optic nerve disease, facial nerve palsy, meningitis, and cerebral granulomas.
    6. Hepatic involvement may occur in about 20% of patients, but rarely produces functional difficulties. Liver function tests may be elevated.
    7. Cardiac involvement is considered common, although often asymptomatic. It may result in congestive heart failure, arrhythmia, or conduction defects.
    8. Other involvement may include granulomatous changes in kidneys, endocrine glands, stomach, bone marrow, spinal cord, and gonads.
C. Cutaneous manifestations.
    1. Erythema nodosum is a nonspecific lesion characterized by firm, red, subcutaneous nodules most commonly found on the anterior tibial surface.
    2. Specific cutaneous lesions (demonstrate noncaseating granulomas on histopathology).
        a. Papular lesions, 3 to 5 mm in diameter, are commonly found on head and neck. Lesions are flesh-colored to red to hyper/hypopigmented and they may coalesce to form annular plaques.
        b. Hutchinson's papillary psoriasis are deeper, cutaneous, plaque-type lesions. They occur anywhere on the body.
            (1) Lupus perino is the term used when these violaceous lesions are found symmetrically on the face and neck and

are telangiectatic.
  c. Scar sarcoidosis involves the infiltration of old scars with granulomatous lesions.
  d. Darier-Roussy sarcoidosis denotes asymptomatic subcutaneous plaques on the trunk and extremities.
D. **Differential diagnosis of cutaneous sarcoidosis includes granuloma annulare, syphilis, cutaneous T-cell lymphoma, lymphoma cutis, lupus erythematosus, and fungal/bacterial infections.**
E. Diagnostic tests.
  1. Chest x-ray.
  2. Skin biopsy demonstrates noncaseating epithelioid cell tubercles.
  3. Tissue biopsy for suspected organ involvement (lung, lymph node, liver, conjunctival, bone marrow, muscle, mediastinum).
  4. Laboratory tests may reveal elevated sedimentation rate, elevated gamma globulins, and increased levels of angiotensin-converting enzyme.

III. COMMON THERAPEUTIC MODALITIES

A. **High-potency topical corticosteroids bid may be helpful. If no effect after 4 weeks, intralesional steroids should be used.**
B. **Intralesional corticosteroids are generally more effective than topical therapy since the medication is more effectively delivered into the dermis.**
C. **Antimalarial agents (hydroxy chloroquine sulfate or chloroquine phosphate) may be helpful in cutaneous sarcoid.**
D. **Systemic corticosteroids are indicated for unresponsive and progressive ocular, pulmonary, neurologic, hypercalcemia, functional endocrine abnormalities, symptomatic cardiac involvement, or disfiguring skin manifestations. Care must be taken during the tapering process to avoid systemic disease flare-ups.**
E. **Other reported therapies that may be helpful include methotrexate, chlorambucil, and isotretinoin.**

IV. COMMON NURSING DIAGNOSES, OUTCOMES, AND INTERVENTIONS

A. **Anxiety related to chronic illness involving multiple body systems and treatment regimens.**
  1. Patient outcomes.
    a. The patient will verbalize decreased feelings of anxiety and demonstrate relaxed facial expression and body language.
    b. The patient reports adequate sleep, dietary, and socialization patterns.
  2. Interventions.
    a. Assess for signs and symptoms of anxiety such as poor appetite, abnormal vital signs,

sleeplessness, sweating, tremors, nervous mannerisms, and verbalizations of excessive anxiety.
    b. Encourage patient to discuss fears and concerns in a calm, nonjudgemental approach.
    c. Point out any unrealistic fears and identify concrete methods to deal with anxiety.
    d. Explain disease process, treatment, and long-term management in a calm, unhurried manner. Encourage patient and family to become active participants in care.
    e. Provide means for patient to gain some control over situation (provide with a thorough orientation to clinic and clinic staff and provide educational material and resources to promote understanding of disease).
    f. When possible, maintain consistency in physicians and staff who are providing direct care.
    g. Encourage questions and clarify information as needed. Encourage the involvement and support of family/significant other.
    h. Assess need for antianxiety agents if above measures are not successful.

V. HOME CARE CONSIDERATIONS

A. **Assess need for social service involvement.**
B. **Ensure appropriate followup care is maintained with multidisciplinary health care members as appropriate.**

GRAFT-VERSUS-HOST DISEASE

I. **OVERVIEW (see Table 3 and Figures 8-6 to 8-14, pages 236-237).**

BEHCET'S DISEASE

I. **OVERVIEW**

A. **Definition: chronic disorder involving mucocutaneous tissues characterized by a triad of oral and genital ulcerations and inflammatory involvement/disease of the eyes and possible systemic inflammatory changes (see Figures 8-15 & 8-16, page 237).**
B. **Etiology/pathophysiology: etiology is unknown.**
  1. Related to abnormalities in humoral and cellular immunity.
  2. Antimucosal antibodies present in serum.
  3. Circulating immune complexes associated in some patients to disease activity but unrelated to duration or affected area.
  4. Cell-mediated hypersensitivity linked to

Table 3.
Graft-Versus-Host Disease (GVHD)

Type and Definition	Etiology/ Pathology	Diagnosis	Skin Changes	Systemic Symptoms	Treatment	Nursing Care/ Comments
Acute GVHD: An immunologic reaction to host tissue that occurs from within 1 week to 3 months of transfer of immuno-competent cells to an immunoin-competent host (most common during a bone marrow transplant or solid organ liver transplant).	More severe reactions and incidence linked to allogeneic (between two people) mismatch of donor marrow or solid organ, older age, and type of preparation for transplant. Skin change is usually most common and earliest effect seen and occurs within first 3 months of transplant, but typically is seen in first 10 to 30 days. Progression of disease occurs over several weeks; liver and GI tract are commonly involved.	Based on onset of clinical lesions, clinical picture, and dif-ferential diag-nosis. Exclusion of: TEN, drug eruption, viral exanthem, and transient acan-tholytic der-matosis. Histopathology may show basal vacuolization, necrotic epider-mal/dermal lym-phocytes and separation, and subepidermal cleft formation.	Erythematous perifollicular or macular rash that commonly starts on pinna, palms, and soles then progresses to trunk and extremities. four stages of skin involvement: Stage 1: <25% Stage 2: >25% Stage 3: Erythroderma Stage 4: Vesicles and bullae Eye and mucous membranes are less commonly affected in acute stage.	Ill-appearing with fever, diarrhea, elevated LFTs, hepatomegaly, +/- jaundice, eyes may be affected.	Prevention: Premedicate with FK506, cyclosporine, and pretrans-plant manipula-tion of the grafted marrow to produce T-lymphocyte depletion. Skin directed: topical steroids, PUVA. Systemic treat-ment for > Stage 1: sys-temic steroids, FK506 or cyclosporine, anti-thymocyte globulin, mon-oclonal anti-bodies.	High risk for sepsis and severe fluid and electrolyte disturbances. Nutritional and fluid management along with intensive skin care are essential. Patient/family education and support.
Chronic lichenoid: As above but usually occurs after 2 to 3 months. Exact adher-ence to time lines in acute vs. chronic is discouraged.	Manifestation of faulty regulation of host immune system. Occurs 60 to 90 days post transplant; usually preceeds chronic sclerodermoid but there is much overlap among GVHD presentations. A graft vs. tumor effect decreases incidence of relapse.	Clinical symp-toms and history: Skin lesions resemble lichen planus. Histopathology commonly involves acan-thosis, ortho-ridges, basal vacuolization, necrotic epider-mal cells, and melanophages in upper der-mis.	Lichen-planus like with red to purple irregular shaped papules on flexor sur-faces. White, lacy patches on oral mucosa. Skin lesions resolve with postinflamma-tory hyperpig-mentation.	Joint contractures. Nutritional deficits.	Systemic: Combinations of steroids, cyclosporine, azathioprine, and thalido-mide. Photochemo-therapy such as PUVA and/or photopheresis may be helpful. May require chronic antibiot-ic prophylaxis.	Severe systemic infections are most common cause of death. Obtain periodic bacterial and fungal cultures. Intensive skin, eye, and mouth care are critical. Requires outpatient support for occupational and physical therapy, nutrition. Patient/family education and support. See also: Nursing Care in Table 2, and as described for sarcoidosis.

Table 3. (continued)
Graft-Versus-Host Disease (GVHD)

Type and Definition	Etiology/ Pathology	Diagnosis	Skin Changes	Systemic Symptoms	Treatment	Nursing Care/ Comments
Chronic sclerodermoid: As above, but usually occurs after 2 to 3 months. Exact adherence to time lines in acute vs. chronic is discouraged.	Manifestation of faulty regulation of host immune system. Occurs 60 to 90 days post transplant. A graft vs. tumor effect decreases incidence of relapse.	Clinical symptoms and history: Abnormal LFTs eosinophilia autoantibody formation, hypergamma-globulinemia. Histopathology commonly involves thick collagen bundles with loss of interstices, eccrine coil entrapment, loss of pilosebaceous anatomy, and lacrimal/salivary gland lymphocyte infiltration.	Resembles scleroderma with plaques of shiny, atrophic, thickened skin and hyper/hypopig-mentation; Erosions due to skin ischemia; Alopecia, nail dystrophy, and recurrent bacterial skin infections. In some cases, the skin may be normal but the underlying tissue (fascia) is hard.	Widespread disease may lead to joint contractures, fasciitis, general wasting, esophagitis, sicca symptoms (dry mouth and eyes), and pulmonary fibrosis.	Systemic and photochemo-therapies as above. Etretinate. May require chronic antibiot-ic prophylaxis. Pentoxifylline may be helpful for chronic skin erosions and ulcerations.	See comments for Chronic Lichenoid.

aphthous ulcers.
5. Characterized by erratic exacerbations.
6. May be genetic inherited component in susceptible individuals (HLA-B51 gene).
7. Repeated bacterial (streptococcal) or viral (herpes simplex I) infections may be linked as causative trigger.

C. **Incidence**
1. Evident worldwide but more prevalent in "Silk Road" regions of Mediterranean basin, Asia, Japan, and Middle East.
2. Disease triad more frequently found in men for mid-east and Asian countries. In the United States and western Europe, it is more common in women.
3. Incidence equalizes in men and women for Behcet's involving only oral and genital mucosa.

D. **Considerations across the life span.**
1. All ages are affected, but more common in 2nd and 3rd decades of life.

II. **ASSESSMENT**

A. **History and physical exam.**
1. Assess for incidence of trauma-induced lesions (pathergy).
2. Typical course starts with aphthous stomatitis

and genital ulceration accompanied by systemic symptoms.
3. Encourage patients to keep log of where and when symptoms occur to assist in diagnosis and treatment as signs and symptoms may not be present at time of clinician examination. Photographs are also helpful.

B. **Differential diagnosis includes aphthous stomatitis, erythema nodosum, erythema multiforme, acute febrile neutrophilic dermatosis, panniculitis, nodular or pustular acne, herpes simplex, acute lupus erythematous, furunculosis, folliculitis, pyoderma gangrenosum, Sweet's disease, Crohn's disease, Reiter's syndrome.**

C. **Diagnosis is based on triad of oral ulcerations accompanied by any two manifestations listed below in 1 to 4.**
1. Genital ulcers (men: scrotum; women: vulva).
2. Eye lesions.
3. Skin lesions.
4. Positive testing for pathergy: trauma-induced papule > 2 mm within 48 hours following 20 to 22 gauge needle prick (most common in Mediterranean and Middle East).
5. Histology is nonspecific but vasculitis is present and there is commonly a majority of help-inducer T-cells over T-suppressor-cytotoxic cells.

D. Skin changes/clinical manifestations.
1. Aphthous lesions begin as vesicles or pustules and generally heal with scar tissue while deeper lesions begin as submucosal or dermal nodules that heal via scar formation.
2. Three typical ulcerative presentations commonly seen on lips, gums, cheeks, and tongue with severe cases also affecting the pharynx and soft palate.
   a. Superficial, gray erosions (similar to canker sores).
   b. Deeply punched-out erosions (similar to periadenitis mucosa necrotica recurrens — Sutton's disease).
   c. Superficial, herpetiform punctate erosions (rare).
3. Other mucosal involvement may include the esophagus, stomach, intestine, and anus, further complicated by perforation.
4. Eye involvement most common cause of morbidity and usually presents unilaterally as iritis or uveitis and hypopyon (uncommon hallmark) but eventually progresses to bilateral disease followed by blindness.
5. Erythematous pustules, papules, and/or erythema nodosum-like lesions (most common) may present on legs, torso, and face may be trauma induced (pathergy).
   a. Trauma-induced lesions less common in United States.
   b. Nodules often ulcerate.
E. Systemic manifestations.
1. Arthralgias.
2. Asymetrical synovitis.
3. Noninflammatory large joint effusions.
4. Superficial and deep thrombophlebitis.
5. Phlebitis of retinal veins, dural sinuses, and superior and inferior vena cavae.
6. Gastrointestinal ulceration.
7. Central nervous system involvement with meningioencephalitis, resulting in headaches, stiff neck, and poor coordination.
8. Lung involvement with artery aneurysm development and/or pleuritis.
9. Renal function abnormalities.
10. Cardiac vessel disease.

III. COMMON THERAPEUTIC MODALITIES

A. Treatment is aimed at controlling symptoms, decreasing discomfort, and preventing complications.
B. Multidisciplinary approach is necessary and includes dermatologist, rheumatologist, urologist, gynecologist, opthamologist, gastroenterologist, and neurologist.
C. Exercise such as swimming or walking is recommended during remissions; rest is required during flare episodes.
D. Surgical intervention may be needed for eye, gastrointestinal, or cardiac involvement.
E. Topical steroids, topical anesthetics, and antibiotic (tetracycline) and anesthetic mouthwashes are helpful for skin and mucosal lesions.
F. Systemic steroids are a mainstay of therapy and are often used in combination with other therapies.
G. Nonsteroidal anti-inflammatory drugs include levamisole, colchicine, dapsone, and sulfapyridine — helpful for mucosal and/or arthritic symptoms.
H. Immunosuppressants.
1. Azathioprine, cyclosporine, and FK506 may be used for eye and CNS involvement.
2. Cyclophosphamide and chlorambucil (alkylating agents).
3. Methotrexate.
I. Immunomodulators include thalidomide for mucosal involvement (cautious use due to its teratogenic effects) and interferon-alpha 2A and B.
J. Anticoagulants for thromboses.
K. Trental® (pentoxifylline) helpful in some cases for vascular symptoms.
L. Sucralfate capsules or slurry helpful in short-term protection of GI mucosal surfaces.

IV. COMMON NURSING DIAGNOSES, OUTCOMES, AND INTERVENTIONS

A. Nursing diagnosis: anxiety related to chronic and variable disease.
B. Outcomes: patient demonstrates decreased anxiety with increased knowledge, well-being, and independence in self-care related to Bechet's disease.
C. Interventions.
1. Provide education on diagnosis and local/systemic treatment.
2. Encourage use of diaries and photographs to document disease changes, especially if the diagnosis is in question.
3. Assist with coordination of multidisciplinary approach and ensure good communication among all health care team members.
4. Assess for depression and need for individual/family counseling related to stressors of living with a chronic illness.
5. Assess pain level and provide adequate pain control measures (see also pyoderma gangrenosum).
6. Encourage involvement with national/community support systems and information sources such as the American Behcet's Disease Association (ABDA), Arthritis

Foundation, and National Arthritis and Musculoskeletal and Skin Diseases Information Clearinghouse (NAMSIC).

7. Encourage an established joint-sparing exercise regimen during periods of remission.

PYODERMA GANGRENOSUM

I. OVERVIEW

A. **Definition: destructive, chronic, inflammatory skin disorder in which painful nodules or pustules break down to form a progressively enlarging ulcer.**

B. **Etiology.**
   1. Exact etiology is unknown.
   2. Autoimmune mechanism and/or an altered response to inflammation is frequently involved.
   3. Associated, in about 50% of cases, with systemic disorders such as Crohn's disease, ulcerative colitis, polyarthritis.
   4. Early lesions are sterile, therefore, it is not an infectious process.

C. **Pathophysiology**
   1. Exaggerated and uncontrolled inflammatory response to nonspecific stimuli.
   2. Gram negative and gram positive organisms may be cultured from ulcerated lesions.
   3. New lesions may develop after minimal trauma in about one-third of patients (pathergy).

D. **Incidence: rare, occurs worldwide, and affects both sexes equally at any age.**

II. ASSESSMENT

A. **History and physical exam.**
   1. Assess for underlying, associated disorders and its current status (active Crohn's disease).
   2. Assess for incidence of trauma-induced lesions.
   3. Assess for hallmark lesions described below.

B. **Diagnostic tests: none are diagnostic; diagnosis is one of exclusion.**
   1. Differential diagnoses include brown recluse spider bite, tropical ulcer, deep fungal or bacterial infection, osteomyelitis, necrotizing vasculitis, tertiary syphilis, and factitial ulcers.
   2. Laboratory tests may show increased sedimentation rate, leukocytosis, anemia, decreased serum iron, and hypo/hyperglobulinemia.
   3. Nonspecific histopathology findings show edema, predominate neutrophilic infiltrates, necrosis, and hemorrhage.

C. **Skin changes/clinical manifestations.**
   1. Hallmark lesion is an irregular ulcer with raised, inflammatory border and boggy, necrotic base.
      a. Ulcers have purple or dusky red, irregular, elevated borders (hallmark sign).
      b. Undermining of ulcers present.
      c. Halo of erythema present at advancing margin.
      d. Base of ulcer may be necrotic.
      e. May extend into the fat or even further into the fascia.
      f. Common sites include lower extremities, abdomen, and buttocks where lesions may develop de novo, at site of previous lesion, scar tissue, stoma, or from trauma.
      g. Lesions heal with a classic cribiform scar.
   2. Evolution of ulcer from primary lesion involves superficial, hemmorhagic pustule or deep-seated, painful nodule.
      a. May arise after tissue trauma. Minor trauma (injections, bug bites) or major trauma (biopsy, surgery) induce lesions (pathergy).
      b. Primary lesions break down and ulcerate.
      c. Lesions exude hemorrhagic and purulent material.
   3. Onset may be explosive with rapid spread, characterized by very painful lesions, fever, hemorrhagic blisters, suppuration, extensive necrosis, and soggy ulcerations with an inflammatory halo.
   4. Indolent form involves massive granulation within ulcer at onset, crusting and hyperkeratosis, slow spread, and spontaneous resolution.
   5. Clinical variants.
      a. Superficial granulomatous pyoderma is localized and limited with vegetative, verrucous, and ulcerative lesions.
      b. Malignant pyoderma is located primarily on the head and neck and is not associated with systemic disease. The lesions also lack erythema and undermining.
      c. Pyostomatitis vegetans is a pustular, vegetative process involving oral mucous membranes. It is associated with ulcerative and vegetative skin lesions and inflammatory bowel disease.
      d. Atypical bullous pyoderma gangrenosum has an acute onset that heralds preleukemic or leukemic states. The lesions are superficial, steadily enlarging soft purple papules and blue-grey, hemorrhagic bullous lesions.
   6. Systemic manifestations include associated toxicity, malaise, pain, and fever.

III. COMMON THERAPEUTIC MODALITIES

A. **Directed at treatment of underlying illness or secondary infection, promotion of healing, prevention of new lesions, and pain management during acute inflammatory periods.**

B. **Local/topical treatment in disease not associated**

with a systemic disease.
1. Intralesional steroids.
2. 2% disodium cromoglycate.
3. Anecdotal therapies such as hyperbaric oxygen, topical nitrogen mustard, thalidomide, potassium iodide, and intralesional cyclosporine are reserved for resistant disease or patient intolerance for standard therapy.
4. Ulcer care includes gentle cleaning, prevention of bacterial overgrowth, saline compresses/whirlpool baths, and judicious use of surgical debridement to avoid trauma induction of new lesions.

C. Systemic treatment.
1. Corticosteroids.
   a. High tapering doses starting at 100 to 200 mg daily to halt progression or prevent new lesions from developing.
   b. Pulse therapy with methylprednisolone.
2. Sulfa drugs (dapsone, sulfapyridine, sulfasalazine).
   a. Use in combination with steroids initially.
   b. Start with 4 to 6 grams tapering to 0.5 to 1.0 grams as maintenance.
3. Immunosuppressants.
   a. Cyclosporine (6 to 10 mg/kg/d) — often combined with steroids.
   b. Azathioprine — moderate success.
   c. 6-mercaptopurine — moderate success.
4. Clofazimine (200 to 300 mg/d).
   a. Stops progression within 1 to 2 weeks.
   b. Complete or partial healing seen in 2 to 5 months.
5. Miscellaneous treatments.
   a. Minocycline.
   b. IV vancomycin and mezlocillin.
   c. Plasma exchange.

IV. COMMON NURSING DIAGNOSES, OUTCOMES, AND INTERVENTIONS

A. Nursing diagnosis: pain related to acute inflammation of ulcerative skin lesions.
B. Patient outcomes.
1. Patient is able to verbalize effective pain control measures.
2. Patient verbalizes increased comfort.
C. Interventions
1. At each patient interaction, assess for potential pain utilizing Joint Commission on Accreditation of Healthcare Organizations (JCAHO) standards.
   a. Pain intensity (based on 0 to 10 scale).
   b. Location.
   c. Quality.
   d. Onset, duration, variation, and patterns.
   e. Alleviating and aggravating factors.
   f. Current pain management regimen and its effectiveness.
   g. Pain management history.
   h. Effects of pain on daily life activities.
   i. Pain relief goal.
   j. Examination of painful site(s).
2. Administer appropriate pain control medications such as nonsteroidal anti-inflammatory agents, acetaminophen, or opioids.
   a. Pain medications may be needed until inflammation subsides.
   b. Assess for effectiveness of pain control.
3. Patient and family member education.
   a. Self-management techniques such as imagery, distraction, and relaxation.
   b. Prescribed medications, expected effects, and patient role in managing/reporting pain.
   c. Injury avoidance strategies for lesion prevention.
   d. Signs and symptoms of inflammation and infection.

Bibliography
Callen, J.P., & Fabre, V.C. (1995). Cutaneous manifestations of systemic diseases. In S.C. Moschella & H.J. Hurley (Eds.), *Dermatology* (pp. 1682-1718). Philadelphia: W.B. Saunders.
Dunwoody, C., McCann, S., & Zumbo, M. (1999). Pyoderma gangrenosum: A case study for pain management in dermatology nursing. *Dermatology Nursing, 11* (4), 1-8.
Gawkrodger, D. (1998). Sarcoidosis. In R. Champion, J. Burton, D. Burns, & S. Breathnach (Eds.), *Textbook of dermatology* (pp. 2679-2702). Oxford, England: Blackwell Science Ltd.
Horn, T. (1999). Graft-versus-host disease. In T.B. Fitzpatrick, A.Z. Eisen, K. Wolff, I. Freedberg, & K. Austen (Eds.), *Dermatology in general medicine* (pp. 1426-1434). New York: McGraw-Hill.
Meador, R., Ehrlich, G., & Von Feldt, J. (2002). Behcet's disease: Immunopathologic and therapeutic aspects. *Current Rheumatology Reports, 4*(1), 47-54.
Weismann, K. & Graham, R. (1998). Systemic disease and the skin. In R. Champion, J. Burton, D. Burns, & S. Breathnach (Eds.), *Textbook of dermatology* (pp. 2703-2757). Oxford, England: Blackwell Science Ltd.
Wolff, K., & Stingl, G. (1999). Pyoderma gangrenosum. In T.B. Fitzpatrick, A.Z. Eisen, K. Wolff, I. Freedberg, & K. Austen (Eds.), *Dermatology in general medicine* (pp. 1140-1147). New York: McGraw-Hill.

1. A possible cutaneous sign of a systemic malignancy includes which of the following?
   a. Rosacea.
   b. Exfoliative erythroderma.
   c. Miliaria rubra.
   d. Onychomycosis.

2. Skin changes in chronic graft-versus-host disease are due to which pathologic feature?
   a. Widespread bacterial infection.
   b. Tumor effect.
   c. Abnormal immune reaction.
   d. Excessive cell turnover.

3. Chronic graft-versus-host disease is characterized by all of the following features except:
   a. Onset within one week of transplant.
   b. May be lichenoid or scerodermoid.
   c. Joints are often affected with contractures.
   d. Sicca symptoms common.

4. Which of the following phrases describing Behcet's disease is false?
   a. More prevalent in "Silk Road" region.
   b. Etiology is related to humoral and cellular immune abnormalities.
   c. Disease course is severe and constant.
   d. Eye involvement is most common cause of morbidity.

5. Behcet's disease is characterized by all of the following except:
   a. Apthous stomatitis.
   b. Coronary artery disease.
   c. Uveitis.
   d. Acanthosis nigricans.

6. A skin finding with sudden onset, associated with abdominal carcinomas and known as the sign of Leser-Trélat is which of the following?
   a. Hypertrichosis.
   b. Multiple abdominal telangiectasia.
   c. Extensive erythema nodusum.
   d. Multiple seborrheic keratoses.

7. The differential diagnosis for skin lesions typically seen in leukemia or lymphoma include which of the following?
   a. Lymphomatoid papulosis.
   b. Actinic reticuloid.
   c. Fungal infection.
   d. All of the above.

8. Common skin, nail, and hair changes in primary hypothyroidism include all of the following except:
   a. Hyperhidrosis.
   b. Xanthomatosis.
   c. Ecchymoses/telagiectasias.
   d. Coarse and brittle hair.

9. Which of the following statements regarding diabetes mellitus Type 1 and 2 is false?
   a. Vascular disease leads to poor circulation, ulcerations, or gangrene.
   b. Skin infections are uncommon since immune system remains intact.
   c. Lipodystrophy may occur related to subcutaneous injection complications.
   d. Acanthosis nigricans may be seen in intertriginous areas.

10. Type 1 neurofibromatosis is characterized by all of the following except:
    a. Axillary or inguinal freckling.
    b. Spenoid bone dysplasia.
    c. Linked to chromosome 22.
    d. Six or more Cafe au lait macules.

11. Common therapeutic modalities for sarcoidosis include all of the following except:
    a. Intralesional steroids.
    b. Systemic antibiotics.
    c. Systemic steroids.
    d. Antimalarial agents.

12. Which of the following statements regarding pyoderma gangrenosum is true?
    a. Etiology is related to an infectious process.
    b. Trauma can induce new lesions.
    c. Primary lesion is a blister.
    d. Lesions are ulcerative and painless.

13. The hallmark lesion in pyoderma gangrenosum is:
    a. Superficial blister with halo of erythema.
    b. Irregular, asymetrical, indurated plaques with bound down dermis.
    c. Cyanotic and clubbed digits.
    d. Ulcer with raised, inflamed borders and necrotic base.

14. Trousseau's syndrome (superficial migratory thrombophlebitis) is associated with which possible malignancy?
    a. Leukemia.
    b. Breast cancer.
    c. Pancreatic cancer.
    d. Ovarian cancer.

Answers to Study Questions

1.	b	6.	d	11.	b
2.	c	7.	d	12.	b
3.	a	8.	a	13.	d
4.	c	9.	b	14.	c
5.	d	10.	c		

DNAP308

CE Answer/Evaluation Form

Chapter 8.
Cutaneous Manifestations of Systemic Disease

Please photocopy this test page and return.

COMPLETE THE FOLLOWING:

Name: _____

Address: _____

City: _____ State: _____ Zip: _____

Preferred telephone: (Home)_____ (Work) _____

State where licensed and license number: _____

CE application fee: DNA member $13.00
                        Nonmember $16.00

POSTTEST INSTRUCTIONS
1. To receive continuing education credit for individual study after reading the article, complete the answer/evaluation form below.
2. Photocopy and send the answer/evaluation form along with a check or money order payable to **Dermatology Nurses' Association** to: **DNA**, East Holly Avenue Box 56, Pitman, NJ 08071-0056.
3. Test returns must be postmarked by December 31, 2008. Upon completion of the answer/evaluation form, a certificate for 3.7 contact hour(s) will be awarded and sent to you.

This chapter was reviewed and formatted for contact hour credit by Marcia J. Hill, MSN, RN, Core Curriculum Editor; and Sally Russell, MN, RN,C, DNA Education Director.

ANSWER FORM

1. Name one new detail (item, issue, or phenomenon) that you learned by completing this activity.

   _____

   _____

   _____

2. How will you apply the information from this learning activity to your practice?
   a. Patient education.
   b. Staff education.
   c. Improve my patient care.
   d. In my education course work.
   e. Other: Please describe _____

   _____

   _____

Evaluation

	Strongly disagree				Strongly agree
3. The offering met the stated objectives.					
a. Identify at least five systemic disorders demonstrating significant cutaneous signs and symptoms.	1	2	3	4	5
b. Describe the cutaneous signs and symptoms common to leukemia/lymphoma.	1	2	3	4	5
c. Discuss the potential skin alterations in the patient with sarcoidosis, hypothyroidism, Behcet's disease, pyoderma gangrenosum, graft-versus-host disease, and diabetes millitus.	1	2	3	4	5
d. List at least five cutaneous signs of possible internal malignancy.	1	2	3	4	5
e. Discuss nursing care for the patient with body image disturbance.	1	2	3	4	5
f. Identify common therapeutic modalities for systemic illness with cutaneous manifestations.	1	2	3	4	5
4. The content was current and relevant.	1	2	3	4	5
5. The content was presented clearly.	1	2	3	4	5
6. The content was covered adequately.	1	2	3	4	5
7. I am more confident of my abilities since completing this material.	1	2	3	4	5

8. The material was (check one) ☐ new, ☐ review for me.

Comments _____

9. Time required to complete reading assignment: _____ minutes

This independent study is provided by the Dermatology Nurses' Association (DNA) for 3.7 contact hours. DNA is accredited as a provider of continuing education in nursing by the American Nurses Credentialing Center's Commission on Accreditation. DNA is approved as a provider of continuing education by the California Board of Registered Nursing Provider #CEP5708.

Connective Tissue Disorders

Lynn A. Babin, MSN, RN, CNS, AAS

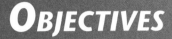

OBJECTIVES

At the end of this chapter, the reader will be able to:
- Identify and differentiate several connective tissue disorders.
- Discuss treatment modalities for the most common connective tissue disorders.
- List several important patient education aspects for each disorder.
- Provide a list of patient resources on connective tissue disorders.

KEY POINTS

- Early diagnosis and treatment may significantly slow the connective tissue disease process and increase patients' quality of life.
- A complete physical exam and physiological assessment should be completed if a collagen vascular disease is suspected due to possible misdiagnosis and to capture any central nervous system involvement.
- Patient education and support are vital to treatment compliance.
- Encourage patients to join support groups and organizations.

Connective Tissue Disorders

Lynn A. Babin, MSN, RN, CNS, AAS

OVERVIEW

Connective tissue disorders (collagen vascular disease) is defined as a group of acquired disorders that have the commonality of immunologic and inflammatory changes in small blood vessels and connective tissue. Common features may include arthritis, skin lesions, iritis and episcleritis, pericarditis, pleuritis, subcutaneous nodules, myocarditis, vasculitis, and nephritis. Lupus, scleroderma, and myositis will be discussed in this chapter.

I. LUPUS

A. Definition: Lupus is a chronic autoimmune disease resulting in inflammation and tissue damage. The name "Lupus," Latin for wolf, was coined in the 10th century possibly because the lesions resembled wolf bites.

B. Etiology.
   1. The exact cause of lupus is unknown; however, current research points to interrelated immunologic, environmental, hormonal, and genetic factors.
   2. 98% of babies born with neonatal lupus erythematosus (NLE) were reported to have anti-Ro antibodies, and approximately one-third with La antibodies. These IgG antibodies pass from the placenta to the fetus.
   3. Recent studies are looking at chromosome 1 for a genetic link; however, only 10% of lupus patients will have a close relative with lupus. About 5% of children born to individuals with lupus will develop the disease.
   4. Often called a "woman's disease," lupus strikes women 10 to 15 times more frequently than men, and occurs most often during childbearing years.
   5. Although the disease occurs worldwide, it is most prevalent in persons with African, American Indian, and Asian origins.

C. Symptoms: (Frequency of occurrence according to the Lupus Foundation of America, Inc.).
   1. Arthralgia (95%).
   2. Fever >100° F (90%).
   3. Arthritis (90%).
   4. Prolonged or extreme fatigue (81%).
   5. Skin rashes (74%).
   6. Anemia (71%).
   7. Kidney involvement (50%).
   8. Pleurisy (45%).
   9. Butterfly-shaped (malar) rash across the cheeks and nose (42%).
   10. Symptoms occurring < 30% include photosensitivity, hair loss, mouth or nose ulcers, abnormal blood clotting problems, Raynaud's phenomenon, and seizures.

D. Four types of lupus.
   1. Cutaneous lupus erythematosus: has many different types including:
      a. Chronic cutaneous lupus erythematosus (CCLE).
         (1) Most common form of CCLE is discoid lupus erythematosus (DLE) (see Figure 9-1, page 238).
            (a) DLE lesions are often red, scaly, and thickened and may produce scarring or discoloration of the skin; usually painless and do not itch.
            (b) *Localized DLE*: lesions limited to head (possible alopecia), ears, and neck.
            (c) *Generalized DLE*: lesions present anywhere on skin.
            (d) Long-standing lesions are at risk for skin cancer.
         (2) Hypertrophic (thickened) or verrucous (wart-like) LE.
         (3) Lupus profundus: DLE lesions occurring in conjunction firm lumps in the fatty tissue (panniculitis).
         (4) Mucosal DLE: lesions that occur in mucous membranes of mouth, nose, and eyes.
      b. Subacute cutaneous lupus erythematosus (SCLE) (see Figure 9-2, page 238).
         (1) Papulosquamous: erythematous plaques.
            (a) May resemble psoriasis.
            (b) Most common on sun-exposed areas of arms, shoulders, neck and trunk; face less frequently involved.
         (2) Erythemic annular lesions.
         (3) Both forms are photosensitive to natural and artificial light.
         (4) Lesions usually do not scar, but may cause discoloration of skin.
      c. Acute cutaneous lupus erythematosus (ACLE).
         (1) Produces flat erythemic areas resembling sunburn.
         (2) *Localized ACLE* involves both cheeks and nose presenting as a butterfly-shaped malar rash.
         (3) *Generalized ACLE* presents with widespread erythemic patches on the arms, legs, and trunk.
   2. Systemic lupus erythematosus (SLE) attacks multiple systems in the body which may

Table 1.
The Criteria for the Diagnosis of Systemic Lupus Erythematosus (SLE).
Four or more must be present during the course of the disease to suspect lupus.
(From the American College of Rheumatology)

❏ Malar or discoiod rash

❏ Photosensitivity

❏ Oral or nasopharyngeal ulcerations

❏ Nonerosive arthritis (of two or more peripheral joints)

❏ Pleuritis or pericarditis

❏ Profuse proteinuria (more than 1.5 g/day) or excessive cellular casts in the urine

❏ Seizures or psychoses

❏ Hemolytic anemia, leukopenia, lymphopenia, or thrombocytopenia

❏ Anti-double-stranded deoxyribonucleic acid or anti-Smith antibody test or positive findings of antiphospholipid antibodies (elevated IgG or IgM anticariolipin antibodies, positive test for lupus anicoagulant, or false-positive serologic test results for syphilis)

❏ Abnormal antinuclear antibody titer

include: the skin (classic butterfly-shaped malar rash most common), liver, joints, lungs, blood vessels, heart, kidneys, liver, brain, and the nervous system (see Figure 9-3, page 238).
3. Drug-induced lupus may develop after taking certain medications. Symptoms usually resolve weeks to months after discontinuation of the drug.
4. Neonatal lupus erythematosus (NLE) (see Figures 1-3).
   a. NLE is rare.
   b. Occurs in neonates with transplacentally acquired maternal anti-Ro (SS-A) and/or anti-La (SS-B) antibodies.
   c. Manifestations may include:
      (1) Congenital heart block.
      (2) Cutaneous lesions.
      (3) Liver disease.
      (4) Thrombocytopenia.
E. **Lupus as a disease continuum.**
   1. CCLE is seen as the mild end of the spectrum with only localized lesions.
   2. SCLE present with mild SLE.
   3. Active SLE with internal organ involvement (possible death), with or without skin lesions, is at the far end of the disease spectrum.
F. **Diagnosis.**
   1. A *complete history and physical* should be performed, including a full-skin assessment.
   2. *Currently, there is no single definitive laboratory test for lupus.*

3. Lupus symptoms can mimic other illnesses and are often vague and transient, resulting in misdiagnosing and under-diagnosing of lupus.
4. The American College of Rheumatology has issued a list of criteria to assist the practioner in diagnosing SLE, and to establish consistency for epidemiologic surveys (see Table 1).
G. **Pregnancy and lupus.**
   1. There is no absolute reason why a woman with lupus should not become pregnant, *unless* she has organ involvement.
   2. There is risk of disease activity during and 3 to 4 weeks after pregnancy; therefore, she should be monitored closely.
   3. Many persons with lupus have antiphospholipid antibodies, which affect coagulation factors and are associated with miscarriage.
H. **Diagnostic testing may include:**
   1. CBC with differential.
   2. Platelet count.
   3. Erythrocyte sedimentation rate.
   4. Serum electrophoresis.
   5. Antinuclear antibodies (ANA) and lupus erythematosus cell tests.
   6. Anti-double-stranded deoxyribonucleic acid antibody (anti-dsDNA): this is the most specific test for lupus and correlates with disease activity.
   7. Urine studies.
   8. C3 and C4 serum studies.
   9. Chest X-rays.

Figure 1.
Neonate with Scaly Annular Lesions of NLE on the Face and Scalp

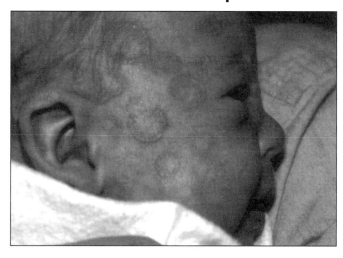

Figure 2.
Close-Up of Scalp Lesion

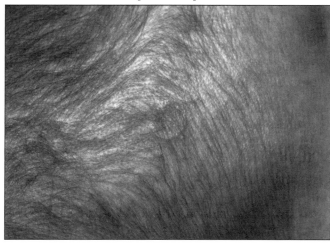

Figure 3.
The Classic "Owl-Eye" Distribution in Neonates with NLE

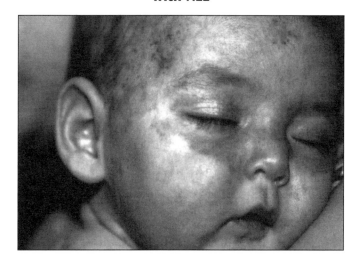

10. Kidney biopsy.
11. Lupus anticoagulant and anticariolipin tests.

I. Treatment.
   1. *Prevention is key* to minimizing symptoms, reducing inflammation, and maintaining normal bodily functions.
      a. Avoid sun exposure/wear sunscreen to prevent rashes.
      b. Exercise regularly to prevent muscle weakness and fatigue.
      c. Participate in support groups, counseling, etc. to reduce stress.
      d. Eliminate negative habits, such as smoking, drinking, etc.
   2. Treatment is individualized and based upon presenting symptoms.
   3. Medications may include:
      a. Nonsteroidal anti-inflammatory drugs (NSAIDs).
      b. Acetaminophen.
      c. Corticosteroids (topical, systemic, or intralesional).
      d. Anticoagulants.
      e. Antihypertensives and/or dietary changes.
      f. Cytotoxic therapy.
      g. Antimalarials.
      h. Dialysis or kidney transplant for renal failure.
      i. Investigational drugs are currently being studied in clinical trials, and include hormone modifiers, more selective immunosuppressive drugs, and biologic agents.

J. Nursing considerations (see Table 2).
   1. Patient education: most significant nursing role.
      a. Provide a comprehensible explanation of disease process/etiology to patient and family.
      b. Discuss possible medication side effects and importance of reporting these to nurse/practitioner. Stress significance of compliance with drug regimen.
      c. Acknowledge emotional stress and provide support.
      d. Provide patient and family with information on support organizations/foundations. (See resource list at end of chapter).
      e. Encourage good nutrition to promote wound healing and well-being.
      f. Reinforce the need for routine evaluations and skin assessments.

II. SCLERODERMA (SYSTEMIC SCLEROSIS)

A. Definition: according to the Scleroderma Foundation, scleroderma (which literally means "hard skin") is a chronic, often progressive autoimmune disease, which can cause thickening and tightening of the skin by excessive collagen

Table 2.
Common Nursing Diagnoses, Outcomes, and Interventions for the Patient with Connective Tissue Disorders

Nusing Diagnoses	Outcomes	Interventions
Impaired skin integrity related to inflammatory process.	Skin integrity is improved/maintained. No evidence of infection.	Assess lesions, obtain debridement as necessary; apply medications/ emollients as indicated. Elevate affected extremity(s). Monitor closely for signs/symptoms of infection.
Pain related to inflammation.	Pain is relieved; inflammation decreased.	Administer anti-inflammatory medications as indicated; assess and record level of discomfort; intervene appropiately (elevation, compresses, rest, medications).
Impaired mobility related to inflammation and pain.	Mobility is increased.	Assess restrictions; administer analgesics/anti-inflammatory medications as indicated; perform ROM exercises; refer to PT if appropriate.
Self-esteem disturbance related to body image changes, decreased self-esteem, and helplessness.	Patient will express positive feelings about himself or herself; patient will have knowledge of support resources.	Provide a climate of acceptance; encourage self-care and independence. Provide patient/ family with written list of available support resources.

production. Scleroderma widely varies in severity; in some cases, internal organs such as lungs, heart, kidneys, esophagus, and GI tract are seriously damaged (see Figures 9-4 to 9-8, pages 238-239).

B. **Etiology/Incidence.**
   1. The exact cause(s) of scleroderma is unknown, but research is pointing to a "susceptible gene."
   2. Most patients do not have a family member with the disease.
   3. Females are affected 4:1 over males.
   4. *Localized* scleroderma is more common in children; whereas *systemic* scleroderma occurs more in adults.

C. **Classifications of scleroderma.**
   1. Localized scleroderma.
     a. Affects the collagen-producing cells in limited skin areas and usually spares the internal organs and blood vessels.
     b. Occurs as patches of thickened skin: *morphea (see special note below)* or as *linear* scleroderma, a line of thickened skin that may extend down an arm or leg. If the line occurs on the forehead it is called *en coup de sabre* ("cut of the saber").
     c. Affects children more often than adults.

     d. *Special note:* Morphea is a mild, mostly benign, and self-limiting disease of the skin with less than a 1% chance of progressing to scleroderma. It is important to use proper terminology and not frighten patients/parents with the term scleroderma unless appropriately diagnosed by the practioner.

   2. Systemic scleroderma (also called progressive systemic sclerosis).
     a. The immune system causes damage to small blood vessels and the collagen-producing cells throughout the body.
     b. The small blood vessels in the hands/fingers narrow or completely close, often causing slow healing and/or spontaneous ulcerations.
     c. Patients are often cold-sensitive.
     d. 95% of patients with systemic scleroderma suffer from Raynaud's phenomenon (intermittent attacks of ischemia of the extremities of the body, especially the fingers, toes, ears, and nose, characterized by severe blanching, cyanosis, redness, numbness, tingling, burning, and often pain).
     e. Scar tissue (sclerosis) many occur in one or

more organs including the heart, lung, skin, kidneys, or GI tract.

   f. Systemic scleroderma is divided into two forms.

     (1) *Limited scleroderma* (often referred to as the CREST form), calcinosis (calcium deposits in the skin), Raynaud's phenomenon (see above), esophageal dysfunction (acid in the esophagus — heartburn), sclerodactyly (tight, thick skin of the fingers), telangiectasias (multiple, small, punctate macules that are particularly prominent on the face and hands).

     (2) *Diffuse scleroderma* has significantly greater organ involvement.

3. Scleroderma-related disorders.

   a. Scleroderma occurs in patients with other autoimmune disorders and may be referred to as an "overlap syndrome."

   b. Some studies suggest that exposure to various drugs (for example, bleomycin) and chemicals can cause lesions similar to those seen in scleroderma. Often these skin changes are indistinguishable from those of systemic sclerosis, and the exposure may be unknown to the patient.

D. Diagnosis of scleroderma.

1. Medical history.

   a. A detailed history of signs/symptoms during general systems review that prompted medical services may indicate progression and severity of disease process.

   b. Question patient as to possible exposure to drugs or chemicals.

2. Physical exam.

   a. Full skin exam: see above for detailed cutaneous manifestations of each category of scleroderma.

     (1) Approximately 98% of patients will present with hardening or thickening of the skin of the fingers.

     (2) Raynaud's phenomenon is present in 95% of patients.

   b. Systemic manifestations identified by a complete physical exam may include:

     (1) Gastrointestinal.

       (a) Decreased motility/absorption.

       (b) Esophageal dysphagia, reflux, and/or strictures.

     (2) Pulmonary fibrosis.

       (a) Decreased pulmonary function, vital capacity.

       (b) Pulmonary hypertension.

       (c) Dyspnea and decreased breath sounds.

     (3) Renal vascular involvement: hypertension, insufficiency or failure.

     (4) Cardiovascular.

       (a) Cardiac fibrosis with possible arrhythmias/myocardial infarction.

       (b) Pericarditis.

     (4) Musculoskeletal.

       (a) Arthralgias.

       (b) Myalgias.

3. Skin biopsy.

   a. Confirms diagnosis of morphea.

4. Laboratory and radiologic tests for systemic scleroderma.

   a. Complete blood count.

   b. Urinalysis.

   c. Renal function tests.

   d. Chest radiograph.

   e. Pulmonary function tests.

   f. Barium swallow.

   g. Antinuclear antibody test.

     (1) Nucleolar staining is associated with mixed connective tissue disease.

     (2) Anticentromere staining is associated with CREST syndrome.

     (3) A positive Scl-70 antibody indicates diffuse scleroderma.

E. Treatment.

1. There is no cure for scleroderma; treatment plans are individualized to each patient's type and severity of symptoms.

2. Medications are prescribed according to treatment goals:

   a. Control high blood pressure.

     (1) ACE inhibitors.

     (2) Angiotensin II inhibitors.

     (3) Others: clonidine, prazosin.

   b. Relieve pericarditis.

     (1) NSAIDS.

     (2) Corticosteroids.

   c. Reduce joint and tendon pain.

     (1) NSAIDS.

     (2) Analgesics.

     (3) Corticosteroids.

   d. Prevent Raynaud's phenomenon.

     (1) Calcium channel blockers.

     (2) Others: nitroglycerine ointment, prazosin, doxazosin, terazosin, and pentoxifylline.

   e. Treat small bowel dysfunction.

     (1) Broad-spectrum antibiotics.

   f. Relieve constipation.

     (1) Bulking agents.

     (2) Softening agent.

     (3) Others: lactulose, bisacodyl.

   g. Prevent heartburn.

     (1) Antacids.

     (2) H-2 blockers.

     (3) Proton pump inhibitors.

     (4) Others: sucralfate, cisapride.

   h. Improve swallowing difficulties.

(1) H-2 blockers.
(2) Proton pump inhibitor.
(3) GI stimulants.
  i. Treat digital ulcerations.
    (1) Oral/topical antibiotics.
    (2) Recommendations from wound care specialist.
  j. Reduce skin itching.
    (1) Skin lotions/emollients.
    (2) Note: diphenhydramine not recommended as it may increase symptoms of dry eyes and dry mouth.
  k. Relieve dry mouth: saliva substitute.
  l. Relieve dry eyes: artificial tears/lubricants.
  m. Treat reactive depression.
    (1) SSRIs.
    (2) Tricyclic antidepressants.
    (3) Others: bupropion, venlafaxine, trazodone.
3. Disease modifiers.
  a. At present, there are no FDA-approved drugs to modify the course of scleroderma; however, there are several drugs currently under study.
  b. Currently, methotrexate, cyclosporin, as well as chemotherapy and immunosuppressants are being used to impair the immune and inflammatory responses.
  c. Interferons (alpha and gamma) have been used to suppress collagen production, but there is no conclusive study to prove effectiveness.
  d. D-penicillamine is used to weaken collagen; however, studies done have been unable to prove effectiveness.
E. Nursing considerations (see Table 2).
  1. Educate patient/family as to reasons for medication protocol, and possible side effects to be reported to nurse/practioner.
  2. Provide patient/family with list of resources for support and education (see resource list on this page).
  3. Continually assess patient for signs /symptoms of diease progression, and encourage routine followups with practioner.

III. INFLAMATORY MYOPATHIES

A. **Definition: inflammatory myopathies are a group of muscle diseases characterized by inflammation of connective tissue and musclefibers which can cause extensive necrosis and destruction of the muscle fibers. They are believed to be autoimmune disorders. The inflammatory myopathies are dermatomyositis (DM), juvenile dermatomyositis (JDMS), polymyositis (PM), and inclusion body myositis (IBM). Each is unique in its development and**

Resources
Coalition of Patient Advocates for Skin Disease Research
PO Box 3784, Crofton, MD 21114-3784
(410)721-2615 fax (410)721-2815
Email: vhwhittemore@aol.com

American Skin Association, Inc.
346 Park Avenue South, 4th floor, New York, NY 10010
(800)499-SKIN fax (212)889-4959
Email: info@skinassn.org
Web-site: www.skinassn.org

Inflammatory Skin Disease Institute
Inflammatory Skin Disorders
PO Box 1074, Newport News, VA 23601
(800)484-6800 ext.6321 fax (757)595-1842
Email: ExDirISDI@aol.com

Lupus Foundation of America, Inc.
1300 Piccard Drive, Suite 200, Rockville, MD 20850
(800)558-0121 fax (301)670-9486
Email: info@lupus.org
Web-site: www.lupus.org

Scleroderma Foundation
12 Kent Way, Suite 101, Byfiled, MA 01922
(978)463-5809 fax (978)463-5809
Email: sfinfo@scleroderma.org
Web-site: www.scleroderma.org

Scleroderma Research Foundation
2320 Bath Street, Suite315, Santa Barbara, CA 93105
(800)441-2873 fax (805)563-2402
Email: charles_spaulding@srfcure.org
Web-site: www.srfcure.org

Myositis Association of America
Web-site: www.myositis.org

treatment (see Figure 9-9, page 239).
B. Etiology/Incidence.
  1. Inflammatory myopathies have been designated as autoimmune diseases because of the presence of autoantibodies in the serum of those affected.
  2. Prevalence rates are approximately 6 per 1,000,000 persons.
  3. Occurs in all ethnic groups.
  4. PM and DM affect females 2:1 over males.
  5. PM rarely affects people under the age of 20.
  6. IBM symptoms usually begin after age 50, and occur in males more frequently than females.
C. Classifications and descriptions of inflammatory myopathies.
  1. Dermatomyositis (DM).
    a. Easily recognized by distinctive rash: apatchy, dusky, reddish or lilac rash on the eyelids with perior bitaledema (heliotrope), cheeks, and bridge of nose. Gottron's

papules, small (<1cm), flat, smooth, reddish/purplish papules found over joints such as, knuckles, fingers, elbows, knees, and medial malleoli.

  b. May also include several of the following signs/symptoms.

    (1) Proximal muscle weakness/pain usually follows rash and typically develops over a period of weeks.

    (2) Elevated serum CK oral dolase levels.

    (3) Polyarthralgia/polyarthritis.

    (4) Positive histadyl tRNA synthetase antibody.

    (5) Raynaud's phenomenon.

    (6) Signs of systemic inflammation (fever:>37° Caxillary, elevated CRP).

    (7) Myogenic EMG changes.

    (8) Muscle biopsy reveals necrosis, inflammation, and degradation.

    (9) Possible malignancy: malignant neoplasms.

2. Polymyositis (PM).

  a. Similar presentation as DM, but without characteristic rash.

  b. Muscle weakness progressess lower than DM effecting proximal muscles; approximatelyone-third of PM patients have muscle pain.

  c. Difficulty swallowing is common.

3. Inclusion body myositis (IBM).

  a. Very similar in presentation to PM.

  b. Only definitive testis muscle biopsy.

  c. Duration of illness > 6 months.

  d. Age of onset > 30 years old.

  e. Affects proximal and distal muscles of arms and legs.

  f. Patient will exhibit one or more of the following:

    (1) Finger flex or weakness.

    (2) Wrist flex or greater than wrist extens or weakness.

    (3) Quadriceps muscle weakness.

  g. Serum CK < 12 times normal.

4. Juvenile dermatomyositis (JDMS).

  a. Juvenile idiopathic inflammatory myopathy (JIIM) or juvenile dermatomyositis (JDMS) usually presents as dermatomyositis (JDM) with the distinctive heliotrope rash (see DM above).

  b. Proximal muscle weakness usually follows rash.

  c. Dysphagia and dysphonia (hoarseness) is common.

  d. Muscle pain occurs in approximately 50% of children.

  e. Abdominal pain and arthralgia canals occur.

D. Treatment

1. There is no known cure for inflammatory myopathies.

2. High doses of immunosuppressants and/or steroids have been effective for many patients.

3. Intravenous immunoglobulins (IVIg) have proven effective for those patients not responding to immunosuppressants.

4. Numerous new drugs are currently being studied.

5. Physical therapy is strongly recommended to maintain mobility.

6. Referral to nutritional therapist recommended-for dysphagia and nutritional assessment.

7. Topical steroids for lesions.

8. Analgesics PRN for pain.

9. Protection from ultraviolet light.

10. Appropriate referrals/treatments for any identified malignancies.

11. Evaluate and treat for possible depression.

E. Nursing considerations (see Table 2).

1. Evaluate and treat complaints of pain routinely.

2. Provide supportive and caring environment to patient/family.

3. Educate patient/family on medications, and encourage immediate reporting of side effects.

4. Assess for dysphagia with each meal/office visit.

Bibliography

American Academy of Dermatology. (2002). *Foundations.* Retrieved from http://www.aad.org/foundations.html

Burch, J.M., Lee, L.A., & Weston, W.L. (2002). Neonatal lupus erythematosus. *Dermatology Nursing, 14*(3), 157-160.

Greenberg, J.E., & Schachner, L.A. (2001). Localized scleroderma or morphea? *Dermatology Nursing, 13*(5), 335-344.

Helm, K.F., & Marks, Jr., J.G. (1998). *Atlas of differential diagnosis in dermatology.* Philadelphia: Churchill Livingstone.

Ignatavicius, D.D., Workman, M.L., & Mishler, M.A. (1995). *Medical-surgical nursing: A nursing process approach* (2nd ed.). Philadelphia: W.B. Saunders Company.

Lookingbill, D.P., & Marks, Jr., J.G. (2000). *Principles of dermatology* (3rd ed.). Philadelphia: W.B. Saunders Company.

Lupus Foundation of America, Inc. (2002). *Lupus disease.* Retrieved from: http://www.lupus.org.

McCance, K.L., & Huether, S.E. (1998). *Pathophysiology: The biologic basis for disease in adults and children* (3rd ed.). St. Louis: Mosby.

Myositis Association of America. (2002). *Resource for inflammatory myopathies.* Retrieved from http://www.myositis.org.

Pullen, Jr., R. L. (2001). Managing subacute cutaneous lupus erythematosus. *Dermatology Nursing, 13*(6), 419-426.

Scleroderma Foundation. (2002). *Scleroderma fact sheet.* Retrieved from http://www.scleroderma.org.

1. All of the following statements about lupus are true *except:*
   a. The exact cause of lupus is unknown.
   b. Lupus is often called a "woman's disease."
   c. The most frequent symptom of lupus is skin rashes.
   d. Currently, there is no single test that can diagnose lupus.
   e. Sun exposure/ultraviolet light will help to eliminate skin lesions.

2. Approximately four times more women than men develop scleroderma.
   a. True
   b. False

3. Morphea is:
   a. Just another name for scleroderma.
   b. A term to refer to discoid lesions associated with cutaneous lupus.
   c. A skin disease with a less than 1% chance of progressing to systemic scleroderma.
   d. A form of inflammatory myopathy which typically occurs in adult men.
   e. A severe form of Raynaud's phenomenon.

4. Which of the following is the incorrect term for the CREST acronym?
   a. Calcinosis.
   b. Raynaud's phenomenon.
   c. Esophageal dysfunction.
   d. Sclerodactyly.
   e. Trigeminal.

5. Which one of the following diseases is associated with a heliotrope rash?
   a. Inclusion body myositis (IBM).
   b. Systemic lupus erythematosus (SLE).
   c. Systemic scleroderma.
   d. Dermatomyositis (DM).
   e. Acne vulgaris.

6. Myositis occurs in all ethnic groups.
   a. True
   b. False

7. Which of the following medication(s) is/are used in the treatment of systemic lupus erythematosus (SLE)?
   a. Anti-inflammatory drugs.
   b. Corticosteroids.
   c. Anti-malarials.
   d. Cytotoxic or immunosuppressive drugs.
   e. All of the above are used to treat SLE.

8. Raynaud's phenomenon can best be described as:
   a. A syndrome in which mothers with SLE pass along the genetic trait for lupus.
   b. Intermittent attacks of ischemia of the extremities of the body, especially the fingers, toes, ears, and nose.
   c. An inflammation involving a spinal nerve root, resulting in pain and hyperesthesia.
   d. Discoid shaped plaques that occur on the trunk in patients suffering from inflammatory diseases.
   e. A condition of abnormally increased muscle tone or strength.

9. Lupus can be viewed as a disease continuum or spectrum with discoid lupus erythematosus (DLE) at the most severe end of the spectrum and patients with active systemic lupus erythematosus (SLE) at the mild end of the spectrum.
   a. True
   b. False

10. The inflammatory myopathies include all of the following *except:*
    a. Coccidioidomycosis.
    b. Inclusion body myositis.
    c. Dermatomyositis.
    d. Polymyositis.
    e. Juvenile dermatomyositis.

Answers to Study Questions

1.	c	5.	d	9.	b
2.	a	6.	a	10.	a
3.	c	7.	e		
4.	e	8.	b		

Chapter 9.
Connective Tissue Disorders

Please photocopy this test page and return.

COMPLETE THE FOLLOWING:

Name: _____

Address: _____

City: _____ State: _____ Zip: _____

Preferred telephone: (Home)_____ (Work) _____

State where licensed and license number: _____

CE application fee: DNA member $7.00
                             Nonmember $10.00

POSTTEST INSTRUCTIONS
1. To receive continuing education credit for individual study after reading the article, complete the answer/evaluation form below.
2. Photocopy and send the answer/evaluation form along with a check or money order payable to **Dermatology Nurses' Association** to: **DNA**, East Holly Avenue Box 56, Pitman, NJ 08071-0056.
3. Test returns must be postmarked by December 31, 2008. Upon completion of the answer/evaluation form, a certificate for 1.5 contact hour(s) will be awarded and sent to you.

This chapter was reviewed and formatted for contact hour credit by Marcia J. Hill, MSN, RN, Core Curriculum Editor; and Sally Russell, MN, RN,C, DNA Education Director.

ANSWER FORM

1. Name one new detail (item, issue, or phenomenon) that you learned by completing this activity.

   _____

   _____

   _____

2. How will you apply the information from this learning activity to your practice?

   a. Patient education.
   b. Staff education.
   c. Improve my patient care.
   d. In my education course work.
   e. Other: Please describe _____

   _____

Evaluation

	Strongly disagree				Strongly agree
3. The offering met the stated objectives.					
a. Identify and differentiate several connective tissue disorders.	1	2	3	4	5
b. Discuss treatment modalities for the most comon connective tissue disorders.	1	2	3	4	5
c. List several important patient education aspects for each disorder.	1	2	3	4	5
d. Provide a list of patient resources on connective tissue disorders.	1	2	3	4	5
4. The content was current and relevant.	1	2	3	4	5
5. The content was presented clearly.	1	2	3	4	5
6. The content was covered adequately.	1	2	3	4	5
7. I am more confident of my abilities since completing this material.	1	2	3	4	5

8. The material was (check one) ☐ new, ☐ review for me.

Comments _____

9. Time required to complete reading assignment: _____ minutes

This independent study is provided by the Dermatology Nurses' Association (DNA) for 1.5 contact hours. DNA is accredited as a provider of continuing education in nursing by the American Nurses Credentialing Center's Commission on Accreditation. DNA is approved as a provider of continuing education by the California Board of Registered Nursing Provider #CEP5708.

Bullous and Vesicular Diseases

Janis S. Johnson, BSN, RN, C, DNC

OBJECTIVES

At the end of this chapter, the reader will be able to:

- Identify the main characteristics of the disease processes of pemphigus vulgaris (PV), bullous pemphigoid (BP), epidermolysis bullosa (EB), Stevens-Johnson syndrome (SJS), and dermatitis herpetiformis (DH).

- Discuss tools used in making the diagnosis of PV, BP, EB, SJS, and DH.

- Define therapeutic interventions used in treating PV, BP, EB, SJS, and DH.

- Identify nursing interventions that assist in providing optimal care to patients.

- List patient/family teaching strategies.

KEY POINTS

- Common therapeutic modalities combine topical treatments, drug therapies, and other medical management.

- Assessment for infection should be included in all phases of care due to impaired skin integrity.

- Close monitoring of the patient on drug therapy, with possible serious side effects, is essential.

- Maintaining adequate nutrition is a challenge, especially for those patients with oral lesions.

- The physician, nurse, and patient/family should develop a plan of care which will provide optimal skin care that the patient/family can accomplish.

Bullous and Vesicular Diseases

Janis S. Johnson, BSN, RN, C, DNC

Vesicular and bullous skin diseases can be acute but are primarily chronic blister-forming diseases. A genetic defect or immunological event causes a break in continuity within the epidermis or epidermal junction.

PEMPHIGUS VULGARIS

I. OVERVIEW

A. **Definition: pemphigus vulagris (PV) is a serious, acute or chronic, bullous, autoimmune disease of the skin and mucous membrane.**
B. **Etiology.**
   1. The cause is unknown. It is characterized by acute exacerbations and remissions.
   2. A genetic association has been proven through immunogenetics. Additionally, various medications have been reported to cause PV.
C. **Pathophysiology.**
   1. PV manifests with flaccid weeping bullous lesions that rupture easily, leaving denuded areas that crust.
   2. Bullae may form from normal looking skin or an erythematous base.
   3. Pemphigus is a disorder due to immunoreactants directed against the intercellular substance (ICS) ("glue connecting the skin cells").
   4. Mucous membranes which can be involved include mouth, vaginal, perianal, and conjunctival areas. The oral mucosa is commonly affected and may be the site of the first lesions.
   5. Symptoms of burning and/or pain occur in affected areas. Conjunctival involvement, which is rare, manifests with photophobia, irritation, and pain.
   6. Two variants of this disease are pemphigus vegetans (a thickened verrucous-like change) and pemphigus foliaceus (a more superficial variant).
   7. Patients may experience weakness, malaise, and weight loss especially if there is prolonged oral mucosal involvement.
   8. The disease process occasionally spontaneously remits after several years, but may often require long-term therapy.
D. **Incidence.**
   1. Usually occurs in 40 to 60-year-old persons.
   2. Equal incidence in males and in females.
   3. Pemphigus vulgaris is the most common type.

II. ASSESSMENT

A. **History and physical examination.**
   1. Vesicles and bullae are flaccid, easily ruptured, weeping, and arise on normal or erythematous skin. Subsequent erosions can bleed easily. Crusts may form and can affect any skin surface including the scalp.
   2. The arrangement is randomly scattered, but there is a high propensity for oral mucosa.
   3. Nikolsky's sign is positive. (Dislodging of the epidermis occurs with the application of lateral finger pressure, which leads to an erosion. This test is no longer used since it is non-specific and because it creates an additional lesion.)
B. **Diagnostic tests.**
   1. Biopsy of an early small bulla or, if not present, the margin of a larger bulla or erosion (perilesional biopsy) for light microscopy. There is loss of intercellular cohesion in the lower part of the epidermis called acantholysis.
   2. Direct immunofluorescence testing is performed on a perilesional skin biopsy looking for immunoreactants directed against ICS.
   3. Serum is used for indirect immunofluorescence testing. This test detects auto-antibodies against ICS. This antibody titer usually correlates with activity of disease and is therefore helpful in directing therapy (doses of medications).
   4. In widespread disease, electrolytes may be altered with sodium, chloride, and calcium decreasing and potassium increasing.
   5. Patients with significant impetiginization of the eroded areas may show an increased WBC count.

III. COMMON THERAPEUTIC MODALITIES

A. **Medical intervention.**
   1. Topical treatment consists of topical antibiotic creams or ointments such as silver sulfadiazine for blisters or erosions. Medicated baths (e.g., potassium permanganate [$KMnO_4$] or oilated oatmeal) and/or wet dressings (aluminum subacetate, $KMnO_4$, or Domeboro® solution) are useful for their antibacterial and cleansing effects. Dressings should be changed every 2 to 3 hours to prevent the dressing material from drying and adhering to the skin. (These "continuous wet" dressings are preferred over "wet to dry" dressings.) Topical corticosteroids are also useful for pruritic and erythematous areas.

Table 1.
Nursing Diagnoses, Outcomes, and Interventions

Nursing Diagnoses	Outcomes	Interventions
Impaired skin integrity: skin lesions	Barrier function will be restored.	1. Body must be protected from micro-organisms by using a temporary barrier with topical medications and dressings. 2. Temperature of wet dressing solution should be slightly above body temperature and the wet dressings should be immediately wrapped with towels or blanket. The dressing materials tend to cool very quickly. 3. Wet dressings should be changed when still slightly damp. Dressings dried to the skin may prematurely debride the lesions. 4. Due to nonintact skin, normal thermoregulation is altered. Increasing the room temperature or additional warmed blankets may be necessary. 5. Do not use tape on the skin. 6. Topical corticosteroids (both as cream/ointment on the skin and as gel or liquid for mucosal lesions) may be beneficial.
Pain: skin erosions	Patient will have pain minimized.	1. Assess pain and administer pain-relief medication as necessary using a numeric scale. 2. Assess need for narcotics with resultant side effects versus non-narcotic analgesia on an around-the-clock regimen. 3. Administer topical anesthetic (viscous lidocaine) prior to each meal by the swish and spit method. Should not be swallowed. 4. For severe pain, apply the creams or lotions to the dressings rather than eroded skin.
Altered nutritional status: oral lesion	Patient will maintain adequate nutrition.	1. Offer mouthwashes containing anesthesia to ease the pain, allowing the patient to eat. 2. Essential to promote good oral hygiene with warm water or saline rinses before and after food to wash away debris. 3. Sponge swabs can be used if patient is unable to use soft bristle toothbrush. 4. Full liquid or mechanical soft diet is better tolerated in the acute phase. High-protein nutritional supplements are easily ingested. 5. Increase fluid intake to replace protein and fluid loss through the open erosions. 6. Calorie counts and daily weights for acute phase patients.
High risk for infection: compromised integument and medical management	Patient will have risk of infection minimized.	1. Assess skin frequently for signs of increased erythema, increased tenderness, and swelling or symptoms of systemic infection (malaise, increased temperature, or confusion). 2. Discourage patient contact with others with infections. 3. Strict handwashing before and after contact with patient. 4. Aseptic technique with wound care, dressing changes, and discarding contaminated materials.
Pruritus: skin lesions	Patient will have pruritus minimized.	1. Assess pruritus and administer an antipruritic to reduce feeling of the need to scratch. 2. Use body temperature dressings and medicated baths for symptom relief to cause vasoconstriction. 3. Topical corticosteroids to pruritic, noneroded skin is beneficial, especially under wet dressings. 4. Relaxation/meditation techniques can be used in conjunction with other therapies.

2. Supportive treatment should be offered to patients unable to tolerate topical creams or ointments. They may be able to tolerate lotions or dusting powders.
3. Patients with severe cases may require hospitalization on an inpatient dermatology unit or burn unit.

B. **Drug therapy.**
1. Systemic corticosteroids are the principal method of treatment with starting doses of 0.5 to 1.0 mg/kg p.o. The dose may be doubled until remission is achieved. Intralesional steroids may be used for resistant localized lesions.
2. Immunosuppressants such as methotrexate, azathioprine (Imuran®), cyclophosphamide (Cytoxan®), or cyclosporine are generally used for remission induction or as an adjunct to steroid therapy.
3. Alternatives to these immunosupressives include sulfones (Dapsone®), tetracycline, or minocycline which are used alone or in combination with high-dose steroids.
4. Less frequently, antimalarial drugs such as chloroquine, hydroxychloroquine, or a combination of both are used.
5. Plasmapheresis can be used in conjunction with corticosteroids for more rapid control in extremely severe cases.
6. Most recently, intravenous immunoglobulin (IVIG) has been used as second-line therapy where the above approaches were ineffective, or had caused significant side effects.

IV. COMMON NURSING DIAGNOSES, OUTCOMES, AND INTERVENTIONS (see Table 1)

V. PATIENT TEACHING

A. **Teach patient/family about disease and its course.**
B. **Explain to patient/family the need for a balanced diet to enhance healing.**
1. Provide a written plan of what constitutes a healthy diet.
   a. Full liquid diet in acute phases with oral lesions.
   b. Progress to a mechanical soft diet when discomfort decreases.
   c. Nutritional supplements are available in flavors to provide variety in the diet over a long period of time.
2. Assess patient/family's financial ability to provide a balanced diet with supplements.
C. **Teach the patient/family about the different types of treatments.**
1. Topical treatment.
   a. Identify if patient is able to care for self or identify a caregiver.

b. Assess patient/family understanding and motivation to perform recommended treatments.
c. Determine availability of bathing facilities, wet dressing materials, and means to purchase creams.
d. Develop a care plan with the patient/family. Include opportunities for return demonstrations, if possible, of cream application by the patient/family.
2. Systemic treatment.
   a. Explain need for regular medical followup, including physician and laboratory visits.
   b. Explain need to monitor any latent infection reactivation or current infection exacerbation.
   c. Review side effects of therapies such as those of corticosteroids (GI bleed, weight change, mood swings, acne, bone density changes, and steroid-induced diabetes).
   d. Explain need to avoid others with infectious processes (flu, colds, coughs, skin infections, etc.) especially since most therapies involve some degree of immunosuppression.
D. **Emphasize the need to comply with all provisions of the treatment regimen.**
1. Provide the nurse's telephone number for patient inquiries and a 24-hour telephone number for emergencies. This will provide greater continuity of care for the patient.
2. Make routine followup calls during the acute phase to decrease incidence of complications with the patient who may be reluctant to call.
3. Assess need for professional home health provider and make referral if necessary.

BULLOUS PEMPHIGOID

I. OVERVIEW

A. **Definition: bullous pemphigoid (BP) is a chronic autoimmune disorder caused by auto-antibodies.**
B. **Etiology.**
1. Presents as a chronic blistering eruption.
2. Manifests with tense, serum-filled bullae that rupture easily.
3. Lesions usually manifest on an inflammatory or urticarial base.
C. **Pathophysiology.**
1. BP can be self-limiting, and may go into remission 2 to 6 years after onset.
2. BP is due to antibodies directed against the basement membrane zone of the epidermis (the "foundation" of the skin).
3. Variants of BP are:
   a. Localized — usually limited to lower

extremities and responds well to treatment; may progress to generalized disease.

    b.   Benign mucosal pemphigoid — synonym for cicatricial pemphigoid, or scarring pemphigoid; recurring bullae on either a mucous membrane or on the skin near an orifice; and has the tendency to scar.

II. ASSESSMENT

A. **History and physical examination.**
1. Erythematous erosions, which may be urticarial lesions, can precede bullae formation by months.
2. The distribution is generalized or localized.
3. The sites of predilection are generally flexural and include axillae, medial aspects of thighs and groin, flexor aspects of forearms, and lower legs.

B. **Diagnostic tests.**
1. Biopsy of a skin lesion shows subepidermal blister with inflammation and edema. The blisters usually contain a mixture of eosinophils and polymorphonuclear leukocytes.
2. Perilesional skin biopsy for direct immunofluorescence shows immunoreactants at the basement membrane.
3. In 70% of patients, circulating anti-basement membrane IgG antibodies are detected by indirect immunofluorescence. Antibody titers typically do not correlate with the course of the disease.

III. COMMON THERAPEUTIC MODALITIES

A. **Medical intervention.**
1. Topical treatment is the same as for pemphigus vulgaris.
2. Admission to an inpatient dermatology unit or burn unit may be indicated in severe cases.

B. **Drug therapy.**
1. Systemic corticosteroids are usually given orally and in lower doses than used in PV unless disease is severe then pulse IV steriods are indicated. Maintenance treatment may extend for years.
2. Other systemic therapies are similar to those used for PV, but they usually require lower doses.

IV. COMMON NURSING DIAGNOSES, OUTCOMES, AND INTERVENTIONS

See Table 1; same as pemphigus vulgaris.

V. PATIENT TEACHING

Same as pemphigus vulgaris.

EPIDERMOLYSIS BULLOSA

I. OVERVIEW

A. **Definition:** epidermolysis bullosa (EB) is a group of heterogeneous, inheritable disorders characterized by abnormal fragility of the skin and mucosa.

B. **Etiology.**
1. The cause of EB is felt to be a genetic defect of the skin structure, such that proper attachment of the epidermis to the dermis does not occur. Other theories of its cause include activation of a cytolytic enzyme or the existence of a mutant, temperature-sensitive protein.
2. Subtypes of EB are classified by inheritance patterns and histologically by bullae location.
3. EB acquisita (EBA) represents a similar disorder acquired (thus, "acquisita") later in life. EBA is an autoimmune condition, where antibodies are directed against Type VII collagen.

B. **Pathophysiology.**
1. At birth or during infancy, patients with EB present with blisters at sites of minor trauma or may appear spontaneously. Patients with EBA have similar manifestations later in life.
2. Depending on the specific type, the patient may only occasionally have blisters with little effect on health or lifestyle. Those patients with severe types have widespread cutaneous and mucosal blisters which can be fatal.
3. The bullae may be non-scarring or scarring. The disorder has been compared to a chronic burn.
4. The most common complications are chronic iron deficiency anemia; malnutrition; growth retardation; and respiratory, GI, and GU blisters and erosions.

C. **Incidences.**
1. Estimates range from 1 in 50,000 to 1 in 100,000 births for types of EB presenting at birth or early childhood.
2. Equal incidence in males and in females.

II. ASSESSMENT

A. **History and physical examination.**
1. Classification of EB is based on the pattern of inheritance and ultrastructural level of blistering. There are over 20 subtypes.
2. Major classifications.
    a.   EB simplex is the most superficial type with mild blistering, rare mucosal involvement, and blisters heal without scarring unless secondarily infected.
    b.   Recessive junctional EB (RJEB) has a wide range of severity; common to all forms of RJEB include oral involvement, atrophy at sites of repeated injury, nail dystrophy, and dysplastic enamel.

c. Dominant dystrophic or dermolytic EB is characterized by repeated blistering and scarring (cigarette paper-like), milia, enamel defects, and dystrophic nails.

d. Recessive dermolytic EB has a wide range of severity; usually present at birth with generalized blistering and erosions; multiple sites of extracutaneous involvement and deformities; increased risk to develop invasive cutaneous squamous cell carcinoma in areas of chronic erosions.

3. Nikolsky's sign is positive.

B. **Diagnostic tests.**

1. Biopsy of a fresh blister (less than 24 hours old) for routine histology, direct immunofluorescence (to rule out other immunobullous diseases), and electron microscopy.

2. Immunochemistry of basement membrane zone antigens to detect some forms of junctional EB.

3. A positive family history is helpful in establishing the diagnosis, but will be negative in patients with types caused by a new mutation and in patients with recessive forms who are born to unaffected parents carrying the disease.

III. COMMON THERAPEUTIC MODALITIES

A. **Medical intervention.**

1. Daily wound care is a major challenge for the EB patient and caregiver. Rotating topical antibiotics will decrease emergence of resistant bacterial strains and decrease incidence of developing a contact sensitivity. Other useful topical agents are silver sulfadiazine and fusidic acid. Non-adhering dressings or Vaseline-impregnated gauze secured by roller gauze will decrease trauma to the affected body part. Only the involved area should be treated.

2. Supportive treatment includes optimal nutritional management with all patients, but especially those patients with oral lesions, esophageal scarring, and gastric outlet obstruction.

3. Pre-medication with mild analgesics such as acetaminophen may be useful for young patients prior to bathing and wound care.

4. Recent studies show phenytoin may be helpful to a subset of patients.

B. **Prenatal diagnosis.**

1. Prenatal diagnosis has been successfully performed on fetuses at risk for all major forms of EB. Diagnosis is made via skin biopsy obtained through fetoscopy from a fetus at risk. DNA in the skin biopsy is analyzed for characteristic abnormalities of EB.

2. Referral to Dystrophic EB Research Association (DEBRA) is helpful as an information clearinghouse for the patient and caregiver.

IV. COMMON NURSING DIAGNOSES, OUTCOMES, AND INTERVENTIONS (see Table 2)

V. PATIENT TEACHING

A. **Teach parents about the disease and its chronic course.**

1. Education of patients with EBA is similar to PV and BP.

2. Referral to a multidisciplinary team of a grief counselor, dietician, social worker, physical therapist, and home nurse may be necessary depending on the severity of the disease.

3. The child must be included in the teaching process, with information provided geared to the child's developmental level.

B. **Explain to parent the need for a balanced diet to enhance healing.**

1. Provide a written plan of what constitutes a healthy diet.

2. Encourage parents to discover ways of feeding the baby that would minimize skin trauma and promote nurturing.

C. **Teach parents about different types of treatments.**

1. Topical treatment.

a. Identify primary caregivers and encourage parents to enlist assistance of others for wound care, bathing, and feeding. This provides opportunities for a respite care for the primary caregivers.

b. Determine availability of bathing facilities, dressing materials, and means to purchase ointments. Encourage parents to organize an area to care for the infant to decrease bathing and wound care time.

c. Develop a care plan that allows for opportunities for the caregivers to perform the bathing and wound care with nursing supervision. This will help increase the level of confidence for the caregivers.

d. Review ways of protecting the infant's skin from trauma. This will become more challenging as the child grows older.

2. Systemic treatment.

a. Explain need for routine medical followup with regular visits to the physician.

b. Explain need to rotate antibiotic ointments and not to treat prophylactically.

D. **Emphasize the need to comply with all provisions of the treatment regimen.**

1. Provide nurse's telephone number for patient inquiries and a 24-hour telephone number for

Table 2.
Nursing Diagnoses, Outcomes, and Interventions

Nursing Diagnoses	Outcomes	Interventions
Impaired skin integrity: skin lesions	Trauma-related blistering will be minimized; temporary barrier function will be provided.	1. Gentle handling of the patient is critical. Well-lubricated gloves help prevent trauma to fragile skin. 2. Intact bullae can be unroofed with iris scissors. 3. It is beneficial to keep bathing and wound care time to a minimum. 4. After the application of an antibiotic ointment, the dressings next to the skin should be nonadhering and also have moisture-wicking properties if there is drainage. Lighter outer dressings should not interfere with range of motion.
Pain: open skin lesions	Patient will be comfortable during wound care.	1. Premedicate 45 minutes prior to bathing and wound care with mild analgesia if needed. 2. Having all care materials organized prior to wound care will assist in minimizing the time the lesions are open to the air. 3. Depending on the age and developmental level, meditation/relaxation techniques may help diminish the effects of pain. Distraction is helpful for the young child.
Altered nutritional state: oral lesions	Patient will increase or maintain weight at acceptable increments relative to age.	1. Daily oral hygiene including soft toothbrush or sponge swab and fluoride mouthwashes for children until adulthood. 2. Low-dose, short-term topical steroid in Orabase® can be used in acute oral trauma that interferes with oral intake. 3. Adequate protein and caloric intake with supplements to maximize growth and healing. 4. Provide soft toys or food for the infant to chew on when teething rather than hard teething cookies to minimize trauma.
High risk for infection: compromised integument	Patient will have risk of an infection minimized.	1. Assess skin frequently for signs of infection. Any infection should be treated aggressively. 2. Discourage patient contact with others with infections. 3. Strict handwashing before and after contact with patient. 4. Aseptic technique with wound care, dressing changes, and discarding contaminated materials.

emergencies. This will help to provide greater continuity of care.
2. Make routine followup calls to parents to decrease incidence of complications.
3. Assess need for professional home health provider and make referral if necessary.

STEVENS-JOHNSON SYNDROME

I. OVERVIEW

A. Definition: Stevens-Johnson syndrome (SJS) is a serious immune-mediated response to an inciting agent, most often a drug or infection.
B. Etiology.
1. The most common inciting drugs include allupurinol, penicillin, phenobarbital, phenytoin, and the sulfonamides. There have been more than 100 medications reported to have caused SJS.
2. Traditionally, SJS has been considered the most severe form of erythema multiforme (EM). However, some researchers propose that SJS

and EM are distinct entities.

3. The mortality rate is 3% to 10%.

C. **Pathophysiology.**

1. With SJS, there is an abrupt development of atypical, target-like and/or bullous lesions. They may be dusky, cyanotic, or purpuric with blisters in the center.

2. The lesions come in crops on the skin, often in a symmetrical pattern.

3. Mucosal involvement with bullae formation may include conjunctiva, oral cavity, nose, gastrointestinal tract, urethra, and genitalia.

4. Lesions are very painful which makes it difficult to perform activities of daily living (ADL).

5. The disease is typically self-limiting and resolves in about 1 month, if there are no complications. Oral lesions may continue for many months.

D. **Incidence.**

1. This syndrome occurs 1 to 6 times per million person years.

2. SJS occurs primarily in children, young adults, and those under 40 years of age.

II. ASSESSMENT

A. **History and physical examination.**

1. A detailed history of recent illnesses and medication use is essential in identifying the causative agent. Particular attention should be given to any new treatments used in the previous weeks. Identifying the causative agent and discontinuing suspect medications can help prevent exacerbations or new episodes.

2. The patient may have fever, sore throat, chills, and malaise.

B. **Diagnostic tests.**

1. A skin biopsy of an early small bulla is performed to exclude other diseases and will help confirm the diagnosis.

2. Direct immunofluorescence may be helpful in atypical cases.

3. In widespread disease, electrolytes may be altered with sodium and calcium decreasing and potassium increasing.

III. COMMON THERAPEUTIC MODALITIES

A. **Medical intervention.**

1. Patients with localized SJS can be treated in an outpatient facility. Serious cases should be admitted to the hospital for observation and supportive care.

2. Cutaneous bullae should be treated with soothing moist compresses. Moist compress solutions which have an antibacterial effect will help prevent secondary infections in the open erosions.

3. Topical steroids can be applied to intact skin for

erythema and pruritus.

4. Pain from oral lesions can be relieved with frequent use of topical anesthetic gels such as viscous lidocaine.

5. Close monitoring of ocular and GI involvement is essential.

B. **Drug therapy.**

1. The value of systemic corticosteroids is debatable. Some clinicians feel the therapeutic effect is limited, especially if the causative agent has been identified and eliminated. Close monitoring of the side effects of systemic corticosteroids is critical.

2. The recovery period depends on how long it takes for the causative agent to be eliminated from the body.

3. Recently, intravenous immunoglobulin (IVIG) 0.75G/Kg per day for 4 days has led to a more rapid response.

4. Antihistamines may be used to control pruritus.

5. Oral antibiotics may be necessary for secondary infection of eroded skin.

IV. COMMON NURSING DIAGNOSIS: OUTCOMES AND INTERVENTIONS (see Table 1)

V. PATIENT TEACHING

Same as pemphigus vulgaris.

DERMATITIS HERPETIFORMIS

I. OVERVIEW

A. **Definition: dermatitis herpetiformis (DH) is a chronic, pruritic, relapsing disease.**

B. **Etiology.**

1. Dermatitis herpetiformis can be grouped, symmetrical, and erythematous.

2. The course of DH is usually life-long but general health is not usually directly affected.

C. **Pathophysiology.**

1. The eruptions may be bullous, papular, papulovesicular, or urticarial.

2. All types of lesions may be present on the same patient.

3. The bullous and vesicular lesions are tense and have clear contents.

4. Gluten sensitive enteropathy (GSE) occurs in approximately 15% of patients with DH.

D. **Incidence.**

1. DH is most common in men.

2. The disease is more common in the descendents of the North European population and is uncommon in blacks.

3. The mean age of onset is in the 4th decade.

II. ASSESSMENT

A. History and physical examination.

1. The grouped erythematous, papulovesicles are sometimes hard to see intact since the pruritic eruption is often rapidly excoriated by the patient.
2. Primary sites are scalp, posterior shoulders, sacral region, buttocks, knees, and extensor areas near the elbows.

B. Diagnostic tests.

1. A punch biopsy of a new red papular lesion that has not blistered is optimal for diagnosis.
2. Direct immunofluorescence studies can be taken from the area adjacent to the lesion (about 1 cm from a lesion).
3. Serologic studies can detect circulating anti-endomysial, anti-reticulum, and anti-gliadin antibodies.
4. A lymphoma workup may be done due to the increased incidence in DH patients.

III. COMMON THERAPEUTIC MODALITIES

A. Medical interventions.

1. Illness, stress, and variations in diet provoke exacerbations.
2. A gluten-free diet, which is difficult for patients to follow, does improve the clinical condition and thus reduces the required dose of medication.

B. Drug therapy.

1. Dapsone is very effective for patients with DH. Pruritus is sometimes relieved within hours of the initial dose. For adults, the typical dose of Dapsone is 100 to 150 mg every day. The dose is adjusted to the lowest dose that provides acceptable relief.
2. Close monitoring of leukocyte count and hemoglobin is critical.
3. Close monitoring of potential side effects of Dapsone is also essential. Peripheral motor neuropathy is one of the most serious side effects. Symptoms slowly improve over months after Dapsone is discontinued.
4. Sulfapyridine may be used as a substitute for Dapsone.
5. Antihistamines may be used for intense pruritus.

IV. COMMON NURSING DIAGNOSIS, OUTCOMES, AND INTERVENTIONS (see Table 1)

V. PATIENT TEACHING

Same as Pemphigus Vulgaris.

Bibliography

Bankston, J., Deshotels, J.M., & Daught, L. (2001). SJS—same trigger, less deadly. *RN, 64*(10), 29-41.

Bello, Y.M., Falabella, A.F., & Schacher, L.A. (2001). Epidermolysis bullose and its treatment. *WOUNDS: A Compendium of Clinical Research and Practice, 13*(3), 113-118.

DeMott, K. (2002). Experimental treatments promising for pemphigus. *Skin and Allergy News, 31.*

Fishman, T.D. (1999). Wound assessment and evaluation. *Dermatology Nursing, 11*(5) 436-437.

Mutasim, D.F. (1999). Autoimmune bullous diseases: Diagnosis and management. *Dermatology Nursing, 11*(5), 15-21.

Rye, B., & Webb, J.M. (1997). Autoimmune bullous diseases. *American Family Physicians, 55*(8), 2709-2718

Sirois, D, Leigh, J., & Sollecito, T. (2000). Oral pemphigus preceding cutaneous lesions. *JADA, 131,* 1156-1160.

STUDY QUESTIONS

1. Causative agents in the development of SJS include:
   a. Anticonvulsants.
   b. Antimalarials.
   c. Antibiotics.
   d. All the above.

2. The earliest symptom of SJS may mimic a nonspecific upper respiratory infection.
   a. True
   b. False

3. The site of the first lesion in pemphigus vulgaris may be:
   a. Perianal.
   b. Face.
   c. Oral mucosa.
   d. Any of the above.

4. There are many different types of pemphigus. The most common form of pemphigus is:
   a. Pemphigus vegetans.
   b. Pemphigus foliaceus.
   c. Pemphigus vulgaris.
   d. Pemphigus erythematosus.

5. Which disease is most characteristically self-limiting and resolves in about 1 month if there are not complications:
   a. PV.
   b. SJS.
   c. DH.
   d. BP.
   e. EB.

6. Lesions such as bullae, vesicles, and erosions may be present in:
   a. SJ.
   b. EB.
   c. PV.
   d. BP.
   e. All of the above.

7. Following a gluten-free diet may reduce the required dose of oral medications in this disease:
   a. BP.
   b. SJS.
   c. PV.
   d. DH.
   e. EB.

8. Of the following diseases, the most likely to be present at birth is:
   a. SJS.
   b. BP.
   c. EB.
   d. PV.
   e. DH.

9. Nikolsky's sign:
   a. Is pathognomonic for PV.
   b. Is defined as dislodging of the epidermis with lataral pressure placed on the skin.
   c. Is often used as a diagnostic test since it is cost effective.
   d. Usually does not result in a cutaneous erosion.

10. The use of systemic steroids is debatable in this disease:
    a. BP.
    b. PV.
    c. SJS.
    d. DH.

11. Illness, variations in diet, and stress may provoke exacerbations of this disease:
    a. EB.
    b. DH.
    c. BP.
    d. PV.
    e. All of the above.

Answers to Study Questions

1. d	5. b	9. b
2. a	6. e	10. c
3. c	7. d	11. b
4. c	8. c	

Acknowledgment: Special thanks to Dr. James A. Yiannas, Associate Professor, Department of Dermatology, Mayo Clinic, Scottsdale, Arizona, for assisting in the perparation of this chapter.

CE Answer/Evaluation Form

Chapter 10.
Bullous and Vesicular Diseases

Please photocopy this test page and return.

COMPLETE THE FOLLOWING:

Name: _____

Address: _____

City: _____ State: _____ Zip: _____

Preferred telephone: (Home)_____ (Work) _____

State where licensed and license number: _____

CE application fee: DNA member $7.00
                        Nonmember $10.00

POSTTEST INSTRUCTIONS
1. To receive continuing education credit for individual study after reading the article, complete the answer/evaluation form below.
2. Photocopy and send the answer/evaluation form along with a check or money order payable to **Dermatology Nurses' Association** to: **DNA**, East Holly Avenue Box 56, Pitman, NJ 08071-0056.
3. Test returns must be postmarked by December 31, 2008. Upon completion of the answer/evaluation form, a certificate for 1.8 contact hour(s) will be awarded and sent to you.

This chapter was reviewed and formatted for contact hour credit by Marcia J. Hill, MSN, RN, Core Curriculum Editor; and Sally Russell, MN, RN,C, DNA Education Director.

ANSWER FORM

1. Name one new detail (item, issue, or phenomenon) that you learned by completing this activity.

_____

_____

_____

_____

2. How will you apply the information from this learning activity to your practice?
   a. Patient education.
   b. Staff education.
   c. Improve my patient care.
   d. In my education course work.
   e. Other: Please describe _____

_____

_____

	Strongly disagree				Strongly agree

Evaluation
3. The offering met the stated objectives.

a. Identify the main characteristics of the disease processes of pemphigus vulgaris (PV), bullous pemphigoid (BP), and epidermolysis bullosa (EB), Stevens-Johnson syndrome (SJS), and dermatitis herpetiformis (DH).	1	2	3	4	5
b. Discuss tools used in making the diagnosis of PV, BP, EB, SJS, and DH.	1	2	3	4	5
c. Define therapeutic interventions used in treating PV, BP, EB, SJS, and DH.	1	2	3	4	5
d. Identify nursing interventions that assist in providing optimal care to patients.	1	2	3	4	5
e. List patient/family teaching strategies.	1	2	3	4	5

4. The content was current and relevant.	1	2	3	4	5
5. The content was presented clearly.	1	2	3	4	5
6. The content was covered adequately.	1	2	3	4	5
7. I am more confident of my abilities since completing this material.	1	2	3	4	5

8. The material was (check one) ☐ new, ☐ review for me.

Comments _____

9. Time required to complete reading assignment: _____ minutes

This independent study is provided by the Dermatology Nurses' Association (DNA) for 1.8 contact hours. DNA is accredited as a provider of continuing education in nursing by the American Nurses Credentialing Center's Commission on Accreditation. DNA is approved as a provider of continuing education by the California Board of Registered Nursing Provider #CEP5708.

Pediatric Dermatology/Acne

Sherrill Jantzi Rudy, MSN, RN, CPNP

OBJECTIVES

At the end of this chapter, the reader will be able to:

- Recognize skin conditions commonly seen in the pediatric population.
- Discuss the therapeutic interventions frequently used in pediatric dermatology.
- Identify important patient teaching issues for common pediatric skin disorders.

KEY POINTS

- Many skin conditions in newborns are transient, self-limited problems that do not require intervention other than to provide reassurance to parents.
- Genetic skin disorders generally present lifelong problems for affected individuals.
- Relief of itching and inflammation is the cornerstone of therapy for atopic dermatitis.
- The two major bacterial pathogens found on children's skin are *Staphylococcus aureus* and *Streptococcus pyogenes.*
- Acne vulgaris is the most prevalent skin condition observed in the pediatric age group.

Pediatric Dermatology/Acne

Sherrill Jantzi Rudy, MSN, RN, CPNP

TRANSIENT CUTANEOUS CONDITIONS IN THE NEWBORN

I. DEFINITION

A. Transient skin conditions that appear and disappear during the first few days to weeks or months of life.

II. ETIOLOGY AND PATHOLOGY

A. Infant skin differs from adult skin in that it seems to reflect bodily changes more readily.

B. These conditions are related to one or several of the following influences:
   1. Events occurring during birth.
   2. Immaturity of various physiologic systems.
   3. Influence of maternal hormones.

III. INCIDENCE

A. Few infants escape this stage without exhibiting one or more of these conditions.

IV. ASSESSMENT

A. Clinical manifestations.
   1. Acne neonatorium (neonatal acne).
      a. Presents as multiple discrete comedones and papules on face, particularly on the cheeks. Occasionally lesions are also present on the chest, back, and/or groin. After a few weeks the papules may develop into pustules.
      b. Appears at 2 to 4 weeks of age and may persist for up to 6 months of age. Present in 20% of infants.
      c. Believed to be the result of transient increases of circulating androgens in the newborn.
   2. Acropustulosis of infancy.
      a. Presents as pustules or vesicles on the palms and soles in recurrent crops and rapidly become pruritic.
      b. Pruritus in the neonate may present as an irritable, fretful child.
      c. Lesions may recur every 2 to 4 weeks until 2 to 3 years of age.
      d. Etiology is unknown.
   3. Erythema toxicum neonatorum.
      a. Transient blotchy, red macules (2 to 3 cm) with or without a papule, vesicle, or yellowish-white pustule (1 to 4 mm) centrally.
      b. Present at 24 to 72 hours of age in 20% to 60% of term infants and clear in 4 to 5 days.
      c. Lesions are seen on the chest, back, face, and proximal extremities.
      d. Etiology is unknown.
   4. Harlequin color change.
      a. Occurs in low-birthweight infants when placed on one side. The dependent skin develops an erythematous flush, with a simultaneous blanching of the upper side.
      b. A distinct line of demarcation runs along the midline of the body.
      c. Usually subsides within a few seconds of placing the baby in the supine position but may persist up to 30 minutes.
      d. Attributed to the immaturity of autonomic vasomotor control.
   5. Milia.
      a. Multiple, pearly white 1 to 2 mm papules on the forehead, cheeks, and nose of infants.
      b. May also occur on the oral mucosa particularly the palate. These are called Epstein's pearls.
      c. Occur on the skin in 40% of newborns and in 60% on the palate.
      d. Papules contain keratin debris that rupture spontaneously and heal during the first months of life.
   6. Cutis marmorata.
      a. A physiologic reaction to cold in the newborn with the development of bluish, reticulated, mottling of the skin on the trunk and extremities.
      b. Disappears on rewarming.
      c. Thought to be caused by immaturity of the autonomic control of skin vascular plexus.
      d. Mottling that persists beyond the 6 months of life may be a sign of hypothyroidism or cutis marmorata telangiectatica congenita.
   7. Sebaceous gland hyperplasia.
      a. Small (1 mm) yellow macules or papules present at the pilosebaceous follicle opening over the nose and cheeks.
      b. Occurs in 50% of infants.
      c. Resolves by 4 to 6 months.
      d. Thought to be the result of maternal androgenic stimulation of the sebaceous glands.
   8. Subcutaneous fat necrosis.
      a. Sharply circumscribed, reddish or purple nodules on the cheeks, buttocks, arms, and/or thighs.

b. Appears within the first 2 weeks of life and resolves over several weeks to months.

c. May heal with atrophy, leaving a skin depression.

d. Results from cold injury to the skin causing crystallization of fatty acids within the subcutaneous fat cells followed by a granulomatous reaction.

9. Sucking blister.

a. Solitary intact blister or erosion on noninflamed skin of the fingers, dorsum of the dominant hand or wrist, or upper lip.

b. Results from vigorous sucking in the prenatal period.

c. Resolves within a few days.

10. Transient pustular melanosis.

a. Presents at birth as vesicles, pustules, or pigmented macules with a collarette of scale.

b. Seen more commonly in infants with darker pigment.

c. Resolves spontaneously over 3 weeks to 3 months.

d. Cause is unknown but thought to be associated with postinflammatory hyperpigmentation.

11. Miliaria.

a. Miliaria crystallina and rubra are the most common forms seen in the neonatal period.

b. Related to the immaturity of the eccrine ducts and retention of sweat.

c. Precipitating factors include warming in incubators, fevers, occlusive clothing, dressings, or devices.

d. Miliaria crystallina is characterized by many 1 to 2 mm easily ruptured vesicles on otherwise normal appearing skin. Older lesions will scale.

e. Miliaria rubra is characterized by discrete and confluent tiny, scaly, erythematous papules or papulovesicular lesions.

B. **Diagnostic tests.**

1. Diagnosis is generally made by the lesions' clinical features.

2. Occasionally a gram stain or Tzanck preparation may be used to rule out infectious causes.

3. In general, due to the benign nature of these conditions, additional diagnostic studies usually are not required.

V. NURSING CONSIDERATIONS (see Table 1)

A. **Interventions.**

1. Maintain an adequate fluid balance and nutrition in the infant.

2. Instruct and demonstrate appropriate skin care

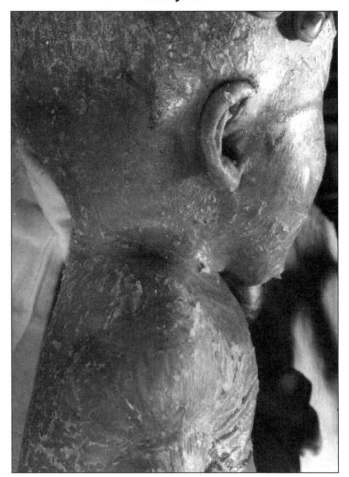

**Figure 1.
Ichthyosis**

techniques that will keep the skin clean, moisturized, and protected.

3. The majority of these conditions resolve spontaneously and do not require treatment.

a. In acne neonatorium, most cases require no treatment. For comedonal lesions azelaic acid 20% cream or mild topical retinoid preparations may be used. For inflammatory lesions, erythromycin 2%, clindamycin 1%, or 2.5% benzoyl peroxide may be used. Systemic therapy is generally avoided.

b. If acropustulosis of infancy is symptomatic, potent topical corticosteroids and/or oral antihistamines (hydroxyzine 2 mg/k/d) may provide relief of itching and may be used in older infants.

B. **Patient education.**

1. Reassure parents regarding the benign nature of these conditions.

2. Assure that the child is kept adequately warm, but avoid over dressing or occlusive clothing.

C. **Followup.**

1. Followup is only necessary if the condition worsens or parents have additional questions.

Table 1.
Nursing Care of a Child with Skin Disorders

Nursing Diagnoses	Goals	Expected Outcomes
Impaired skin integrity related to: 1. Environmental agents 2. Somatic factors	Promote healing. Eradicate source of skin injury.	Affected area displays signs of healing. Avoids precipitating agents.
Potential impaired skin integrity related to: 1. Mechanical trauma 2. Body secretions 3. Infection susceptibility 4. Allergenic factors	Maintain skin integrity. Prevent skin breakdown. Protect healthy skin. Prevent secondary infection. Promote general health.	Skin remains clean, dry, and intact. Infection remains confined to primary location. Complies with general hygienic measures.
Pain related to skin lesions and/or pruritus.	Relieve discomfort. Prevent or minimize scratching. Promote rest.	Displays no evidence of discomfort. Affected areas remain free of excoriation. Child receives adequate rest.
Potential for infection related to presence of microorganisms.	Prevent spread of infection to self and others.	Infection remains confined to primary location.
Body image disturbance related to perception of appearance.	Promotion of a positive self-image. Provide tactile contact. Support child. Encourage self-care. Educate child on home care.	Verbalizes concerns and feelings. Displays signs of comfort. Positive response to tactile stimulation. Identifies ways to improve appearance. Assumes responsibility for care when appropriate. Maintains usual activities and relationships.
Altered family process related to having a child with a skin condition: 1. Child's discomfort. 2. Time intensive and lengthy therapy.	Support family. Educate family on home care.	Family demonstrates necessary skills. Family demonstrates understanding of skin problem and supports child.

GENODERMATOSES

I. ICHTHYOSIS

A. **Definition.**
  1. Excessive scaling of the skin (see Figure 1). The scale may be "fish scale-like."
  2. Four major hereditary types have been described.
    a. Lamellar ichthyosis and congenital nonbullous ichthyosiform erythroderma.
    b. Bullous ichthyosis (also called congenital bullous ichthyosiform erythroderma or epidermolytic hyperkeratosis).
    c. Ichthyosis vulgaris.
    d. X-linked ichthyosis.
B. **Etiology and pathology.**
  1. Ichthyosis vulgaris (IV) is inherited as an autosomal dominant disease
  2. X-linked ichthyosis (XLI) is inherited as a X-linked recessive trait that is due to a deficiency of the enzyme, steroid sulfatase. Female carriers are asymptomatic.
  3. Lamellar ichthyosis (LI) and congenital

nonbullous ichthyosiform erythroderma (CNIE) are inherited in an autosomal recessive trait pattern.

4. Bullous ichthyosis (BI) is inherited as an autosomal dominant disorder.

5. Increased epidermal turnover with excessive production of stratum corneum cells has been demonstrated in LI and BI.

6. In XLI and IV, there appears to be normal epidermal turnover, and the accumulated scale is thought to be due to faulty shedding of the stratum corneum.

C. **Incidence.**
1. IV is extremely common with 1:250 children having some variant of this disorder from mild to severe.
2. XLI is estimated to occur in 1 in 60,000 males.
3. LI and CNIE appear to occur in approximately 1 per 100,000 live births.
4. Incidence of BI is unknown.

D. **Assessment.**
1. Clinical manifestations.
   a. Ichthyosis vulgaris.
      (1) The skin of the newborn with IV usually remains normal throughout the newborn period.
      (2) Manifestations are limited to the skin with fine scales predominately over the legs and buttocks that may be evident by 6 months to 2 years of age.
      (3) Dry, follicular, horny plugs (keratosis pilaris) are present on the extensor surface of extremities and may become widespread.
      (4) The entire surface of the skin is dry and may be associated with atopic dermatitis.
   b. X-linked ichthyosis.
      (1) Presents in infancy with scales over the posterior neck, upper trunk, and extensor surfaces of the extremities.
      (2) Scaling is usually mild during the first 30 days of life and the skin is a normal color.
      (3) As the child ages, the scales become thicker and dirty-yellow/brown in color. Antecubital and popliteal areas are often spared as well as the palms and soles.
      (4) Corneal opacities are a clinical marker in XLI, but are usually not present until adulthood.
      (5) Cryptorchidism may occur in as many as 25% of males with XLI and there is an associated increased risk of testicular cancer.
   c. Lamellar ichthyosis and congenital nonbullous ichthyosiform erythroderma.
      (1) Large, plate-like, dark scales with or

without erythematous skin are present in LI.
      (2) In CNIE, generalized fine scales on erythematous skin are present. The erythema may fade as the child ages.
      (3) With either condition, the affected infant may be born with a collodion membrane.
      (4) Facial tautness commonly produces ectropion and eclabium that appears shortly after birth in children with LI.
      (5) The skin of the palms and soles are generally thickened.
      (6) Cicatricial alopecia may develop as well as thickening of the nails and inflammation of the nail folds.
      (7) Heat intolerance is common and due to obstruction of the eccrine glands.
   d. Bullous ichthyosis.
      (1) Presents at birth with extensive scaling, erythroderma, and recurrent episodes of bullous formation.
      (2) The bullae frequently become infected with *Staphylococcus aureus* causing problems in the neonatal and infant periods.
      (3) With age, the involvement is more limited in extent and by school age, thick, warty, malodorous, dirty-yellow/brown scales will have developed on the palms, soles, elbows, and knees.
      (4) Flexure areas tend to have greater involvement and frequently become macerated and secondarily colonized with bacteria producing a foul body odor.
      (5) After the neonatal period the mechano-bullous component becomes less prominent; however, focal blistering continues.
      (6) Facial involvement is common, but ectropion does not occur. Nails may become dystrophic due to nail fold inflammation.
2. Diagnostic tests.
   a. Skin biopsy helps to demonstrate the histologic changes in the epidermis and hyperkeratosis.
   b. Measurement of steroid sulfatase activity in red blood cells may be useful in the diagnosis of X-linked ichthyosis.
   c. Molecular genetic diagnosis is useful to distinguish the various forms of ichthyosis.

E. **Nursing considerations (see Table 1).**
1. Interventions.
   a. Skin hydration one to two times daily.
   b. Daily use of emollients.
      (1) Bland emollients such as petrolatum or

mineral oil. For example, Vaseline®, Aquaphor®, Eucerin®, Vanicream®, or Johnson's Ultra Sensitive® product line.

   c. Keratolytics.

     (1) Alpha-hydroxy acid (lactic acid, urea, glycolic acid) in cream of ointment vehicles. Commercial preparations include Eucerin Plus®, Lacticare®, LacHydrin®, AmLactin®, Aqua Glycolic®, or Carmol®.

     (2) If available, compounding products of varying concentration is also an option.

   d. Topical retinoids are helpful to some people to remove scaling. These include tretinoin and tazarotene.

   e. Oral retinoids may be used to alleviate the hyperkeratosis. Due to their toxicity their use is warranted only in patients with severe physical or emotional complications.

   f. Adequate provision of calories in diet, especially protein and monitoring of child's iron status due to the metabolic drain of erythroderma on a growing child and substantial iron loss in hyperproliferative states.

   g. Infants with widespread blistering or colloidian membrane are cared for in the NICU with precautions to avoid further trauma to the skin, regulate skin temperature and hydration, as well as prevent infection.

   h. Psychosocial support to deal with issues related to body image, social relationships, and demanding complex therapy.

2. Patient education.

   a. Prevent heat prostration particularly during strenuous physical activity and/or warm temperatures.

   b. Bath with antibacterial soaps to decrease bacterial colonization of scales.

   c. Consideration of choice of clothing and shoe wear for children with mechanically induced blisters.

   d. Blistering after infancy often signifies a bacterial infection requiring treatment with an oral antibiotic effective against *S. aureus*.

   e. Referral to the Ichthyosis Foundation for family support.

3. Followup.

   a. One week after discharge from the newborn nursery.

   b. Routine visits for pediatric care and additional visits may be necessary, depending on the severity of the ichthyosis.

II. EPIDERMOLYSIS BULLOSA

A. **Definition.**

1. A group of diseases linked by the formation of vesicular-bullous lesions of various depths, which usually appear in response to mechanical trauma.

2. At least 18 distinct hereditary types of epidermolysis bullosa (EB) have been described and are classified according to the site of blister formation.

   a. Epidermolytic (simplex) group — epidermis.

   b. Junctional group — epidermal/dermal junction.

   c. Dermolytic (scarring) group — dermis.

B. **Etiology and pathology.**

1. EB disorders are inherited as either autosomal dominant (see Figures 11-1 & 11-2, page 239) or recessive (see Figures 11-3 to 11-7, pages 239-240) traits.

2. Children born with EB have genetically weakened anchoring structures of the skin. Therefore, when friction is applied to the skin, especially in the presence of heat and moisture, blisters are formed.

C. **Incidence.**

1. It is estimated that 25,000 to 50,000 Americans have some form of EB.

2. Recessive dystrophic cases are estimated to occur in 1:45,000.

D. **Assessment.**

1. Clinical manifestations.

   a. Epidermolysis bullosa simplex (EBS).

     (1) Most common form is localized to hands and feet.

     (2) Blisters are formed in the intra-epidermal layers and are usually not scarring.

     (3) Onset is in childhood or adolescence with minor frictional trauma particularly in warm weather.

     (4) May be generalized with lesions present at birth or appearing by 6 to 12 months of age.

     (5) Blisters are more numerous on distal extremities but may also be seen on elbows and knees.

   b. Junctional epidermolysis bullosa (JEB).

     (1) Two forms are recognized.

       (a) Generalized, often fatal form.

       (b) Milder form.

     (2) Presents at birth with a few lesions.

     (3) Mucous membrane lesions appear within the first month of life in the lethal form and are absent in the milder form. Severely affected oral mucosa results in failure to thrive. The gastrointestinal, genitourinary, and respiratory tracts may

also be involved.
   (4) The majority of lesions heal without scarring, but lateral extension of large bullae and complications such as infection or hemorrhage can result in scarring.
   c. Dystrophic epidermolysis bullosa (DEB).
   (1) Hemorrhagic bullae appear on the skin at birth or shortly thereafter. Mucous membranes may also be involved.
   (2) Removal of the blister roof leaves a raw, bleeding base that heals with scar formation. Healing scars entrap islands of epithelium, producing milia within the scars. After prolonged and repeated trauma, squamous cell carcinoma may develop.
   (3) Scarring frequently results in replacement of nails and pseudo-webbing of digits, leading to a club-like appearance of hands and feet.
   (4) Scarring also can result in alopecia, immobilization of the tongue, esophageal stricture, or respiratory stridor.
   (5) Anemia and malnutrition often occur and may lead to failure to thrive.
   (6) Secondary infection with Candida or bacteria is common.
   (7) The dominant type of DEB is not as debilitating as the recessive type due to less involvement of the mucous membranes.
   2. Diagnostic tests.
   a. Skin biopsy examined by electron microscopy will differentiate the various forms of EB.
E. **Nursing considerations (see Table 1).**
   1. Interventions.
   a. Minimize trauma to skin.
   (1) Handle gently.
   (2) Do not apply adhesives to the skin.
   (3) Do not rub the skin.
   (4) Dress in loose-fitting clothes.
   (5) Avoid over-heating.
   (6) Thoroughly soak materials that are stuck to the skin before removing.
   (7) Lubricate the skin to decrease friction.
   (8) Drain blisters.
   (9) Pad bony prominences with dressings.
   (10) Avoid rectal temperatures or other invasive procedures (catheterization, endoscopic examination, naso-gastric tubes, etc.) that may cause trauma to mucous membranes.
   b. Provide moist wound healing environment.
   (1) Use only nonadherent dressings such as white petrolatum gauze, hydrogels,

fenestrated silicone dressing, or absorbent foam silicone dressing covered with a nonadherent pad and secured in place with soft roller gauze bandages and elastic tubular dressings.
   (2) Additional topical ointment may be applied to promote moist wound healing.
   c. Prevent bacterial superinfection of wounds or sepsis.
   (1) Observe wounds for signs of infection.
   (2) Monitor colonization with occasional wound cultures.
   (3) Apply topical antibiotics (bacitracin, polymyxin, silvadene, gentamycin, or mupirocin) only when there is evidence or strong suspicion of an infection.
   (4) In cases of chronic infection, rotate the topical antibiotics every 3 months to prevent the development of resistant organisms.
   (5) Cleanse skin daily with a hydrophilic agent such as Cetaphil® or with a very mild soap such as Neutrogena® or Dove®.
   (6) Change outer dressings daily. Some contact layer dressings such as the fenestrated silicone dressings may be left in place for several days.
   d. Maximize nutrition.
   (1) Breastfeed if possible.
   (2) If unable to breastfeed, pump breast milk and bottle feed with a Habermann feeder, soft nipples, or if sucking causes too much trauma with a medicine dropper.
   (3) Vitamin and nutritional supplements in cases of anemia and malnourishment.
   e. Treatment is symptomatic and supportive and often requires a multidisciplinary approach.
   (1) Primary care.
   (2) Gastroenterology.
   (3) Nutrition.
   (4) Dermatology.
   (5) Plastic surgery.
   (6) Dental.
   (7) Ophthalmology.
   (8) Respiratory.
   (9) Urology.
   (10) Genetics.
   (11) Physical/Occupational therapy.
   (12) Speech therapy.
   (13) Social services.
   f. Psychosocial support should be provided to the child and family with education provided for caregivers on prevention and care of blisters and complications.

Dermatologic Nursing Essentials: A Core Curriculum 2nd Edition © DNA 2003

2. Patient education.
   a. Skin care techniques.
   b. Steps to reduce friction.
   c. Referral to the lay support group —
      Dystrophic Epidermolysis Bullosa Research
      Association of America, Inc (DEBRA).
3. Followup.
   a. After birth, visits should be weekly or
      biweekly.
   b. Once the condition is stabilized and parents
      are comfortable with care
      recommendations, regular visits are
      scheduled to monitor skin condition,
      wound healing, infection, malignancy, and
      nutrition.

DERMATITIS

I. ATOPIC DERMATITIS

A. **Definition.**
   1. A hereditary disorder associated with
      inflammation of the skin leading to pruritus and
      disruption of the skin surface.
   2. Seen commonly in children.
      a. Fifty percent clear by 2 years of age.
      b. Of the remaining 50%, half clear by
         adolescence.
      c. The rest persist into adulthood.
B. **Etiology and pathology.**
   1. The exact pathogenesis is unknown.
   2. Is associated with an exaggerated response to
      inflammatory stimuli, dysfunction of the
      cutaneous barrier, and hyperproduction of
      proinflammatory cytokines by keratinocytes.
   3. Several theories have proposed a relationship to
      immunodeficiency, abnormal β-adrenergic
      receptors, food allergies, or other
      environmental allergies. However, these
      theories have not been substantiated.
   4. Commonly there is a family history of atopic
      dermatitis, asthma, and/or allergic rhinitis.
C. **Incidence.**
   1. A very common disorder with onset in infancy.
   2. Approximately 50% of children with atopic
      dermatitis also have asthma or allergic rhinitis.
D. **Assessment.**
   1. Clinical manifestations.
      a. Characterized by:
         (1) Xerosis.
         (2) "Sensitive" skin.
         (3) Inflammation.
         (4) Pruritus.
      b. Severity ranges from mild to severe; tends
         to wax and wain with seasonal variation,
         frequently worsening in the winter.
      c. Precipitating factors.
         (1) Extremes in temperature and humidity:

hot/humid or cold/dry.
         (2) Sweating.
         (3) Course clothing such as wool and some
             synthetic fabrics.
         (4) Drying soaps (vs soaps in general).
         (5) Emotional stress.
         (6) Allergies (food and environmental).
      d. Primary lesions.
         (1) Some believe no primary lesion can be
             identified and that all visible skin lesions
             in AD are secondary to scratching.
         (2) Erythematous papules that may
             coalesce.
      e. Secondary lesions.
         (1) Scale.
         (2) Excoriations.
         (3) Lichenification.
         (4) White dermatographism.
      f. Distribution.
         (1) Tends to be symmetrical.
         (2) Is often more pronounced in areas not
             covered by clothing.
         (3) The extensor surfaces and face tend to
             have greater involvement in infants.
             Diaper area is generally clear.
         (4) The flexor surfaces tend to have greater
             involvement in older children.
      g. Complications.
         (1) Secondary infection usually caused by *S.
             aureus.*
         (2) Eczema herpeticum when exposed to
             someone with herpes simplex.
   2. Diagnostic tests.
      a. IgE tests are frequently elevated but are not
         helpful diagnostically.
      b. Allergy testing if allergies are strongly
         suspected, but may not be helpful in
         changing disease course.
      c. Skin cultures in cases of suspected
         secondary infection.
E. **Nursing considerations (see Table 1).**
   1. Interventions.
      a. Relief of xerosis.
         (1) Bathe in warm, plain water (avoid bath
             water additives). Soaking in water for up
             to 20 minutes is helpful for some
             children.
         (2) Use mild, fragrence-free, dye-free soap
             such as Dove®, Basis®, Aveeno®,
             Johnson's Ultra Sensitive® products, and
             Johnson's Head-to-Toe Baby Wash®.
         (3) Daily use of fragrance-free emollients
             that are either in the form of lotions,
             creams, or ointments depending on the
             severity of the xerosis. May need to
             apply several times a day.
         (4) Wet dressing with occlusion several
             times a day or overnight to treat

children with multiple excoriations, crusting, and weeping lesions.
- (a) Wet one pair of cotton sleepers in warm water, wring out until damp, and put damp sleepers on child.
- (b) Place a pair of dry sleepers on top of the damp ones.
- (c) Keep the room warm to avoid chilling.
- b. Decrease inflammation.
  - (1) Mild-to-moderate strength, topical corticosteroids twice a day as needed.
  - (2) Topical corticosteroids may be used in combination with wet dressings in severe cases.
    - (a) Use overnight for 5 to 10 nights.
    - (b) Change every 6 hours for 24 to 72 hours.
  - (3) Topical immunomodulator (tacrolimus or pimecrolimus) may be used twice a day in patients requiring frequent use of topical corticosteroids, those failing conventional therapy, and is indicated as first-line therapy for facial dermatitis.
  - (4) Cream or ointment vehicle may be used. Some children with AD are sensitive to the ingredients of creams.
  - (5) Short-course systemic corticosteroids are used in extreme cases only. Rebound flaring occurs when systemic corticosteroids are discontinued.
  - (6) Ultraviolet light therapy or low-dose cyclosporin A may be used in severe cases of atopic dermatitis that do not respond to conventional therapies.
- c. Relief of pruritus.
  - (1) Antihistamines such as diphenhydramine (3 to 5 mg/kg/day) or hydroxyzine (1 to 2 mg/kg/day) may help to relieve pruritus because of their sedative effect.
  - (2) Use antihistamines at bedtime for itching and to promote more restful sleep.
  - (3) Other antihistamines such as cetirizine or loratadine may be used to provide relief from pruritus in children 2 years and older. Fexofenadine may used in children 6 years and older.
  - (4) Cool soaks followed by emollients or topical corticosteroids also help to relieve pruritus.
- d. Treatment of infections.
  - (1) Topical antibiotic — mupirocin 2% ointment may be applied 3 times a day to small areas of impetigo.
  - (2) For more widespread infection, use an antistaphylococcal oral antibiotic (for example, dicloxacillin 12 to 25

mg/kg/day, erythromycin 30 to 50 mg/kg/day, or cephalexin 25 to 50 mg/kg/day).
- e. Environmental control.
  - (1) Decrease exposure to predisposing factors.
  - (2) Avoid exposure to anyone with active herpes lesions.
2. Patient education.
  - a. Methods of skin hydration.
  - b. Proper methods of application of medications.
  - c. Signs of skin infection.
  - d. Ways to incorporate treatments into daily routines.
  - e. Sources of psychosocial support such as the National Eczema Association for Science and Education (NEASE).
3. Followup.
  - a. First followup visit in 10 to 14 days to assess treatment effectiveness.
  - b. Monthly visits until child is using lubricants only.
  - c. When skin condition is stable visits every 3 to 4 months for re-evaluation.
  - d. As needed for flares and failure to respond to treatment.

II. SEBORRHEIC DERMATITIS

A. Definition.
1. Common chronic dermatitis occurring primarily in areas of increased sebaceous gland concentration resulting in an overproduction of sebum.
2. Occurs in two age groups — the neonate and the adolescent.

B. Etiology and pathology.
1. Etiology: Inflammatory response to the presence of yeast.
2. Occurrence in the neonate is believed to be related to intrauterine exposure to maternal hormones.
3. Occasionally may be associated with serious illness and failure to thrive. In HIV-infected patients it may be an early sign of AIDS.

C. Incidence.
1. The incidence in the general population is 2% to 5%.
2. In infants, tends to regress by 5 to 6 months of age.
3. In adolescents, may improve with age, tends to wax and wain.

D. Assessment.
1. Clinical manifestations.
  - a. Minimal to no pruritus in infancy. Adolescents may complain of pruritus.
  - b. Lesions are symmetric and typically red

with greasy yellow to salmon-colored scale.

   c. Areas of involvement are primarily the scalp, medial eyebrows, central face, retroauricular area, presternal, and groin.

   d. Varies from minimal to widespread involvement.

   e. Primary lesions — erythematous papules/patches, poorly marginated.

   f. Secondary lesions — greasy scale, excoriations if pruritic.

  2. Diagnostic tests.

   a. Not helpful unless severe systemic disease is suspected.

E. Nursing considerations (see Table 1).

  1. Interventions.

   a. Topical anti-fungals and low-potency corticosteroid creams applied twice daily for several days will usually clear the dermatitis and then used occasionally will control recurrences.

   b. Frequently in infants, tear-free shampoos are adequate to loosen the scales when allowed to remain on the scalp for several minutes and lightly scrubbed with a soft brush to remove the scale.

   c. Keratolytic/antiseborrheic shampoos may be helpful for adolescents to control scalp scaling. For more stubborn cases, use ketoconazole (Nizoral®) shampoo.

   d. Diaper involvement may result in secondary Candida infection which should be treated with an antifungal cream.

  2. Patient teaching.

   a. Review the expected course of the disorder.

   b. Encourage gentle therapy in removal of the scales.

   c. Instruct on proper use of the medication.

  3. Followup.

   a. One week visit to evaluate response.

   b. Thereafter, the child is seen only if the dermatitis does not resolve.

III. DIAPER DERMATITIS

A. Definition.

  1. A cutaneous eruption in the diaper area caused by wearing a diaper.

B. Etiology and pathology.

  1. Is caused by an interaction between several factors.

   a. Frequent and prolonged skin wetness from occlusion and urine trapping close to the skin.

   b. Friction by movement of the skin against skin, the diaper, plastic leg gathers, or fastening tape.

   c. Fecal enzymes causing cutaneous irritation.

   d. Bacterial or yeast growth in a dark moist environment on inflamed damaged skin.

  2. Administration of oral antibiotic medication may predispose a child to develop diaper dermatitis.

  3. Other conditions that may be associated with diaper dermatitis.

   a. Impetigo.

   b. Staphylococcal scalded skin.

   c. Scarlet fever.

   d. Streptococcal perianal cellulitis.

   e. Kawasaki disease.

   f. Congenital syphilis.

   g. HIV infection.

   h. Langerhans' cell histiocytosis.

   i. Psoriasis.

C. Incidence.

  1. Diaper dermatitis is a common problem in infants.

  2. May occur in any child who is incontinent of urine or stool.

D. Assessment.

  1. Clinical manifestations.

   a. Erythema with or without papules, erosions, scale and/or maceration on the lower abdomen, groin, perineum, buttocks, labia majora, scrotum, penis, or upper thigh that initially spares skin creases.

   b. If diaper dermatitis is present for longer than 3 days there is likely to be secondary *Candida albicans* infection. This presents as confluent erythema with satellite papules and often involves skin creases.

   c. Fragile bulla or erosions with a collarette of scale may indicate bullous impetigo.

  2. Diagnostic tests.

   a. KOH preparation to identify Candida infection.

   b. Bacterial culture may be needed to rule out bacterial infection.

   c. Skin biopsy may be required in diaper dermatitis that is unresponsive to therapy to rule out other associated problems.

E. Nursing considerations (see Table 1).

  1. Interventions.

   a. Most irritant diaper dermatitis is self-limited and may resolve quickly with the following steps.

    (1) Airing of the diaper area.

    (2) Application of barrier creams and ointments (such as petrolatum or zinc oxide).

    (3) Frequent diaper changes.

   b. Candida diaper dermatitis is treated with a topical antiyeast cream such as nystatin applied TID or with each diaper change.

   c. In severe dermatitis, hydrocortisone 1% cream twice daily for 1 or 2 days may help to decrease discomfort.

2. Patient education.
   a. Diaper dermatitis is less prevalent in children whose diapers are changed at least 8 times a day.
   b. Use of barrier ointments.
   c. Signs of Candida infection.
3. Followup.
   a. Routine visits for pediatric care is sufficient followup.
   b. In severe diaper dermatitis, a return visit in 2 days to assess response is recommended.

BACTERIAL SKIN INFECTIONS

I. IMPETIGO CONTAGIOSA AND ECTHYMA

A. **Definition.**
   1. Impetigo.
      a. A highly contagious, superficial bacterial skin infection seen frequently in children.
      b. Presents as a primary pyoderma or a secondary pyoderma complicating pre-existing skin conditions such as insect bites, atopic dermatitis, or varicella lesions.
   2. Ecthyma.
      a. A deeper type of pyoderma involving the entire epidermis and into the dermis.
      b. Frequently follows skin trauma from an insect bite, cut, or varicella.

B. **Etiology and pathology.**
   1. *S. aureus* causes bullous impetigo.
   2. Group A streptococci cause nonbullous impetigo.
   3. Currently, in many areas of North America, penicillinase-producing staphylococci are believed to be responsible for 70% to 80% of childhood impetigo.
   4. Poststreptococcal glomerulonephritis may follow streptococcal skin infections if nephritogenic strains of streptococci are involved.
   5. The following factors predispose children to developing impetigo.
      a. Impaired skin barrier.
      b. Poor hygiene.
      c. Malnutrition.
      d. Warm climates.

C. **Incidence.**
   1. Very common in children.
   2. Incidence increases in warm humid climates and with poor skin hygiene.

D. **Assessment.**
   1. Clinical manifestations of impetigo.
      a. Often begins as an area of localized erythema. A small vesicle, bullae, or pustule may develop; however, the intact primary lesion is rarely seen.
      b. The lesions seen clinically most commonly

are erosions covered with moist honey-colored crusts.
   c. The vesicles of bullous impetigo quickly lose the fragile roof leaving an outer rim of desquamation.
   d. Single or multiple lesions commonly appear on areas such as the face, nares, and extremities.
   2. Clinical manifestations of ecthyma.
      a. Begins as an erythematous vesicle or pustule.
      b. Develops a firm, dry, dark crust with surrounding erythema and induration.
      c. Purulent material may be expressed with direct pressure on the crust.
      d. Most commonly located on the lower extremity or buttocks.
      e. Usually painful.
   3. Diagnostic tests.
      a. Frequently impetigo and ecthyma are diagnosed by their typical presentations and do not require culture.
      b. Bacterial culture of the serous or purulent material beneath the crust may be obtained for confirmation of the organism and to obtain antibiotic sensitivities, in less typical presentations, or in persistent infections.
      c. Gram stain of the fluid or scrapings from the floor of the erosion or ulcer yields gram-positive clusters.

E. **Nursing considerations (see Table 1).**
   1. Interventions.
      a. A small localized impetigo infection not involving mucous membranes may be effectively treated with topical mupirocin ointment applied TID.
      b. To treat both pathogens orally:
         (1) Cephalexin 25 to 50 mg/kg/day for 10 days.
         (2) Dicloxacillin, 15 to 50 mg/kg/day for 10 days. The liquid form has an unappealing taste and compliance is poor in children requiring liquid medication.
         (3) Erythromycin 40 mg/kg/day for 10 days may be used as an alternative; however, in certain areas of North America strains of erythromycin-resistant staphylococci have been identified.
         (4) Azithromycin or clarithromycin are alternative treatments
      c. If streptococci only are cultured, penicillin V 250 to 500 mg 4 times a day for 10 days may be given.
   2. Patient education.
      a. Instruct on how to administer topical or oral antibiotics.
      b. Instruct on the application of warm tap

water compresses 3 to 4 times daily until lesion is no longer weepy or crusted.

   c. Review good handwashing techniques and good general personal hygiene to prevent further infection of contacts and reduce recurrence.

   d. Instruct that the child may return to school or daycare after having used the antibiotic for 24 hours.

3. Followup.

   a. Ten days to 2 weeks after therapy has begun to evaluate response.

II. CELLULITIS

A. Definition.

1. Full-thickness infection of the skin involving the dermis and subcutaneous tissue which may subsequently spread to the lymphatics.

B. Etiology and pathology.

1. Group A streptococci account for most cases of cellulitis.
2. *Haemophilus influenzae* and *S. aureus* also may be responsible.
3. The bacteria invade into the deep dermis and subcutaneous fat, with subsequent spread via the lymphatics.

C. Incidence.

1. Not as prevalent as impetigo, but is not an uncommon diagnosis in children.
2. Eighty-four percent of cases involve the limbs and facial cellulitis accounts for 16% of cases.

D. Assessment.

1. Clinical manifestations.

   a. A preceding puncture wound or other penetrating trauma is often noted.

   b. Streptococcal cellulitis spreads rapidly, within hours, as compared to staphylococcal cellulitis.

   c. May be accompanied by symptoms of fever, chills, and malaise.

   d. Manifests as erythematous or violaceous plaques with ill-defined borders that are tender and warm to touch.

   e. Occasionally linear red macules proximal to the large plaque are seen.

   f. Desquamation and scale may be present.

   g. Tender regional lymphadenopathy is a common finding.

2. Diagnostic tests.

   a. Blood cultures are most likely to reveal the responsible bacteria.

   b. Cultures of the nasopharynx, conjunctiva, and possibly the middle ear or cerebrospinal fluid may be indicated with facial cellulitis.

   c. Aspiration of the advancing border of the cellulitis is rarely positive.

E. Nursing considerations (see Table 1).

1. Interventions.

   a. In acutely ill children or children with periorbital cellulitis, hospitalization with IV administration of antibiotics is often required.

   b. If a streptococcal infection is suspected, systemic penicillin is given, either as benzathine penicillin, 600,000 to 1,200,000 U IM or oral penicillin V 30 to 60 mg/kg/day for 10 days.

   c. If staphylococcal infection is suspected, oral dicloxacillin 15 to 50 mg/kg/day or cephalexin 25 to 50 mg/kg/day.

   d. If *H. influenzae* is suspected, ampicillin is given IV with chloramphenicol or a third-generation cephalosporin such as cefotaxime or ceftriaxone after obtaining blood cultures.

2. Patient education.

   a. Instruct on the life-threatening potential of cellulitis.

   b. Review proper wound cleansing procedures.

   c. Importance of followup.

3. Followup.

   a. Daily visits until improvement in the cellulitis is observed to assess response to therapy.

III. STAPHYLOCOCCAL SCALDED SKIN SYNDROME (SSSS)

A. Definition.

1. A erythematous condition that may be generalized or limited to the upper body.
2. Occurs following an upper respiratory tract infection, purulent conjunctivitis, or impetigo.

B. Etiology and pathology.

1. Caused by *S. aureus* of phage group II which produces a toxin (*S. exfoliatin A*).
2. This toxin is carried to the skin by the circulation causing injury to the epidermal granular cells resulting in separation of the cells and subsequent shedding of the entire granular layer and stratum corneum when minor trauma to the skin occurs.

C. Incidence.

1. Seen in infants and children under the age of 5 years.
2. Occurs rarely in children over 5 years of age unless immunocompromised.
3. Mortality rate is 3% to 7%.

D. Assessment.

1. Clinical manifestations.

   a. A faint erythematous eruption begins on the central face, neck, axillae, and groin and gradually spreads.

b. The skin rapidly becomes acutely tender, with crusting around the mouth, eyes, and neck.

c. The child becomes feverish, irritable with malaise.

d. In 12 to 14 hours the epidermis may form vesicles, bullae, and easily desquamate in large sheets revealing bright red moist underlying skin.

e. Over the next 2 to 3 days the moist skin dries with crusts, fissuring, scaling, and desquamation.

2. Diagnostic tests.
   a. Skin biopsy to differentiate SSSS from toxic epidermal necrolysis.
   b. Nikolsky's sign is positive.
   c. Cultures of the nose, nasopharynx, throat, and/or conjunctiva reveal the responsible organisms.

E. **Nursing considerations (see Table 1).**
   1. Interventions.
      a. Children are frequently hospitalized for IV administration of antistaphylococcal antibiotics.
      b. Oral cephalexin 25 to 50 mg/kg/d or dicloxacillin 15 to 50 mg/kg/day may be used to treat less-severe cases.
      c. Infants may require burn therapy protocols for care of the skin as well as fluid and electrolyte replacement.
      d. Bland ointments several times a day will help in restoring the skin and reduce pain during the desquamation stage.
   2. Patient education.
      a. Healing will occur without scarring.
      b. May need to investigate for asymptomatic household carriers.
      c. Skin care procedures.
   3. Followup.
      a. One to two weeks after hospital discharge.
      b. Then routine followup care in regular pediatric visits.

FUNGAL/YEAST INFECTIONS

I. DERMATOPHYTE INFECTION (TINEA, RINGWORM)

A. **Definition.**
   1. Superficial fungal infection of the stratum corneum.
   2. Some species may also invade the hair and nails.
   3. Fungal infections are classified according to the area of the body involved.
      a. Tinea capitis — infection of the hair.
      b. Tinea corporis — infection of the skin.
      c. Tinea pedis — infection of the feet.

d. Tinea faciei — infection of the face.

e. Tinea cruris — infection of the inner thighs and inguinal creases.

B. **Etiology and pathology.**
   1. *Trichophyton tonsurans* and *Microsporum canis* cause almost all cases of tinea capitis. *T. tonsurans* accounts for 95% of tinea capitis in North America.
   2. Tinea corporis is caused by *M. canis, T. mentagrophytes, T. tonsurans,* or *T. rubrum.*
   3. Tinea pedis is caused by *T. mentagrophytes* or *T. rubrum.*
   4. Tinea faciei is caused by *M. canis* or *T. verrucosum.*
   5. *T. mentagrophytes* or *Epidermophyton floccosum* are the organisms most often responsible for tinea cruris.
   6. Transmission occurs by direct contact with the infected source or by indirect contact with inanimate objects contaminated with fungal spores (combs, brushes, clothing, shower floors, etc.).
   7. *M. canis* is harbored by cats, dogs, and certain rodents and children handling such animals are susceptible to infection. Human-to-human transmission of this organism does not seem to occur.

C. **Incidence.**
   1. Tinea capitis is quite prevalent in North America, especially in urban areas.
   2. Fungal infections, particularly tinea capitis and tinea corporis, are very common infections in childhood.

D. **Assessment.**
   1. Clinical manifestations.
      a. Tinea capitis is seen usually in prepubertal children and evidenced by patchy hair loss. Broken hairs may be evident at follicular orifice. White scale is frequently present.
      b. Kerion, a boggy inflammatory nodule with superficial pustules, may appear in tinea capitis 2 to 8 weeks after infection and can result in scarring and permanent hair loss if not treated.
      c. Regional lymphadenopathy with the presence of enlarged suboccipital and posterior cervical lymph nodes in association with tinea capitis is common.
      d. Tinea corporis often presents with one or several annular erythematous patches with scale, especially at the border, and central clearing or inflammation throughout the lesion.
      e. Tinea pedis is seen almost exclusively in postpubertal adolescents and presents with vesicles and erosions on the instep of one or both feet. Occasionally fissuring and scaling between the toes is seen.

f. Tinea faciei occurs commonly in children as erythematous scaly lesions that may have a butterfly distribution.

g. Tinea cruris is unusual before adolescence and presents as an erythematous, scaly eruption on the inner thighs and inguinal creases.

2. Diagnostic tests.

a. KOH examination of broken hairs or scale from the borders of lesions will confirm the diagnosis.

b. Fungal culture of broken hairs or scale.

E. **Nursing considerations (see Table 1).**

1. Intervention.

a. Tinea capitis.

(1) Griseofulvin (microsized) 20 to 25 mg/kg/day orally with high-fat foods for a minimum of 6 weeks. Treatment for 2 to 3 months may be required.

(2) Topical antifungal medication is ineffective in tinea capitis.

(3) Oral fluconazole, terbinafine, or itraconazole are second alternatives to griseofulvin. Side effects are more frequent with these agents than with griseofulvin.

(4) Selenium sulfide 2.5% or Nizoral® 2% shampoos, applied 3 times a week to the scalp reduces shedding and the potential spread of the infection.

(5) Usually kerions respond well to griseofulvin. Occasionally in long-standing kerions, a short course of oral steroids to reduce inflammation and prevent scarring is recommended. Prednisone 1 to 2 mg/kg/day for 5 to 10 days.

b. Tinea corporis, tinea pedis, tinea faciei, tinea cruris.

(1) Topical therapy is efficacious against 90% of dermatophyte species.

(a) Ciclopirox, clotrimazole, econazole, haloprogin, ketoconazole, miconazole, oxiconazole, sulconazole, terbinafine, tolnaftate creams or solutions are all effective.

(b) Applied once or twice daily until lesions have cleared.

(2) Rarely are oral terbinafine, itraconazole, fluconazole, griseofulvin, or other systemic agents required.

2. Patient education.

a. Methods of transmission and identification of likely contacts.

b. Environmental control measures.

c. Proper use of topical medications.

d. May need to take griseofulvin for 6 to 8 weeks with tinea capitis.

e. Griseofulvin absorption is improved when taken with high-fat foods.

3. Followup.

a. Children with tinea capitis should be reassessed monthly to evaluate response to therapy and to culture scalp. Treatment is continued until a negative culture is obtained.

b. Children with tinea capitis may return to school after oral and shampoo treatments are started.

c. Children with tinea corporis, pedis, faciei, and cruris should be seen in 2 weeks to evaluate response to therapy.

d. Children requiring griseofulvin for longer than 3 months should have liver function studies.

II. CANDIDIASIS

A. **Definition.**

1. Invasion of the skin or mucous membrane in regions of the body where warmth and moisture lead to maceration.

2. Candidiasis in different body sites has distinct clinical features.

a. Thrush — infection of the oral cavity.

b. Diaper candidiasis — infection of the diaper area.

c. Intertriginous candidiasis — infection of the inframammary, axillary, neck, and inguinal body folds.

d. Paronychia — infection at the base of nails.

e. Congenital candidiasis — generalized infection in a newborn.

f. Vulvovaginal candidiasis — infection of the vulva and/or vagina.

B. **Etiology and pathology.**

1. Candida albicans, considered part of the normal flora of the skin and mucous membranes, overgrows and invades the epidermis that has broken down due to moisture, warmth, or contact with irritating substances.

C. **Incidence.**

1. Very common infection in neonates and infants.

2. May be seen in children on long-term corticosteroid, antibiotic, or oral contraceptive therapy.

3. Immunodeficient children and children with diabetes mellitus and reticuloendothelial neoplasms are predisposed to candidiasis.

D. **Assessment.**

1. Clinical manifestations.

a. White plaques on an erythematous base on the buccal, tongue, or palate mucosa are seen in thrush.

b. Beefy erythema involving the skin folds

with elevated margins and satellite lesions are seen in cutaneous candidiasis.
    c. Diaper area candidiasis may present with erosions, pustules, or vesicles.
    d. Nontender erythema with swelling around the base of the nail occurs with paronychia.
    e. Vulvovaginal candidiasis appears as a cheesy vaginal discharge with erythematous vaginal mucosa and pruritus.
    f. Congenital candidiasis presents with generalized erythema with scaling and pustule formation.
  2. Diagnostic tests.
    a. KOH examination of scrapings of skin or mucosal lesions reveals budding yeast.
    b. *C. albicans* is easily cultured on Sabouraud dextrose agar or cornmeal agar.

E. Nursing considerations (see Table 1).
  1. Interventions.
    a. Thrush is treated with nystatin oral suspension 4 times daily for 5 days.
    b. Cutaneous candidiasis is treated with nystatin, miconazole, or clotrimazole in a cream vehicle applied 3 to 4 times a day. In the diaper area, the cream may be applied at each diaper change until clearing is achieved.
    c. Cases that are resistant to topical therapy may be treated with fluconazole 6 to 12 mg/k/d.
  2. Patient education.
    a. Sterilize nipples and pacifiers in infants with thrush.
    b. If breastfeeding, may need simultaneous treatment of mother's nipples or vulvovaginal candidiasis to adequately treat thrush.
    c. Proper diaper area care to prevent skin breakdown.
  3. Followup.
    a. A visit in 5 to 7 days to evaluate response to therapy.

VIRAL INFECTIONS

I. VIRAL EXANTHEMS

A. Definition.
  1. Any cutaneous eruption associated with an acute viral syndrome.
  2. Classified according to the type of eruption that occurs.
    a. Morbilliform eruptions — maculopapular eruptions that mimic measles.
    b. Vesiculobullous eruptions.

B. Etiology and pathology.
  1. A variety of viruses are known to cause viral exanthems.

    a. Measles virus.
    b. Rubella virus.
    c. Herpesvirus.
    d. Echovirus.
    e. Parvovirus.
    f. Epstein-Barr virus.
    g. Coxsackie virus.
  2. The clinical lesions are a result of a host response to the virus within the skin.

C. Incidence.
  1. The exact incidence is unknown.
  2. Despite immunization, measles have not been eradicated because of children who are not immunized or vaccine failure.
  3. The annual incidence of infectious mononucleosis is estimated a 50 per 100,000 children with the highest incidence in adolescents and young adults.
  4. Varicella is very common; however, the incidence is declining with the recent introduction of the varicella live virus vaccine.

D. Assessment.
  1. Clinical manifestations.
    a. Morbilliform eruptions.
      (1) Measles (rubeola).
        (a) The classic features include a severe prodrome of high fever, cough, rhinitis, and conjunctivitis lasting for 3 to 5 days followed by a cutaneous eruption.
        (b) The cutaneous eruption is preceded by intense erythema of the mucous membranes with focal 1 mm white areas that are called Koplik's spots.
        (c) The exanthem begins on the forehead as blotchy erythema and progresses to involve the face, trunk, and extremities with multiple discrete macules and papules.
        (d) Complications of measles include bacterial otitis media, pneumonia, encephalitis, myocarditis, thrombocytopenia, hepatitis, acute glomerulonephritis, and Stevens-Johnson syndrome.
      (2) Rubella.
        (a) Up to 50% of rubella infections may be entirely asymptomatic.
        (b) Mild lymphadenopathy may precede the cutaneous eruption by several days.
        (c) A faint pink macular eruption appears first on the face and spreads to the trunk and proximal extremities. Within 48 hours, the face and trunk have cleared and the eruption involves the distal extremities.

Dermatologic Nursing Essentials: A Core Curriculum 2nd Edition © DNA 2003

(d) The child usually appears well.

(e) Congenital rubella acquired during the first trimester of pregnancy may result in neonatal purpura, petechiae, thrombocytopenia, deafness, congenital heart defects, cataracts, glaucoma, growth retardation, and psychomotor retardation.

(3) Roseola.

(a) Occurs predominantly in infants under 2 years of age.

(b) Infants commonly have 2 or 3 days of sustained fever, followed by a fall in their temperature often to a subnormal level and then the development of a pink, morbilliform, cutaneous eruption which then fades in 24 hours.

(c) Mild edema of the eyelids and posterior cervical lymphadenopathy may be seen.

(4) Erythema infectiosum (fifth disease).

(a) Eruptions classically begin with an intense, confluent redness of both cheeks. It may then spread to involve the arms, legs, and abdomen with a lacy pink to dull-red macular rash.

(b) Eruption tends to last from 3 to 5 days; however, it may reappear up to 4 months with cutaneous vasodilatation.

(c) Twenty percent of children develop a mild fever.

(5) Echovirus exanthems.

(a) Result in morbilliform eruptions associated with two predominant clinical patterns.

i. A roseola-like pattern caused by echovirus 16 with a morbilliform cutaneous eruption appearing after the end of 2 or 3 days of fever.

ii. A petechial pattern caused by echovirus 9 results in a morbilliform eruption with acral petechiae.

(b) Seen more commonly in infants and toddlers than in older children.

(c) Skin rash tends to last 2 to 7 days.

(d) Usually occur in the summer with an incubation period of 3 to 5 days and is spread by the enteric route.

(6) Infectious mononucleosis.

(a) Has an incideous onset with fatigue, fever, generalized lymphadenopathy, sore throat with exudate, headache, splenomegaly, and hepatomegaly.

(b) A pink fleeting morbilliform eruption occurs in 15% of patients and lasts 1 to 5 days.

(c) Treatment with penicillin frequently results in an increased incidence of the rash.

(d) Fever and sore throat may last 1 to 3 weeks with fatigue and lethargy persisting for 3 months.

(e) The incubation period is 4 to 8 weeks.

(7) Papular acrodermatitis (Gianotti-Crosti syndrome).

(a) Characterized by groups of large, flat-topped, nonpruritic papules that appear in acral areas. Cheeks and buttocks may also be involved.

(b) Skin eruption may be preceded by low-grade fever and mild upper respiratory symptoms.

(c) The eruption may persist for 2 to 8 weeks and may be recurrent.

(d) In Europe, 30% of patients have mild viral hepatitis B; however, EBV, CMV, and Coxsackie virus A16 are more common etiologic agents in the United States.

b. Vesiculobullous eruptions.

(1) Herpes simplex virus (HSV).

(a) In infants and children, 60% of HSV infections appear as gingivostomatitis. The initial episode is frequently accompanied by extensive erosions of the oral cavity, pain, fever, and irritability.

(b) The most common sites of involvement in recurrent HSV in children are the lips, eyes, cheeks, and hands. The skin lesions are more typical of the classic grouped vesicles on an erythematous base.

(c) For more extensive discussion of HSV, see Chapter 19.

(2) Varicella (chicken pox).

(a) Incubation is 10 to 27 days and averages 14 days. Is highly contagious, spread by respiratory droplets.

(b) Characterized by an abrupt onset of crops of skin lesions that begin as erythematous macules progressing to papules and then to vesicles in 24 to 48 hours.

(c) The vesicles then develop moist crusts that dry and are shed.

(d) Distribution is generalized and mucous membranes are frequently involved.

    (e) Pruritus is common and can be severe.

    (f) Low-grade fever, rhinorrhea, and cough may accompany the rash.

    (g) Duration is 7 to 10 days. Severity varies from a few lesions to many.

    (h) Complications include secondary bacterial infection and pneumonia.

   (3) Varicella zoster.

    (a) Characterized by 2 or 3 groups of vesicles on an erythematous base appearing within several adjacent dermatomes.

    (b) May be accompanied by pain and post-zoster neuralgia.

    (c) Pruritus is often severe.

   (4) Coxsackie virus infection (hand, foot, and mouth disease).

    (a) Incubation is 3 to 5 days.

    (b) Scattered papules and oval or linear vesicles in an acral distribution.

    (c) Discrete oral lesions may be present as shallow oval erosions.

    (d) Children are usually afebrile and lesions are not pruritic.

2. Diagnostic tests.

  a. Generally diagnostic testing is not required. Diagnoses is made by clinical manifestations.

  b. Rubella may be cultured from nasal mucosa.

  c. Viral cultures of vesicle fluid may be obtained in vesiculobullous disorders if the diagnosis is in question.

  d. Diagnosis of erythema infectiosum may be confirmed by serum analysis for immunoglobulin M B19 antibodies within 30 days on onset.

  e. Coxsackie virus and Epstein-Barr virus can be isolated from oropharynx secretions.

E. **Nursing considerations (see Table 1).**

  1. Interventions.

    a. No specific treatment is available for measles, rubella, and roseola. Symptomatic treatment should be provided and children monitored closely for complications.

    b. The management of rubella embryopathy requires a multidisciplinary effort that includes ophthalmologists, cardiologists, and developmental specialists.

    c. Treatment of varicella and varicella zoster are symptomatic with wet dressings, soothing baths, oral antihistamines, and antipyretics.

    d. Systemic antiviral agents may be administered to children with varicella who are likely to have complications such as

those with chronic pulmonary disease, immunosuppression, or receiving chronic salicylate therapy.

    e. Oral acyclovir or famciclovir may be used to treat cutaneous herpes simplex infections; however, in cases where infection is limited to small areas of skin, systemic treatment is not required.

    f. Prevent varicella, measles, mumps, and rubella by administering the vaccine to children 12 months or older.

2. Patient education.

  a. Isolation during contagious periods.

   (1) Measles — from onset of respiratory symptoms through the 3rd day of the cutaneous rash.

   (2) Rubella patients should be isolated from pregnant women for 7 days after the rash has appeared.

   (3) Children with erythema infectiosum should be kept away from pregnant women, immunosuppressed patients, and patients with chronic hemolytic anemia for 2 weeks.

   (4) Children with chickenpox should be isolated until all lesions are crusted and contact with the elderly, neonates, and immunocompromised individuals should be avoided.

  b. Unvaccinated normal infants and children exposed to measles should receive a preventive dose of immune serum globulin, 0.25 ml/kg IM as soon as possible after exposure. Eight weeks later they should be vaccinated with the live attenuated measles vaccine provided they are at least 15 months of age.

  c. Instruct the family on the contagious nature of viral infections and isolation requirements.

  d. Review proper handwashing techniques and care of contaminated inanimate objects to prevent spread of viruses.

  e. Children with mononucleosis should avoid contact sports or other vigorous activity in which abdominal injury is likely for 3 to 4 months.

3. Followup.

  a. Close contact should be maintained with the child with rubeola to watch for bacterial superinfection, development of pneumonia, and encephalitis.

  b. For most of the viral exanthems, followup visits are unnecessary unless complications develop.

  c. Careful ophthalmologic followup is required in herpes keratitis.

II. WARTS

A. Definition.
1. Epithelial tumors induced by human papillomavirus (HPV) that manifest in a variety of clinical lesions known as warts.

B. Etiology and pathology.
1. HPV induces keratinocyte proliferation with relatively normal differentiation giving rise to the epithelial tumor.
2. The HPV virus is spread by contact with infected skin.

C. Incidence.
1. Warts are very common in children.
2. Condyloma acuminata are more commonly seen in adults and are considered a sexually transmitted infection.

D. Assessment.
1. Clinical manifestations.
   a. Common warts — appear as a solitary papule with an irregular, rough surface that may enlarge into a plaque. They are commonly found on the extremities, particularly the hands, but may appear anywhere including the trunk and scalp.
   b. Plantar warts — appear as papules on the plantar or palmar surfaces. Dermal ridges are disrupted by these lesions that are frequently grouped and painful when occurring on weight-bearing surfaces.
   c. Flat warts — appear as multiple flat-topped, smooth surface, skin-colored papules less than 5 mm in size. They most commonly occur on the extremities and face.
   d. Condyloma acuminata — also known as venereal warts, appear as multiple, discrete, or confluent papules with rough or smooth surfaces that occur on the genital mucosa, adjacent dry skin, or both.
2. Diagnostic tests.
   a. Diagnosis can be established by biopsy and HPV molecular typing, but these procedures are rarely required and warts are diagnosed by their clinical appearance.
   b. To assist in visualizing condyloma, apply 3% to 5% acetic acid to vulva, penial, and perianal area to reveal acetowhitening.
   c. Perform a Pap smear to detect cervical dysplasia with condyloma in female adolescents who are sexually active.

E. Nursing considerations (see Table 1).
1. Interventions.
   a. Therapy is aimed at boosting the body's immune response and/or destroying the skin in which the HPV is living.
   b. Imiquimod 5% cream applied 3 to 7 times a week may be helpful for enhancing the normal immune response. Although this drug is currently approved for treatment of genital warts, recent published reports have supported its use in treating all forms of warts.
   c. Cryotherapy.
      (1) Liquid nitrogen is applied to the center of the lesion until the wart turns white extending 1 to 3 mm beyond the margin of the wart. The freeze is maintained for 10 to 30 seconds.
      (2) Warts greater than 7 mm should not be frozen with liquid nitrogen because scarring is likely to occur.
      (3) In 1 to 2 days a blister forms. Removing the blister roof in 1 week and refreezing may be necessary.
   d. Salicylic acid plasters/paints.
      (1) Plasters impregnated with 40% salicylic acid or solutions containing salicylic acid may be applied to the wart lesion. The plasters are taped into place and tape or adhesive bandage is applied over warts treated with the solution.
      (2) Once a day the tape and plaster are removed and the wart is soaked in water for 45 minutes. The dead skin is rubbed off and a new plaster or fresh solution is applied and covered. This process is repeated until the wart is resolved.
      (3) If the lesion becomes painful, treatment may be held until the pain has resolved and then resumed.
      (4) This treatment is used with plantar warts, common warts (especially periungual warts), and flat warts.
   e. Retinoic acid 0.025% or 0.05% cream may be applied once or twice daily for 4 to 6 weeks for flat warts.
   f. Podophyllum and trichloroacetic acid can be effective against genital and common warts. They are carefully applied by the health care provider. Podophyllum should be washed off in 4 hours.
      (1) Condylox (a purified podophyllotoxin) is now available for application by the patient twice daily for 3 days, then 4 days later reapplied for 3 days if the warts remain.
   g. Surgery — CO_2 lasers, electrodesiccation, and surgical excision may also be used but frequently result in scarring.
   h. Oral cimetidine has been reported to be helpful in some cases.
2. Patient education.
   a. One treatment is unlikely to cure the wart.
   b. The effects of imiquimod may take 8 to 16 weeks to occur.
   c. Most warts spontaneously resolve in 12 to

24 months, but may persist longer in some children.

d. When genital warts occur in young children, the possibility of sexual abuse must be considered; however, this is not the only method of transmission.

3. Followup.

a. A visit in 2 weeks to determine the effectiveness of treatment and if retreatment is required.

III. MOLLUSCUM CONTAGIOSUM

A. **Definition.**

1. Benign epidermal tumors that may appear on any skin surface caused by a virus and have distinct clinical features.

B. **Etiology and pathology.**

1. Caused by a poxvirus that induces epidermal cell proliferation.

2. Three types of poxvirus are recognized.

a. Type 1 is believed to be responsible for common lesions on the extremities, head, and neck.

b. Types 2 and 3 are most often associated with genital lesions in the adolescent or young adult.

3. Incubation period is 2 to 7 weeks.

C. **Incidence.**

1. Commonly occur in children.

2. Children with atopic dermatitis may develop dozens of lesions.

3. Children with AIDS may develop hundreds of lesions and some may be very large.

D. **Assessment.**

1. Clinical manifestations.

a. White or yellow-white usually 1 to 6 mm discrete papules.

b. Papules have a central umbilication.

c. Most lesions contain white keratinous material in which the poxvirus thrives.

d. Larger lesions may have a surrounding area of dermatitis.

2. Diagnostic tests.

a. Extrusion of the papule contents onto a glass slide and Wright's stain will reveal the characteristic viral inclusions.

b. Generally, the diagnosis is made based on the clinical characteristics of the lesions.

E. **Nursing considerations (see Table 1).**

1. Interventions.

a. Imiquimod 5% cream applied 3 to 7 times weekly is effective in boosting the natural immune response.

b. Removal of the papule with a sharp curette is curative.

c. Applying a drop of cantharidin with a wooden toothpick to the papule is less

traumatic for children than curetting. Cover the lesions with tape after application. Remove tape in 4 to 6 hours.

d. Cryotherapy may also be used; however, may be more painful and not tolerated by small children.

e. Oral cimetidine has been reported to be successful in some cases.

2. Patient education.

a. The highly contagious nature of molluscum and the mode of transmission.

b. Wash skin thoroughly after removal of the tape.

c. Recurrences are common.

3. Followup.

a. A visit 1 to 2 weeks to determine if retreatment is necessary.

ACNE

I. DEFINITION

A. **A disease of the pilosebaceous unit where abnormally adherent keratinocytes cause plugging of the follicular duct followed by accumulation of sebum and keratinous debris.**

II. ETIOLOGY AND PATHOLOGY

A. **Contributing factors to acne.**

1. Development of a keratin plug at the sebaceous follicle opening.

2. Increased sebum production.

3. Proliferation of gram-positive bacteria such as *Propionibacterium acnes* or *S. epidermidis*.

4. Inflammation.

B. **Neonatal acne is a response to maternal androgens.**

C. **Persistence of neonatal acne beyond 12 months of age may be associated with endocrine abnormalities.**

D. **Drugs (such as androgens, ACTH, glucocorticoids, phenytoin, lithium, and isoniazid) and hyperandrogenism may also induce acne.**

E. **Frictional acne can occur from headbands, football helmets, hats, tight bras, etc.**

F. **Oil-based cosmetics and hair products can also be responsible for predominantly comedonal acne.**

III. INCIDENCE

A. **Acne is the most prevalent skin condition observed in the pediatric population.**

B. **Seen most frequently in adolescents and the newborn. Eighty-five percent of adolescents develop acne.**

IV. ASSESSMENT

A. Clinical manifestations.

1. Neonatal acne.
   a. Appears at 2 to 4 weeks of age and lasts until 4 to 6 months.
   b. Lesions are seen primarily of the face, particularly the cheeks, and occasionally on the upper chest and back.
   c. An oily face or scalp may be observed.
   d. Individual lesions are similar to adolescent acne lesions.
2. Adolescent acne.
   a. May first appear at the age of 8 to 10 years, peaks in late adolescence and may continue until the late 20s or early 30s.
   b. Distribution occurs in areas of high sebaceous activity, such as the face, upper chest, and back.
   c. Types of lesions.
      (1) Noninflammatory microcomedones.
      (2) Noninflammatory comedones.
         (a) Closed comedones.
         (b) Open comedones.
      (3) Inflammatory papules.
      (4) Inflammatory pustules.
      (5) Inflammatory nodules.
   d. Classification of inflammatory acne.
      (1) Mild — consists of few to several inflammatory papules or pustules, no nodules.
      (2) Moderate — several to many inflammatory papules, pustules, and a few nodules.
      (3) Severe — numerous extensive inflammatory papules, pustules, and many nodules.
   e. Scarring is common in inflammatory nodular acne and with frequent manipulation of the acne lesions.
2. Diagnostic tests.
   a. No diagnostic testing is generally required and diagnosis is based on the clinical appearance of the lesions.
   b. Hyperandrogenism is evaluated by obtaining blood levels of free testosterone, DHEA, and androstenedione.
   c. Patients being prescribed isotretinoin require the following evaluations pretreatment and monthly during treatment; complete blood count, platelets, liver function studies, fasting lipid profile, BUN, creatinine.
   d. Females being prescribed isotretinoin need two negative pregnancy tests prior to initiation of treatment and monthly pregnancy tests during treatment.

V. NURSING CONSIDERATIONS (see Table 1)

A. Interventions.

1. Gentle skin cleansing techniques that use mild soap and water twice a day. Avoid abrasive soaps and cleansers.
2. Topical medications.
   a. Benzoyl peroxide (2.5%, 5%, 10%) 1 to 2 times daily.
   b. Azelaic acid 20% 1 to 2 times daily.
   c. Adapalene 0.1% q hours.
   d. Tretinoin (0.025%, 0.05%) q hours.
   e. Tazarotene (0.05%, 0.1%) q hours.
   f. Antibiotics (erythromycin, clindamycin, sodium sulfacetamide) 1 to 2 times daily.
3. Systemic medications.
   a. Antibiotics.
      (1) Tetracycline 500 mg bid for 3 to 6 weeks in patients over 14 years old.
      (2) With the increased bacterial resistance to tetracycline, doxycycline 50 to 100 mg bid or minocycline 50 to 100 mg bid are frequently prescribed.
   b. Isotretinoin (Accutane®) 1mg/k/d is prescribed for severe nonresponsive nodular acne.
   c. Dexamethasone for patients with congenital adrenal hyperplasia.
   d. Low-progesterone containing oral contraceptives for patients with ovarian cysts or acne flares associated with their menstrual cycle.
   f. Antiandrogens for patients with high-circulating androgens.
4. Combination therapy.
   a. The combination of benzoyl peroxide every morning and a topical retinoid (tretinoin, adapalene, tazarotene) every evening is often effective.
   b. Frequently systemic antibiotics are combined with topical medications.
   c. Combination of topical benzoyl peroxide with both topical and systemic antibiotics is recommended to reduce the development of antibiotic-resistant organisms.

B. Patient education.

1. Precipitating factors in acne.
2. Application techniques for topical medications.
3. Avoid manual manipulation of lesions and keep hands away from face.
4. Use noncomedogenic cosmetic and skin care products.
5. Keep hair oils, spray, and mousse away from face.
6. It may take 4 to 6 weeks before effect of treatment is seen.
7. Side effects associated with prescribed treatment. If isotretinoin is being prescribed,

written and signed consent is required by parent, legal guardian or patient if 18 years or older.

8. Pregnancy prevention measures with female patients using oral antibiotics or isotretinoin. If isotretinoin is being prescribed, written and signed consent regarding pregnancy prevention measures is required by parent, legal guardian, or patient if 18 years or older.
9. Measures to manage dryness associated with treatment with isotretinoin.
10. Sun-protection measures.

C. Followup visits.
1. Every 4 to 6 weeks until control is obtained.
2. Then every 1 to 3 months particularly if being treated with systemic medication.
3. Patients on isotretinoin are seen monthly during the course of treatment.

HEMANGIOMAS

I. DEFINITION

A. Benign tumors of capillary endothelium (see Figure 11-8, page 240).

II. ETIOLOGY AND PATHOLOGY

A. The underlying cause of hemangiomas is unknown.
B. Proliferating hemangiomas are associated with capillary endothelial cell proliferation and an overabundance of mast cells.

III. INCIDENCE

A. By 1 year of age 10% to 12% of children will have a hemangioma.
B. By 5 years of age 50% of hemangiomas have maximally regressed.
C. By 9 years of age 90% have reached maximal regression.

IV. ASSESSMENT

A. Clinical manifestations.
1. Only 20% of hemangiomas are present at birth.
2. Classification of hemangiomas.
   a. Superficial hemangiomas — bright red papular hemangiomas.
   b. Deep hemangiomas — blue nodular hemangiomas.
   c. Mixed hemangiomas — contain both a superficial and a deep component.
3. Characteristics of growth.
   a. Rapid growth phase — at 4 to 8 weeks of age, hemangiomas undergo rapid growth that continues until the infant is 8 to 12 months. Growth at this time exceeds the growth rate of the infant.
   b. Stabilization phase — the hemangioma growth slows and approximates the growth rate of the child.
   c. Regression phase — this phase tends to begin sometime in the 2nd year of life with paling of the hemangioma, followed by flattening of the tumor. This phase slowly continues over a 3 to 10 year period.
4. Associated complications.
   a. Obstruction of a vital function, such as vision, urination, breathing, eating, or defecation.
   b. Platelet trapping with consumption coagulopathy (Kasabach-Merritt syndrome).
   c. High output cardiac failure.
   d. Ulceration.
   e. Infection.

B. Diagnostic tests.
1. Generally none. Diagnosed by clinical appearance.
2. MRI may be required for lesions that overlie the midline sutures of the head or the spinal column to rule out extension into central nervous system.
3. Imaging and biopsy may be required to differentiate hemangiomas from other vascular malformations, lymphatic malformations, or subcutaneous sarcomas.

V. NURSING CONSIDERATIONS (see Table 1)

A. Interventions.
1. In most uncomplicated hemangiomas, the lesions are observed and treated only if complications arise.
2. Measurement of the size of the hemangioma, along with photographs of the lesions at each visit, will document growth and regression.
3. Lesions on the face and in the diaper area are often treated due to disfigurement and high risk of complications.
4. Oral corticosteroids at 2 mg/kg and then adjusted depending on the response of the hemangioma.
5. Occasionally, interlesional steroids may be used.
6. Interferon alpha-2a may be used in lesions unresponsive to corticosteroids.
7. Vascular-specific pulsed-dye laser is an effective treatment for ulcerated, facial, or diaper area hemangiomas. This may be used in conjunction with corticosteroids.
8. Hemangiomas that are superficial before or early in the rapid growth phase respond well to laser treatment.

B. Patient education.
1. Review the natural history of hemangiomas.
2. Difficulty in predicting the eventual size, type, final outcome, and need for treatment during

the rapid growth phase of the hemangioma.
3. Potential complications.

C. Followup.

1. Follow closely during rapid growth phase, possibly may need to be seen every 2 to 8 weeks.
2. Once growth is stabilized, time between visits can be lengthened.
3. Children with periorbital hemangiomas should be referred for ophthalmologic evaluation.

Bibliography

Allen, A.L., & Siegfried, E.C. (2000). What's new in human papillomavirus infection. *Current Opinion in Pediatrics, 12*(4), 365-369.

Aly, R., Forney, R., & Bayles, C. (2001). Treatments for common superficial fungal infections. *Dermatology Nursing, 13*(2), 91-99.

Bello, Y.M., Falabella A.F., & Schachner, L.A. (2001). Epidermolysis bullosa and its treatment. *Wounds: A Compendium of Clinical Research and Practice, 13*(3),113-118.

Boiko, S. (1997). Diapers and diaper rashes. *Dermatology Nursing, 9*(1), 33-47.

Brust, M.D., & Lin A.N. (1996). Epidermal bullosa: Practical management and clinical update. *Dermatology Nursing, 8*(2), 81-90.

Buchanan, P.I., (2001). Behavior modification: A nursing approach for young children with atopic eczema. *Dermatology Nursing, 13*(1), 15-23.

Bunikowski, R., Stabb, D., Kussebi, F., Brautigam, M., Weidinger, G., Renz, H., & Wahn, U. (2001). Low-dose cyclosporin A microemulsion in children with severe atopic dermatitis: Clinical and immunological effects. *Pediatric Allergy and Immunology, 12*(4), 216-223.

Cooper, A.J. (1998). Systemic review of Propionibacterium acnes resistance to systemic antibiotics. *Medical Journal of Australia, 169*(5), 259-261.

Darmstadt, G.L. (1997, May). A guide to superficial strep and staph skin infections. *Contemporary Pediatrics, 293- 303.*

Darmstadt, G.L. (1997). Oral antibiotic therapy for uncomplicated bacterial skin infections in children. *Pediatric Infectious Disease Journal, 16*(2), 227-240.

Eady, E.A. (1998). Bacterial resistance in acne. *Dermatology, 196*(1), 59-66.

Edwards, L. (2000). Imiquimod in clinical practice. *Journal of the American Academy of Dermatology, 43*(1)(Part2), S12-S17.

Eichenfield, L.F., Frieden, I.J., & Esterly, N.B. (2001). *Textbook of neonatal dermatology.* Philadelphia: W.B. Saunders Co.

Enjolras, O. (1997). Management of hemangiomas. *Dermatology Nursing, 9*(1), 11-17.

Feingold, D.S. (1993). Staphylococcal and streptococcal pyodermas (Review). *Seminars in Dermatology, 12*(4), 331-335.

Hanifin, J.M., & Tofte, S.J. (1999). Patient education in the long-term management of atopic dermatitis. *Dermatology Nursing, 11*(4), 284-289.

Hengge, U.R., Esser, S., Schultewolter, T., Behrendt, C., Meyer, T., Stockfleth, E., & Goos, M., (2000). Self-adminstered topical 5% imiquimod for the treatment of common warts and molluscum contagiosum. *British Journal of Dermatology, 143*(5), 1026-1031.

Klein, P.A. & Clarck R.A.F. (1999). An evidence-based review of the efficacy of antihistamines in relieving pruritis in atopic dermatitis. *Archives of Dermatology, 135*(12), 1522-1525.

Koo, J. (1995). The psychosocial impact of acne: Patients' perceptions. *Journal of the American Academy of Dermatology, 32,* S26-S30.

Layton, A.M. (2001). Optimal management of acne to prevent scarring and psychological sequelae. *American Journal of Clinical Dermatology, 2*(3),135-141.

Leyden, J.J. (2001). Are two combined antimicrobial mechanisms better than one for the treatment of acne vulgaris? *Cutis, 67*(Suppl. 2), 5-7.

Lucky, A.W. (1998). A review of infantile and pediatric acne. *Dermatology, 196*(1), 95-97.

Lucky, A.W. (1997). Predictors of severity of acne vulgaris in young adolescent girls: A five-year longitudinal study. *Journal of Pediatrics, 130,* 30-39.

Meynadier, J. & Alirezai, M., (1998). Systemic antibiotics for acne. *Dermatology, 196*(1), 135-139.

O'Donoghue, M.N. (1999). Update on acne therapy. *Dermatology Nursing, 11*(3), 205-208.

Oprica, C., Emtestam, L., & Nord, C.E. (2002). Overview of treatment for acne. *Dermatology Nursing, 14*(4), 242-246.

Park, K.C. & Han, W.S. (2002). Viral skin infections: Diagnosis and treatment considerations. *Drugs, 62*(3), 479-490.

Rudy, S.J. (1999). Superficial fungal infections in children and adolescents. *Nurse Practitioner Forum, 10*(2), 56-66.

Rudy, S.J., Pinto, C., & Townsend-Akpan, C. (2001). Guidelines for practice: Caring for women of childbearing potential taking teratogenic drugs in dermatology. *Dermatology Nursing, 13*(1), (Suppl.), 5-13.

Schachner, L.A., & Hansen, R.C. (1995). *Pediatric Dermatology* (2nd ed.). New York: Churchill Livingstone.

Schober-Flores, C. (1999). Epidermolysis bullosa: A nursing perspective. *Dermatology Nursing, 11,* 243-248, 253-256.

Shires, G.I., & Mallory, S.B. (1995). Diaper dermatitis: How to treat and prevent. *Postgraduate Medicine, 98*(6), 79-84, 86.

Tofte, S.J., & Hanifin, J.M. (2001). Current management and therapy of atopic dermatitis. *Journal of the American Academy of Dermatology, 44*(1) (Suppl.), S13-S16.

Toyoda, M., & Morohashi, M., (1998). An overview of topical antibiotics for acne treatment. *Dermatology, 196*(1), 130-134.

Van Praag, M., Van Rooij, R., Folkers, E., Spritzwer, R., Menke, H., & Oranje, A. (1997). Diagnosis and treatment of pustular disorders in the neonate. *Pediatric Dermatology, 14*(2), 131-143.

Ward, D.B., Fleischer, A.B. Jr., Feldman, S.R., & Krowchuk, D.P., (2000). Characterization of diaper dermatitis in the United States. *Archives of Pediatrics & Adolescent Medicine, 154*(9), 943-946.

Weston, W.L., Lane, A.T., & Morelli, J.G. (2002). *Color textbook of pediatric dermatology* (2nd ed.). St. Louis: Mosby Year Book, Inc.

Wolverton, S.E. (2001). *Comprehensive dermatologic drug therapy.* Philadelphia: W.B. Saunders Co.

STUDY QUESTIONS

1. Erythema toxicum neonatorum and transient neonatal pustular melanosis share which one of the following features?
   a. Evanescent rash that disappears in 1 to 2 days.
   b. Lack of systemic symptoms.
   c. More common in African-American infants.
   d. Presence of hyperpigmented macules.

2. The most common form of ichthyosis seen in children is:
   a. Bullous ichthyosis.
   b. Congenital nonbullous ichthyosiform erythroderma.
   c. Ichthyosis vulgaris.
   d. Lamellar ichthyosis.

3. The clinical hallmark of all forms of epidermolysis bullosa is:
   a. Hearing loss.
   b. Hyperkeratosis of the palms and soles.
   c. Mechanical fragility of the skin.
   d. Mottled skin pigmentation.

4. The cutaneous manifestations of atopic dermatitis are the same at any age.
   a. True
   b. False

5. The infant with seborrheic dermatitis generally presents with all of the following signs and symptoms *except:*
   a. Erythematous papules.
   b. Greasy yellow scale.
   c. Intense pruritus.
   d. Rash on scalp and forehead.

6. A parent can best prevent irritant diaper dermatitis in a healthy 6-month-old infant by:
   a. Changing diapers frequently.
   b. Increasing dietary vitamin C intake.
   c. Using cloth diapers only.
   d. Using commercial diaper wipes regularly.

7. Teaching topics to be emphasized with families suffering from tinea capitis include all of the following *except:*
   a. Children may return to school after treatment is started.
   b. Do not share items such as hats, combs, hair clips, or brushes.
   c. Griseofulvin absorption is improved when taken with high-fat foods.
   d. Griseofulvin should be taken for 10 to 14 days.

8. Appropriate systemic antibiotic therapy for impetigo includes which of the following drugs?
   a. Dicloxacillin
   b. Griseofulvin
   c. Mupirocin
   d. Penicillin VK

9. A goal in the treatment of warts is aimed at:
   a. Decreasing the pruritus.
   b. Destruction of the skin infected with human papilloma virus.
   c. Killing only the human papilloma virus.
   d. Preventing bleeding.

10. The skin infection that manifests itself with white to whitish-yellow umbilicated papules is called:
    a. Acne
    b. Milia
    c. Molluscum contagiosum
    d. Warts

11. Patient education about acne treatments should include all of the following *except:*
    a. Abrasive skin-cleansing techniques.
    b. Application techniques for topical medications.
    c. Noncomedogenic skin care products.
    d. Sun-protection measures.

12. Characteristics of hemangiomas that would indicate the need for pharmacologic or surgical intervention include:
    a. Small deep hemangioma on the abdomen.
    b. Large superficial hemangioma on the forearm.
    c. Small hemangioma immediately adjacent to the rectal orifice.
    d. Mixed hemangioma on the scalp.

Answers to Study Questions

1.	a	5.	c	9.	b
2.	c	6.	a	10.	c
3.	c	7.	d	11.	a
4.	b	8.	a	12.	c

Dermatologic Nursing Essentials: A Core Curriculum 2nd Edition © DNA 2003

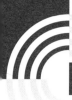

Chapter 11.
Pediatric Dermatology/Acne

Please photocopy this test page and return.

COMPLETE THE FOLLOWING:

Name: _____

Address: _____

City: _____ State: _____ Zip: _____

Preferred telephone: (Home)_____ (Work) _____

State where licensed and license number: _____

CE application fee: DNA member $15.00
                        Nonmember $20.00

POSTTEST INSTRUCTIONS
1. To receive continuing education credit for individual study after reading the article, complete the answer/evaluation form below.
2. Photocopy and send the answer/evaluation form along with a check or money order payable to **Dermatology Nurses' Association** to: **DNA**, East Holly Avenue Box 56, Pitman, NJ 08071-0056.
3. Test returns must be postmarked by December 31, 2008. Upon completion of the answer/evaluation form, a certificate for 5.6 contact hour(s) will be awarded and sent to you.

This chapter was reviewed and formatted for contact hour credit by Marcia J. Hill, MSN, RN, Core Curriculum Editor; and Sally Russell, MN, RN,C, DNA Education Director.

ANSWER FORM

1. Name one new detail (item, issue, or phenomenon) that you learned by completing this activity.

   _____

   _____

   _____

   _____

2. How will you apply the information from this learning activity to your practice?
   a. Patient education.
   b. Staff education.
   c. Improve my patient care.
   d. In my education course work.
   e. Other: Please describe _____

   _____

   _____

Evaluation

	Strongly disagree				Strongly agree
3. The offering met the stated objectives.					
a. Recognize skin conditions commonly seen in the pediatric population.	1	2	3	4	5
b. Discuss the therapeutic interventions frequently used in pediatric dermatology.	1	2	3	4	5
c. Identify important patient teaching issues for common pediatric skin disorders.	1	2	3	4	5
4. The content was current and relevant.	1	2	3	4	5
5. The content was presented clearly.	1	2	3	4	5
6. The content was covered adequately.	1	2	3	4	5
7. I am more confident of my abilities since completing this material.	1	2	3	4	5

8. The material was (check one) ☐ new, ☐ review for me.

Comments _____

9. Time required to complete reading assignment: _____ minutes

Figure 2-1.
Microscope, KOH Solution, and Slide

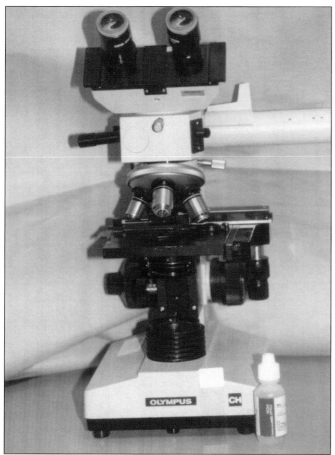

Figure 2-3.
Dewar and Cryac for Liq N2

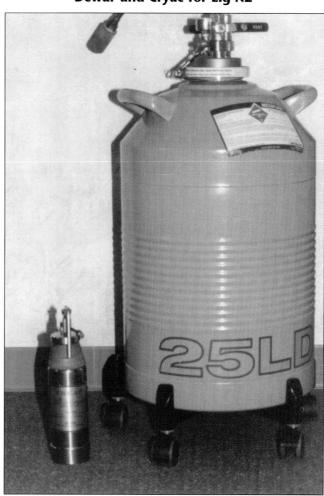

Figure 2-2.
Wood's Lamp

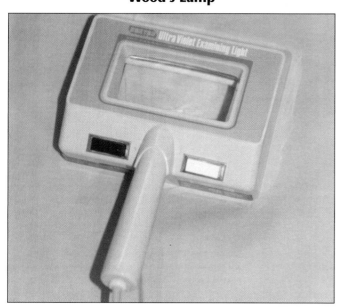

Figure 2-4.
Blade and Punch Tool

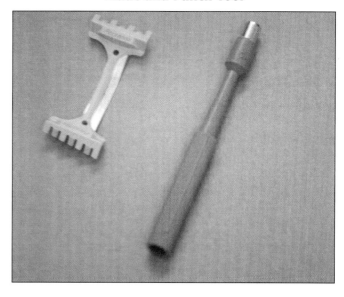

Figure 4-1.
Koebner's Phenomenon

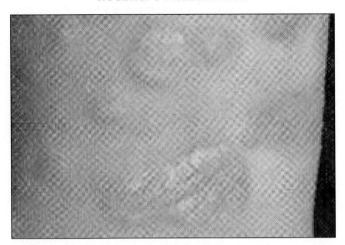

Figure 4-2.
Plaque with Silver Scale

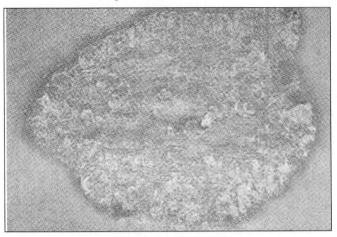

Figure 4-3.
Orchestration of Cutaneous T Cell During Immune Response

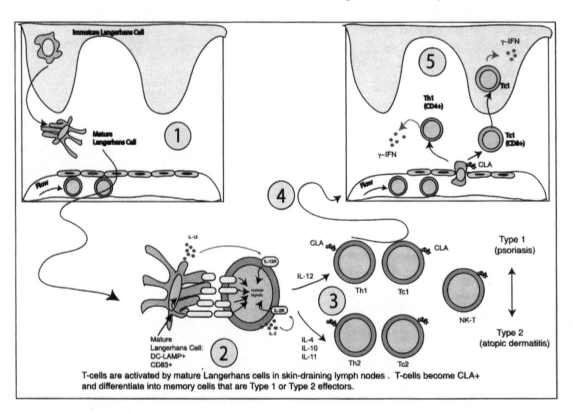

T-cells are activated by mature Langerhans cells in skin-draining lymph nodes. T-cells become CLA+ and differentiate into memory cells that are Type 1 or Type 2 effectors.

Generation of a cutaneous T-cell immune response de novo. This figure diagrams the sequence of cellular immune activation and trafficking pathways of Langerhans' cells and T lymphocytes during an immune response. Stages in this response are (1) antigen capture by immature Langerhans' cells in the epidermis, which then activates maturation and migration of cells to lymph nodes draining skin sites; (2) molecular interactions between a mature Langerhans' cell and a naive T cell in a lymph node that activates the T lymphocyte; (3) activated lumphocytes acquire the skin-homing receptor CLA and differentiate into type 1 or type 2 effector lymphocytes; (4) CLA+ memory T cells enter the circulation and exit cutaneous blood vessels at sites of inflammation; and (5) T lymphocytes in the dermis or epidermis become activated to release cytokines (or exert other effector actions) upon encountering the initiating antigen. Psoriasis is a disease in which type 1 T lymphocytes are expanded and effector actions in skin involve the release of IFN-γ, as diagrammed. In normal immune responses, antigens are eliminated by T-cell-stimulated pathways in the skin and then the immune response ceases. In psoriasis, T-cell infiltration and effector responses persist chronically. For expansion of abbreviations. See Table 1 page 85.

Reprinted with permission from Lookingbill, D.P., & Marks, J.G. (2000). *Principles of dermatology* (3rd ed.). Philadelphia: W.B. Saunders, Co.

Figure 4-4.
T Cells Interact With Mature Langerhans' Cell to Become Activated

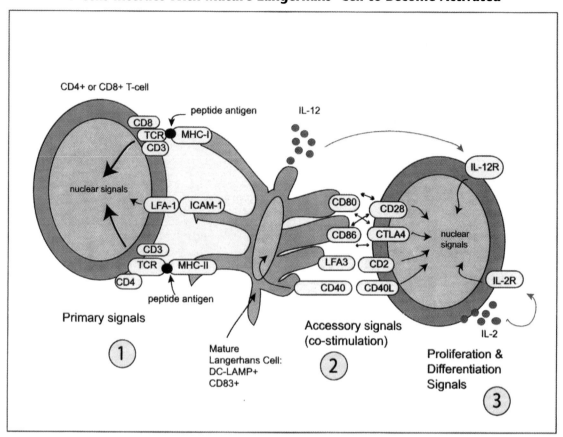

A T cell interacts with a mature Langerhans' cell to become activated. The T cell receives 3 sets of signals from counter-receptors expressed by the Langerhans' cells or by soluble cytokines released during cellular activation. Psoriasis lesions contain mature Langerhan's cells that express activation-related molecules diagrammed in this figure. For expansion of abbreviations, see Table 1, page 85.

Reprinted with permission from Lookingbill, D.P., & Marks, J.G. (2000). Principles of dermatology (3rd ed.). Philadelphia: W.B. Saunders, Co.

Figure 4-5.
The Migration Pathway for Skin-Homing T Cells in Psoriasis

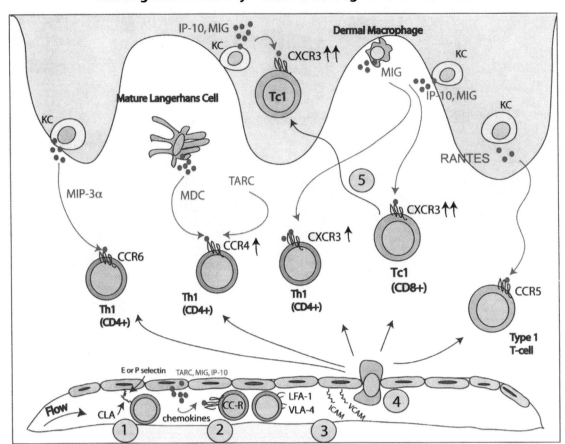

CLA+ T cells roll after tethering to selectins (step 1), where chemokines activate cells via specific cell-surface receptors (step 2). Chemokine activation enables integrins to bind to intercellular adhesion molecules and vascular cell adhesion molecules, which mediate firm adhesion to the endothelium (step 3). T cells migrate across endothelium into the dermis (step 4) in response to chemokines that are synthesized in psoriatic lesions. Chemokines and receptors that mediate trafficking of type 1 T cells are indicated. Tc1 lymphocytes then migrate into epidermis (step 5) according to chemokine gradients and adhesion molecules expressed on this T-cell subset. Chemokines and binding pathways are drawn in red, while cell migration pathways in response are drawn in blue. RANTES, Regulated upon expression, normal T-cell expressed and secreted; for other abbreviations, see Table 1, page 85.

Reprinted with permission from Lookingbill, D.P., & Marks, J.G. (2000). *Principles of dermatology* (3rd ed.). Philadelphia: W.B. Saunders, Co.

Figure 4-6.
T-Cell Mediated Inflammatory Pathways That Stimulate Pathogenic
Pathways in Psoriasis Vulgaris Lesions

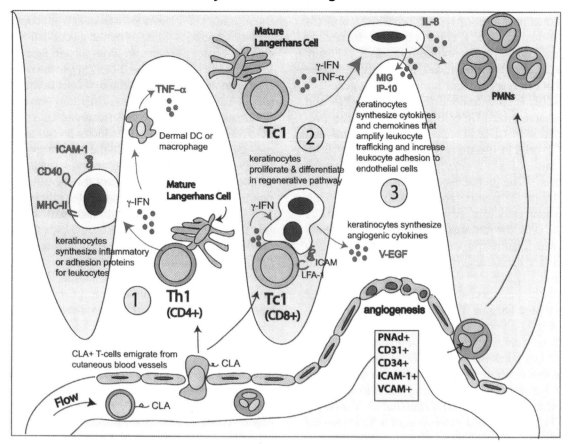

Dermal type 1 helper T (TH1) cells (1) or epidermal type 1 cytotoxic T (Tc1) cells (2) release IFN-γ and other cytokines that cause increased expression of inflammatory proteins on keratinocytes. Tc1 cells produce epidermal damage by mechanisms shown in Figure 4-7. Cytokine-activated keratinocytes produce chemokines and various other growth factors (3) that then stimulate neutrophil influx, vascular alterations, and keratinocyte hyperplasia, as detailed in the text. PNAd, Peripheral lymph node addressin; for other abbreviations, see Table 1, page 85.

Reprinted with permission from Lookingbill, D.P., & Marks, J.G. (2000). *Principles of dermatology* (3rd ed.). Philadelphia: W.B. Saunders, Co.

Figure 4-7.
Schematic Drawings of Antibodies and Fusion Proteins Used as Immunotherapeutics

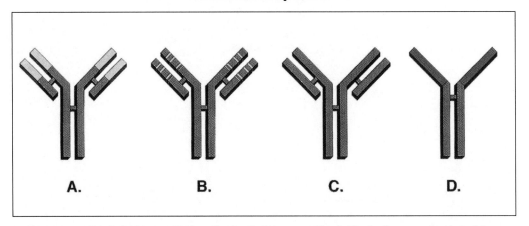

A, Chimeric antibody. B, Humanized antibody. C, Human antibody. D, Fusion protein. A and B, Murine-derived amino acids are indicated by yellow, whereas human sequences are shown in gray. D, Receptor domains (blue) are shown fused to constant-region sequences of human IgG (gray). The region of each molecule that binds to a target antigen is shown by a light-gray back-ground shading.

Reprinted with permission from Lookingbill, D.P., & Marks, J.G. (2000). *Principles of dermatology* (3rd ed.). Philadelphia: W.B. Saunders, Co.

Figure 4-8.
Large Psoriatic Plaques; Anterior Torso

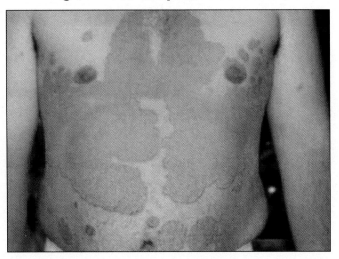

Figure 4-9.
Large Psoriatic Plaques; Posterior Torso

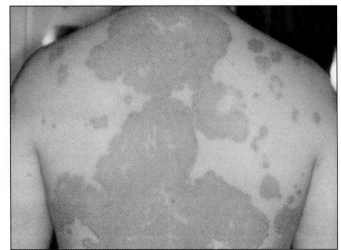

Dermatologic Nursing Essentials: A Core Curriculum 2nd Edition © DNA 2003

Figure 4-10.
Large Plaques Coalescing

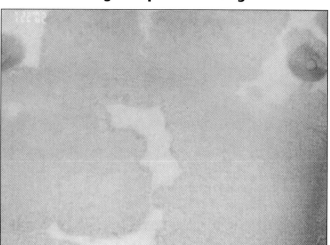

Figure 4-11.
Scalp Psoriasis

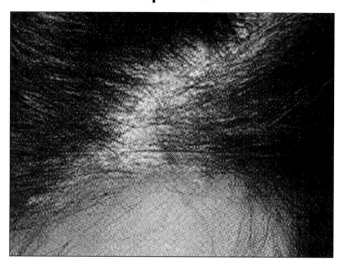

Figure 4-12a & 12b.
Pitting in Nail Psoriasis/Schematic; Pitting in Nail Psoriasis

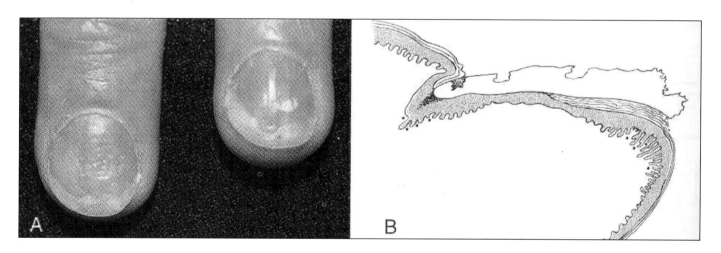

Figure 4-13a & 13b.
Herald Patch/Schematic; Herald Patch

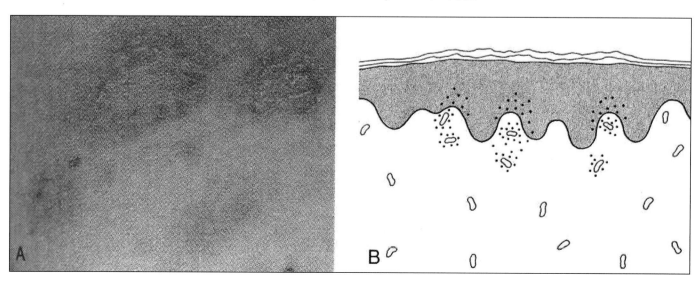

Figure 4-14a & 14b.
Lichen Planus/Schematic; Lichen Planus

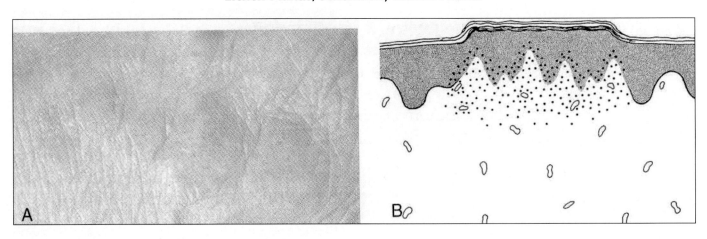

Figure 4-15.
Keratosis Pilaris

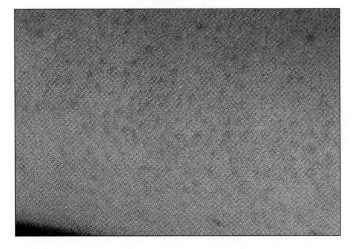

Dermatologic Nursing Essentials: A Core Curriculum 2nd Edition © DNA 2003

Figure 6-1.
Nodular BCC

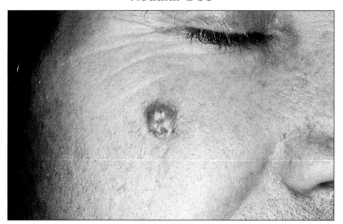

Figure 6-2.
Superficial BCC

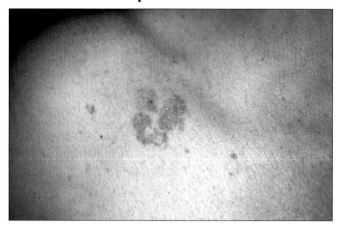

Figure 6-3.
Morpheaform BCC

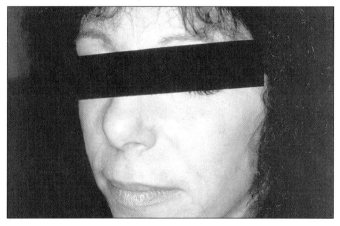

Figure 6-4.
Pigmented BCC

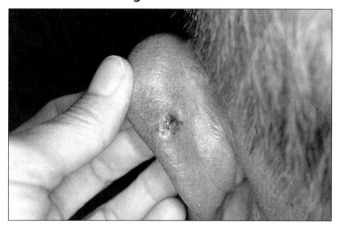

Figure 6-5.
SCC in Actinic Skin

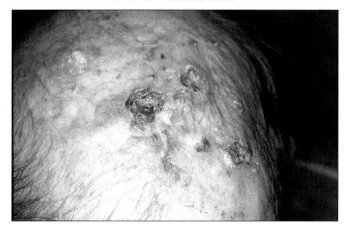

Figure 6-6.
Verrucous Carcinoma

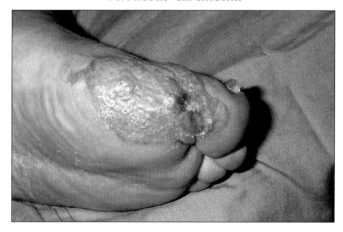

Figure 6-7.
Bowenoid SCC

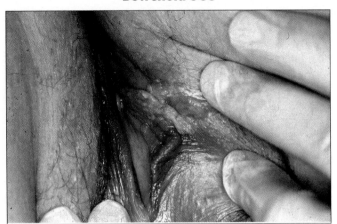

Figure 6-8.
Invasive SCC

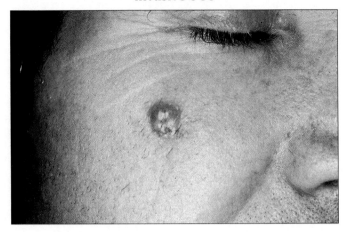

Figure 6-9.
Melanoma In Situ

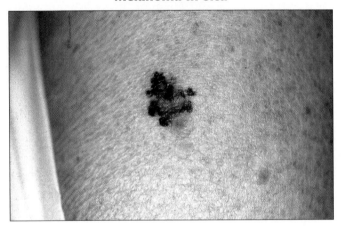

Figure 6-10.
Lentigo Maligna Melanoma

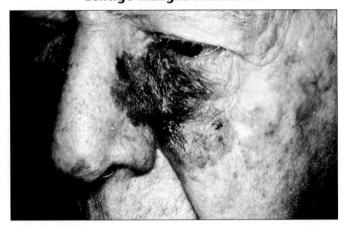

Figure 6-11.
Superficial Spreading Melanoma

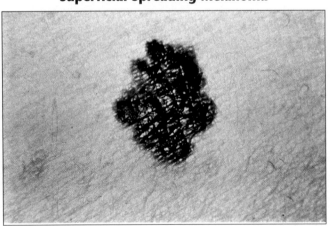

Figure 6-12.
Nodular Melanoma

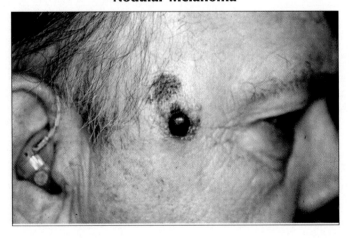

Dermatologic Nursing Essentials: A Core Curriculum 2nd Edition © DNA 2003

Figure 6-13.
Acral-Lentigenous Melanoma

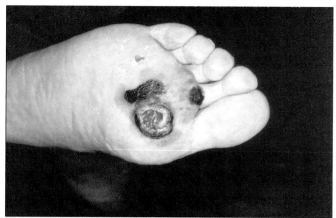

Figure 6-14.
Keratoacanthoma

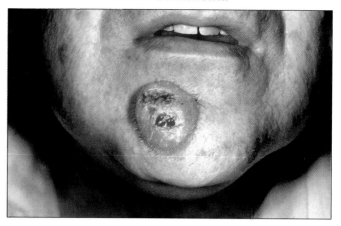

Figure 6-15.
CTCL Patch Phase

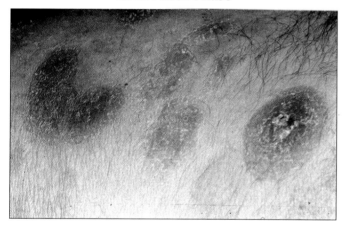

Figure 6-16.
CTCL Plaque and Tumor Phase

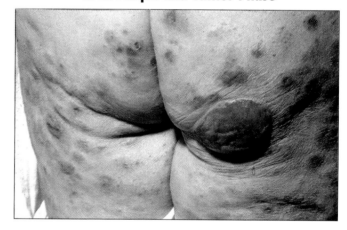

Figure 6-17.
Classic Kaposi's Sarcoma

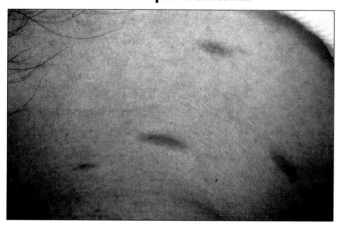

Figure 6-18.
Kaposi's in an AIDS Patient

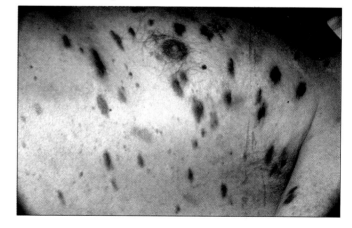

Figure 7-1.
Achrocordon

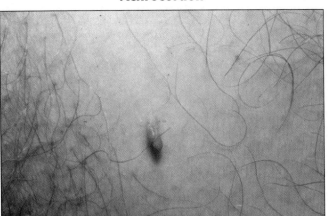

Figure 7-2a.
Callus

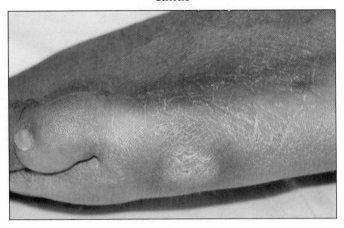

Figure 7-2b.
Callus

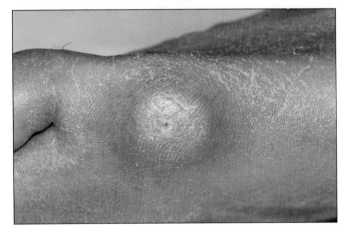

Figure 7-2c.
Callus

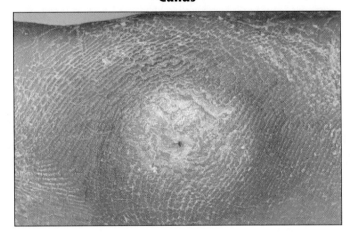

Figure 7-3a.
Corn (clavi)

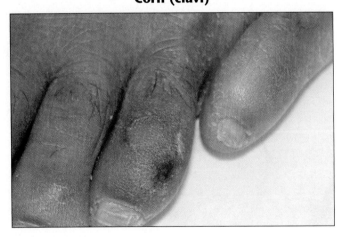

Figure 7-3b.
Corn (calvi)

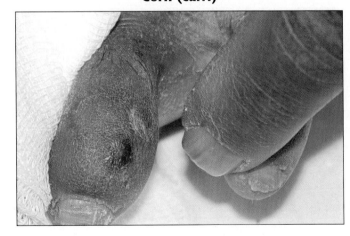

Dermatologic Nursing Essentials: A Core Curriculum 2nd Edition © DNA 2003

Figure 7-3c.
Corn (calvi)

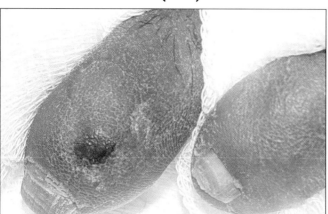

Figure 7-3d.
Corn (calvi)

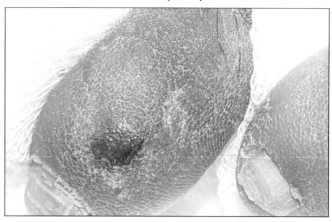

Figure 7-4.
Epidermal Cyst

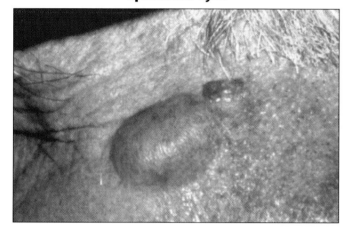

Figure 7-5.
Pilar Cyst

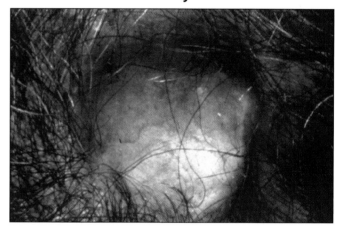

Figure 7-6.
Dermatofibroma

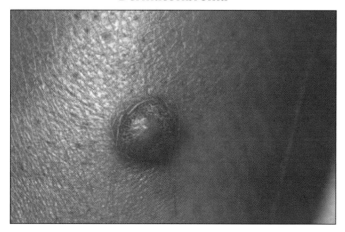

Figure 7-7.
Keliod

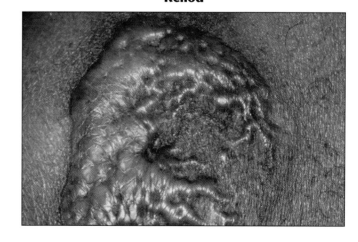

Figure 7-8.
Lipoma

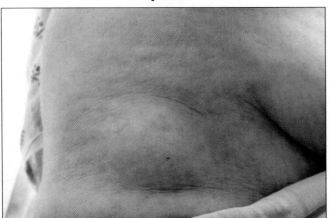

Figure 7-9.
Lipoma

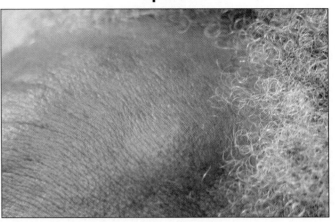

Figure 7-10.
Sebaceous Hyperplasia

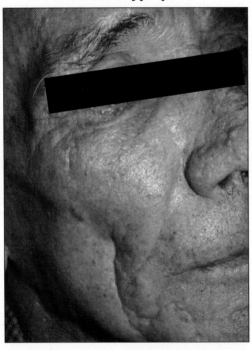

Figure 7-11.
Seborrheic Keratosis

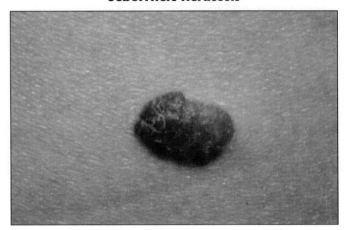

Figures 7-1, 7-4, 7-5, 7-6, 7-7, 7-8, 7-10, and 7-11 courtesy of Theodore Rosen.

Figures 7-2, 7-3, and 7-9 courtesy of Shawn D. James.

Figure 8-1.
Lymphoma/Leukemia
Purple/Red Plaques and Papules

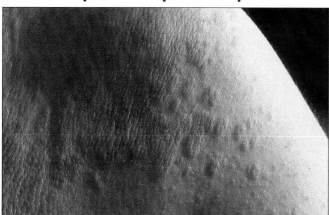

Figure 8-2.
Diabetes Mellitus
Diabetic Bullae of Foot

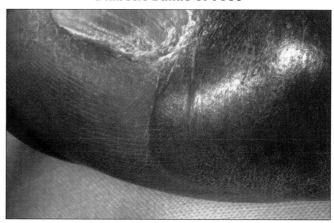

Figure 8-3.
Xanthomas of Diabetes

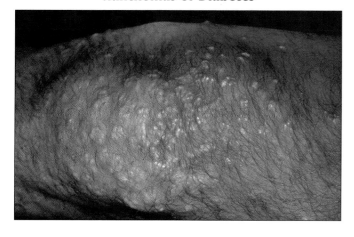

Figure 8-4.
Neurofibromatosis
Cafe´ Au Lait Spots of Neurofibromatosis

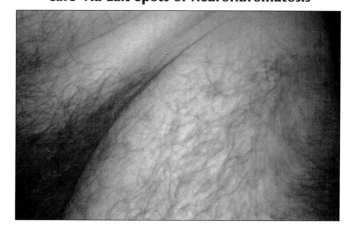

Figure 8-5.
Tumors of Neurofibromatosis

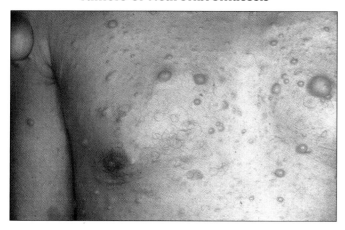

Figures 8-1 to 8-5 courtesy of Brian V. Jegasothy, MD

Figure 8-6.
**Chronic GVHD with Bronze Tone,
Scleroderma-like Changes of Arm**

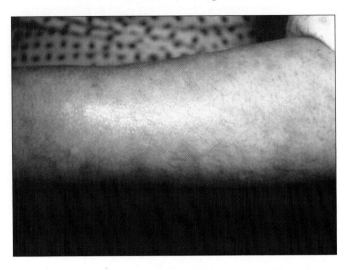

Figure 8-7.
**Chronic GVHD with Early Symptom of
Maculo-Papular Rash of Hand**

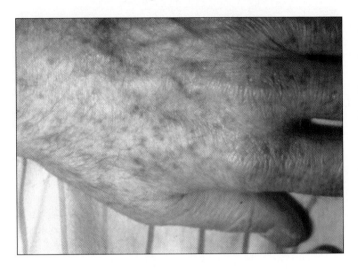

Figure 8-8.
**Chronic GVHD with Scaling and Erythema
of the Sole**

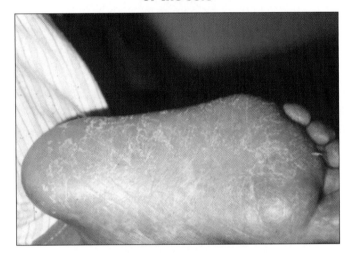

Figure 8-9.
**Chronic GVHD Demonstrating Ocular
Involvement with Erythema and Irritation**

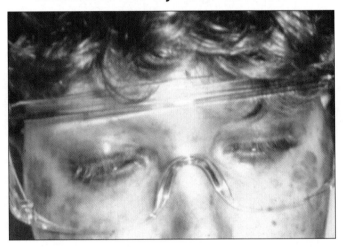

Figure 8-10.
**Chronic GVHD with Extensive Oral
Ulceration and Erosion**

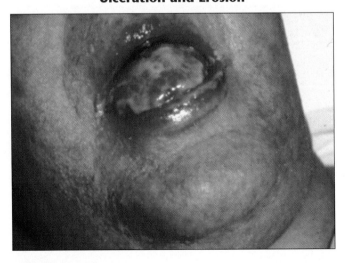

Figure 8-11.
Chronic GVHD with Nail Pitting and Ridging

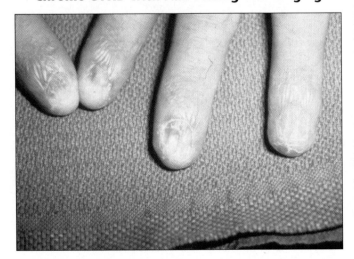

Dermatologic Nursing Essentials: A Core Curriculum 2nd Edition © DNA 2003

Figure 8-12.
Chronic GVHD with Scalp Alopecia

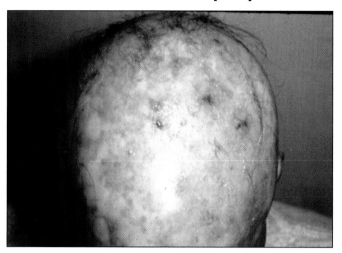

Figure 8-13.
Chronic GVHD Demonstrating Muscular Atrophy and Ankle Joint Contractures

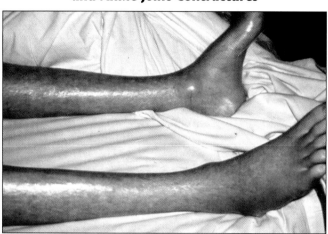

Figure 8-14.
Chronic GVHD with Diffuse Hypo/Hyperpigmentation of Trunk

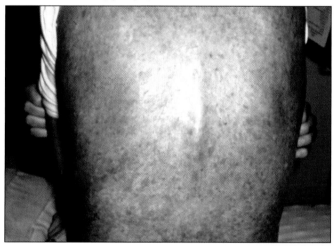

Figure 8-15.
Behcet's Oral Apthous Ulcer Lower Lip

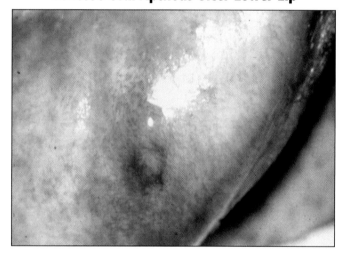

Figure 8-16.
Behcet's of Hard Plate

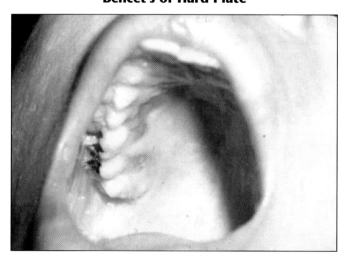

Figure 9-1.
Discoid Lesions

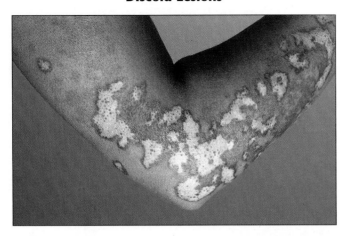

Figure 9-2.
Subacute Cutaneous Lupus Erythematosus

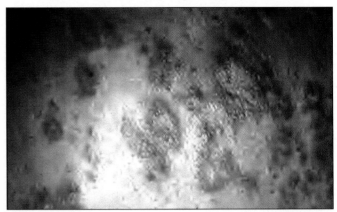

Courtesy of Antoinette M. Hood, MD, Indiana University School of Medicine.

Figure 9-3.
Lupus Erythematosus
Facial Rash of Systemic Lupus Erythematosis

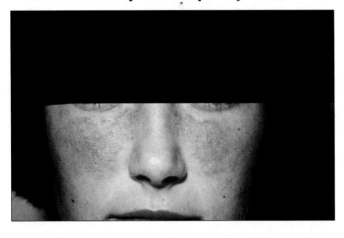

Figure 9-4.
Systemic Sclerosis
Raynaud's Reaction in Scleroderma

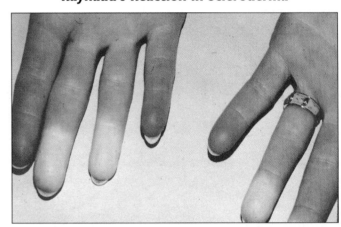

Figure 9-5.
Sclerodactyly and Raynaud's Reaction in Scleroderma

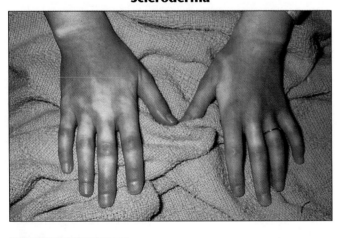

Figure 9-6.
Digital Pitting and Ulceration in Scleroderma

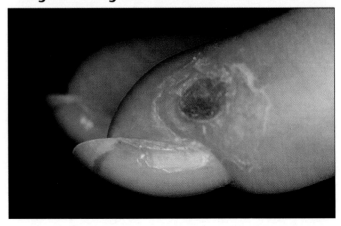

Dermatologic Nursing Essentials: A Core Curriculum 2nd Edition © DNA 2003

Figure 9-7.
Tautness, Hyper/Hypopigmentation

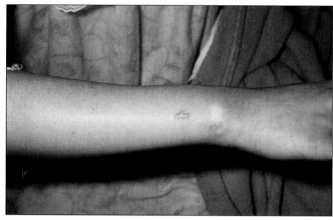

Figure 9-8.
Facial Telangiectasias

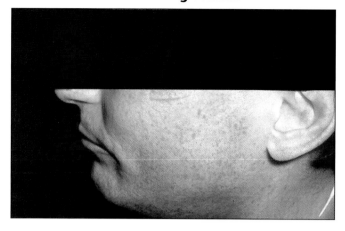

Figure 9-9.
Dermatomyositis
Gottron's Papules and Periungal involvement

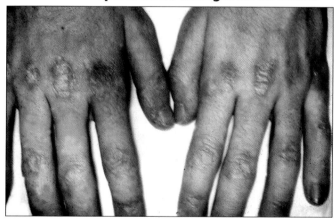

Figure 11-1.
Milium after Healing in Dominant Dystrophic EB

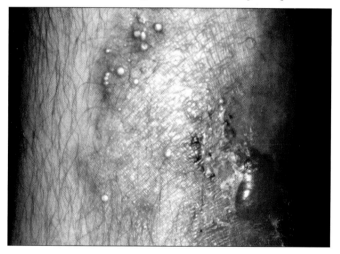

Figure 11-2.
Dominant Dystrophic EB

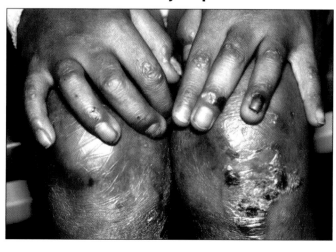

Figure 11-3.
Recessive Dystrophic EB: Losing and Loss of Nails

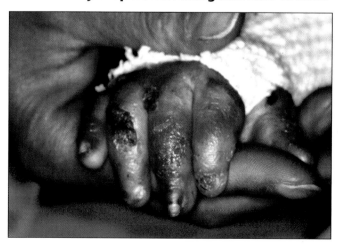

Figure 11-4.
Oral Lesion with Recessive Dystrophic EB

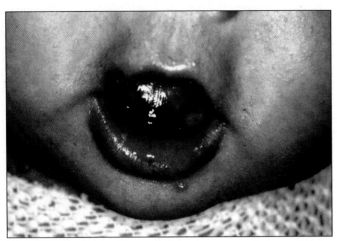

Figure 11-5.
Newborn Infant with Recessive Dystrophic EB:
Intrauterine Blistering

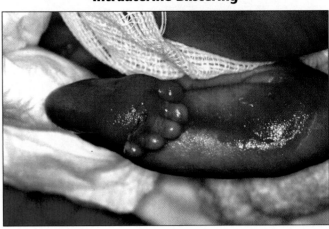

Figure 11-6.
Contractures with Recessive Dystrophic EB

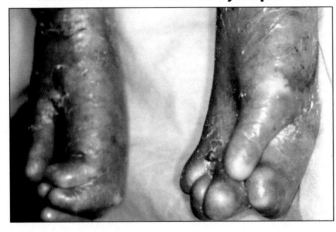

Figure 11-7.
Recessive Dystrophic EB:
Mitten Deformity of Left Foot

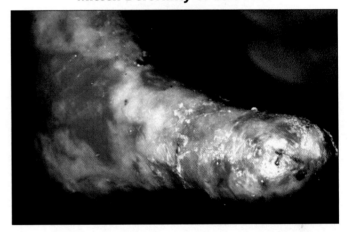

Figure 11-8.
Oral Lesion with Recessive Dystrophic EB

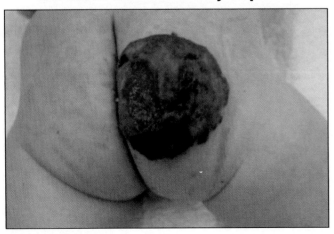

Dermatologic Nursing Essentials: A Core Curriculum 2nd Edition © DNA 2003

Figure 15-1.
Urticaria
The light pink color with central pallor due to edema of these gyrate coalescing plaques is characteristic of urticaria.

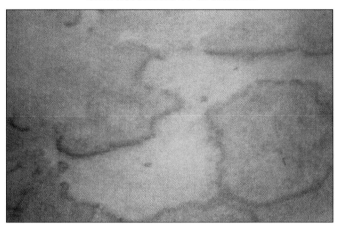

Figure 15-2.
Erythema Multiforme
Although these red, nonscaling papules with a more deeply erythematous center are classic for erythema multiforme, papules of erythema multiforme often don't show this "target" shape.

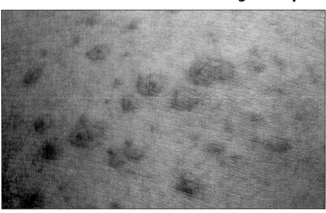

Figure 15-3.
Stevens-Johnson Syndrome
When erythema multiforme exhibits remarkable central inflammation, epidermal necrosis can occur, resulting in the blistering of Stevens-Johnson syndrome.

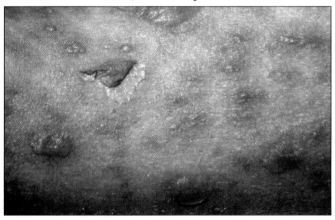

Figure 15-4.
Toxic Epidermal Necrosis
Widespread sheets of blistering rather than discrete blistering papules distinguishes TEN from blistering erythema multiforme or SJS.

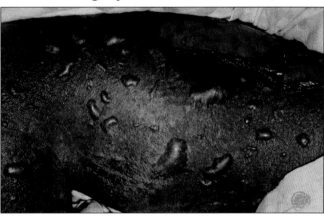

Figure 15-5.
Erythema Nodosum
Erythema nodosum appears as a dusky red, poorly demarcated plaque, most often located on the lower extremity.

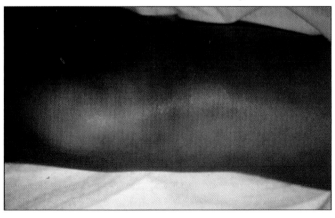

Figure 19-1.
Kaposi's Sarcoma

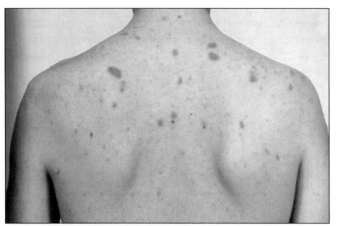

http://aidshistory.nih.gov/imgarchive/index.html#HIV

Figure 19-2.
Herpes Simplex

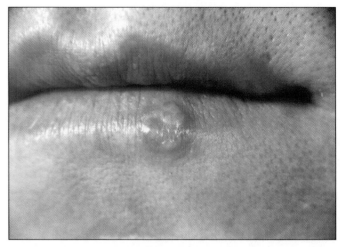

CDC Public Health Library,
http://phil.cdc.gov/phil/search_page.asp

Figure 19-3.
Oral Thrush

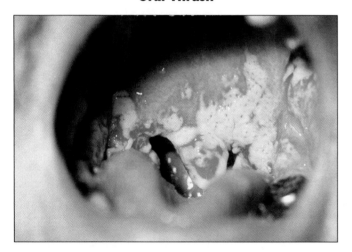

Figure 19-4.
Tinea Unguium (Onychomycosis) Onychomycosis due to *Trychophyton Rubrum*, Right and Left Great Toe. Tinea Unguium

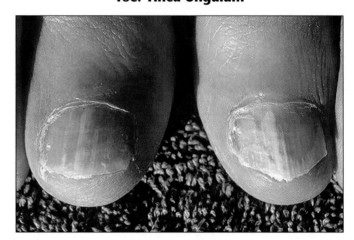

Figure 20-1.
Acute Skin Tear with Inflammation and Hematoma Formation

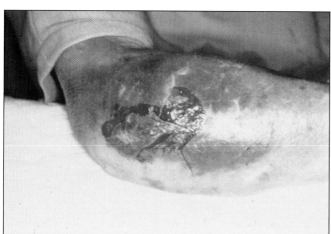

Figure 20-2.
Wound Healing by Secondary Intention with New Epithelial Growth at Margins

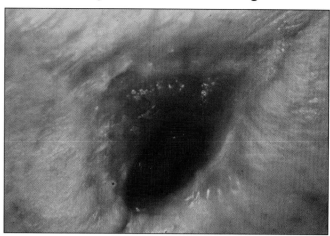

Figure 20-3.
Burn Wound with Epithelial Buds

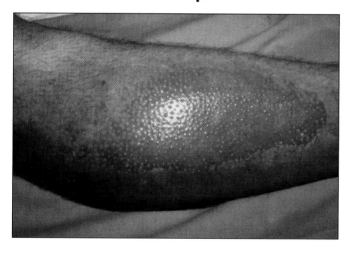

Figure 20-4.
Healthy Granulation Tissue

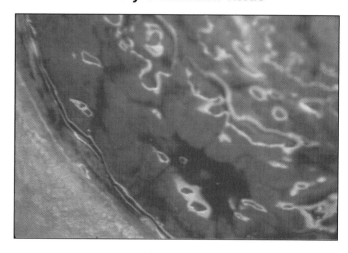

Figure 20-5.
Contracting Wound

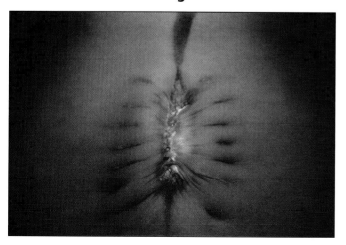

Figure 20-6.
Hypertrophic Scar

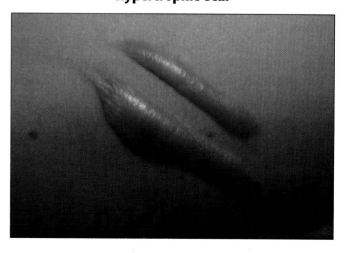

Figure 20-7.
Red Wound Infected with Streptococcus

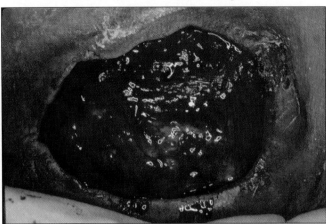

Figure 25-1.
Erythema Multiforme

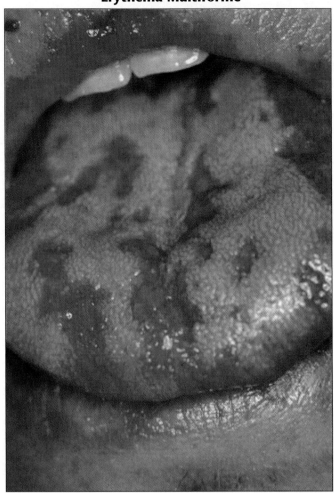

Photo courtesy of Dr. Drore Eisen,
Dermatology Research Associates

Figure 20-8.
Yellow Wound with Slough

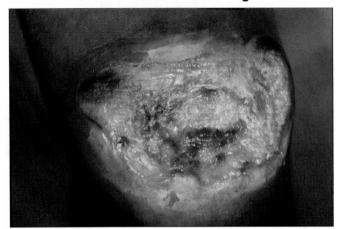

Figure 25-2.
Oral Lichen Planus

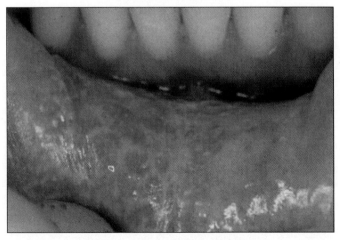

Photo courtesy of Dr. Drore Eisen,
Dermatology Research Associates

Infections

Marcia J. Hill, MSN, RN

OBJECTIVES

At the end of this chapter, the reader will be able to:

- Describe the cutaneous presentation of bacterial, viral, and fungal infections.
- Discuss factors that precipitate certain infections.
- List fungal infections by body region.
- Understand the pathology of cutaneous infection.

KEY POINTS

- Infection compromises the barrier function of the skin.
- Immunocompromised patients are at higher risk for dissemination of cutaneous infection.
- Cutaneous infections can be caused by both extrinsic and intrinsic factors.
- Appropriate treatment of cutaneous infections depends upon accurate recognition and diagnosis.

Infections

Marcia J. Hill, MSN, RN

OVERVIEW

Infections in the skin may range from superficial to deep, and may be caused by bacteria, fungi, or viruses. These infections may occur in otherwise healthy individuals.

BACTERIAL INFECTIONS

I. IMPETIGO (impetigo contagiosa)

A. Definition: a common, contagious, superficial skin infection caused by streptococci, staphylococci, or both.
1. Bullous impetigo.
   a. Etiology.
      (1) Caused by group II *Staphylococcus aureus.*
      (2) Usually not secondarily contaminated by streptococci.
      (3) Colonization of the respiratory tract precedes colonization of skin by days.
   b. Pathophysiology.
      (1) Begins as small vesicles.
      (2) Evolves into sharply demarcated bullae without erythematous halo; which eventually rupture.
      (3) Nikolsky's sign not present.
      (4) Shallow erosions result within 1 to 2 days.
      (5) Typically occurs on the face in infants and children, but may infect any body surface and any age group.
      (6) May resemble poison ivy.
      (7) Heals with hyperpigmentation in dark-skinned individuals.
      (8) Characteristic honey-colored (or white-brown) crust.
2. Vesicular impetigo.
   a. Etiology.
      (1) Caused by beta-hemolytic streptococci.
      (2) Begins with exposure to Streptococcus which enters the skin via areas of minor trauma.
   b. Pathophysiology.
      (1) Begins as a small vesicle or pustule.
      (2) After rupture a moist, red base is exposed.
      (3) Characteristic honey-colored (or white-brown) crust.
      (4) Satellite lesions may appear beyond the periphery.
      (5) Generally asymptomatic.
      (6) Generally heals without scarring.

Table 1.
Taking the History in the Patient with Cutaneous Infection

In addition to a routine history and physical, the following issues must be explored:

1. Time of onset of lesions (exacerbations, remissions, and recurrences).

2. Site of onset (pattern of spread or dissemination is important to making correct diagnosis).

3. Change (evolution) in lesions (lesions seen on exam may not be the primary lesion).

4. Cutaneous symptoms (burning, pruritus, or other discomfort).

5. Precipitating factors.

6. Previous treatment (self-treatment may alter presentation).

7. Occupation/hobbies — important to rule out exposure to specific infections.

B. Assessment.
1. History (see Table 1).
2. Current health status.
3. Physical exam.
   a. Clinical presentation.
   b. Evidence of trauma (bites, abrasions, lacerations).
   c. Gram stain.
   d. Culture for causative organism(s).
C. Prevention/Treatment.
1. Topical antibiotic, Bactroban® (mupirocin) is recommended.
2. Treatment of infection.
   a. Wash with antibacterial soap.
   b. Mechanical debridement of crusts.
   c. Apply topical antibacterial preparation; mupirocin is the recommended topical antibiotic for treatment of the infection.
   d. Parenteral treatment for 10 days with oral antibiotics (for example, cloxacillin, dicloxacillin, or cephalexin) or IM benzathine penicillin (erythromycin for patients with penicillin allergy) for noncompliant patients.
   e. Prevention — infected children should be isolated briefly until treatment is under way. Mupirocin® should be applied to the nares in patient's who are Staphylococcus carriers.
D. Nursing considerations (see Table 2).

Table 2.
Nursing Considerations for Patients with Cutaneous Infections

Nursing Diagnoses	Outcomes	Interventions
Impaired skin integrity related to inflammatory process.	Skin integrity has been improved or maintained.	Assess lesions, remove crusts or necrotic material before applying medication; elevate and immobilize affected extremity as indicated (cellulitis/erysipelas).
High risk for impaired skin integrity related to exudates.	Skin integrity is preserved.	Instruct patient and significant others regarding good handwashing technique; contain and eliminate exudates with appropriate dressings.
High risk for infection related to inadequate primary or secondary defenses.	No evidence of infection spread.	Instruct patient and significant other regarding importance of using good handwashing technique and appropriate disposal of dressings to avoid spread of infection; observe for signs of spreading infection; maintain good nutritional status.
Body image disturbance related to presence of lesions.	Patient exhibits improved/positive body image.	Assess patient's perception of body image; allow verbalization; give positive feedback.
Pain related to infection.	Pain is relieved; need for analgesics is decreased.	Assess level of discomfort; intervene appropriately to relieve any discomfort (medications, elevation and immobilization, compresses).
Impaired mobility related to pain and edema.	Mobility is increased.	Assess restriction in mobility and cause; elevate to help relieve edema.

II. CELLULITIS

A. Definition: a diffuse, acute bacterial infection of the skin and subcutaneous tissue.
B. Etiology.
   1. Group A beta-hemolytic streptococci (erysipelas), or *S. aureus* most common cause.
   2. Non-group A streptococcus, *Haemophilus influenza* type B, *Pseudomonas aeruginosa,* or *Camplyobacter* fetus may be the etiology in patients with underlying abnormalities of the lymphatics or venous drainage.
C. Pathophysiology.

   1. Most commonly seen in lower extremities (secondary to beta-hemolytic streptococci).
   2. Infection spreads locally secondary to release of enzymes.
   3. Erythema and edema seen.
   4. Skin hot and tender to the touch.
   5. Lymphangitic streaks may develop (common in erysipelas).
   6. Typically occurs near surgical wounds, cutaneous ulcers, or may occur in normal skin; may occur anywhere in immunocompromised patients.
D. Assessment.
   1. History (see Table 1).

2. Evaluate patient's overall health status.
3. Physical exam.
   a. Pain.
   b. Erythema.
   c. Warmth.
   d. Edema.
   e. Fever.
   f. May have pre-existing lesion.
   g. Lymphadenopathy.
4. Diagnostic tests.
   a. CBC with differential.
      (1) Mild leukocytosis with shift to the left.
      (2) Mildly elevated sedimentation rate.
   b. Bacterial culture.
E. **Treatment.**
1. Staphylococcal or Streptococcal cellulitis — penicillinase-resistant penicillin, dicloxacillin, or cephalosporin.
2. Recurrent disease — prophylactic antibiotics.
3. Burow's compresses for pain.
4. Surgical debridement if gas formation or pockets of purulent material present.
5. Intravenous antibiotics may be used in advanced infections.
F. **Prevention — long-term oral antibiotics of recurrent infections.**
G. **Nursing considerations (see Table 2).**

III. FURUNCLE/CARBUNCLE

A. **Furuncle (boil).**
1. Etiology.
   a. Staphylococcal infection (coagulase-positive *S. aureus*).
   b. May be secondary to ingrown hair or obstruction of sebaceous gland.
2. Pathophysiology.
   a. Abscess of the skin and subcutaneous tissue.
   b. Central necrosis and suppuration seen.
   c. Associated with hair follicle or sebaceous glands.
   d. Secondary factors that may induce infection.
      (1) Scratching.
      (2) Friction.
      (3) Infestation.
      (4) Pressure from restrictive clothing.
      (5) Chemical irritation.
      (6) Hyperhidrosis.
      (7) Occlusion of follicle with ointments, etc.
   e. Lesions.
      (1) Primary lesion — small, painful, indurated nodules.
      (2) Evolves to elevated, tender lesion with shiny erythema and intense pain.
      (3) Mature lesion.
         (a) Fluctuant.

(b) Yellow or creamy white discharge.
(c) Central necrosis.
   (4) May spontaneously rupture.
   (5) Single or multiple lesions may be present.
   f. Systemic signs.
      (1) Fever.
      (2) Malaise.
      (3) Regional adenopathy.
3. Assessment.
   a. History (see Table 1).
   b. Physical exam.
   c. Distinguish between furuncle and ruptured epidermal cyst.
   d. Note location — lesions commonly seen on the back of the neck, face, buttocks, thighs, perineum, breasts, or in axillae.
   e. Evaluate the appearance of the lesion(s).
   f. Predisposing conditions.
      (1) Occlusion especially in hyperhidrosis.
      (2) Follicular abnormalities.
      (3) Colonized skin in patients with atopic dermatitis, eczema, and scabies.
   g. Diagnostic tests.
      (1) Gram stain.
      (2) Bacterial culture.
4. Diseases manifesting as furunculosis (differential diagnosis).
   a. Bacterial furunculosis — any body surface.
   b. Recurrent furunclosis in scarred tissue — buttocks or any location.
   c. Ruptured epidermal cyst — pre-/postauricular areas, back, face, chest.
   d. Hidradenitis supprativa — axillae, groin, buttocks, under breasts.
   e. Cystic acne — face, chest.
   f. Primary immunodeficiency — any body surface.
   g. Diabetes, alcoholism, malnutrition, severe anemia, debilitation — any surface.
5. Treatment.
   a. Warm compresses.
   b. Incision, drainage, and packing to promote continuous drainage.
   c. Antibiotics aimed at organism cultured.
B. **Carbuncle: a carbuncle is an aggregation of interconnected furuncles that drain through several openings in the skin.**

VIRAL INFECTIONS

I. WARTS: BENIGN EPIDERMAL GROWTHS (see Chapter 11 for further information)

A. **Etiology/Pathophysiology.**
1. Human papillomavirus (HPV).
2. Most common in children and young adults, but can occur at any age.

3. Variable course.
4. Spontaneous resolution is common.
5. Generally seen at sites of previous trauma.
   a. Hands.
   b. Periungual area (generally secondary to nail biting) .
   c. Plantar surfaces.
6. Can be transmitted by touch.
7. More severe in patients with impaired immunity (see Chapter 19).

B. **Common warts: verruca vulgaris.**
   1. Elevated.
   2. Well circumscribed.
   3. Irregular in shape with hyperkeratotic surfaces; minute papillary projections may be seen.
   4. Vary in size from pinhead to 10 mm.
   5. May proliferate and coalesce.
   6. May be brown, gray, or flesh colored.
   7. Found on dorsa of hands, fingers; may be seen on any body surface
   8. Generally manifest as multiple lesions.

C. **Assessment (see Table 1).**

D. **Treatment.**
   1. Topical salicylic acid preparations.
   2. Liquid nitrogen.
   3. Light electrocautery.
   4. Blunt dissection for large or resistant lesions.
   5. Intralesional bleomycin sulfate when other treatments fail (used most commonly in plantar warts).

E. **Plane warts (verruca plana, flat warts, juvenile warts).**
   1. Slightly raised.
   2. Irregular, smooth, or slightly hyperkeratotic.
   3. Characteristically multiple lesions with irregular distribution.
      a. Dorsa of the hands.
      b. Face.
   4. Flesh colored.
   5. Prevalent in patients with compromised immunity.

F. **Treatment.**
   1. Tretinoin cream, 0.025%, 0.05%, or 0.1% applied at bedtime; may require weeks to months to resolve.
   2. Liquid nitrogen.
   3. Light touch electrocautery.
   4. 5-fluorouracil cream — may take 3 to 5 weeks of treatment.
   5. Aldara® gel.

G. **Nursing considerations (see Chapters 11 and 19).**

II. MOLLUSCUM CONTAGIOSUM

A. **Etiology/Pathophysiology.**
   1. Benign tumor seen in skin and mucous membranes.

2. Caused by an unassigned pox virus.
3. May be spread through sexual or casual contact.
4. Widespread distribution of lesions is characteristic in patients with impaired immunity.
5. Smooth, firm, spherical lesions with central umbilication.
6. Cheesy white material may be expressed upon manipulation (this material contains virus).
7. Seen around the eyes and mouth in children (see Chapter 9). When seen in genital/anal areas of children, sexual abuse should be suspected.
8. In adults it is seen on the face, trunk, and extremities.
9. Linear presentation represents autoinoculation with the virus.
10. Atopics at risk for dissemination of lesions.
11. Generally resolve spontaneously.

B. **Treatment.**
   1. Curettage.
   2. Cryosurgery.
   3. Tretinoin cream (0.025%, 0.05%, 0.1%) or gel (0.01% or 0.025%); may take weeks or months for resolution.
   4. Salicylic acid.
   5. Cantharidin.
   6. Laser therapy.
   7. Aldara gel.

C. **Assessment (see Table 1).**

D. **Nursing considerations (see Chapters 11 and 19).**

III. CONDYLOMATA ACUMINATA (anogenital/venereal warts)

A. **Definition: highly contagious; sexually transmitted; often seen in conjunction with other sexually transmitted diseases (STDs).**

B. **Etiology/Pathophysiology.**
   1. Caused by human papillomavirus (HPV).
   2. Genitalia and anorectal area, urethral, bladder, and oral mucosa may be affected.
   3. Asymptomatic infection.
   4. Minor trauma during intercourse may allow virus to enter.
   5. Immunosuppressed, pregnant, and diabetic patients most susceptible.
   6. Lesions.
      a. Discrete single or multiple papillary growths.
      b. White or gray in color.
      c. May coalesce forming large cauliflower-like masses.
      d. Seen on penis, scrotum, around the anus or in urethra.
      e. In females lesions seen on vulva, vagina,

cervix, and perianal area.

    f.   Lesions grow rapidly during pregnancy.

    g.   Virus can be transmitted to newborn during delivery.

D. Assessment.

    1. History (see Table 1).

    2. Distinguish from condylomata lata of secondary syphilis, carcinoma, or benign neoplasm.

        a.   Serologic tests.

        b.   Cytologic tests.

        c.   PAP smear.

        d.   Biopsy if PAP is dysplastic.

        e.   VIRAPAP — uses DNA hybridization technique to determine presence of some types of HPV.

E. Treatment: difficult to treat.

    1. 80% to 90% trichloracetic acid applied directly to surface of the wart.

    2. Podophyllin (10% to 25%) recommended for small warts on external genital.

    3. Cryotherapy.

    4. Electrocautery.

    5. Laser.

    6. 5-fluorouracil.

    7. Surgical excision.

    8. Aldara® gel.

    9. Recurrence/reinfection possible; therefore long-term followup recommended.

F. Nursing considerations (see Table 2).

III. HERPES SIMPLEX VIRUS (Herpesvirus hominis)

A. Definition: cold sores, fever blisters, genital herpes, and herpetic whitlow caused by a specific virus and having both primary and secondary presentations.

B. Etiology.

    1. Types — distinguished in the laboratory.

        a.   Herpes simplex virus type I (HSV-I) — generally associated with oral lesions.

        b.   Herpes simplex virus type II (HSV-II) — generally associated with genital infections.

    2. Virus remains in nerve root ganglion, returning to skin producing recurrence when exacerbated.

C. Pathophysiology.

    1. Primary infection.

        a.   May be asymptomatic.

        b.   Elevated IgG antibody titer.

        c.   Severity increases with age and decreased immune status.

        d.   May be spread by respiratory droplet, direct contact, virus-containing fluid (saliva, cervical secretions).

        e.   Symptoms occur 3 to 7 days after contact.

            (1) Tenderness, pain, mild parasthesias, burning prior to appearance of clinical lesions.

            (2) Localized pain, tender lymphadenopathy, flu-like symptoms (may or may not occur); more common with initial infection.

    2. Recurrent infections.

        a.   Exacerbating factors.

            (1) Sunlight.

            (2) Trauma.

            (3) Menses.

            (4) Stress.

            (5) Systemic infection.

        b.   Not every individual has recurrences.

        c.   Prodrome.

            (1) Lasts 2 to 24 hours.

            (2) Resembles prodrome of primary infection.

        d.   Recurrent lesions may be seen within 12 hours of prodromal symptoms.

        e.   Higher frequency of recurrences in HSV-2 infections.

D. Assessment.

    1. History (see Table 1).

    2. Overall general health of patient should be evaluated.

    3. Diagnosis is generally made on clinical presentation:

        a.   Grouped vesicles on an erythematous base.

        b.   Subsequent erosions.

        c.   Crusting may occur except on mucosal lesions.

        d.   Last 2 to 6 weeks.

        e.   Heals without scarring.

    4. Laboratory tests — sensitivity of tests depends on stage of lesion (higher sensitivity in vesicular lesions when an intact vesicle can be cultured, and in primary lesions).

        a.   Tzanck smear.

        b.   PAP smear.

        c.   Viral culture.

        d.   Biopsy of intact vesicle.

        e.   Serology — herpes simplex IgG and IgM serum antibodies.

E. Treatment.

    1. Symptomatic.

        a.   Cool, moist compresses; astringent compresses (Burow's solution).

        b.   To control secondary infections.

            (1) Moisture barrier creams (zinc oxide base).

            (2) Topical antimicrobials for genital erosions exposed to feces (particularly in immunocompromised patients).

    2. Drug therapy.

        a.   Acyclovir (topical, oral, IV), valcyclovir (Valtrex®), or famciclovir (Famvin®)

        b.   L-lysine has been used to prevent recurrent episodes (no data regarding benefit available).

F. Nursing considerations (see Chapter 17).

IV. HERPES ZOSTER (shingles)

A. Definition: an acute vesicobullous eruption seen in a dermatomal distribution with sharp demarcation at the midline.
B. Etiology.
1. Caused by reactivation of varicella virus acquired during an episode of (or exposure to) chicken pox.
2. Virus lies dormant in nerve root ganglion until reactivated.
3. Occurs in 10% to 20% of all persons; can occur in all ages with incidence increasing with age.
C. Pathophysiology.
1. Factors that reactivate virus.
   a. Age.
   b. Immunosuppressive drugs.
   c. Lymphoma.
   d. Fatigue.
   e. Emotional upset (stress).
   f. Radiation.
2. Pre-eruption symptoms (localized to dermatome) — precede eruption 4 to 5 days.
   a. Pain — may be severe, simulating pleurisy, myocardial infraction, abdominal disease, or migraine headache.
   b. Pruritus or burning.
   c. Tenderness or hyperesthesia.
   d. Urinary hesitancy or retention if S2, S3, S4 nerves involved
   e. Flu-like symptoms.
   f. Regional lymphadenopathy may be present.
3. Eruptive phase.
   a. Generally limited to a single dermatome.
   b. Rare bilateral symmetrical or asymmetrical dermatomes (may signal presence of underlying malignancy).
   c. Viremia (appearance of 20 to 30 scattered vesicles, outside the dermatome); seen in approximately 50% of patients.
   d. Eruption.
      (1) Begins with erythematous, swollen plaques of various sizes.
      (2) Spreads to involve dermatome.
      (3) Vesicles with purulent fluid form 3 to 4 days after appearance of erythema.
      (4) Vesicular eruption may continue for up to 7 days.
      (5) Rupture of vesicles leads to erosion and crusting.
      (6) Elderly or debilitated patients may have a prolonged and difficult course of infection and may also have prolonged pain (postherpetic neuralgia) for several months.

D. Assessment (see Chapter 19).
1. History (see Table 1).
2. Current health status of patient.
3. Clinical presentation of lesions (particularly if atypical presentation).
E. Treatment (see Chapter 19).
1. Acyclovir®, Valtrex®, Famvir®.
2. Vidarabine (Vira-A®) given IV for severe infections and infections in immunocompromised patients.
3. Systemic corticosteroids to reduce postherpetic neuralgia.
4. Analgesics.
5. Cool compresses.
6. Astringent compresses.
7. Zinc oxide shake lotions with menthol to help relieve pain and enhance drying of lesions.
8. Zostrix®.
F. Nursing considerations (see Chapter 19).

FUNGAL INFECTIONS

I. DERMATOPHYTES

A. Definition: known as tineas and are superficial infections of the skin, and responsible for the vast majority of skin, hair, and nail infections.
B. Etiology.
1. Invade the skin and survive on dead keratin (stratum corneum).
2. Cannot survive on mucosal surfaces which are devoid of keratin.
3. Rarely undergo deep invasion except in immunocompromised patients.
4. Some patients may have genetic predisposition to dermatophyte infections.
C. Pathophysiology.
1. Lesions vary in presentation.
2. Lesions may resemble other dermatoses leading to misdiagnosis.
3. Classifications.
   a. Genera.
      (1) Microsporum.
      (2) Trichophyton.
      (3) Epidermophyton.
   b. Anthropophilic.
      (1) Grow on human hair, nails, or skin.
      (2) Mild inflammatory response seen with infection.
   c. Geophilic.
      (1) Originate in soil.
      (2) Elicit brisk inflammatory response.
   d. Zoophilic.
      (1) Originate from animals; may infect humans.
      (2) Brisk inflammatory response.
4. Classification by body region (see Chapters 11, 16, and 19).

a. Tinea corporis — nonhairy parts of body, face, neck, extremities.
b. Tinea cruris — groin, inner thighs.
c. Tinea capitis — scalp.
d. Tinea pedis — feet.
e. Tinea unguium — toenails, fingernails (less common).

5. Characterized by an annular lesion with active border of infection and central clearing.
6. Vesicles are present in severe inflammation.

D. **Assessment.**
1. Current health status.
2. Inspect skin and mucous membranes.
3. Diagnostic tests.
   a. Potassium hydroxide wet mount (KOH); take specimen from active border of lesion.
   b. Wood's lamp to detect *Microsporum canis* or *Microsporum audouinii*.
   c. Fungal culture.

E. **Treatment (see Chapters 11, 18, and 19).**
1. Anti-infectives.
2. Topical agents.

F. **Nursing considerations (see Chapters 16 and 17).**

II. TINEA VERSICOLOR (pityriasis versicolor; tinea flava)

A. **Definition: superficial, chronic fungal infection seen on upper trunk, arms, or neck.**

B. **Etiology.**
1. Caused by *Pityrosporum orbiculare* (*Malassezia furfur*).
   a. Part of normal skin flora.
   b. Concentrated in areas with increased sebaceous activity.
2. Factors contributing to fungal proliferation.
   a. Heat/humidity.
   b. Cushing's disease.
   c. Pregnancy.
   d. Malnutrition.
   e. Burns.
   f. Corticosteroid therapy.
   g. Immunosuppression.
   h. Oral contraception.

C. **Pathophysiology.**
1. Characteristic lesions and distribution.
2. Postpubertal and mature individuals more susceptible.
3. Pruritus may be present.
4. Lesions more prominent in summer due to tanning of noninvolved skin.

D. **Assessment.**
1. History (see Table 1).
2. Current health status.
3. Evaluate affected skin sites.
4. Clinical manifestations.
   a. Multiple, small, circular macules of varying color.
   b. Lesions enlarge radially.
   c. Red to fawn-colored macules, patches, or follicular papules.
   d. Slightly scaly.
   e. Papular, nummular, of confluent.
5. Diagnostic tests.
   a. KOH.
   b. Wood's lamp.
   c. Fungal culture rarely necessary.

E. **Treatment.**
1. Topical.
   a. Selenium sulfide shampoo.
   b. Sodium thiosulfate.
   c. Miconazole, ketoconazole.
   d. Sulfur-salicylic shampoo.
   e. Zinc pyrithione shampoo.
   f. Keratolytic soaps.
2. Systemic — ketoconazole.

F. **Nursing considerations (see Table 2).**

III. CANDIDIASIS (moniliasis, thrush)

A. **Definition: skin, mucous membrane, and internal infection caused by proliferation of normal flora in mouth, vaginal tract, and gut.**

B. **Etiology.**
1. *Candida albicans* — yeast-like fungus; most common cause of superificial and systemic fungal infections.
2. Factors predisposing to proliferation of organisms.
   a. Pregnancy.
   b. Oral contraceptives.
   c. Antibiotic therapy.
   d. Diabetes.
   e. Skin maceration.
   f. Topical steroids.
   g. Some endocrinopathies.
   h. Immunocompromised states.
3. Infects outer layers of epithelium of mucous membranes and stratum corneum of skin.

C. **Pathophysiology.**
1. Candidiasis of moist areas.
   a. Vulvovaginitis.
      (1) Heat/moisture increase risk of infection.
      (2) Menstruation may worsen symptoms.
      (3) May coexist with Trichomonas.
   b. Oral candidiasis.
      (1) Seen in infants (see Chapter 11) and adults.
      (2) Causative factors — diabetes, depressed cell-mediated immunity, advanced age, cancer, prolonged steroid therapy, chemotherapy, broad-spectrum antibiotics, AIDS (see Chapter 19).
      (3) Tongue involved in a acute infection — extending into esophagus and trachea.

(4) Localized, firmly adherent plaques characteristic of chronic infections.

C. Intertrigo.
1. Occurs in large skin folds.
2. Heat and moisture provide environment for proliferation of organisms.
3. Poor hygiene and inflammatory diseases also increase risk of infection.

D. Assessment (see Chapters 11 and 19).
1. Current health status.
2. Evaluate skin and mucous membranes.
3. Clinical presentation.
   a. Pustules (satellite lesions).
   b. Erythematous, moist, glistening plaques extending beyond the limits of opposing skin folds.
   c. Painful fissuring.
4. Pruritus and discharge initial signs of infection.
5. Edema, erythema, and erosion of mucous membranes and external genitalia.
6. Satellite lesions may develop.
7. Diagnostic tests.
   a. KOH.
   b. Wood's lamp.
   c. Fungal culture.

E. Treatment.
1. Vulvovaginitis.
   a. Miconazole, clotrimazole, terconazole, or butoconazole vaginal cream.
   b. Oral azoles.
   c. Nystatin vaginal tabs.
   d. Gentian violet.
   e. Oral azoles.
2. Oral candidiasis.
   a. Nystatin oral suspension.
   b. Clotriamazole troche.
   c. Gentian violet.
   d. Azoles orally.
3. Intertrigo.
   a. Maintain dryness.
   b. Burow's compresses.
   c. Antifungal creams.
   d. Absorbent powders.
   e. Oral azoles.

F. Nursing considerations (see Table 2).

Bibliography

Habif, T.P. (2001). *Skin disease: Diagnosis and treatment.* St. Louis, MO: The CV Mosby Company.

Habif, T.P. (1996). *Clinical dermatology: A color guide to diagnosis and therapy* (3rd ed.). St. Louis, MO: The CV Mosby Company.

Hill, M.J. (1994). *Skin disorders.* St. Louis, MO: Mosby.

Leach, E.E., & Ruszkowski A.M. (1996). Nursing role in the management of integumentary problems. In S.M. Lewis, I.C. Collier, & M.M. Heitkemper (Eds.), *Medical-surgical nursing: Assessment and management of clinical problems* (pp. 496-526). St. Louis, MO: Mosby.

Nesbit, L.T. (1995). Evaluating the patient with a skin infection — general considerations. In C.V. Sanders, & L.T. Nesbitt (Eds.). *The skin and infection: A color atlas and text* (pp. 104-118). Philadelphia: Williams and Wilkins.

1. Bullous impetigo is caused group II *Staphylococcus aureus.*
   a. True.
   b. False.

2. Erysipelas is a form of cellulitis caused by:
   a. *Staphylococcus aureus.*
   b. *Pseudomonas aeruginosa.*
   c. Group A beta-hemolytic streptococci.
   d. Non-group A streptococcus.

3. Condyloma acuminata *are not considered to be* contagious.
   a. True.
   b. False.

4. Prodromal symptoms of HSV infection include all of the following except:
   a. Flu-like symptoms.
   b. Nausea.
   c. Mild parasthesias.
   d. Burning.

5. Recurrent lesions of HSV may be seen within 12 hours of prodromal symptoms.
   a. True.
   b. False.

6. Factors that may reactivate herpes zoster include:
   a. Immunosuppressive drugs.
   b. Fatigue.
   c. Stress.
   d. Smoking.
   e. a, b, c only.
   f. a, c, d only.

7. Dermatophytes are responsible for the majority of skin, hair, and nail infections.
   a. True.
   b. False.

8. All the following describe dermatophyte infection *except:*
   a. Invade skin and survive on dead keratin.
   b. Undergo deep invasion.
   c. Cannot survive on mucosal surfaces.

9. Factors contributing to fungal proliferation include all of the following *except:*
   a. Heat/humidity.
   b. Pregnancy.
   c. Corticosteroid therapy.
   d. Age.
   e. Malnutrition.

10. Lesions of tinea versicolor are more prominent during the winter.
    a. True.
    b. False.

11. Intertrigo is caused by *Candida albicans.*
    a. True.
    b. False.

12. Factors contributing to the formation of a furuncle include all of the following *except:*
    a. Friction.
    b. Hyperhidrosis.
    c. Nutritional status.
    d. Scratching.
    e. Pressure from restrictive clothing.

Answers to Study Questions

1.	a	5.	a	9.	d
2.	c	6.	e	10.	b
3.	b	7.	a	11.	a
4.	b	8.	b	12.	c

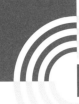

CE Answer/Evaluation Form

Chapter 12.
Infections

Please photocopy this test page and return.

COMPLETE THE FOLLOWING:

Name: _____

Address: _____

City: _____ State: _____ Zip: _____

Preferred telephone: (Home)_____ (Work) _____

State where licensed and license number: _____

CE application fee: DNA member $10.00
                        Nonmember $13.00

POSTTEST INSTRUCTIONS
1. To receive continuing education credit for individual study after reading the article, complete the answer/evaluation form below.
2. Photocopy and send the answer/evaluation form along with a check or money order payable to **Dermatology Nurses' Association** to: *DNA*, East Holly Avenue Box 56, Pitman, NJ 08071-0056.
3. Test returns must be postmarked by December 31, 2008. Upon completion of the answer/evaluation form, a certificate for 2.8 contact hour(s) will be awarded and sent to you.

This chapter was reviewed and formatted for contact hour credit by Marcia J. Hill, MSN, RN, Core Curriculum Editor; and Sally Russell, MN, RN,C, DNA Education Director.

ANSWER FORM

1. Name one new detail (item, issue, or phenomenon) that you learned by completing this activity.

   _____
   _____
   _____
   _____

2. How will you apply the information from this learning activity to your practice?
   a. Patient education.
   b. Staff education.
   c. Improve my patient care.
   d. In my education course work.
   e. Other: Please describe _____

   _____

Evaluation

	Strongly disagree				Strongly agree
3. The offering met the stated objectives.					
a. Describe the cutaneous presentation of bacterial, viral, and fungal infections.	1	2	3	4	5
b. Discuss factors that precipitate certain infections.	1	2	3	4	5
c. List fungal infections by body region.	1	2	3	4	5
d. Understand the pathology of cutaneous infection.	1	2	3	4	5
4. The content was current and relevant.	1	2	3	4	5
5. The content was presented clearly.	1	2	3	4	5
6. The content was covered adequately.	1	2	3	4	5
7. I am more confident of my abilities since completing this material.	1	2	3	4	5

8. The material was (check one) ☐ new, ☐ review for me.

Comments _____

9. Time required to complete reading assignment: _____ minutes

Photodermatoses, Photodamage, and Aging Skin

Sharon M. Simpson, BS, RN, DNC

OBJECTIVES

At the end of this chapter, the reader will be able to:
- Identify the symptoms, discuss the etiology, and support the treatment of the major types of photodermatoses.
- Discuss with patients and the public the various treatments available to correct photodamage to the skin.
- List and promote at least three widely available methods of protecting the skin from damage by the sun.

KEY POINTS

- It is important to have clinical knowledge and a teaching perspective on the various degrees of risk that accompany many common skin diseases, their behavioral, genetic, and environmental causes, and effective treatments that have proven successful in resolving them.
- It is important for a patient to see a dermatologist when rashes, questionable lesions, or other observable symptoms of skin disorders occur, and to rely on proven clinical analysis and a wide modality of treatments to correct them.
- Educating everyone, especially parents regarding the guidance of their children, regardless of skin color, age, or genetic inheritance, is important in protecting skin from the sun's damaging rays.

Photodermatoses, Photodamage, and Aging Skin

Sharon M. Simpson, BS, RN, DNC

PHOTODAMAGE

I. OVERVIEW

Exposure of the skin to the sun's rays causes cumulative damage to people of all skin colors from childhood through adult years. Variations in susceptibility, kinds of damage, presentation, and pathologies can be traced to climate conditions, genetic inheritance, and personal behavior patterns. Systematic treatment options include surgery, a wide variety of chemical applications and injections, cosmetic and laser therapies, and patient education to change the choices that induce preventable damage.

A. Definition: a term describing the skin of middle age and elderly adults who have been chronically exposed to the sun. The condition is identified by clinical and histological findings.

B. Etiology.
   1. The damage caused by the ultraviolet radiation starts as early as childhood.
   2. Since the promotion of sun protection is a relatively recent campaign, many individuals were unprotected and vulnerable to sunburn.
   3. Both UVA and UVB rays play a part in damaging the skin, but the erythema and tanning of the skin are more significant with UVB rays.
   4. Other influences on photodamage are wind, smoke, and chemical exposure.

C. Pathophysiology.
   1. Melanin is the basic physiologic sunscreen in man. Because of less melanin, people with Type I, II, and III skin are more susceptible to burns and damage from the sun; people with types IV, V, and VI can also be damaged by ultraviolet rays (see Table 1).
   2. Changes that occur because of sunburn and tanning include:
      a. Impaired immune response because of epidermal cell necrosis.
      b. Skin pigment darkening quickly with UVB rays, whereas delayed darkening occurs with UVA rays.
      c. Erythema that is caused by release of inflammatory mediators, such as cytokines and prostaglandins.
   3. Early in childhood or the teenage years, the skin absorbs the sun's rays while children play outdoors, bask on the beach, or are otherwise exposed. The sunburns or tans are only temporary, but the damage remains.
   4. As middle age approaches, the skin becomes leathery, dry, and nodular.
   5. The skin also appears blotchy, sometimes yellowing and forming deep wrinkles (see Table 2).
   6. Histologically, the sun-damaged epidermis is generally thicker than unexposed skin and shows some cellular atypia.
   7. There is a marked elastosis and a decrease in collagen fibers and bundles in the dermis.
   8. There are instances of telangiectasia and solar lentigines in prolonged sun-damaged skin.

D. Treatment options.
   1. Surgical treatment.
      a. Dermabrasion is a standard method that has been successfully used for many years.
         (1) It can be used for the total face or smaller local areas where trichloracetic acid (TCA) peels and other methods have not been effective.
         (2) Some physicians believe that elderly skin tends not to heal as well, causing greater incidence of hypertrophic scarring.
         (3) The older person tends to heal more slowly, leaving the skin open to a greater chance of infection.
      b. Aluminum oxide crystal microdermabrasion is a relatively new and popular treatment for facial rejuvenation for damage caused by ultraviolet light.
         (1) It is a simple, noninvasive procedure that can be repeated as often as every week for 4 to 12 weeks.
         (2) The aluminum oxide crystals are used to abrade the skin.

Table 1.
Fitzpatrick's Sun-Reactive Skin Types

Skin Type	Skin Color	Tanning Response
Type I	White	Always burn, never tan
Type II	White	Usually burn, tan with difficulty
Type III	White	Sometimes mild burn, tan average
Type IV	Brown	Rarely burn, tan with ease
Type V	Dark brown	Very rarely burn, tan very easily
Type VI	Black	No burn, tan very easily

Table 2.
Glogau Photoaging Classification

Type I: No Wrinkles	Type II: Wrinkles in Motion	Type III: Wrinkles at Rest	Type IV: Only Wrinkles
Early photoaging	Early to moderate photoaging	Advanced photoaging	Severe photoaging
Mild pigmentary changes No keratoses Minimal wrinkles	Early senile lentigines visible Keratoses palpable but not visible Parallel smile lines beginning to appear	Obvious dyschromia and telangiectasia Visible keratoses Wrinkles even when not moving	Yellow-gray color of skin Prior skin malignancies Wrinkled throughout, no normal skin
Patient age, 20s or 30s Minimal or no makeup	Patient age, late 30s or 40s Usually wears some foundation	Patient age, 50s or older Always wears heavy foundation	Patient age, 6th or 7th Cannot wear makeup – "cakes and cracks"

(3) Following the procedure a mild, transient erythema may occur.

c. Chemical peels.

   (1) Phenol or various formulations containing phenol is a method of deep peeling photodamaged skin that is preferred by some physicians.

     (a) Side effects: there is a risk of renal toxicity and cardiac arrhythmias from phenol.

     (b) But very good results have been obtained from careful use by well-trained physicians.

   (2) TCA is a medium-depth peel. TCA is used in various concentrations, 20% to 50%, to obtain good results in photodamaged skin.

     (a) It is sometimes used with other agents such as Jessner's solution.

     (b) Side effects of TCA peels are hypo or hyperpigmentation, scarring, and infection. The erythema may be persistent.

     (c) Because of potential side effects, physicians may use a light concentration of the peel or a series of peels for better and safer results.

   (3) Alpha hydroxy acids (the most common being glycolic acid) are found in natural sources.

     (a) Lactic acid is found in sour milk, tartaric acid in grapes, and glycolic acid is found in sugar cane, although cosmetic manufacturers primarily use synthetic glycolic acid.

     (b) The smaller the molecular structure of the acid, the more penetrable it is in the skin. With its two-carbon atom, glycolic acid is more penetrable than lactic acid or tartaric acid with three and four carbon atoms respectively.

     (c) Glycolic acid comes in concentrations of 5% to 99%; 50% to 70% solutions are most commonly used in the physician's office, and 10% to 20% solutions are most commonly used in home applications.

     (d) The best results of glycolic peels are seen after several months of increased concentration.

     (e) Glycolic acid is less sun sensitizing, but a patient should use a good sunscreen when receiving these peels.

d. Collagen injections may be used on the expressive lines and fine-line wrinkles caused by photoaging.

   (1) The patient must have 1 to 2 skin tests prior to starting the injections, to check for any allergic reactions.

   (2) The effects of the collagen injections are not permanent and must be repeated every 6 to 18 months for sustained results.

e. Hylan B gels are derived from hyluronan, a component of all connective tissues.

   (1) Because they are biocompatible, there is no need for skin tests.

   (2) Hylan B gels are water insoluble, they resist degradation, and they are unlikely to migrate.

   (3) There are three hylan B gels with increasingly greater viscosities, so that each is suitable for a different contour, from fine wrinkles to common wrinkles to deep folds.

(4) Hylan B gels are pending FDA approval, as of June 2002.

f. Lipotransfer is the transfer of the patient's own fat from the buttocks or abdomen, and injection into the facial expression lines.

    (1) It is a relatively simple procedure done under local anesthesia.

    (2) No skin tests are needed.

    (3) The most commonly injected area is the naso-labial fold.

    (4) Like collagen, it lasts only 6 to 18 months.

    (5) An advantage is that extra fat may be withdrawn and frozen to be injected several months later.

2. Topical retinoids.

a. Tretinoin, a retinoid, applied topically helps to even skin coloring, soften fine wrinkle lines, and increase the formation of the blood vessels.

b. Tretinoin acts by gently peeling the skin and also by normalizing the epidermal turnover.

c. The patient may experience some skin irritation or dryness at first, but this usually subsides.

d. When a patient is on tretinoin, a sunscreen with SPF of 15 or more must be used, as this medication makes the skin very sun sensitive. A cream or lotion is preferred, since gels contain alcohol.

e. Tretinoin should be applied to cleansed, slightly damp skin in a thin layer, avoiding the corners of the eyes and the eyelids. It should also be feathered down the neck for a smoother look.

f. Because of increased sun sensitivity, tretinoin should be applied at night, and a sunscreen should be applied in the morning.

g. Women who are pregnant, or may be pregnant, should not use tretinoin.

3. Cosmetic treatment.

a. Alpha hydroxy acids are found in many creams, cleansers, and lotions for application at home.

b. Vitamin C, in an aqueous base, applied topically, may provide some protection from ultraviolet damage, although no significant clinical trials have been completed for evaluation.

4. Lasers.

a. Telangiectasia of the face, a result of photodamaged skin, may be treated with vascular lesion lasers, such as the pulsed dye, copper bromide, and krypton laser. This technique is relatively new, but the results are promising.

    (1) The treated veins appear reddish-purple or exhibit a light bruising after the treatment.

    (2) Scabbing rarely occurs.

    (3) Makeup should not be applied for several days after the laser treatment, or at least until the deep purple fades, as the skin is fragile after the treatment, and rubbing the area could cause skin damage.

    (4) Discoloration fades and disappears in 8 to 14 days.

    (5) Some slight discoloration may remain, but this is rarely seen on the face.

b. Brown macular lesions (solar lentigines) may be treated with excellent results with several lasers, one of which is the Q-switched ruby laser.

    (1) The areas treated may appear frosty white immediately after treatment, then erythematous, lastly forming flat reddish-brown scabs, which flake off after 7 to 12 days.

    (2) The only discomfort felt is an initial "snap of the rubber band" sensation.

    (3) The treated areas should be cleansed and dried gently so as not to remove the scabs before healing. A gentle cleanser that is chemical free should be used.

    (4) The treated area may be covered with makeup, but applied and removed very gently so as not to disturb the scabs. A delay of 2 to 3 days is preferable.

c. Short-pulsed and scanned CO_2 resurfacing lasers are used for spot areas, fine lines around the eyes or upper lip, or the total face. Patients with lupus or scleroderma are not candidates for this treatment.

    (1) Two weeks prior to treatment, patients begin a daily application of tretinoin cream and a bleaching agent to prep the skin. Two days prior to the laser treatment the patient is placed on antiviral medication and antibiotics. These are continued for 5 days after the treatment.

    (2) Small areas may be treated with a local anesthetic only, but for full face and around the eyes an anesthesiologist is present to administer IV sedation.

    (3) There can be a fair amount of discomfort for 2 to 3 days following laser treatment and a pain medication is often prescribed.

    (4) Treated areas will be crusty and quite red for 7 to 14 days. The patient will apply Vaseline® frequently during the day and

Table 3.
Laser Treatments

Condition	Laser	Preparation	Post-Procedure Care
Telangiectasia; pigmented lesions	Krypton	Cleanse face	Gentle cleansing; thin layer bacitracin or polysporin ointment to scab area; make-up after 4 to 5 days.
Pigmented lesions	Q switch; Ruby laser Yag	Cleanse face	Gentle cleansing and drying of skin; make-up applied very gently the following day, if necessary.
Telangiectasia, hemangiomas, scars	Sclerolaser Pulsed dye V-beam	Cleanse face	(Scabs do not appear, but skin is very fragile); gentle cleansing and drying of skin; make-up may be applied and removed very gently the same day; if necessary, moisturizer may be applied for dryness.
Rhytides (fine wrinkles and expression lines), atrophic scars	Pulsed CO_2 Cutaneous laser Erbium	Some physicians apply a tretinoin cream and bleaching agent is applied 2 weeks prior to treatment; NPO after midnight if IV sedation.	Vaseline® applied several times per day; some physicians use Vigilon® dressing; cleanse twice daily with Dial® liquid or Basis® liquid soap; make-up may be applied after scabs are gone, 7 to 14 days; tretinoin cream and bleaching agent resumed after 2 weeks.

night, cleansing the skin twice a day with a gentle liquid soap and rinsing thoroughly.

(5) The red to pink skin may remain for several months.

(6) Make-up can be applied after 1 to 2 weeks, after the skin has re-epithelialized.

(7) After 2 weeks the daily application of tretinoin cream and a bleaching agent may be resumed to decrease the chance of pigmentation.

(8) Patients should avoid direct sunlight and other sources of ultraviolet rays for several months and always wear a sunblock.

d. Lasers are also being developed for hair removal (see Table 3).

E. **Patient education.**

1. Sunscreens, sunscreens, sunscreens!

a. Definition: sunscreens reflect the sun's UVB rays, whereas sunblocks block out UVB and UVA rays. Examples of total blocks are titanium dioxide and zinc oxide (see Table 4).

b. SPF (sun-protective factor) identifies the

multiple of protection time compared to no protection. SPF 15 protects the skin from UV rays 15 times longer than unprotected skin.

c. Fair-skinned individuals, because of their susceptibility to sun damage, should use a sun block. Patients with darkly pigmented skin should use sunscreens, as their skin can be damaged by UV rays, although to a lesser degree.

d. Sunscreens are available in creams, lotions, and gels. Many people prefer the gels because they leave less of a greasy sensation.

e. Parents must be encouraged to put broad-spectrum sunscreen on their children starting with 6 months of age. There are special sunscreens for children.

f. If children are taught early to use sunscreen, they are more likely to continue using it as teenagers.

g. Middle-aged and elderly adults should use sunscreen faithfully. They are never too old to slow down the skin damage. And don't forget the ears and lips.

h. The best sunscreens are those that block

Table 4.
Characteristics of Sunscreens and Sunblocks

Sun Protection	Formulation	Skin Type	Application	Medical Effect	Cosmetic Effect
Broad-spectrum sunscreen	Lotion, cream, or gel	IV, V, VI	All sun-exposed skin including lips	Reflects UVB rays	Slows burning, tanning, and wrinkling
Sunblock	Lotion, cream, or gel	I, II, III	All sun-exposed skin including lips	Reflects UVB and UVA rays	Slows burning, tanning, and wrinkling

UVA and UVB rays. Several are available on the market (see Table 5).
2. Protective clothing.
   a. Patients should be taught to wear long sleeves to protect their arms when out in the bright sun or on the water. The cloth should be tightly woven to allow little UV ray penetration.
   b. Wide-brimmed hats for men, women, and children are highly recommended. Infants should wear bonnets.
   c. There are several companies that sell specifically designed sun-protective clothing.
3. Patients should be advised to avoid being outside between 10 am and 2 pm, when the sun is strongest.
4. Avoid tanning booths.
5. Sunglasses should be worn by children and adults to protect the eyes.

PHOTODERMATOSES

I. ACTINIC KERATOSES (AKs)

A. Definition: actinic keratoses or solar keratoses are lesions caused by sun damage, and are commonly found in the elderly population with skin types I, II and III. They are made up of aggregates of anaplastic keratinocytes confined to the epidermis.
B. Etiology.
1. Sun exposure begins at a very early age, but AKs are not commonly seen in children or teenagers, except in albinism.
2. AKs are found more in men than women, and greatly increase in number as the population ages.
3. Although they can appear on any sun-exposed area, AKs are most frequently seen in the face, scalps, and ears of men, and arms.
4. People with blue eyes, fair skin, and albinos are at higher risk to develop AKs, whereas they are rarely seen in people with black skin.
5. If left untreated, 10% to 20% may grow

Table 5.
Sunscreen Agents

UVB absorbers
Para-Amino benzoic acid
Clinoxate
Homosalate
Octocrylene
Octyl methoxycinnamate
Octyl salicylate
Padimate O
Phenylbenzimidazole sulfonic acid
Trolamine salicylate

UVA absorbers
Avobenzone (Parsol 1789®)
Oxybenzone
Sulisobenzone
Dioxybenzone
Methyl anthranilate

UVA/UVB absorbers
Titanium dioxide
Zinc oxide

through the basement membranes of the epidermal-dermal junction and become squamous cell carcinomas.
C. Pathophysiology.
1. Clinically AKs are small, measuring from a few millimeters to 1-2 centimeters, and may range in number from 1 to more than 100. This generally depends on the type of skin and the amount of sun exposure.
   a. AKs can vary in color from a tan to a reddish tone.
   b. Occasionally they appear the same color as the skin and must be palpated.
   c. AKs appear as individual, scaly, or rough papules on the epidermis.
   d. A higher percentage of AKs are found in men than in women. Perhaps there is a

higher percentage of sun exposure for men.

2. A rare variation of the AK is the spreading pigmented AK.
   a. These lesions are large in size, over 1 cm.
   b. They may be smooth on the surface, slightly scaly or warty in texture, and be variable in color.
   c. There is a tendency for centrifugal spread.
   d. The spreading pigmented AK is found mostly on the face, and can mimic the lentigo maligna in appearance.

3. The lichenoid keratosis resembles a solitary lesion of lichen planus. There is learned discussion whether this is a totally benign lesion or an inflamed AK.
   a. It begins small but can increase in size to 3 to 4 cm, and has uneven borders.
   b. The color tends toward red, and it is scaly in texture.

4. Histologically, AKs are well-defined aggregates of abnormal keratinocytes. The epidermis is generally hyperkeratotic.
   a. The nucleus of the keratinocyte is enlarged, hyperchromatic, and irregular in shape. The keratinocyte may be multinucleated.
   b. Cells of the sweat gland ducts and hair follicles tend to be normal.
   c. Changes of solar elastosis often appear in the underlying dermis.

D. Treatment.

1. 5-fluorouracil (5-FU) in a light 1% to 5% cream or solution is effective for patients with moderate to extensive actinic damage.
   a. It also treats subclinical lesions.
   b. 5-FU is applied twice a day for an average of 2 weeks, followed by 2 weeks of application of a gentle cortisone cream.
   c. The skin may become very red and irritated. Therefore, in cases with severe actinic damage the 5-FU is applied in sections, such as the forehead or left cheek. This routine, however, takes several weeks longer, and the patient requires a good deal of support during these times.
   d. Complications of 5-FU treatment are scarring, infection, loss of pigmentation, and recurrence. Also a color difference remains between the normal skin and the actinic-damaged skin after treatment.
   e. Retreatment with 5-FU may be necessary every 3 to 5 years for patients with severe damage, as the AKs will continue to develop.
   f. Fluorouracil cream 0.5% is a newer treatment.
      (1) It is applied only once a day, therefore patients are more compliant.
      (2) The cream is applied for 4 weeks.
      (3) Side effects are the same as with 5-FU, plus redness, dryness, burning, and swelling.

2. Several other methods for treating AKs are cryosurgery, electrodesiccation, and chemical cauterization, using TCA or glycolic acid. Phenol is less commonly employed in this setting.
   a. These methods have cure rates of up to 95%.
   b. They are excellent methods for discrete lesions and less diffuse actinically damaged skin.
   c. Cryosurgery and electrodesiccation are more commonly used for all areas of the body.
   d. Complications of these treatments are hypopigmentation, scarring, infection, and recurrence.

3. Dermabrasion is another very effective method of removing multiple AKs.
   a. The patient is generally not incapacitated as long as with the use of 5-FU.
   b. Because dermabrasion removes the skin uniformly, the skin heals uniformly, and the results are cosmetically appealing.
   c. Some dermatologists believe that dermabrasion is more effective in long-term prevention of new AKs forming than treatment with 5-FU.
   d. Complications are hypertrophic scarring, hypopigmentation, and infection.

4. Topical isotretinoin has been used in several studies to eradicate AKs from the face and upper extremities.
   a. It has some benefit on early facial AKs, but little effect on extremities.
   b. There is little response by advanced lesions, even after twice a day application of 0.1% isotretinoin.
   c. Although there may be some local irritation at the time of treatment, there are no serious or permanent side effects.

5. Photo-dynamic therapy (PDT) is the newest treatment available.
   a. It is useful for treating multiple lesions.
   b. PDT requires two visits to the dermatologist's office.
      (1) A topical medicine, aminolevulinic acid (ALA), is applied to the AK lesions on the first visit.
      (2) The second visit should be 14 to 18 hours after the application of ALA, when the lesions are exposed to a special blue light for less than 20 minutes.
      (3) The blue light activates the ALA, causing a chemical reaction in the skin that kills

the AK cells.

(4) In between visits it is important to avoid all sun and ultraviolet light exposure.

E. **Patient education.**
1. Sunscreens and sunblockers should be used from early childhood. Teenagers must be strongly encouraged to use them.
2. Sun-protective clothing such as tightly woven cotton shirts should be worn. Wearing wide-brim hats that protect the ears and nose should be encouraged.
3. Any patient who has sun-damaged skin or has a history of AKs should see a dermatologist every 6 to 12 months for a full body exam.
4. The patient should be persuaded that the risk of ignoring these lesions is that AKs may develop into squamous cell carcinomas.

II. LENTIGINES

A. **Definition: generally pigmented macules that measure 1 to 5 mm. They are rarely seen larger than 1 cm. They are found on normal skin.**
B. **There are many different varieties of lentigines, but three of the more common ones will be discussed here. These are not sun induced or associated with any systemic disease.**
1. The lentigo simplex (juvenile lentigo) appears commonly in children, as the name suggests. But it can appear on a person at any age.
   a. Clinical features:
      (1) These lesions may occur anywhere on the body and have no particular affinity to the sun-exposed areas of skin.
      (2) They remain small, usually 1 to 5 mm, and few in number.
      (3) The color of the lesions varies from brown to black and is evenly pigmented.
      (4) These lesions are flat and therefore not palpable.
   b. Histological features:
      (1) The rete ridges are moderately elongated.
      (2) There is increased epidermal hyperplasia and hyperpigmentation.
      (3) The number of melanocytes is increased in the basal cell layer.
      (4) Solar elastosis is absent.
   c. Treatment: juvenile lentigines are benign and may be left untreated.
2. Freckles (ephelides) are found on sun-exposed areas, such as the face, arms, and back of the hands.
   a. Clinical features:
      (1) Freckles are yellow to light brown macules found most frequently in people with light skin and red hair.
      (2) They are found in people with blond, brown, and black hair, but are fewer in number.
      (3) Although they commonly appear in the summer months, freckles may last all year or throughout the person's life.
      (4) Freckles may measure up to 5 mm, and have irregular or well-defined borders.
      (5) Whether their numbers are many or few, they are symmetrical in distribution.
   b. Histological features:
      (1) The rete ridges are not elongated in freckles.
      (2) Although there is an increase in pigment in the basal cell layer, there does not appear to be an increase in melanocytes.
   c. Treatment: freckles may be left untreated, or they can be removed with the ruby, alexandrite, or Q-switched YAG laser.
3. Lentigines profusa (generalized lentigines) usually appear without any associated abnormality. But they can rarely occur as a cutaneous sign of a systemic disorder (such as LEOPARD, NAME, or LAMB syndrome), lentigo plus cardiac, pulmonary and endocrinologic defects.
   a. Clinical features:
      (1) The lesions usually are present at birth, but may not appear until early childhood to early adulthood.
      (2) They appear as 1 mm to 2 cm pigmented lesions that occur anywhere on the body except for the soles of the feet and the buccal mucosa.
      (3) The color varies from dark brown to black.
      (4) The texture of the skin is normal, and the lesions are flat and nonpalpable.
      (5) Lentigines profusa are similar to freckles except for the widespread distribution of the lesion.
   b. Histological features:
      (1) The rete ridges are slightly elongated.
      (2) There is increased pigment in the melanocytes and an increase in the number of keratinocytes and melanocytes.
      (3) There is no solar elastosis.
   c. Treatment: like all lentigines, these lesions are benign and may be left untreated.
C. **Patient education: although these lentigines are not sun induced, the sun can darken them, and in the case of freckles, increase their number. Sunblocks or the use of protective clothing should be recommended at all times as a means of prevention.**

III. POLYMORPHOUS LIGHT ERUPTION (PMLE)

A. **Definition: PMLE is a sun-induced allergic reaction to a yet unknown photosensitizer.**

B. **Etiology.**
   1. Studies are showing some genetic predisposition, but there are no definitive percentages.
   2. PMLE can appear anytime, but it is most common before the age of 30 years.
   3. In North American and Latin American Indians, it commonly appears in childhood.
   4. Although it is present in both sexes, several studies show a greater prevalence in women.
   5. It affects all skin types from I through VI.
   6. 10% to 15% are found in the caucasian population.
   7. PMLE tends to become less seasonal and more extensive through time in severe cases.
   8. Occasionally there is a complete disappearance.

C. **Clinical.**
   1. Generally there is intense pruritus followed by the eruptions of skin lesions.
   2. The eruptions may occur several hours or several days after exposure, making diagnosis more difficult.
   3. The lesions usually remain 2 to 3 days, with extremes of 24 hours to 10 or more days.
   4. The lesions range from small papules and papulovesicles to eczematous reactions, or coalescent papules, which may merge to form plaques.
   5. The large papules are pink or red to erythema multiforme-like lesions, and usually occur on the face.
   6. PMLE lesions are confined to sun-exposed areas.
      a. If conditions are such that one involved area is exposed to enough radiation from the sun or artificial sources, another involved area may flare, even if unexposed.
      b. Although there may be an autosensitization response that results in the extension of the eruptions to an unexposed area, the sun-exposed surfaces remain more severe.
   7. The clinical action spectrum of sun exposure is UVB in the range of 290 to 320 nm. Much less common are reactions from UVA or visible rays.

D. **Histopathology.**
   1. The small papules and eczematous lesions show epidermal edema, spongiosis of interfollicular epidermis, and occasional vesicle formation. Parakeratosis and acanthosis are frequently present.
   2. The large papular lesions show very little epidermal response, but parakeratosis and acanthosis are frequently present.
   3. Some edema of the basal cell layer has been noted with both lesions.
   4. Both small and large papular lesions show a superficial and deep lymphocytic infiltration in the upper and middle dermis.

E. **Treatment.**
   1. Systemic drugs have mixed results.
      a. Beta carotene has been used with little positive response.
      b. Chloroquine and hydroxychloroquin are more effective.
         (1) Both are quite effective in large papule reactions and in very early small papule-type variants.
         (2) Frequent eye exams are recommended for those taking these drugs more than 2 months beyond the base line exam.
         (3) Extreme caution must be taken when using these drugs with children, as they are very sensitive.
      c. Some studies have been done using thalidomide, with no definitive results yet.
   2. Topical therapy with high-potency corticosteroids bring some relief, but cannot be used long term because of atrophy, telangiectasia, and dependency.
   3. Studies have been done using PUVA with 8-MOP as a prophylactic to tan and thicken the stratum corneum, with positive results.
   4. BB-UVB and NB-UVB have also proved to be effective prophylactic treatments.

F. **Patient education.**
   1. First, patients must be educated about the dangers of sun exposure.
   2. The importance of avoiding direct exposure to the sun and protection from solar radiation must be emphasized.
      a. Sunblocks and broad-spectrum sunscreens must be used freely.
      b. Sun-protective clothing, such as tightly woven cotton garments, hats, and long sleeves should be worn.
      c. Patients must be persuaded to avoid outdoor sports or activities during the hours of 9 am to 3 pm.
      d. Tanning machines must be avoided.

IV. PHOTOTOXICITY AND PHOTOALLERGY

A. **Definition: photosensitivity reactions are created by combining light, generally UVA, with a photosensitizing chemical. The two types of photosensitivity reactions are phototoxicity and photoallergy (see Table 6).**

B. **Pathophysiology.**
   1. In order for a reaction to occur, light must be absorbed by the chemical.
   2. The chemical may be systemic within the body, or introduced externally to the skin.
   3. Although direct sunlight is the major source of

Table 6.
Common Phototoxic Agents, Photoallergens, and Phototoxins

Common Systemic Phototoxic Agents by Generic Name	Common Photoallergens	Common Phototoxins In the Environment
Amiodarone	Sunscreens:	Coal tar
Benoxaprofen	PABA	Psoralens
Chloroquine	Sulisobenzone (BZP-4)	Tar Pitch
Chlorpromazine	Oxygensone (BZP-3)	
Chlorpropamide	Cinoxate	
Chlorothiazide	Octyl methoxyinnamate	
Ciprofloxacin	Homosalate	
Decarbazine	Octyl salicylate	
Desipramine		
Diphenhydramine	Fragrances:	
5-Flourouracil	Musk ambrette	
Furosemide	6-methylcoumarin	
Griseofulvin	Sandalwood oil	
Imipramine		
Ketoprofen	Antibacterials:	
Naladixic acid	Bithionol	
Naproxen	Fenticlor	
Nifedipine	Triclosan	
Piroxicam	Dichlorophene	
Promethazine	Tribromasalicylanilide	
Psoralens	Hexachlorophene	
Quinidine	Chlorhexidene diacetate	
Quinine		
Sulfanilamide		
Tetracyclines	Others:	
Thiazides	Chloropomazine	
Tiaprofenic acid	Hydrochloride	
Tolbutamide	Promethazin	
Vinblastine	Thiourea	

light, fluorescent light may also cause response.

4. The clinical pattern of photosensitivity reaction appears on exposed areas of skin such as the face, particularly the nose and cheeks, ears, the backs of hands, and the neck area.

5. The most common cause of photoallergic reactions is external exposure to chemicals in the workplace, and in rare cases to chemicals in the general environment or in commercially purchased goods.

6. The two photosensitivity reactions differ (see Table 7).

V. SUNBURN

A. **Webster's definition is superficial inflammation of the skin caused by direct exposure to the sun's rays.**

B. **Etiology.**
   1. Sunburn is not caused by a disease but is the result of indiscretion.

   2. People who are skin types I and II and III have very little melanin and tend to burn more readily than those with skin types IV and V and VI.

   3. Almost anyone, regardless of skin type or melanin content, can burn if they expose their skin long enough to the ultraviolet rays of the sun or to artificial sources.

   4. Some drugs, such as tetracycline, sulfonamides, Diabinese® and griseofulvin are photosensitizing. Exposure to ultraviolet rays should be avoided while taking them.

   5. Erythema usually develops 2 to 12 hours after exposure, and reaches its greatest severity at 24 hours.

C. **Pathophysiology.**
   1. In more severe cases vesiculation appears.

   2. There can be extreme burning discomfort accompanying a deeper burn.

Table 7.
Phototoxicity and Photoallergy

Phototoxicity	Photoallergy
1. Individual must be exposed to a sufficient amount of photosensitizing chemical at the same time as to the causal wavelength of light.	1. Individual must be exposed to a sufficient amount of photosensitizing chemical at the same time as to the causal wavelength of light.
2. Reaction occurs minutes to hours after the first exposure to the sensitizing agent.	2. Due to a need for prior sensitization, reaction will not occur upon first exposure; a minimum of 24 to 72 hours is required after the combined exposure before the first reaction occurs.
3. Nonimmunologic reaction.	3. This is an immunologic reaction.
4. Because of differences in penetration, absorption, and the metabolism of the chemicals in the patient, the reaction can be sporadic.	4. Photoallergy reactions are less frequent in most patients. The amount of chemical needed to induce a reaction is minimal, and cross-reactivity to other agents is always possible.
5. Clinically the patient shows a sunburn which may even blister. There is peeling and there may be hyperpigmentation. Burning or stinging may be experienced with the reaction.	5. Clinically the patient has acute pruritic eruptions or vesicles and papules in areas exposed to light. In patients with chronic reactions, excoriated and lichenified plaques occur.
6. Pathophysiology: a. The phototoxic molecules absorb energy, which is transferred to oxygen molecules; this creates a reactive oxygen species that causes cellular damage. b. A photosensitizer may bind with a biologic substrate so with the exposure to radiation, the structure of the substrate is altered. Psoralen binding with pyrimidine bases of DNA molecules is an example of this reaction. c. Radiation interacting with phototoxic substances may cause a release of inflammatory mediators. d. A chemical that absorbs radiation may form a photoproduct, which in turn may react with a biologic substrate. Chlorpiomazine-induced phototoxicity is an example	6. Pathophysiology: a. The systemic or topical chemical absorbs radiation, producing a photoallergen. b. The antigen-presenting cells, such as macrophages and Langerhans', process the photo-allergen and introduce it to helper T-cells and class II molecules. c. The consequent reaction is the classic type IV delayed hypersensitivity response. d. Photoallergies are most commonly caused by external chemicals, and rarely by systemic drugs
7. Diagnoses may be facilitated by phototesting. A small area of non-sun-exposed skin is irradiated with gradually increasing amounts of UVB or UVA, until a minimal erythema appears. Usually a lesser dose of UVA irradiation is needed in the phototoxic patient than in the general population where the amount of UVB is the same.	7. Photopatch testing is a method of confirming photoallergic contact dermatitis. a. Day 1: duplicate sets of photoallergens are applied to the back and covered with an opaque tape. b. Day 2: one set of patches is removed and sites are exposed to 10J/cm^2 of UVA, or 50% of minimal erythema does (MED). c. Day 3: both sites uncovered and the reactions are graded. d. Both sites are graded for delayed reaction.

3. Other symptoms are chills, malaise, and generalized weakness.
4. After a few days, the vesicles dry, the skin tightens and peels.
5. The peeling leaves a mottled and sensitive skin underneath.
D. Treatment.
1. Cool water or skimmed milk compresses can be applied.
2. Burrows solution compresses (1% to 5%) are

helpful if vesicles are present.
3. The application of steroid lotions can be helpful.
4. Systematic analgesics will help decrease the pain.
5. In extremely severe cases of sunburn, oral steroids might be necessary.
6. If there has been any damage to the cornea of the eye, an ophthalmologist must be consulted.
E. Patient education.

Dermatologic Nursing Essentials: A Core Curriculum 2nd Edition © DNA 2003

1. The prophylactic use of sunblocks and broad-spectrum sunscreens is the best protection.
2. If the patient is at the beach or lives in a very sunny climate, he/she should be instructed to reapply sunscreen every few hours.
3. If the patient has already suffered a sunburn, the exposed skin will be extra sensitive to the UV rays. Further exposure should be absolutely avoided.
4. Stay away from tanning booths.

VI. PORPHYRIA CUTANEA TARDA (PCT)

A. **Definition: a porphyrin-induced photosensitive disorder, usually acquired, but which can be autosomal dominant.**
B. **Etiology.**
   1. Except for the rarer inherited autosomal dominant form (less than 10%), PCT usually appears after 40 years of age.
   2. The inherited PCT occurs under the age of 20.
   3. The disorder may occur sporadically, or be induced by drugs or toxic chemicals, mostly hydrocarbons.
   4. Originally PCT was a male-dominated disorder due to alcohol consumption, but with the widespread use of estrogen, a large increase in the female population has been noted, so that now the distribution is more equal.
   5. The reason for the increase caused by estrogen is unknown.
   6. PCT is a chronic disorder and unrelated to sun exposure. It is mildly photosensitive.
   7. There are a few diseases which commonly accompany PCT. A few examples are viral infection, hepatitis C, and HIV.
   8. Certain porphyrias have neurologic and visceral symptoms, and a positive family history.
   9. Patients with PCT usually do not complain of sensitivity to sunlight.
C. **Clinical.**
   1. There is hypo and hyperpigmentation of the sun-exposed areas, particularly the face.
   2. Hypertrichoses (hirsutism) is noted in most cases, and found generally in the face and the limbs.
   3. The exposed skin is abnormally fragile, causing blisters and erosions.
   4. The bullae heal with erythema, scarring and milia formation.
   5. Periocular erythema and a ruddy tone to the face are often noted.
   6. Sclerodermal thickening of the skin may occur in unexposed areas and the face.
D. **Pathophysiology.**
   1. Laboratory findings show:
      a. A greatly elevated uroporphyrin excretion (>500 g/24 hrs) in the urine.

b. Total iron stores that are often twice the normal amount in the hepatocytes.
c. H and E reveals subepidermal bullae with little inflammation.
   2. PCT is one of several porphyrias associated with defective enzymes in the heme biosynthetic pathway.
      a. Heme is used in the formation of hemoglobin, cytochromes, and other substances.
      b. Porphyrinogens are used in the production of heme.
      c. When the metabolic pathway is blocked by a deficiency in the enzyme uroporphyrinogen decarboxylase, the porphyrinogens break up or are oxidized into porphyrins.
      d. When there is light absorption, the porphyrin becomes greatly agitated, creating an unstable state.
      e. In this unstable state it causes damage to cells and cell membranes, releasing chemicals that cause inflammation and further tissue damage.
E. **Treatment.**
   1. Abstinence from alcohol is advised.
   2. Avoiding Dilantin®, diethylstilbestrol, and unnecessary iron intake is recommended, as they can aggravate the disease. And they should never be combined with alcohol.
   3. Phlebotomy is the most common treatment for PCT, as it appears to deplete the hepatic iron overload. The recommended procedure is removing 500 cc of blood every 2 weeks, 3 to 4 times. Then 500 cc are removed every 3 to 6 weeks, for a total of 10 to 15 pints of blood.
   4. Chloroquine in doses of 125 mg twice weekly for 8 to 18 months can help.
      a. Because chloroquin can be hepatotoxic, it is used in low doses and requires base line and biweekly liver function tests and urinary porphyrin analysis until the uroporphyrin level is less than 100 g/24 hours.
      b. Although it is not known exactly why this works, it may be that the chloroquin bonds with the hepatic porphyrins, causing them to become more water soluble, and increasing the urinary output of uroporphyrins.
   5. Using the combination of both phlebotomy and chloroquin may work better than either alone.
F. **Patient education.**
   1. The patient must be encouraged to avoid alcohol absolutely.
   2. The patient should be aware that the use of drugs named above can trigger the disease, so

as to avoid them.
3. Using sunblocks and avoiding the sun when possible should be encouraged.

VII. SOLAR URTICARIA (SU)

A. **Definition: an uncommon photodermatosis in which UV or visible irradiation causes whealing of some or all exposed skin.**
B. **Etiology.**
1. SU occurs in all races and at any age.
2. Generally it appears in young adults.
3. It is slightly more common in females age 10 to 50 years.
4. Susceptibility to his condition may occasionally disappear spontaneously.
C. **Clinical.**
1. It appears within a few minutes of sun exposure.
2. The symptoms of SU are itching, erythema, burning, and whealing.
3. After 24 hours, if there is no more exposure to the sun, the lesions and symptoms usually disappear.
4. The lesions are usually found on the V area of the neck and on the arms.
5. UVA, UVB, and/or visible light can cause SU.
D. **Pathophysiology.**
1. Phototesting is used to confirm SU by determining the smallest irradiation dose that causes whealing.
2. This is referred to as the minimal urticarial dose (MUD).
3. To determine the MUD, readings must be taken immediately after exposure and 6 hours later.
4. The effectiveness of therapy can be seen in the change of the MUD.
E. **Treatment.**
1. The initial method of treating SU is with antihistamines, specifically, H-1 receptor antagonists.
    a. Sunlight-induced histamine release is inhibited by antihistamines.
    b. This leads to a decrease in pruritus and prevention of the wheal and flare response.
    c. H-1 receptor blockers are prescribed in higher doses than for common allergies.
2. Less-effective therapies, used when the patient is unresponsive to antihistamines, include antimalarials, doxepin, indomethacin, and beta-carotene.
3. PUVA alone, or combined with plasmapheresis, has shown good results.
4. In recalcitrant cases, cyclosporine and plasmapheresis may be beneficial.
F. **Patient education.**
1. Broad-spectrum sunscreens and sunblock

should be applied to the skin before sun exposure.
2. Protective clothing should be worn.
    a. Dark-colored dyes reduce UV transmission more effectively than light-colored dyes.
    b. Wide brim hats should be worn.
    c. Long sleeves and long pants of cotton or polyester/cotton blend should be worn.
    d. Sunglasses.
3. Avoidance of sun exposure between 10 am and 4 pm.

VIII. CHRONIC ACTINIC DERMATITIS (CAD)

A. **Definition: CAD is a syndrome of persistent light reactivity defined by three criteria:**
1. There is commonly an eruption of eczematous character.
2. Histologically, its appearance is consistent with chronic eczema, with or without lymphoma-like changes.
3. Photobiologic: there is a reduction in the MED to UVB irradiation.
B. **Etiology.**
1. CAD is found more often in males age 63 to 65 years.
2. It has occurred occasionally in young people.
3. CAD is more prevalent in temperate climates.
C. **Clinical.**
1. CAD appears as hyperpigmented patches and scaly, pruritic lichenified plaques.
2. Generally they appear on sun-exposed areas, but in acute exacerbation covered skin may be involved.
3. In severe cases of CAD eczematous eruptions may appear.
D. **Pathophysiology.**
1. Atypical mononuclear cells may be found in the dermis and epidermis.
2. There is lymphocytic infiltrate confined to the upper dermis, causing epidermal spongiosis, acanthosis, and sometimes hyperplasia.
3. The patient with CAD will have abnormal phototest results to ultraviolet, UVB, UVA, and/or visible light.
E. **Treatment.**
1. Broad-spectrum sunscreens and protective clothing are helpful, but not always sufficient.
2. Avoidance of ultraviolet light and sun, where possible, should be a rule.
3. Topical steroids and emollients are used to control acute dermatitis.
4. Occasionally a short course of oral steroids is given.
5. In severe cases of CAD, it may be treated with PUVA, or immuno-suppressive agents such as cyclosporine, azathioprine, and systemic corticosteroids.

F. Patient education.
1. Broad-spectrum sunscreens and sunblocks should be applied to the skin before sun exposure.
2. Avoidance of sun exposure between 10 am and 4 pm should be practiced.
3. Wear protective clothing:
   a. Wide brim hats.
   b. Long sleeve shirts and long pants.
   c. Sunglasses.

AGING

I. OVERVIEW

A. **Intrinsic aging of the skin differs from photoaging in that it is genetic in origin.**
B. **Etiology.**
1. Skin that has been protected from the sun over the years remains smooth and unblemished.
2. Due to gravity, hormonal changes, and facial expressions, the facial lines tend to deepen and widen.
3. There is also atrophy of dermal and subcutaneous tissue.
4. In comparison, intrinsic aging is exemplified by atrophy whereas photoaging is hypertrophic.
C. **Treatment options.**
1. Collagen injections and lipotransfer can be used on the facial lines.
2. Resurfacing laser used to soften the facial lines around the eyes and upper lip gives very satisfactory results.
3. Plastic surgery procedures such as rhytidectomy (face lifts) and blepharoplasty are available.

II. XEROSIS

A. **Definition: xerosis is dry skin that appears when there is dehydration of the stratum corneum.**
B. **Pathophysiology.**
1. Older people have an accelerating decrease in epidermal free fatty acids, compared to younger individuals with similar skin conditions.
2. Xerotic skin has a reduced amino acid content.
3. The lower legs and feet are more commonly affected than the arms among older people.
4. The skin appears dry and scaly.
5. The patient usually complains of dryness and itching.
6. The systemic drying of the skin acids with age is a genetic inheritance.
C. **Treatment.**
1. The goal of all treatment is to add water to the skin and its environment.
2. Room temperatures should be kept cool, and the use of humidifiers encouraged.
3. Warm to cool baths and showers should be taken, not hot; and bathing should be every

2 to 3 days instead of daily.
4. Bath oils may be added to the water.
5. Excessive use of soaps should be avoided, as well as solvents and drying compounds.
6. Patients should be encouraged to use emollients. Petroleum may be tolerated best by the elderly, and should always be applied to moist skin.
7. Where possible, warmer, humid climates are preferable to cold dry regions.
8. For symptomatic xeroses, topical corticosteroid ointments can bring rapid and effective relief.
D. **Education.**
1. Patients should be taught or explained effective ways to keep the air at home humidified.
2. Taking cool baths and applying lubricating agents to the skin are very important.
3. Wearing rough or constricting clothing is to be avoided, as it can traumatize dry skin. If the patient is using corticosteroid ointments, emphasis must be placed on the need for cool water compresses 10 to 15 minutes prior to the application of the medication.

III. SEBORRHEIC KERATOSIS

A. **Definition: seborrheic keratosis is a benign epithelial lesion.**
B. **Etiology.**
1. Heredity is the most important factor in determining who will develop these keratoses and how many will occur.
2. Age is the second important factor. Lesions can start to develop as early as the late 20s or early 30s.
3. Lesions are more commonly seen in people with oily or acne seborrheic skin types.
C. **Pathophysiology.**
1. The lesions occur mostly on the scalp, face, neck, and upper trunk, and are less common on the appendages.
2. The color varies from a flesh color to a coal black.
3. They may be as small as a few millimeters, or up to 3 cm in size.
4. The lesions are usually raised and are papules or plaques, occasionally appearing as macules.
5. They can be greasy or warty to the touch.
6. As they age they become larger and darker in color.
7. Occasionally the keratosis is irritated by clothing or jewelry and becomes inflamed.
8. Histologically, the melanocytes are small and restricted to the basal cell layer.
9. There is hyperplasia of the epidermis and adnexal epithelium.
10. There may be an increase of melanin in the keratinocytes, and the granular layer is not prominent.

D. Treatment.

1. The seborrheic keratosis is a benign lesion, and may be left untreated.
2. When one becomes inflamed or irritated, it should be removed, usually by a simple shave or curettage biopsy.
3. Often patients want them removed for cosmetic reasons, or because clothing irritates them, or they interfere with shaving.
4. Complications of removing these lesions are hypopigmentation, hypertrophic scarring, and infection.

E. Patient education.

1. The patient should understand that these lesions are benign and can be left untreated.
2. If the lesions become irritated, or if the patient is concerned about melanomas, the dermatologist should be consulted for a thorough exam.

Bibliography

Alirezai, M., Dupuy, P., Amblard, P., Kalis, B., Souteyrand, P., Frappaz, A., & Sendagorta, E., (1994). Clinical evaluation of topical isotretinoin in the treatment of actinic keratoses. *Journal of the American Academy of Dermatology, 30,* 447-451.

Arndt, K.A. (1995). *Manual of dermatologic therapeutics* (5th ed.). Boston: Little, Brown & Co.

Balin, A.K., Lin, A.N., & Pratt, L. (1988). Actinic keratoses. *Journal of Cutaneous Aging and Cosmetic Dermatology, 1,* 77-84.

Colven, R.M., & Pinnell, S.R. (1966). Topical vitamin C in aging. *Clinics in Dermatology, 14,* 227-234.

Elson, M.L. (1994). Treatment of photoaging: Examining the options. *Journal of Geriatric Dermatology, 2,* 45-53.

Epstein, J.H. (1980). Polymorphous light eruption. *Journal of the American Academy of Dermatology, 3,* 329-343.

Eubanks, S.W., Patterson, J.W., May, D.I., & Aeling, J.L. (1983). The porphyrias. *International Journal of Dermatology, 22,* 337-347.

Fazel, N., & Lim, H.W., (2002). Evaluation and management of the patient with photosensitivity. *Dermatology Nursing, 14*(1), 23-30.

Fenske, N.A., & Lober, C.W. (1986). Structural and functional changes of normal aging skin. *Journal of the American Academy of Dermatology, 15,* 571-583.

Gilchrist, B.A. (1989). Skin aging and photoaging: An overview. *Journal of the American Academy of Dermatology, 21,* 610-613.

Gilchrist, B.A., (1990). Skin aging and photoaging. *Dermatology Nursing, 2*(2), 79-82.

Glogau, R.G. (1996). Aesthetic and anatomic analysis of the aging skin. *Seminars in Cutaneous Medicine and Surgery, 15,* 134-138.

Glogau, R.G., (2001). Aesthetic analysis of the aging face. In R.S. Narins (Ed.), *Cosmetic surgery, an interdisciplinary approach.* (pp. 17-26). New York: Basel, Marcel Dekker, Inc.

Hawk, J.L.M., & Norris, P.G., (1999). Abnormal responses to ultraviolet radiation: Ideopathic. In I. Freedburg, A.Z. Eisen, K. Wolff, K.F. Austen, L.A. Goldsmith, S.I. Katz, & T.B. Fitzpatrick, (Eds.), *Fitzpatrick's dermatology in general medicine.* (5th ed.). New York: McGraw Hill.

Holzle, E., Plewig, G., Hofmann, C., & Roser_Maass, E. (1982). Polymorphous light eruption. *Journal of the American Academy of Dermatology, 7,* 111-125.

International Medical News Group. (2001). Treatment of actinic keratosis. *Skin and Allergy News,* 1.

Kligman, A.M., & Larker, M. (1988). Cutaneous aging: The differences between intrinsic aging and photoaging. *Journal of Cutaneous Aging and Cosmetic Dermatology, 1*(1), 5-12.

Kligman, L.H. (1989). Prevention and repair of photoaging: Sunscreens and retinoids. *Cutis, 43,* 458-465.

Lavker, R.M. (1994). Topical therapy of aging skin. *Journal of Geriatric Dermatology, 2,* 20-23.

Lewis, A.B., & Gendler, E.C. (1996). Resurfacing with topical agents. *Seminars in Cutaneous Medicine and Surgery, 15,* 139-144.

Lim, H.W., & Murphy, G.M. (1996). The porphyrias. *Clinics in Dermatology, 14,* 375-388.

Nehal, K.S., & Lim, H.W. (1995). Phototoxicity and photoallergy. *Dermatology Nursing, 7*(4), 227-234.

Pollack, S.V. (2002). Facial rejuvenation: Fillers old and new. *Dermatology Nursing Association Convention Proceedings, pp.* 137-144.

Rahman, S.B., & Bhawan, J. (1996). Lentigo. *International Journal of Dermatology, 35,* 229-238.

Roenigk, H.H. Jr. (1994). Dermabrasion and aging skin. *Journal of Geriatric Dermatology, 1,* 24-29.

Sauer, G.C. (1980). *Manual of skin diseases.* Philadelphia and Toronto: J.B. Lippincott.

Schwartz, R.A. (1996). Premalignant keratinocytic neoplasms. *Journal of the American Academy of Dermatology, 35,* 223-242.

Sendagorta, E., Lesiewicz, J., & Armstrong, R.B., (1992). Topical isotretinoin for photodamaged skin. *Journal of the American Academy of Dermatology, 27,* S15-S18.

Tan, M., Spencer, J., Pires, L.M., Ajmeri, J., & Skoven, G. (2001). The evaluation of aluminum oxide crystal microderm abrasion for photodamage. *Dermatology Surgery, 27,* 943-949.

Van Praag, M.C.G., Boom, B.W., & Vermeer, B.J. (1994). Diagnosis and treatment of polymorphous light eruption. *International Journal of Dermatology, 33,* 233-239.

Young, J.W., & Conte, E.T. (1991). Porphyrias and porphyrins. *International Journal of Dermatology, 30,* 399-406.

1. Sunprotection is important for:
   a. Skin types V and VI.
   b. Only redheads.
   c. Everyone.
   d. Only skin Types I, II and III.

2. A tanning response of mild burn to tan average is likely to be:
   a. Skin Type II.
   b. Skin Type VI.
   c. Skin Type IV.
   d. Skin Type III.

3. Type III of the photoaging classification includes:
   a. Wrinkles in motion.
   b. Wrinkles at rest.
   c. Prior skin malignancies.
   d. Early senile lentigines.

4. The pulsed-dye laser is used to remove:
   a. Telangiectasia.
   b. Lentigines.
   c. Tattoos.
   d. Keratosis.

5. Preventive photodamage education should include:
   a. Broad-spectrum sunscreens and sunblocks.
   b. Solar-protective clothing.
   c. Avoiding the sun between 10 am and 2 pm.
   d. All of the above.

6. Actinic keratoses appear as:
   a. Coal black plaques.
   b. Round purple papules.
   c. Scaly or rough papules.
   d. Yellow vesicles.

7. PMLE lesions:
   a. Are confined to sun exposed areas.
   b. Occur immediately after sun exposure.
   c. Usually disappear within 12 hours.
   d. Present as small vesicles.

8. Photoallergy is:
   a. A nonimmunologic reaction.
   b. An immediate response to a sensitizing agent.
   c. A sporadic reaction to a chemical.
   d. An immunologic reaction.

9. Clinically PCT patients are seen with:
   a. Hypertrichoses on the face and limbs.
   b. Peeling and flaking of the skin.
   c. Intense pruritus of sun exposed skin.
   d. Pigmented lesions of the soles of the feet.

10. CAD most often presents in:
    a. Male alcoholics.
    b. Females of age 50 to 60 years on estrogen.
    c. Males of age 63 to 65.
    d. All of the above.

11. Treatment for solar urticaria includes:
    a. High doses of antihistamines.
    b. High doses of antibiotics.
    c. Burow's solution (1% to 5%) compresses.
    d. Cool baths daily.

12. Xerosis tends to affect:
    a. The legs and feet of middle age people.
    b. The arms and hands of people age 50 to 60 years.
    c. The trunk of older people.
    d. The legs and feet of older people.

Answers to Study Questions

1. c	5. d	9. a
2. d	6. c	10. c
3. b	7. a	11. a
4. a	8. d	12. d

Chapter 13.
Photodermatoses, Photodamage, and Aging Skin

Please photocopy this test page and return.

COMPLETE THE FOLLOWING:

Name: _____

Address: _____

City: _____ State: _____ Zip: _____

Preferred telephone: (Home)_____ (Work) _____

State where licensed and license number: _____

CE application fee: DNA member $13.00
                        Nonmember $16.00

POSTTEST INSTRUCTIONS
1. To receive continuing education credit for individual study after reading the article, complete the answer/evaluation form below.
2. Photocopy and send the answer/evaluation form along with a check or money order payable to **Dermatology Nurses' Association** to: *DNA*, East Holly Avenue Box 56, Pitman, NJ 08071-0056.
3. Test returns must be postmarked by December 31, 2008. Upon completion of the answer/evaluation form, a certificate for 4.0 contact hour(s) will be awarded and sent to you.

This chapter was reviewed and formatted for contact hour credit by Marcia J. Hill, MSN, RN, Core Curriculum Editor; and Sally Russell, MN, RN,C, DNA Education Director.

ANSWER FORM

1. Name one new detail (item, issue, or phenomenon) that you learned by completing this activity.

   _____

   _____

   _____

2. How will you apply the information from this learning activity to your practice?
   a. Patient education.
   b. Staff education.
   c. Improve my patient care.
   d. In my education course work.
   e. Other: Please describe _____

Evaluation

	Strongly disagree				Strongly agree
3. The offering met the stated objectives.					
a. Identify the symptoms, discuss the etiology, and support the treatment of the major types of photodermatoses.	1	2	3	4	5
b. Discuss with patients and the public the various treatments available to correct photodamage to the skin.	1	2	3	4	5
c. List and promote at least three widely available methods of protecting the skin from damage by the sun.	1	2	3	4	5
4. The content was current and relevant.	1	2	3	4	5
5. The content was presented clearly.	1	2	3	4	5
6. The content was covered adequately.	1	2	3	4	5
7. I am more confident of my abilities since completing this material.	1	2	3	4	5

8. The material was (check one) ☐ new, ☐ review for me.

Comments _____

9. Time required to complete reading assignment: _____ minutes

This independent study is provided by the Dermatology Nurses' Association (DNA) for 4.0 contact hours. DNA is accredited as a provider of continuing education in nursing by the American Nurses Credentialing Center's Commission on Accreditation. DNA is approved as a provider of continuing education by the California Board of Registered Nursing Provider #CEP5708.

Disorders of Pigmentation

Marcia J. Hill, MSN, RN

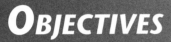

OBJECTIVES

At the end of this chapter, the reader will be able to:
- Distinguish disorders of hypo and hyperpigmentation.
- Describe current treatment modalities used to treat pigment disorders.
- Differentiate different types of nevi.
- Discuss health maintenance issues related to vitiligo.

KEY POINTS

- Both hypo and hyperpigmentation can have tremendous impact on patients from both a cosmetic and health standpoint.
- Dermatology nurses must be knowledgeable of disorders of pigmentation and nevi to effectively care for patients and improve their outcomes.
- Patients with hypopigmentation, hyperpigmentation, and nevi will require emotional support and education to assist with coping processes.

Disorders of Pigmentation

Marcia J. Hill, MSN, RN

THE MELANOCYTE

I. OVERVIEW

The melanocyte composes approximately 50% of the cellular component of the interfollicular epidermis and an equal component of the hair bulb.
A. Characteristics of the melanocyte.
  1. Limited in number.
  2. Major synthetic product is melanin.
    a. Melanin is the primary determinant of skin and hair color.
    b. Accounts for racial and ethnic skin pigmentation differences.
    c. Functions to:
      (1) Absorb ultraviolet light; protecting genome of dividing basal keratinocytes and melanocytes.
      (2) Scavenge free-oxygen radicals.
  3. Melanocytes can up or down-regulate pigmentation in response to:
    a. Physiologic stimuli.
    b. Environmental stimuli.
    c. Pathologic stimuli.
B. Theorized to contribute to epidermal homeostasis during inflammation.

II. DISORDERS OF PIGMENTATION

A. Overview: disorders of pigmentation may present as either hypo or hyperpigmentation and can be either acquired or congenital.
B. Acquired hypopigmentation.
  1. Vitiligo.
  2. Postinflammatory or secondary to neoplasms.
  3. Inflammatory disorders (for example, resolving psoriasis, atopic dermatitis).
    b. Neoplasms (for example, mycosis fungoides).
  4. Postinfection.
    a. Bacteria — *Treponema pertenue, Treponema carateum, Mycobacterium leprae.*
    b. Yeast — *Pityrosporum orbiculare.*
    c. Protozoan — *Leishmania donovani.*
    d. Helminth — *Onchocerca volvulus.*
    e. Fungus — tinea versicolor.
C. Congenital hypopigmentation.
  1. Albinism.
  2. Piebaldism.
  3. Tuberous sclerosis.
D. Acquired hyperpigmentation.
  1. Melasma.
  2. Chemically induced.
  3. Melanocytic nevi.
  4. Freckles (ephelides) — small red or light-brown macules promoted by sun exposure, fading in winter months; usually on face, arms, and back; autosomal dominant inheritance; benign.
  5. Fixed drug eruptions.
  6. Café-au-lait spots — uniformly pale-brown macules seen on any cutaneous surface; present at birth; six or more macules of greater than 1.5 cm would warrant a work-up for neurofibromatosis (von Recklinghausen's disease).
E. Diffuse brown hyperpigmentation: Addison's disease.

DISORDERS OF HYPOPIGMENTATION: VITILIGO

I. OVERVIEW

A distinctive disorder of hypopigmentation in which the epidermis is devoid of one of its three main cell types leading to abnormal functioning.
A. Definition.
  1. An acquired loss of pigmentation characterized histologically by absence of melanocytes.
B. Etiology.
  1. Unknown.
  2. Thought to be an autoimmune disease associated with antibodies (vitiligo antibodies) to melanocytes.
  3. May be genetic (a predisposing factor), over 30% of affected individuals have reported vitiligo in a parent, sibling, or child.
  4. No definitive precipitating factor has been established; anecdotal correlation with the following environmental factors.
    a. Psychologic stress.
    b. Physical trauma.
    c. Pregnancy.
    d. Oral contraceptives.
    e. Sunlight and artificial ultraviolet light.
    f. Illness.
    Note: These associations are frequently observed in a high percentage of normal individuals and have not been epidemiologically shown to occur more frequently in patients with vitiligo.
C. Pathophysiology.
  1. Caused by a loss of melanin from the epidermis.
  2. A decrease in the number of melanocytes in affected areas.
  3. Pigment loss may be localized or generalized.
D. Incidence.
  1. Approximately 1% of the population is affected.

2. Fifty percent of cases begin before the age of 20 (between ages of 2 to 40).

II. ASSESSMENT

A. **History.**
   1. Ask about initial presentation.
   2. Ask about any somatic complaints that may be associated with vitiligo.
      a. Migraines.
      b. Decrease in hearing.
   3. Assess other diseases associated with vitiligo.
      a. Thyroid disease (hypo and hyperthyroidism, Grave's disease).
      b. Diabetes mellitus.
      c. Pernicious anemia.
      d. Addison's disease.
      e. Multiglandular insufficiency syndrome.
      f. Alopecia areata.
   4. Diseases that have been reported in patients with vitiligo.
      a. Hodgkin's.
      b. Multiple myeloma.
      c. Dysgammaglobulinemia.
      d. Cutaneous T-cell lymphoma (CTCL).
      e. Thymoma.
      f. Immune deficiency diseases.

B. **Clinical manifestations.**
   1. Initial presentation and progression — variable; but genital, anal, and axillary are first areas affected.
   2. Usually a snow-white macule or patch (1 to 3 cm).
   3. Distinct margins.
   4. Variations in color and margins can occur (margin may be hyperpigmented or exhibit erythema which is suggestive of an inflammatory process).
   5. Face, joints, hands, and legs most commonly affected areas.
   6. Mucous membranes may be affected.
   7. Often symmetrical in presentation.
   8. Classification of patterns of distribution.
      a. Localized.
         (1) Focal — one or more macules in one area.
         (2) Segmental — dermatomal pattern.
         (3) Mucosal — localized on mucous membranes.
         (4) "Lip-tip" pattern — involves skin around the mouth as well on distal fingers and toes; lips, nipples, and genitalia (tip of penis).
      b. Generalized often remarkable symmetrical.
         (1) Acrofacial — distal extremities and face.
         (2) Vulgaris — diffuse presentation.
         (3) Mixed — combination of acrofacial and vulgaris.

      c. Universal.
   9. Associated cutaneous findings.
      a. White and prematurely gray hair.
      b. Alopecia areata.
      c. Halo nevi.

C. **Differential diagnosis.**
   1. Piebaldism.
   2. Lupus erythematous.
   3. Tinea versicolor.
   4. Pityriasis alba.
   5. Pityriasis versicolor alba.
   6. Lichen sclerosus et atrophicus.
   7. CTCL.
   8. Sarcoidosis.
   9. Scleroderma.
   10. Postinflammatory hypopigmentation.
   11. Tuberous sclerosis.

III. COMMON THERAPEUTIC MODALITIES

A. **Goals of treatment.**
   1. Restore normal function to epidermis.
   2. Cosmesis.

B. **Medical therapy: aimed at stimulating proliferation and migration of melanocytes.**
   1. Topical steroids.
      a. Low-potency steroids are employed.
      b. Applied daily for several months or longer.
      c. If pigmentation not seen within 3 months, steroid should be stopped for approximately 6 months and then may be reinstituted or another treatment modality used.
   2. Phototherapy.
      a. PUVA (see Chapter 3) either topical or systemic.
      b. Topical PUVA is used for 3 months after erythema dose reached; if no results discontinue for at least 6 months before trying again.
      c. Systemic PUVA is used for 3 to 4 months; if no response, stop treatment for at least 6 months before trying again.
      d. Narrow-band UVB may be effective.
   3. Depigmentation.
      a. Used when there is involvement of more than 50% of the skin surface.
      b. Monobenzone is applied to skin twice daily.
      c. Requires informed consent from the patient since depigmentation is permanent and increases photosensitivity.

C. **Surgical therapy.**
   1. Punch grafts — technique similar to hair transplants.
      a. Donor sites are pigmented areas of the skin.
      b. Transplanted into depigmented areas of the skin.
      c. Held in place with pressure dressings.

Table 1.
Common Nursing Diagnoses, Outcomes, and Interventions for Patients with Disorders of Pigmentation or Nevi

Nursing Diagnoses	Outcomes	Interventions
Body image alteration related to skin changes.	Patient accepts appearance; verbalizes positive feelings and realistic expectations of any cosmetic interventions employed.	Assess perception of self-image and allow/assist patient to express feelings related to skin changes and impact on daily life.
Impaired skin integrity related to hypopigmentation.	Patient will not suffer disruption of integument secondary to sun exposure.	Educate patient about the necessity for sunscreens to avoid burn in hypopigmented areas.
Increased risk for damage to the eye secondary to hypopigmentation.	Patient will not suffer any eye complications secondary to ultraviolet light.	Educate patient about the necessity for use of sunglasses that will decrease both UVA and UVB radiation in the eye.
Increased risk for developing skin cancer secondary to hypo or hyperpigmentation.	Patient will be free of skin cancer, or early detection will occur.	Emphasize need for sunscreen use, and regular skin inspection for early detection of skin cancer.
Hyperpigmentation related to chemical exposure.	Patient will be able to identify and verbalize possible causative agents; will have understanding of need to remove causative agent.	Identify causative agent by taking a thorough history from the patient; remove causative agent.
Increased risk for infection related to surgical interventions.	Patient will remain free of infection in surgical sites.	Assess surgical area(s) for signs of infection; intervene appropriately with topical or oral antibiotics; instruct patient on signs and symptoms. of infection and appropriate postoperative care.
High risk for altered health maintenance related to lack of knowledge of disorder.	Patient will have a good understanding of disorder; patient will feel comfortable in asking questions for clarification.	Thoroughly explain disorder to the patient allowing time for questions and correcting any misinformation.

    d. Repigmentation seen in 4 to 6 weeks after transplantation.

    e. Residual pebbled skin may result which is cosmetically unacceptable.

2. Minigrafts — variant of the punch graft using smaller donor grafts to minimize pebbling.

3. Suction blisters.

    a. Epidermal grafts are obtained by vacuum suction.

    b. Blister roof is removed intact and grafted to depigmented site.

    c. Good for large areas of depigmentation.

    d. Repigmentation using this method may cause a mottled appearance.

4. Autologous cultures.

    a. Use cultured melanocytes and keratinocytes.

    b. Applied to sites that have had epidermis removed by suction, freezing, or dermabrasion.

    c. Color tends to be mottled.

5. Autologous melanocyte grafts.

    a. Variant of autologous cultures.

    b. Injected into the depigmented site or used on superficially dermabraded skin.

    c. Culturing melanocytes requires expertise and several months.

    d. Spread of pigmentation is minimal.

6. Problems with surgical therapies.

    a. Graft failure.

    b. Donor sites may become depigmented (isomorphic response).

c. Risk of infection.
d. Risk of scarring in donor sites.
e. May be cost prohibitive.

Note: Five general options for management are sunscreens, coverup, repigmentation, minigrafting, and depigmentation.

IV. NURSING CONSIDERATIONS (see Table 1)

A. Alteration in body image.
B. Increased risk for developing skin cancer.
C. Increased risk for infection related to surgical interventions.
D. Impaired skin integrity due to lack of melanin.
E. High risk for altered health maintenance related to lack of knowledge.

ALBINISM

I. OVERVIEW

A disorder of hypopigmentation secondary to a defect in the melanocyte.
A. Definition.
1. A genetically defined defect in the melanocyte system of the eye, skin, or both.
B. Etiology.
1. Genetic.
C. Pathophysiology.
1. Failure of melanocytes to produce normal amounts of melanin; probably a metabolic defect.
2. Two classifications.
a. Oculocutaneous albinism (OCA).
b. Ocular albinism (OA).
D. Incidence.
1. OCA — 1:5,000 to 1:25,000.
2. OA — not established.

II. ASSESSMENT

A. History.
B. Clinical manifestations.
1. OCA — diluted skin/hair pigmentation.
a. Skin.
(1) In Caucasians skin is very light.
(2) In darkly pigmented individuals large pigmented freckles in light-exposed areas are seen.
b. Hair.
(1) In darkly pigmented individuals hair is yellow to yellowish-brown.
(2) In Caucasians hair may range from white to cream; yellow to yellow-red to vibrant red.
c. Eye.
(1) Iris — blue/gray and translucent.
(2) Retina and choroid — paucity of pigment.

(3) In darkly pigmented individuals the iris will be pale blue to cinnamon brown.
(4) Photophobia a problem in all races.
(5) Visual acuity is decreased.
2. OA.
a. Decrease or absence of melanin in iris and retinal pigment epithelium.
b. Nystagmus present.
c. Iris translucency may occur.
d. Decrease in visual acuity.
e. Hair and skin color are normal.

III. COMMON THERAPEUTIC MODALITIES

A. Treatment goals are surveillance and preventing complications.
B. Sunscreen use.
C. Regular skin inspection for early detection of skin cancers.
D. Appropriate eye protection.

IV. NURSING CONSIDERATIONS (see Table 1)

A. Body image alteration.
B. Impaired skin integrity due to lack of melanin.
C. Increased risk for ocular complications related to hypopigmentation of the eye.
D. Increased risk for developing skin cancer.
E. High risk for altered health maintenance related to lack of knowledge.

PIEBALDISM

I. OVERVIEW

Congenital leukoderma (depigmentation) that may have spontaneous expansion and contraction.
A. Definition: disorder of hypopigmentation which involves skin and hair only.
B. Etiology.
1. Autosomal dominant.
2. Does not appear at birth in Caucasians.
C. Pathophysiology.
1. Hypomelanosis.
2. Histologically, absence or markedly decreased melanocytes in amelanotic areas.
D. Incidence: appears to be more common in Caucasians.

II. ASSESSMENT

A. History.
1. Screen for deafness.
2. Screen for congenital megacolon particularly in infants.
B. Clinical manifestations.
1. Distinctive pattern.
a. White forelock.
b. Occasionally white macule on chin.
c. Lack of pigmentation.

(1) Trunk.
(2) Anterior thorax.
(3) Abdomen.
(4) Midarm to wrist.
(5) Midthigh to midcalf (anterior and posterior).
(6) Normal pigmentation of hands, upper part of arm, shoulders, upper thighs, and feet to midcalf.
2. Two features to distinguish piebaldism from vitiligo.
   a. Presence of islands of normal pigmentation in areas of hypomelanosis.
   b. Characteristic distribution.

III. COMMON THERAPEUTIC MODALITIES

A. Minigrafts: most successful.
B. Culture grafts: not always cosmetically acceptable.
C. PUVA: not always cosmetically acceptable.

IV. NURSING CONSIDERATIONS (see Table 1)

A. Body image alteration.
B. Impaired skin integrity related to lack of melanin.
C. Increased risk for developing skin cancer.
D. High risk for altered health maintenance related to lack of knowledge.

TUBEROUS SCLEROSIS

I. OVERVIEW

Hypopigmentation is one of the earliest clinical signs of tuberous sclerosis.
A. Definition.
   1. Disorder of hypomelanosis exhibiting with a variety of lesions in skin, nervous system, heart, kidney, and other organs; exhibits with adenoma sebaceum, epilepsy, and mental retardation.
B. Etiology.
   1. Genetic.
C. Pathophysiology.
   1. Melanocytes present.
   2. Melanosomes in melanocytes decreased and poorly melanized.
D. Incidence.
   1. In institutions, 1:100 to 1:300; in general population, 1:20,000 to 1:100,000.

II. ASSESSMENT

A. History.
B. Clinical manifestations.
   1. Common locations.
      a. Trunk.
      b. Lower extremities.

2. Configurations.
   a. Ash-leaf spot — lance-ovate (round at one end and pointed at the other); considered as a tertiary feature of tuberous sclerosis.
   b. Oval.
   c. Polygonal.
3. May see multiple 1 to 3 mm macules ("confetti-like") poliosis of scalp, hair, eyebrows, and eyelashes.
4. Hypopigmented spots of the iris and fundus.
5. Wood's lamp enhances lesions in light-skinned individuals.

III. COMMON THERAPEUTIC MODALITIES

None for skin lesions.

IV. NURSING CONSIDERATIONS (see Table 1)

A. High risk for health maintenance related to lack of knowledge.

DISORDERS OF HYPERPIGMENTATION: MELASMA

I. OVERVIEW

Disorders of hyperpigmentation can be caused by the following factors: hereditary/developmental, metabolic, endocrine, inflammatory, chemically induced, nutritional, or neoplastic. Melasma is one of the most commonly seen disorders of hyperpigmentation.
A. Definition: acquired, brown hypermelanosis of the face.
B. Etiology.
   1. Secondary to an increase in the number and activity of melanocytes.
   2. Factors affecting melanocytes in melasma.
      a. Oral contraceptives.
      b. Pregnancy.
      c. Cosmetics (usually a phototoxic reaction).
      d. Genetic.
      e. Endocrine (progesterone and estrogen both have an effect on melanogenesis).
      f. Racial.
      g. Nutritional.
      h. Metabolic.
      i. Sunlight.
C. Pathophysiology.
   1. Epidermal type — melanin is deposited in the basal and suprabasal layers of the epidermis.
   2. Dermal type — melanophages in the superficial and deep dermis in addition to epidermal hyperpigmentation.
D. Incidence.
   1. More common in women.
   2. More common in persons of Latino origin living in tropical areas.
   3. 50% to 70% of pregnant women (more

common in summer and in southern latitudes).
4. 8% to 29% of nonpregnant women on birth control pills (more common in summer and in southern latitudes).
5. Is seen in men, but without hormonal factors.

II. ASSESSMENT

A. **History: always take a complete history.**
B. **Clinical manifestations.**
1. Symmetrical.
2. Irregular light to dark-brown hyperpigmentation.
3. Seen on the face.
   a. Centrofacial.
      (1) Most common presentation.
      (2) Involves cheeks, forehead, upper lip, nose, and chin.
   b. Malar.
      (1) Localized to cheeks and nose.
      (2) Second most common presentation.
   c. Mandibular.
      (1) Involves the ramus of the mandible.
      (2) Least common presentation.
4. Four types (distinguished with the use of Wood's light).
   a. Epidermal — shows enhancement of pigmentation (most common type).
   b. Dermal — no enhancement of color.
   c. Mixed — shows no or slight enhancement of color.
   d. A type seen in skin types V to VI in which lesions are not discernible under Wood's light.
5. Differential diagnosis (partial list).
   a. Drug-induced hyperpigmentation.
   b. Pigmented contact dermatitis.
   c. Postinflammatory hyperpigmentation.
   d. Exogenous ochronosis (pigment changes secondary to prolonged topical application of hydroquinone, phenol, or resorcinol).

III. COMMON THERAPEUTIC MODALITIES

A. **Identify and eliminate causative factors.**
B. **Medications.**
1. Hydroquinone alone (concentrations of >3% for patients with extensive involvement).
2. Hydroquinone with retinoic acid (retinoic acid enhances epidermal penetration of hydroquinone and reduces the activity of the melanocytes).
3. Broad-spectrum sunscreen.
4. Topical steroids (alone or in conjunction with hydroquinone, or hydroquinone plus retinoids).
5. 5-Fluorouracil (effective particularly if patients have actinically damaged skin).
6. 4-Isopropylcatechol (high incidence of irritant and allergic contact dermatitis).

7. Azelaic acid (causes reversible inhibition of tyrosinase; may be used in conjunction with 2% hydroquinone).
C. **Possible side effects of topical medications.**
1. Hydroquinone therapy.
   a. Irritant contact dermatitis.
   b. Exogenous ochronosis.
   c. Brown discoloration of the nails secondary to deposition of hydroquinone oxidation products.
2. Topical steroids — hypopigmentation.
3. 4-Isopropylcatechol — irritant and allergic contact dermatitis.
D. **Limited chemical peel (25% trichloroacetic acid or 95% phenol solution).**
E. **Laser (Q-switched ruby laser most effective).**

IV. NURSING CONSIDERATIONS (see Table 1)

A. **Body image alteration.**
B. **High risk for health maintenance related to lack of knowledge.**

CHEMICALLY INDUCED HYPERPIGMENTATION

I. OVERVIEW

Hyperpigmentation has long been associated with exposure to a variety of chemicals.
A. **Definition.**
1. Unusual darkening of the skin as a direct result of exposure to chemicals.
B. **Etiology.**
1. Direct deposition of the chemical into the skin.
2. Stimulation of melanin formation.
3. Binding of chemical to melanin.
4. Production of metabolites or nonmelanin pigments.
5. Hyperpigmentation may be enhanced by exposure to ultraviolet light.
6. Offending agents.
   a. Antimalarials.
   b. Antibiotics.
   c. Heavy metals.
   d. Chemotherapeutic agents.
   e. Topical preparations (for example, tar-containing compounds).
C. **Pathophysiology.**
1. Dependent on etiologic agent.
2. Antimalarials — hyperpigmentation appears in dermis; may be combination of melanin and hemosiderin.
3. Antibiotics — pigmentation depends on presentation; minocycline is used as an example here.
   a. In acne scars, hemosiderin and ferritin are present in macrophages.

Table 2.
Types of Nevi

Type	Morphology	Comments
Junction	Initially 1 to 2 mm, expanding to 4 to 6 mm; flat, slightly elevated smooth surface; sharply circumscribed; uniformly brown, tan, or black.	Progression slow — over decades; may change into compound nevi; rare at birth, develop after 2 years of age; degeneration into melanoma rare.
Compound	Slightly elevated, dome-shaped, papule; flesh, brown, "halo nevus;" cells at dermo-epidermal junction and upper dermis; hair may be present.	Generally benign, only a cosmetic issue.
Dermal	Brown or black but may lighten with age; vary in size maybe a few millimeters up to a centimeter; dome-shaped nevi most common; symmetric with smooth surface; white or translucent; surface telangiectasia may make lesion difficult to distinguish from a basal cell carcinoma; may be polypoid or warty in appearance; found on trunk, neck, axilla, groin.	Elevated lesions should be removed due to being prone to trauma; white border may present making nevus look like a halo nevus; rarely degenerate into a melanoma but should be monitored carefully.
Congenital (Birthmark)	Present at birth; vary in size from a few millimeters to several centimeters; may cover wide areas of the trunk (bathing trunk nevi), extremity, or face; giant hairy nevus are the largest form; may see coarse hair in the body of the nevus; uniformly brown or black, but may be red or pink; surface flat at birth and becomes verrucous or nodular over time; high risk of degeneration into melanoma in very large lesions.	Large, thick lesions should be removed as soon as possible due to tendency to become malignant; removal should be be done by a plastic surgeon; all congenital nevi should be checked frequently by a dermatologist.
Nevus spilus	Oval or irregular; hairless lesion that is brown with dots of darker pigmentation present; flat surface with the darker dots with some elevation; range in size from 1 to 20 centimeters; appear at any age.	Degeneration into melanoma not documented; excision for cosmetic purposes requires surgery with closure.
Halo nevi	Can be a compound or dermal nevus which exhibits a white border (halo); sharply demarcated borders that are round or oval; generally located on trunk, may occur on palms and soles; develop spontaneously and frequently in adolescence; may be singular or multiple; incidence of vitiligo may be increased in individuals with halo nevi.	Removal indicated if atypical features develop; removal may be accomplished by shave or excision.
Becker's nevus	Lacks nevus cells; developmental anomaly; presents as a brown macule with a patch of hair, or both; usually seen in adolescent males; seen on the shoulder, submammary area, upper and lower back; vary in size; irregular border that is sharply demarcated.	Malignant degeneration has not been reported; lesions are generally too large to remove; hair may be shaved or permanently removed.
Benign juvenile melanoma (Spitz's nevus)	Common in children, but can be seen in adults; hairless, red or reddish-brown; domed shaped; surface may be smooth or warty; range in size from 0.3 to 1.5 cm; vascular and may bleed with trauma; usually solitary but may be multiple; appear suddenly.	Should be removed for histologic examination to rule out malignancy.
Blue nevus	Common on extremities and dorsum of hands; small, round lesions, slightly elevated; blue in color; appear in childhood.	Large lesions may degenerate into a malignant lesion.
Labial melanotic macule	Located on the lower lip; exhibit as brown macules; commonly seen in young adult women; do not darken with exposure to sunlight.	Do not require removal even for cosmetic reasons.

Table 3.
Aplastic Mole Syndrome
(Familial Dysplastic Nevus Syndrome)

The identification of the dysplastic nevus (DN) in melanoma-prone families led to the determination that DN are cutaneous markers that identify family members who are at increased risk for melanoma. DN may be the single most important precursor lesion of melanoma occurring in persons with melanoma-prone families and in persons who lack both a family history of melanoma and a personal history of melanoma.

Characteristics
- Autosomal dominant.
- Develop melanoma at an early age.
- Predisposition to multiple primary melanomas.
- Tendency to develop superficial spreading melanomas.
- Distinctive large melanocytic nevi present (larger than common moles).
- Mixture of colors including tan, brown, pink, and black.
- Irregular and indistinct border, may fade into surrounding skin.
- Surface may be both macular and papular.
- Characteristic presentation — pigmented papule surrounded by a macular collar of pigmentation ("fried egg lesion").
- Nevi not present at birth; present in mid-childhood as common moles which change appearance at puberty.
- Lesions may continue to appear after age of 40.
- Lesions occur in sun-exposed areas as well as scalp, buttocks, and breasts.

Management
- History — document sun exposure, evolution of nevi, family history of melanoma or presence of large number of moles (particularly large moles).
- Physical exam — entire integument should be examined including scalp and eyes; examinations should be done at a minimum of twice a year.
- Excisional biopsy should be done of one or more DN; total excisional biopsy to avoid recurrence; consider excision of all new nevi particularly those in the scalp.
- Photograph of total body surface as a baseline for comparison on followup.
- Patient education is paramount to compliance with surveillance, treatment, and followup; self-exam should be emphasized.
- All family members should be examined on a regular basis for early detection.

b. Blue-gray patches on extremities have pigmented macrophages that stain for both melanin and iron.
c. Muddy brown pigmentation affecting entire skin surface due to basilar epidermal melanin.

II. ASSESSMENT

A. History with emphasis on chemical exposure.
B. Physical exam.
C. Clinical manifestations.
   1. May vary.
   2. Skin biopsy may be indicated to confirm diagnosis.

III. COMMON THERAPEUTIC MODALITIES

A. Often persistent.
B. Stop offending agent if known (particularly drug).
C. Prevent exposure.
D. Use sunscreens.

IV. NURSING CONSIDERATIONS (see Table 1)

A. Body image alteration.
B. Hyperpigmentation related to chemical exposure.
C. High risk for health maintenance related to lack of knowledge.

NEVI: MELANOCYTIC NEVI

I. OVERVIEW

Nevi, or moles, are benign tumors composed of nevus cells that are derived from melanocytes and can occur anywhere on the cutaneous surface, and except for certain types (large congenital and dysplastic) most nevi have low-malignancy potential.

A. **Definition.**
 1. Nevus cell — larger than melanocyte, lacks dendrites; has more abundant cytoplasm and coarse granules; aggregate in groups or proliferate in basal region at dermoepidermal junction.
 2. Types of nevi (see Table 2).
   a. Common nevi — classified based on location.
     (1) Junction.
     (2) Compound.
     (3) Intradermal
   b. Special forms.
     (1) Congenital.
     (2) Halo nevus.
     (3) Nevus spilus.
     (4) Becker's nevus.
     (5) Benign juvenile melanoma (Spitz nevus).
     (6) Blue nevus.
     (7) Labial melanotic nevus.

B. **Etiology.**
 1. Dependent on type.

C. **Pathophysiology.**
 1. Junctional — nevus cells at dermoepidermal junction.
 2. Compound — nevus cells at dermoepidermal junction and upper dermis.
 3. Dermal — nevus cells in dermis, sometimes among fat cells.

D. **Incidence.**
 1. Very common.
 2. Present in 1% of newborns with incidence increasing throughout infancy and childhood, peaking at puberty.

II. ASSESSMENT

A. History.
B. Clinical manifestations (see Table 2).

III. COMMON THERAPEUTIC MODALITIES

A. **Common nevi.**
 1. Suspicious lesions.
   a. Should be biopsied (punch or excisional); then appropriate intervention taken after histology established.
   b. Removal for cosmetic purposes (shave or simple excision).
 2. Special forms.
   a. Large congenital nevi — at risk for development of melanoma; surgical removal indicated.
   b. Nevus spilus — cosmetic surgical excision.
   c. Halo nevi — removal unnecessary unless atypical; shave or excisional removal; if seen in patients with history of, or at high risk

for melanoma, the lesion should be biopsied.
   d. Becker's nevus — usually too large to remove.
   e. Benign juvenile melanoma (Spitz's nevus)— requires removal and biopsy to rule out melanoma.
   f. Blue nevus — biopsy and removal due to possible malignant degeneration.
   g. Labial melanotic macule — removal not necessary.

B. **Dysplastic nevus syndrome (see Table 3).**
 1. Excisional biopsy.
 2. Photograph for comparison and followup.

IV. NURSING CONSIDERATIONS (see Table 1).

A. Body image alteration.
B. Increased risk for developing skin cancer.
C. High risk for altered health maintenance related to lack of knowledge.

Bibliography

Boissy, R.E., & Nordlund, J.J. (1996). Biology of melanocytes. In K.A. Arndt, P.E. LeBoit, J.K. Robinson, & B.U. Wintroub (Eds.), *Cutaneous medicine and surgery, an integrated program in dermatology* (pp. 1203-1209). Philadelphia: W.B. Saunders Company.

Boissy, R.E., & Nordlund, J.J. (1996). Vitiligo. In K.A. Arndt, P.E. LeBoit, J.K. Robinson, & B.U. Wintroub (Eds.), *Cutaneous medicine and surgery, an integrated program in dermatology* (pp. 1210-1218). Phildelphia: W.B. Saunders Company.

Bolognia, J.L., & Shapiro, P.E. (1996). Albinism and other disorders of pigmentation. In K.A. Arndt, P.E. LeBoit, J.K. Robinson, & B.U. Wintroub (Eds.), *Cutaneous medicine and surgery, an integrated program in dermatology* (pp. 1219-1232). Philadelphia: W.B. Saunders Company.

Fitzpatrick, T.B., & Mihm, M.C. (1971). Abnormalities of the melanin pigmentary system. In T.B. Fitzpatrick, K.A. Arndt, W.H. Clark, A.Z. Eisen, E.J. Van Scott, & J.H. Vaughan (Eds.), *Dermatology in general medicine* (pp. 1591-1637). New York: McGraw-Hill Book Company.

Habif, T.P. (1990). *Clinical dermatology, a color guide to diagnosis and therapy* (2nd ed.). St. Louis: The CV Mosby Company.

Habif, T.P. (2001). Skin disease: diagnosis and treatment. St. Louis: The CV Mosby Company.

Halder, R.M. (1991). Topical PUVA therapy for vitiligo. *Dermatology Nursing, 3*(3), 178-182.

Thompson, F.V. (1993). Management of a vitiligo patient: A case study. *Dermatology Nursing, 5*(2), 139-144.

Torres, J.E., & Sanchez, J.L. (1996). Melasma and other disorders of hyperpigmentation. In K.A. Arndt, P.E. LeBoit, J.K. Robinson, & B.U. Wintroub (Eds.), *Cutaneous medicine and surgery, an integrated program in dermatology* (pp. 1233-1241). Philadelphia: W.B. Saunders Company.

1. Vitiligo is characterized by:
   a. Loss of melanin from the epidermis.
   b. Decrease of melanin from the epidermis.
   c. Increase risk of sunburn in hypopigmented areas.
   d. A localized or general presentation of hypopigmentation.
   e. All of the above.
   f. a, c, & d.

2. Albinism is a disorder of hypopigmentation secondary to a defect in the melanocyte.
   a. True.
   b. False.

3. Melasma is characterized by all of the following *except:*
   a. An increased number and activity of melanocytes.
   b. A relation to oral contraceptives.
   c. An increased incidence in men with hormonal dysfunction.
   d. Deposition of melanin in the basal and suprabasal layers of the epidermis.

4. A Wood's light is beneficial in distinguishing the types of melasma.
   a. True.
   b. False.

5. Hyperpigmentation may be caused by the following:
   a. Antimalarials.
   b. Heavy metals.
   c. Infection.
   d. Topical tar-containing preparations.
   e. a, b, & c.
   f. a & c.
   g. All of the above.

6. Becker's nevus is easily removed with surgery.
   a. True.
   b. False.

7. It is documented that nevus spilus may degenerate into melanoma.
   a. True.
   b. False.

8. Patients with familial dysplastic nevus syndrome generally develop melanoma at a young age.
   a. True.
   b. False.

9. The following are all part of the management plan for patients with familial dysplastic nevus syndrome except:
   a. Thorough physical exam, including scalp and eyes.
   b. Thorough history of evolution of lesions, family disposition.
   c. Dermabrasion of any suspicious lesions.
   d. Photographs of lesions for surveillance and followup.

10. Dysplastic nevi are generally present at birth.
    a. True.
    b. False.

Answers to Study Questions

1.	f	5.	g	9.	c
2.	a	6.	b	10.	b
3.	c	7.	b		
4.	a	8.	a		

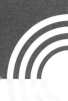
Chapter 14.
Disorders of Pigmentation

Please photocopy this test page and return.

COMPLETE THE FOLLOWING:

Name: _____

Address: _____

City: _____ State: _____ Zip: _____

Preferred telephone: (Home)_____ (Work) _____

State where licensed and license number: _____

CE application fee: DNA member $7.00
Nonmember $10.00

POSTTEST INSTRUCTIONS
1. To receive continuing education credit for individual study after reading the article, complete the answer/evaluation form below.
2. Photocopy and send the answer/evaluation form along with a check or money order payable to **Dermatology Nurses' Association** to: **DNA**, East Holly Avenue Box 56, Pitman, NJ 08071-0056.
3. Test returns must be postmarked by December 31, 2008. Upon completion of the answer/evaluation form, a certificate for 1.6 contact hour(s) will be awarded and sent to you.

This chapter was reviewed and formatted for contact hour credit by Marcia J. Hill, MSN, RN, Core Curriculum Editor; and Sally Russell, MN, RN,C, DNA Education Director.

ANSWER FORM

1. Name one new detail (item, issue, or phenomenon) that you learned by completing this activity.

_____

_____

_____

_____

2. How will you apply the information from this learning activity to your practice?
   a. Patient education.
   b. Staff education.
   c. Improve my patient care.
   d. In my education course work.
   e. Other: Please describe _____

_____

_____

Evaluation

	Strongly disagree				Strongly agree
3. The offering met the stated objectives.					
a. Distinguish disorders of hypo and hyperpigmentation.	1	2	3	4	5
b. Describe current treatment modalities used to treat pigment disorders.	1	2	3	4	5
c. Differentiate different types of nevi.	1	2	3	4	5
d. Discuss health maintenance issues related to vitiligo.	1	2	3	4	5
4. The content was current and relevant.	1	2	3	4	5
5. The content was presented clearly.	1	2	3	4	5
6. The content was covered adequately.	1	2	3	4	5
7. I am more confident of my abilities since completing this material.	1	2	3	4	5

8. The material was (check one) ☐ new, ☐ review for me.

Comments _____

_____

9. Time required to complete reading assignment: _____ minutes

This independent study is provided by the Dermatology Nurses' Association (DNA) for 1.6 contact hours. DNA is accredited as a provider of continuing education in nursing by the American Nurses Credentialing Center's Commission on Accreditation. DNA is approved as a provider of continuing education by the California Board of Registered Nursing Provider #CEP5708.

Hypersensitivities, Vasculitides, and Miscellaneous Inflammatory Disorders

Marrise M. Phillips, BS, RN, CCRC, DNC

OBJECTIVES

At the end of this chapter, the reader will be able to:

- Describe the major events in the formation of antibodies against a specific antigen.
- List the four general types of hypersensitivity reactions.
- Differentiate between immediate and delayed-type hypersensitivities.
- Define the major hypersensitivities and vascular reactions.
- Identify diagnostic and therapeutic interventions used to diagnose and treat hypersensitivities, vasculitides, and miscellaneous inflammatory disorders.

KEY POINTS

- The immune system is designed to protect the host but may fail.
- Hypersensitivity reactions are transient whereas vasculitides are persistent.
- Diagnosis of hypersensitivities and vasculitides is one of exclusion.
- Assessment and history-taking skills are of paramount importance.
- Prevention is a major aspect of therapy related to hypersensitivities and vasculitides.

Hypersensitivities, Vasculitides, and Miscellaneous Inflammatory Disorders

Marrise M. Phillips, BS, RN, CCRC, DNC

I. OVERVIEW

The immune response to an antigen is designed to protect the host. However, if the system overreacts to an allergen, mistaking an ordinarily harmless substance for a dangerous enemy, the host may be harmed. The most important biological function of the immune system is recognition and elimination of infectious agents and foreign antigens. Regardless of the system intent, re-exposure of previously sensitized individuals to the same antigen may bring about an exaggerated or misdirected immune response that results in minor local tissue injury or major systemic involvement which may eventually lead to death. Immune responses that result in pathophysiologic changes are called allergic/immunopathologic reactions (hypersensitivities).

A. The manifestations of the allergic response may be the result of:
   1. Release of vasoactive substances.
   2. Phagocytosis or other cellular destruction.
   3. Activation of components of the complement system.
   4. Release of proteolytic enzymes, cytokines, and other mediators of tissue injury and inflammation from inflammatory cells.

B. Hypersensitivity reactions are generally classified into four types:
   1. Type I — mediated by IgE antibodies, called immediate hypersensitivity, and includes hay fever, allergies to dust and animal dander, and anaphylaxis.
   2. Type II — mediated by IgG or IgM antibodies resulting in phagocytosis and cell lysis. Response time is minutes to hours and includes transfusion reactions, drug-induced anemias, and hemolytic disease of the newborn.
   3. Type III — mediated by IgG or IgM antibodies in immune complexes, which deposit in blood vessels and tissues, activate complement and attract leukocytes leading to release of destructive molecules resulting in normal tissue destruction as in autoimmune diseases such as RA, lupus, and serum sickness.
   4. Type IV — cell mediated/delayed, initiated by T cells that secrete cytokines attracting macrophages, which mediate inflammation and tissue damage; response time is 1 to 3 days; for example, poison ivy, metal contact sensitivity, TB.

C. Nursing diagnoses, outcomes, and interventions (see Table 1).

URTICARIA AND ANGIOEDEMA

I. OVERVIEW

Approximately 1 out of 5 people will experience urticaria (hives). Urticaria is typically an allergic response. In response to an irritant, histamine and other chemicals are released into the bloodstream resulting in the familiar itching, localized swelling, and other symptoms associated with urticaria. Occasionally, urticaria is associated with deeper less well-demarcated edema referred to as angioedema. Angioedema, however, is more often associated with systemic signs of anaphylaxis, including life-threatening bronchoconstriction and hypotension. The eyelids and lips are the areas most typically affected by angioedema.

II. DEFINITION

A. Urticaria is a common cutaneous vascular reaction, involving the upper dermis, caused by diverse and multiple factors. It is usually transient, demonstrating localized edema caused by dilation and increased permeability of the capillaries, and marked by the development of wheals.

B. Angioedema is a swelling similar to urticaria, but the swelling is beneath the skin rather than on the surface. Angioedema is an allergic response associated with the release of histamine and other chemicals into the bloodstream, as is urticaria, therefore open to similar causative factors. Angioedema is usually located on the eyes and mouth but may also occur on the hands and feet or in the throat. Lesions are red and deep rather than superficial and blanch and swell if irritated. Complications include abdominal cramping, anaphylactic reactions, and in the case of hereditary angioedema, airway obstruction from laryngeal edema. Laryngeal edema does not usually occur with urticaria or simple angioedema. There may be a hereditary tendency toward the development of both angioedema and urticaria.

C. Physical urticarias are different from other urticarias in that a physical stimulus can reproduce the characteristic wheals.

III. ETIOLOGY

A. Contact with allergens.
   1. Inhalation, ingestion, or other contacts with an allergen can trigger an allergic response presenting clinically as urticaria (hives) or

angioedema. Common allergens include:

a. Medications — penicillin, sulfa-related medications, thiazide diuretics, sulfonylureas, phenothiazines, and procainamide.

b. Foods (shellfish, fish, nuts, eggs, milk, chocolate, and berries), especially in infants.

c. Food dyes (tartrazine; other azo dyes).

d. Food preservatives (monosodium glutamate).

e. Pollen and animal dander, especially cats.

f. Insect bites and infestations (scabies).

B. **Nonallergen induced.**

1. Hives may also be caused by nonallergenic agents and develop after infections or illnesses such as streptococcal infection, acute viral syndromes, hepatitis B, coccidioidomycosis, lupus erythematosus, chronic inflammatory bowel disease, cryoglobulinemia, and leukemia.

2. Endocrinopathy — hypothyroidism or hyperthyroidism, diabetes mellitus, and menopause.

3. Cholinergic urticaria occurs with exposure to variations in temperature, sunlight, and water.

4. Psychogenic and emotional factors.

5. Dermographism — wheals occur within 5 to 10 minutes in response to simple rubbing of the skin and usually resolve in 15 to 20 minutes.

6. Delayed pressure urticaria — edema, itching, and pain lasting 30 minutes to 48 hours in response to pressure from an external source (belts, bra straps, etc.) on soft tissue.

7. Vibratory urticaria — a rare familial condition consisting of edema and erythema following the stretching of skin as in massage and towel drying. Sometimes symptoms may last for days.

IV. EPIDEMIOLOGY

A. **Incidence.**

1. Urticaria occurs in approximately 15% to 25% of the general population.

2. The decrease in environmental purity increases the number and type of allergens; thus, increasing risk of hypersensitivity reactions.

B. **Considerations across the life span.**

C. **Urticaria can occur at any age.**

2. Usually concentrated in the 2nd through 6th decade of life, with a peak incidence between the ages of 20 to 35.

V. PATHOPHYSIOLOGY

Urticaria is characterized by transient, erythematous, blanchable papules or plaques, also called "wheals" or "hives," and accompanied by a subjec-tive sensation of itching. Urticaria can be classified as an immediate hypersensitivity reaction mediated by IgE antibodies.

A. **Prototypic explanation for the development of urticaria.**

1. During the process of sensitization, IgE antibodies are synthesized and attached to the cytoplasmic membrane of mast cells. Subsequent exposure to the sensitizing agent results in the attachment of an antigen to two adjacent antibody molecules on the mast cell. This "bridging" attachment then results in mast cell degranulation and release of various chemicals which serve as inflammatory mediators.

2. Major mediators include histamine, eosinophil chemotactic factor A, and heparin (an acidic proteoglycan that forms the granule matrix, also an anticoagulant). Basophiles have also been identified as a source of inflammatory mediators. Specifically, histamine which increases the permeability of the blood vessels permitting fluid to escape, resulting in the production of the characteristic wheals and itching noted with the typical outbreak of hives.

VI. DIAGNOSES

The diagnosis of urticaria is one of exclusion. It is essential to rule out the presence of serious illnesses of which recurring hives and/or edema can be a symptom. Examples of such illnesses may include hepatitis, hyperthyroidism, lymphomas, lupus, and cancers of the rectum, kidneys, and gastrointestinal tract.

A. **Assessment.**

1. History and physical exams are the most important parts of the initial evaluation, and should include an evaluation of the following factors.

a. Association with any specific substance or activity.

b. Character of the primary lesion in urticaria is an edematous papule or plaque called a wheal (see Figure 15-1, page 241). Wheals are sharply marginated and predominantly flat topped. Their color varies from light pink to dark red depending on the amount of fluid present between the skin surface and the underlying dilated vascular bed. Wheals frequently have a dimpled surface because of the anchoring effect of hair follicles as fluid fills the papillary dermis surrounding them.

c. Location of the lesions — itchy lesions that come and go, located anywhere on the skin.

Table 1.
Nursing Diagnoses, Outcomes, and Interventions for Hypersensitivities and Vasculitides

Diagnoses	Outcomes	Interventions
Impaired skin integrity to disease process.	Skin integrity will improve; further trauma to skin will be avoided.	Assess lesions accurately; administer antipruritics as indicated to decrease pruritus, scratching, and decrease trauma to skin; apply topical medications as indicated to areas of impairment to provide artificial barrier, enhancing healing.
Increased risk for infection related to compromised integrity and secondary to to scratching.	Patient will remain infection-free.	Continually assess the skin for signs of breakdown (excoriation); assess whether antipruritics are alleviating symptoms, adjust as necessary.
Body image disturbance related disease to disease and impaired integrity.	Patient will have improved body image.	Assess patient's perceptions and feelings regarding disease process; allow patient to express feelings; give patient support.
High risk for altered health maintenance related to knowledge deficit.	Patient will be educated about causative or or exacerbating factors; patient will understand interventions and importance of compliance.	Assess knowledge or understanding of causative or exacerbating factors related to disease process; allow time for patient to ask questions; correct any misinformation or treatment misunderstanding.

d. Length of response — individual lesions do not last for more than 24 hours.
e. Assessment of previous incidence of symptoms related to common causes of urticaria.
f. Evaluation of recent exposure to possible allergens.
g. Assessment of common subtypes of urticaria.
h. Evaluate the role that occupation can play in establishing the diagnosis of urticaria.
i. Differentiation of angioedema from urticaria is of utmost importance related to the life-threatening possibilities associated with angioedema. Urticarial lesions are superficial and widespread, while lesions associated with angioedema are deep and the eyelids and lips are the areas most typically affected.

B. **Diagnostic tests.**
1. Complete blood count (CBC) with differential.
2. Liver and thyroid function tests.
3. Urine analysis.
4. Erythrocyte sedimentation rate (ESR).
5. C-reactive protein (CRP) and throat culture.
6. Rheumatoid factors, hepatitis screen, antinuclear antibody (ANA).
7. Skin biopsies.

VII. COMMON THERAPEUTIC MODALITIES

A. **Preventative: eliminate or modify physical factors and reactive agents.**
B. **Treat any underlying disease.**
C. **Symptomatic care.**
1. Antihistamines for the relief of pruritus.
   a. H1 blockers — there are approximately 30 H1 antagonists which are subdivided into several groups. The most common and widely used antihistamine is diphenhydramine (Benadryl®) in dosages of 150 to 200 mg per day. It is quite potent and creates considerable sedation. The key to the successful use of H1 blockers is related to gradual dose adjustment. Most success is seen when the dose is increased until clinical improvement occurs. When subsequent sedation or anticholinergic side effects (dry mouth, blurred vision, and impairment in voiding) become troublesome, discontinuation must be considered.
   b. The two H2 antagonists available are cimetidine (Tagamet®) and ranitidine (Zantac®). H2 receptors are found in blood vessels of the skin. Treatment with H2 blockers alone is not usually successful.

Some studies have demonstrated beneficial synergistic effect in treatment when H2 blockers are used in conjunction with standard H1 blockers.

2. Topical and systemic corticosteroids.
   a. Primary desired pharmacologic effect is the reduction of inflammation. In response to the decrease in inflammation these drugs produce a secondary antipruritic effect as well.
   b. In using topical steroids the clinician must determine the brand, strength, vehicle, and quantity of medication necessary to achieve the desired effects.
   c. Limitations — topical steroids can take up to 48 hours to be of benefit and are of no benefit in noninflammatory diseases.
   d. Systemic corticosteroids are useful in situations where the severity or extensiveness of a cutaneous disease prevents topical application. Systemic steroids may be administered orally or intramuscularly. Prednisone is the most commonly used oral corticosteroid. It is inexpensive, relatively short acting, and available in a variety of doses.

3. Immunotherapy (allergy shots).
   a. Uses — desensitization of the body's reaction to allergens, thus reducing allergic responses and the need for other medications.
   b. Limitations — requires frequent regularly scheduled injections in increasing potency until maintenance dose is reached, then frequency is decreased. Desensitization can be a lengthy process.

4. Antipruritic agents.
   a. Anesthetics — topically applied anesthetics act quickly to reduce pain associated with the allergic responses. Some of the more commonly used anesthetics are benzocaine, dibucaine, lidocaine, and pramoxine. Allergic contact is less likely to occur with lidocaine and pramoxine.
   b. Antihistamines — topically applied antihistamines, probably because of their emollient effect, are also frequently used. Benadryl mixed with calamine lotion (Caladryl®) is a common example. This combination does present a high risk of allergic sensitization.
   c. Other — a hodgepodge of antipruritic products containing menthol, phenol, and camphor. The actual mechanism by which these agents work is not clearly understood. However, in the case of phenol it is probably due to the necrotizing effect on nerve endings.

5. Emollients, skin care, bathing, and hydration.

D. Nursing diasnosis, outcomes, and interventions (see Table 1).

VASCULITIDES

I. OVERVIEW

Unlike the transient erythemas of urticaria and angioedema, the persistent and purpuric erythemas involve various degrees of vessel and structural damage which leads to leakage of lymphocytes as well as plasma. The purpuric erythemas involve partial destruction of vessel walls by neutrophils with subsequent red blood cell escape. Separate discussion of vascular reactions is very difficult because they exist on a spectrum in which there is overlap in clinical features, etiology, and pathophysiology.

A. Definition: reactions characterized by the presence of smooth surfaced, nonscaling erythematous or purpuric papules and plaques. These reactions are directly related to integrity of blood vessel walls.

II. ETIOLOGY.

A. Definition: specific etiology is found in about 10% of cases and can be grouped into six categories: medications, infections, immune diseases, malignancies, food, food dyes, and preservatives. In older patients, medications are the most common cause of vascular reactions.

B. Types.
   1. Erythema multiforme is a very common hypersensitivity reaction. The more common and milder form, erythema multiforme minor, is relatively asymptomatic and short lived (see Figure 15-2, page 241). Erythema multiforme major or Stevens-Johnson Syndrome (SJS)/Toxic Epidermal Necrolysis (TEN, very severe blistering reactions) can be extremely painful and life threatening (see Figures 15-3 and 15-4, page 241). In about one-third of cases of TEN (erythema multiforme major), the cause is unclear because of concomitant serious disease (for example, graft-vs.-host disease) and treatment with drugs. In most of the remaining cases, the cause is unknown.
   2. The most frequently identified causes of erythema multiforme are:
      a. Sulfa-related medications, penicillins, tetracyclines, anticonvulsants, NSAIDs, and allopurinol.
      b. Streptococcal infection.
      c. HSV infection which accounts for almost all cases of recurrent erythema multiforme and the related herpes virus EBV (Epstein Barr virus).
      d. Mycoplasma pneumonia.

e.   Coccidioidomycosis.
f.   Histoplasmosis.
g.   Lupus erythematosus.
h.   Chronic inflammatory bowel disease.
3.   Erythema nodosum is a hypersensitivity reaction characterized by the presence of large, up to 10 cm, nonscaling, red, painful lesions on the anterior surface of the lower legs (see Figure 15-5, page 241). The reaction of erythema nodosum occurs in the subcutaneous fat. No obvious cause is found in approximately one-half of the cases. The most commonly identified causes of erythema nodosum include:
a.   Sulfa-related medications.
b.   Infections, especially streptococcal disease in children.
c.   Oral contraceptives and oral estrogens are particular well-known causes.
d.   Pregnancy.
e.   Yersinial enterocolitis.
f.   Tuberculosis.
g.   Chronic inflammatory diseases such as sarcoidosis and inflammatory bowel disease.
4.   Leukocytoclastic vasculitis is a hypersensitivity reaction that occurs when blood vessels are infiltrated and destroyed by polymorphonuclear leukocytes. Red blood cells leak out of the vessels into the surrounding tissue, producing purpura. Unlike the purpuric lesions caused by trauma or coagulopathies, leukocytoclastic purpura is palpable because of the inflammation and edema associated with the reaction. The most commonly identified causes of leukocytoclastic vasculitis include:
a.   Sulfa-related medications, penicillin, aspirin, quinidine, and allopurinol.
b.   Infections, most commonly streptococcus, hepatitis B, the herpes viruses, EBV, CMV, influenza, and tuberculosis.
c.   Autoimmune diseases, lupus erythematosus, rheumatoid arthritis, chronic inflammatory bowel disease, and polyarteritis nodosum.
d.   Leukemia and myeloma.
5.   Henoch-Schonlein purpura or anaphylactoid purpura is a neutrophilic vasculitic disease occurring primarily in children, but can affect people of any age. The incidence in males is greater than females. The skin lesions, up to 3 cm plaques, are usually intermingled with the more classical purpuric papules. Additionally, immunoglobulin A (IgA) rather than immunoglobulin G (IgG) is present around the cutaneous blood vessels. Renal and gastrointestinal lesions are not uncommon.
C.   Pathophysiology.
1.   Erythema multiform — the specific

immunologic mechanism is unknown. Circulating immune complexes are frequently present and, at least in those instances resulting from herpes simplex infection, may be deposited at the site of the lesion. Mediator release as a result of mast cell degranulation probably occurs, but the mechanism is unknown.
2.   Erythema nodosum — essentially nothing is known about the pathway(s) through which the lesions of erythema nodosum arise. Histologically, the process is a mixed lymphocyte-histiocyte-mediated panniculitis; some minor degree of lymphocytic vasculitis is often present.
3.   Leukocytoclastic vasculitis — nearly all examples develop as a result of immune complex formation and deposition. Circulating immune complexes are deposited on the basement membrane of venules. In response to some disturbance of the endothelial cells (possibly occurs as a result of mediator release from mast cells) the immune complexes gain direct exposure to the underlying basement membrane. As part of the complement cascade, chemo-attractant molecules are released that draw neutrophils into the area. These neutrophils attempt to phagocytize the deposited immune complexes and in so doing release destructive proteolytic lysosomal enzymes. The vascular wall damage done by these enzymes allows for fibrin deposition in the vessels, fragmentation of neutrophil nuclei, and extravasation of erythrocytes. This entire process takes 24 to 72 hours.
4.   Henoch-Schonlein purpura — as with other vascular reactions it is idiopathic. The exact method of activation is unknown. Studies have revealed this reaction to be IgA rather than IgG mediated.

III. DIAGNOSIS

A.   History and physical exam.
1.   Erythema multiforme is characterized by the presence of flat-topped, sharply marginated papules 1 to 2 cm in diameter. Typically, at least a few of the larger papules will be of the "target" type in which three concentric rings are found: an outermost red ring, a lighter-colored intermediate ring, and a central, dusky-colored bull's-eye. Diagnostic hallmarks for erythema multiforme are:
a.   Distribution — trunk, but palm and sole involvement is characteristic when present.
b.   Target lesions.
c.   Papules and plaques are similar but less transient than those in urticaria.

2. Stevens-Johnson and TEN (erythema multiforme major). Clinical onset consistent with medication history and characteristic skin lesions. General erythema with detachment of the epidermis producing bullae, erosions, and large areas of unattached skin. TEN typically begins with painful localized erythema that disseminates rapidly. At the sites of erythema, flaccid blisters occur or the epidermis peels off. It may peel off in large sheets with gentle touching or pulling. Malaise, chills, myalgias, and fever accompany the denudation. Widespread areas of erosion, including all mucous membranes (eyes, mouth, genitalia) occur within 24 to 72 hours and the patient may become gravely ill. Affected areas of skin often look like second-degree burns. Mortality is caused by fluid and electrolyte imbalance, multi-organ sequelae (for example, pneumonia, GI bleeding), and infection.

3. Erythema nodosum — characterized by the presence of large (up to 10 cm) nonscaling, red, painful lesions on the anterior surface of the lower legs. The smaller lesions appear as slope-shouldered nodules, whereas the larger lesions appear as flat-topped plaques. On palpation the lesions are slightly warm and very tender. Generally no more than six lesions are present at any one time. Lesions usually occur on the anterior shins or around the ankles. Lesions may develop above the knee, on the thigh, or posteriorly on the calf. Diagnostic hallmarks include:
   a. Distribution — anterior lower legs.
   b. One or several palm-sized plaques.
   c. Lesional pain, warmth, and tenderness.
   d. Differentiation from cellulitis is obtained by presence of more than a single lesion, a duration of more than several days, and the failure to respond to antibiotics.
   e. Superficial thrombophlebitis also mimics erythema nodosum, but it is rarely if ever bilateral.

4. Leukocytoclastic vasculitis — the purpuric lesions consist entirely of petechiae; ecchymoses are not found. Because of the association with perivascular inflammatory infiltrate, the petechiae are usually at least slightly palpable. The smallest lesions occur as pinpoint dots that, early in the course of the disease, are bright red. As the lesions age, they become increasingly violaceous even blue-black. Diagnostic hallmarks include:
   a. Distribution — marked predilection for the lower legs.
   b. Nonblanchable petechiae.
   c. Slightly palpable petechiae.
   d. Absence of ecchymoses.

5. Henoch-Schonlein purpura — lesions are large (up to 3 cm) purpuric plaques, usually over the buttocks, lower legs, and elbows. Diagnostic hallmarks include:
   a. Joint pains, abdominal pain, hematuria, nausea, vomiting.
   b. Glomerulonephritis.

B. **Diagnostic tests.**
   1. Skin biopsies.
   2. Cultures, bacterial and viral.
   3. Laboratory evaluations as is relevant.

C. **Nursing diagnosis, outcomes, and interventions (see Table 1).**

GRANULOMA, ANNULARE, AND PYOGENIC

I. OVERVIEW

A. **Definition.**
   1. Granuloma annulare (GA) is a benign, fairly common condition which usually affects children and young adults. GA is characterized by a raised annular configuration consisting of papules or nodules arranged in a ring-like or circinate distribution. Lesions may be generalized in children or in immunocompromised patients but most often, patches occur on only one or two sites of the body, often bony areas such as the backs of the hands, elbows, and ankles or in close proximity to joints. GA is self-limiting and usually does not produce any medical complications.
   2. Pyogenic granuloma (PG) is misnamed, being neither pyogenic nor granuloma. Purplish, pulpy, vascular lesions of PG often involve the gum and other mucous membranes of the mouth.

B. **Etiology/Pathophysiology.**
   1. The cause of granuloma annulare is unknown. Various studies have shown latent diabetes to be present in a third of patients with this disorder. In some individuals granuloma annulare has been noted following trauma, insect bites, sun exposure, viral infections, and PUVA.
   2. PG is a disorder of angiogenesis whose underlying etiology remains unknown. A predilection exists for the head and neck, although lesions may appear on any part of the body.

C. **Clinical manifestations.**
   1. Granuloma annulare.
      a. Localized lesions.
         (1) Occur more commonly in children and young adults.
         (2) Annular, skin-colored, erythematous, or violaceous plaque.
         (3) May be papular.

    (4) Asymptomatic.

    (5) Telangiectasia may be present.

    (6) Common on dorsa of hands and feet; may be seen on forearms, arms, legs, and thighs.

  b. Generalized lesions.

    (1) 1 to 2 mm, commonly skin-colored papules (may be violaceous, pink, yellow or grey).

    (2) May arise on any cutaneous surface; common on neck and extensor surface of elbows.

    (3) May be annular, discrete papules or arcuate (seen when uneven spontaneous resolution occurs).

  c. Subcutaneous lesions.

    (1) Large, painless, deep dermal or subcutaneous nodules.

    (2) Skin colored.

    (3) Seen in children and young adults.

    (4) Occurs on palms, legs, buttocks, fingers, toes, or scalp.

    (5) May be solitary or multiple.

  d. Perforating lesions.

    (1) Small papules (may have central umbilication, plugs, or crusts).

    (2) Superficial.

    (3) Most common on hands/fingers.

2. Granuloma pyogenic.

  a. Acquired vascular proliferations occurring on the skin and mucous membranes.

    (1) Lesions are soft, dusky red or violaceous papules.

    (2) Lesions range in size from 5 mm to 1 cm to 2 cm.

    (3) Both sexes are affected equally.

    (4) Lesions can occur at all ages but, mostly in childhood.

    (5) Has no respect to racial heritage.

    (6) Approximately one-third of lesions appear following minor trauma.

  b. Histologically, the basic lesion is a proliferation of capillaries.

    (1) Each lobule is made of a central feeder vessel surrounded by smaller, less well-formed capillaries.

    (2) The overlying epithelium is often flattened with peripheral acanthosis and hyperkeratosis, giving the lesion a "cuffed" appearance.

    (3) Constriction of the base of the lesion results in the characteristic "balloon" or pedunculated appearance.

    (4) These lesions may bleed extensively if biopsied.

  c. GA is self-limiting, cosmetic, usually without any systemic complications.

    (1) Rarely it may involve fascia and tendons; resulting in sclerosis, lymphedema, and deformities such as joint ankylosis.

    (2) On rare occasions lesions have been associated with malignancy.

    (3) Intraoral lesions can have an appearance and behavior of Kaposi sarcoma.

D. **Nursing diagnosis, outcomes, and interventions (see Table 1).**

CUTANEOUS DRUG REACTIONS

I. OVERVIEW

A cutaneous reaction caused by a chemical substance or combination of substances that are ingested, injected, inhaled, inserted, instilled, or topically applied to the skin or mucous membranes is among the most frequently observed reaction. Adverse reactions may result from overdose, accumulation, pharmacologic side effect, drug-drug interactions, idiosyncrasy, microbiologic imbalance, exacerbation of existing latent or overt disease, hypersensitivity, autoimmune-like reaction, teratogenic effect interaction of the drug and sunlight or other light sources or other unknown mechanisms. Drug reactions are common; data on incidence differs. The most common causative agents are aspirin, penicillin, sulfa, and blood products.

A. **Definition.**

1. An adverse cutaneous reaction caused by a drug is any undesirable change in the structure or function of the skin its appendages, or mucous membranes.

B. **Classification of drug reactions.**

1. Dose-related.

  a. Excessive therapeutic effect (miscalculation).

  b. Secondary reactions (side effects).

  c. Hypersusceptibility to pharmacologic actions.

  d. Overdose toxicity.

  e. Iatrogenic drug effects (mimic pathologic disorders).

2. Sensitivity-related.

  a. Drug allergy.

  b. Idiosyncratic response.

C. **Etiology.**

1. Immunologic reaction (drug allergies).

  a. IgE dependent.

  b. Immune complex dependent.

  c. Cytotoxic.

  d. Cell mediated.

2. Nonimmunologic.

  a. Overdosage.

  b. Cumulative toxicity.

  c. Side effects.

  d. Ecologic disturbances.

e. Interactions with other drugs.

f. Metabolic changes.

g. Exacerbation of pre-existing dermatologic conditions.

3. Predisposing factors: patient-related.

a. Extremes of age.

b. Extremes of body weight.

c. Genetic variations.

d. Patient's temperament and attitude (personal values/beliefs; noncompliance; self-medication).

e. Circadian rhythms.

f. Changes associated with disease.

g. Pregnancy.

4. Predisposing factors: drug-related.

a. Dosage.

b. Route of administration and techniques.

c. Speed of administration.

d. Number of drugs being administered.

5. Exogenous factors.

a. Dietary.

b. Environmental.

II. MORPHOLOGIC CLASSIFICATIONS

A. Characteristic morphology and known mechanism.

1. Urticaria.

a. Characterized by red, pruritic wheals.

b. Rarely last longer than 24 hours.

c. Angioedema — severe life threatening urticarial presentation.

2. Photosensitivity eruptions.

a. Resemble sunburn.

b. Can occur with first exposure to the drug.

c. May induce photosensitivity diseases.

(1) Hexachlorobenzene — may induce porphria cutanea tarda.

(2) Procainamide — may induce LE.

(3) Isoniazid — may induce pellagra.

3. Pigmentation changes.

a. Heavy metals — stimulation of melanocyte activity.

b. Phenothiazines — cause slate grey pigmentation.

c. Antimalarials — cause slate grey or yellow pigmentation.

d. Inorganic arsenic — diffuse macular pigmentation.

e. Long-term use of hydantoin derivatives — cholasma-like pigmentation in females.

f. Oral mucosa may discolor with heavy metals, copper, antimalarials, arsenical agents, and ACTH.

4. Nail changes.

a. Onycholysis secondary to systemic fluorouracil.

b. Blue or brown pigmentation seen with

antimalarials.

c. Zidovudine — brown pigmentation.

5. Vasculitis.

6. Dilantin hypersensitivity reaction.

a. Hypersensitivity syndrome.

(1) Cutaneous eruption.

(2) Fever.

(3) Facial edema.

(4) Lymphadenopathy.

(5) Leukocytosis.

(6) Nephritis.

(7) Pneumonitis.

b. Skin signs range from mild morbilliform eruption to toxic epidermal necrolysis.

B. Reactions with characteristic morphology and suspected mechanism.

1. Morbilliform reactions (exanthems).

a. Most frequent of all cutaneous drug reactions.

b. Indistinguishable from viral exanthems (laboratory test fail to distinguish the two).

c. Most common causative agents: ampicillin (classic reaction pattern to this drug), barbiturates, phenytoin, gentamicin, isoniazid, phenothiazines, quinidine, sulfonamides, thiazides, thiouracil, trimethoprin-sulfamethoxazole, phenylbutazone, meclofenamate.

d. Lesions develop 7 to 10 days after starting the drug; may last for 1 to 2 weeks after drug discontinued.

e. Mildly pruritic, erythematous maculopapular rash begins on trunk; spreads in symmetrical pattern to face and extremities (usually within hours).

f. Spares palms, soles, and mucous membranes.

2. Erythema multiforme.

3. Fixed drug.

a. Clinical manifestations.

(1) Recurs at same site each time drug is ingested.

(a) Reactivation 30 minutes to 8 hours after re-exposure.

(b) Cross-sensitivity possible.

(2) Single or multiple dusky-red sharply demarcated plaque.

(3) Pruritus/burning might precede lesions.

(4) Blister formation with subsequent erosion, desquamation, or crusting.

(5) Hyperpigmentation after healing.

(6) Lesions can occur on any skin surface or mucous membrane except glans penis.

b. Diagnosis.

(1) Careful history asking specifically about over-the-counter products.

(2) Provoke reaction with suspected agent (use less than therapeutic dose).

(3) Biopsy.
4. Erythema nodosum.
   a. Tender, subcutaneous, erythematous nodules.
   b. Generally seen on extensor surfaces of extremities.
   c. Individual lesions will resolve in 1 to 2 weeks; new lesions may continue to appear for 3 to 6 weeks.
   d. Prodrome of fatigue and malaise or symptoms of urinary tract infection may precede cutaneous signs; arthralgias have been reported.
   e. Common causative agents — iodides, oral contraceptives, sulfonamides, bromides.
   f. Self-limiting; symptomatic treatment with salicylates (or NSAIDs) and bed rest.
C. **Drug eruptions of unknown mechanisms.**
   1. Toxic epidermal necrolysis (see Chapter 19).
   2. Lichenoid.
      a. Mimic generalized lichen planus and heals with brown pigmentation.
      b. Common causative agents — antimalarials, arsenicals, beta-blockers, captopril, gold salts, methyldopa, penicillamine, quinidine, and thiazides.

III. COMMON THERAPEUTIC MODALITIES

A. **Preventative, when possible eliminate the reactive agent.**
B. **Treat any underlying disease.**
C. **Provide symptomatic relief as necessary.**
D. **Removal of the affected area.**
   1. Erythema multiforme: oral corticosteroids administered early may help alleviate the tenderness.
      a. Recurrent erythema multiforme may respond to oral acyclovir by preventing HSV infections.
   2. Erythema nodosum responds to the institution of NSAIDs and the use of elastic wraps to minimize discomfort. Bed rest helps to relieve painful nodules. If an underlying streptococcal infection is suspected, antibiotic therapy is beneficial (for example, penicillin long-term — at least 1 year). If symptoms are severe without evidence of underlying infection or drug etiology, aspirin may be helpful, although the lesions often recur. When there are few lesions, intralesional triamcinolone acetonide (2.5 to 5 mg/ml) may provide symptomatic relief. Systemic corticosteroids are often the only means of controlling the lesions. They reduce the lesions but may mask an underlying systemic disease. Other possible therapies include oral potassium iodide or a short burst of oral prednisone.

3. Leukocytoclastic vasculitis: management includes investigation for and elimination of the causative agent.
   a. Corticosteroids for patients with more severe skin disease.
   b. Very ill patients my require hospitalization and intravenous corticosteroids.
4. Henoch-Schonlein purpura: there is no specific treatment. Most cases resolve spontaneously without treatment. If symptoms persist, therapy with corticosteroids is implemented.
5. Granuloma annulare: in general, GA rarely requires any treatment since spontaneous resolution is common. Multiple medicinal therapies have been tried including potassium iodide, dapsone, niacinamide, chlorambucil, and isotretinoin, but none have been shown to be particularly efficacious. Corticosteroids decrease inflammation by suppressing the migration of polymorphonuclear leukocytes and reversing capillary permeability.
6. Pyogenic granuloma: effective treatment includes excision, electrodesiccation, curettage, chemical cauterization, and injection sclerotherapy. CO_2 and argon lasers have been used successfully for treating PGs when lesions are superficial and of less than 0.5 cm thickness. Vascular packing may be needed in some cases.
7. Prevention through identification of drugs that frequently cause adverse reactions and screening them out of therapy whenever possible.
   a. Actual withdrawal of drugs if possible.
   b. Use of antihistamines.
   c. Local and systemic corticosteroids as indicated.
   d. Baths, soaks, and application of topicals for relief of pruritus.
E. **Nursing diagnosis, outcomes, and interventions (see Table 1).**

Bibliography

Assier, H., Gastuji-Garin, S., Revuz, J., & Roujeau, J.C. (1995). Erythema multiforme with mucous membrane involvement and Stevens-Johnson syndrome are clinically different disorders with distinct causes. *Archives of Dermatology, 131,* 539-543.

Bystryn, J.C. (1996). Erythema multiforme with mucous membrane involvement and Stevens-Johnson syndrome are clinically different disorders. *Archives of Dermatology, 132,* 711-713.

Daoud, M.D., et al. (1998). Recognizing cutaneous drug eruptions. *Post Graduate Medicine, 104*(1), 101-115.

Edwards, L. (1997). *Dermatology in emergency care.* New York: Churchill Livingstone.

Felner, E.L., Steinberg, J.B., & Weinberg, A.G. (1997). Subcutaneous granuloma annulare: A review of 47 cases. *Pediatrics, 100*(6).

Huang, S.W., & Borum, P.R.(1998). Study of skin rashes after antibiotic use in young children. *Clinical Pediatrics, 37*(10), 601-607.

Heller, H.M. (2000). Adverse cutaneous drug reactions in patients with human immunodeficiency virus-1 infection. *Clinical Dermatology, 18*(4), 485-489.

Houch, H.E., Kauffman, L., & Casey, D.L. (1997). Minocycline treatment for leukocytoclastic vasculitis associated with rheumatoid arthritis. *Archives of Dermatology, 133,* 19.

Lynch, P.J. (1994). *Dermatology house officer series* (3rd ed.). Baltimore: Williams & Wilkins.

Oppenheimer, J., & Kirkpatrick, C. (1991). Chronic urticaria. *Medical/Scientific Update, 9*(6).

Pomeranz, A.J., & Fairley, J.A. (1998). The systematic evaluation of the skin in children. *Pediatric Clinic of North America, 45*(1).

Rasmussen, J.E. (1995). Erythema multiforme: Should anyone care about the standards of care? *Archives of Dermatology, 131,* 726-729.

Roujeau, J.C. (1999). Treatment of severe drug eruptions. *Journal of Dermatology, 26*(11), 718-722.

Tay, Y.K., Weston, W.L., & Morelli, J.G. (1997). Treatment of pyogenic granuloma in children with the flashlamp-pumped pulsed dye laser. *Pediatrics, 99*(3).

Zurcher, K., & Krebs, A. (1992). *Cutaneous drug reactions.* New York: S. Karger.

Wolkenstein, P., Charue, D., Laurent, P., et al. (1995). Metabolic predisposition to cutaneous adverse drug reactions. *Archives of Dermatology, 131,* 544-51.

Dermatologic Nursing Essentials: A Core Curriculum 2nd Edition © DNA 2003

1. Characteristic of the primary lesion in urticaria is an edematous papule or plaque called a:
   a. Lesion.
   b. Mass.
   c. Wheal.
   d. Whelp.

2. The areas most typically affected with angioedema are:
   a. Scalp, arms, and legs.
   b. Lips and scalp.
   c. Lips and eyelids.
   d. Mucous membranes.

3. Anesthetics act quickly to:
   a. Stop itching.
   b. Reduce pain.
   c. Reduce swelling.
   d. a & b

4. In older patients with vasculitic reactions, the most common cause is:
   a. Food.
   b. Dyes.
   c. Medication.
   d. Immune disease.

5. Histoplasmosis, NSAIDs, and sulfa-related medications are in a group of frequently identified causes of erythema multiforme.
   a. True
   b. False

6. The reaction of erythema nodosum occurs in the subcutaneous fat.
   a. True
   b. False

7. Children with granuloma annulare are otherwise healthy and have the lesions for several months without any other symptoms.
   a. True
   b. False

8. In granuloma annulare the papules are flesh-colored or slightly pink and:
   a. 5 to 10 cm in size.
   b. 1 to 2 mm in size.
   c. 5 mm to 2 cm in size.
   d. None of the above.

9. The following drugs may produce photosensitivy diseases:
   a. Ampicillin.
   b. Procainamide.
   c. Isoniazid.
   d. All of the above.
   e. b & c.

10. Patient-related predisposing factors to cutaneous drug reactions include circadian rhythms.
    a. True
    b. False

11. Dilantin hypersensitivity syndrome includes:
    a. Cutaneous eruption.
    b. Fever.
    c. Facial edema.
    d. Lymphadenopathy.
    e. a, c, & d
    f. All of the above.

12. Morbilliform reactions are:
    a. Exanthems.
    b. Shaking syndrome much like Parkinson's disease.
    c. Most commonly produced by ampicillin.
    d. a & c
    e. All of the above.

13. Which of the following are examples of predisposing factors, patient related, for cutaneous drug reactions.
    a. Extremes of body weight.
    b. Race.
    c. Skin thickness.
    d. All of the above.

14. A subjective sensation of itching is characteristic of urticaria.
    a. True
    b. False

15. Granuloma annulare is a benign and self-limiting disorder.
    a. True
    b. False

16. The most common form of cutaneous drug reaction is urticaria.
    a. True
    b. False

Answers to Study Questions

1.	c	7.	a	13.	a
2.	c	8.	c	14.	a
3.	d	9.	e	15.	a
4.	c	10.	a	16.	a
5.	b	11.	f		
6.	a	12.	d		

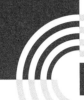

CE Answer/Evaluation Form

Chapter 15.
Hypersensitivities, Vasculitides, and Miscellaneous Inflammatory Disorders

Please photocopy this test page and return.

COMPLETE THE OLLOWING:

Name: _____

Address: _____

City: _____ State: _____ Zip: _____

Preferred telephone: (Home)_____ (Work) _____

State where licensed and license number: _____

CE application fee: DNA member $10.00
                       Nonmember $13.00

POSTTEST INSTRUCTIONS
1. To receive continuing education credit for individual study after reading the article, complete the answer/evaluation form below.
2. Photocopy and send the answer/evaluation form along with a check or money order payable to **Dermatology Nurses' Association** to: **DNA**, East Holly Avenue Box 56, Pitman, NJ 08071-0056.
3. Test returns must be postmarked by December 31, 2008. Upon completion of the answer/evaluation form, a certificate for 2.6 contact hour(s) will be awarded and sent to you.

This chapter was reviewed and formatted for contact hour credit by Marcia J. Hill, MSN, RN, Core Curriculum Editor; and Sally Russell, MN, RN,C, DNA Education Director.

ANSWER FORM

1. Name one new detail (item, issue, or phenomenon) that you learned by completing this activity.

_____
_____
_____
_____

2. How will you apply the information from this learning activity to your practice?
   a. Patient education.
   b. Staff education.
   c. Improve my patient care.
   d. In my education course work.
   e. Other: Please describe _____

_____

Evaluation

	Strongly disagree				Strongly agree
3. The offering met the stated objectives.					
a. Describe the major events in the formation of antibody against a specific antigen.	1	2	3	4	5
b. List the four general types of hypersensitivity reactions.	1	2	3	4	5
c. Differentiate between immediate and delayed-type hypersensitivities.	1	2	3	4	5
d. Define the major hypersensitivities and vascular reations.	1	2	3	4	5
e. Identify diagnostic and therapeutic interventions used to diagnose and treat hypersensitities, vasculitides, and miscellaneous inflammatory disorders.	1	2	3	4	5
4. The content was current and relevant.	1	2	3	4	5
5. The content was presented clearly.	1	2	3	4	5
6. The content was covered adequately.	1	2	3	4	5
7. I am more confident of my abilities since completing this material.	1	2	3	4	5

8. The material was (check one) ☐ new, ☐ review for me.

Comments _____

9. Time required to complete reading assignment: _____ minutes

This independent study is provided by the Dermatology Nurses' Association (DNA) for 2.6 contact hours. DNA is accredited as a provider of continuing education in nursing by the American Nurses Credentialing Center's Commission on Accreditation. DNA is approved as a provider of continuing education by the California Board of Registered Nursing Provider #CEP5708.

Bites, Stings, and Infestations

Marcia J. Hill, MSN, RN

Part I: Bites and Stings

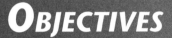

OBJECTIVES

At the end of this chapter, the reader will be able to:

- Identify the common skin manifestations of biting and stinging insects.
- List appropriate avoidance behaviors that may reduce exposure to biting and stinging insects.
- Describe common therapeutic interventions used to return the skin and tissues to pre-exposure condition.

KEY POINTS

- Understanding how humans interface with insects helps to avoid bites and stings.
- Topical application of OTC and household therapies will reduce much of the pain and discomfort of many bites or stings.
- Careful handwashing and reducing scratching will greatly lessen the chance of secondary infections after insect bites.
- Prompt emergency treatment is indicated for some bites or stings and any anaphylactic reaction.
- Patient and family education must include precautions to be used when sensitivity reactions are identified.

Bites and Stings

Marcia J. Hill, MSN, RN

ARTHROPODA

I. OVERVIEW

Humans come in frequent contact with varying numbers of the more than one million varieties of insects that inhabit this earth. A very limited number of these cause more than fleeting annoyance or discomfort. Some insects inject venom into humans as a means of self-protection. Others use the human animal for a blood meal, most often when a four-legged animal is not readily available. Although almost everyone has experienced a bite or sting, only about 0.4% of our population experiences allergic reactions each year. The insects vary in their ability to transmit disease.

A. Arachnida: class of eight-legged insects that includes scorpions, spiders, ticks, and mites.
   1. Scorpion: *centruroides sculpturatus.*
      a. Found in Arizona and surrounding states and northern Mexico.
      b. Obtaining a length of 3 to 5 inches, it has a forebody, six projecting legs, and a hindbody with a hooked caudal stinger which it uses to inject venom into its prey.
      c. Major function is control of insect population.
      d. Stings occur most frequently on the legs, thighs, and buttocks of its human victims, often the result of sitting or walking in the scorpion's territory.
      e. The sting produces an immediate sharp, burning sensation. Local edema soon surrounds the small puncture wound often followed by skin discoloration. Numbness may extend beyond the puncture site.
      f. Avoidance behaviors include careful attention to where you sit or walk when in the natural habitat of the scorpion.
         (1) Children, because of their size, tend to have severe reactions and must be observed to prevent them from sitting on a scorpion.
         (2) A debilitated adult is also at increased risk for complications of a bite.
   2. Black widow spider: *latrodectus mactans.*
      a. Found in the entire continental United States except Alaska.
      b. The 0.5-inch female is glossy black with a characteristic red hourglass on the underside of the abdomen. The male of the species is smaller with four pairs of red markings on the abdomen.
      c. Diet consists of insects, centipedes, and other spiders. After mating, the female often ensnares and devours her mate, from which she derives the name, black widow.
      d. Generally not aggressive, the venomous bite occurs most frequently when the female is guarding an egg sac.
      e. The local reaction of the black widow spider bite is generally not the most likely reason to seek medical attention.
         (1) The injected venom is a neurotoxin which may cause severe muscle spasms making breathing difficult.
         (2) An autonomic response to the venom produces diaphoresis and hypertension.
         (3) The local reaction manifests as a 3 to 4 mm reddish papule with a puncture wound in the center.
      f. Avoiding bites depends greatly on observing presence of webs as the spider may be present inside structures as well as out of doors.
   3. Brown recluse spider: *loxosceles reclusa.*
      a. Found in all states with the highest concentration in the southern regions of the United States, especially in Arkansas, Kansas, Missouri, and Tennessee.
      b. The spider has a cephalothorax with a characteristic violin-shaped marking, joined to abdomen, and is light to medium brown in color.
      c. Like most spiders, the brown recluse prefers an insect diet.
      d. Bites occur most frequently to the extremity of its victim.
      e. The initial bite, which injects a coagulotoxin that can remain biologically active for up to 12 days, may go unnoticed.
         (1) Pain develops 2 to 8 hours after the initial bite.
         (2) The presentation is very unpredictable, often with the presence of a gray-blue halo surrounding the puncture site.
         (3) Local tissue response may include erythema, edema, a wheal or purpura, and cyanosis with development of an eroding central region.
         (4) Systemic reactions may vary from a mild flu-like presentation to anaphylactic shock. Symptoms caused by the coagulotoxin may include deep vein thrombosis, renal failure, pulmonary edema and hemolysis, and cardiac arrhythmia.

Table 1.
Rocky Mountain Spotted Fever

Rocky Mountain spotted fever (RMSF) is an infectious disease spread to humans by the bite of a deer or dog tick. Severe headache and fever generally appear after a 2 to 16 day incubation period following the transfer of the organism *Rickettsia rickettsii* from the tick. Several days later, as the organism invades the lining of the blood vessels, causing thrombosis, a patchy, rose-colored rash develops on the wrist and ankles. As it spreads centrally, the rash deepens in color from dark red to brown. Treatment is aimed at destroying the organism by use of tetracycline or chloramphenicol. RMSF has been reported in all states of the United States. Prevention is aimed at control of tick populations, avoidance behaviors, and early tick removal.

Table 2.
Lyme Disease

Lyme disease is caused by the transfer of the spirochete *Borrelia burgdorferi* to humans by feeding of the deer tick, *Ixodes dammini,* and certain other tick species. The tick is capable of transmitting the disease during any of its stages of development when it varies from poppy seed to sesame seed size. The characteristic rash, erythema migrans (EM), occurs in about 60% of patients within 3 days to 4 weeks of the tick bite. The classical presentation is a large circular or oval rash with central clearing and irregular margin of redness surrounding the tick bite. Satellite lesions may occur with spread of the spirochete. Flu-like symptoms, fever, chills, aches and pains, and arthritis symptoms may be present. Heart block and various neuropathies are observed in 10% to 15% of cases. Tetracycline is the drug treatment of choice. High-dose penicillin may be required for treating arthritis or meningitis.

    f.   Caution when putting on any article which has been stored in drawers, closets, or attics will reduce the chance of a bite. The spider may also be found under woodpiles and in sheds.

4.   Ticks (see Tables 1 and 2).

    a.   This parasite is widespread, preferring thick vegetation or grasses on which to cling when not in contact with animals or humans.

    b.   The tick is mite-like, varies in size by species, and has four pairs of clawed legs. The mouth parts are specialized for grasping and slicing a hole in the skin of its victim so it is able to suck blood. Diseases may be transmitted during this process so it is important NOT to squeeze the tick in an effort to remove it from the skin.

       (1) When attempting to remove a tick, protect the hands from organisms and grasp the tick with tweezers or forceps and apply steady pull until the tick releases its grasp.

       (2) Cleanse the wound to reduce secondary infection.

       (3) Observe for development of vector disease, especially if the tick was squeezed or crushed during removal or has been attached for greater than 24 hours.

    c.   Some species of ticks require only three blood meals during their life cycle of 2 years.

    d.   A tick will attach itself to any exposed skin but often travels under clothing or around body parts until it reaches a constricted area.

    e.   Avoidance behavior includes caution in tick-infested areas and the meticulous search for ticks on the skin after exposure. Light-colored clothing increases the visibility of the tick. Removing the tick within 3 hours of attaching reduces the risk of vector disease (see Table 3).

5.   Chiggers.

    a.   Present in most grain-growing regions of the United States, they are most prevalent in the south during the summer and fall. They may be known by many other names such as red bugs, jiggers, harvest mites, harvest lice, and harvest bugs.

    b.   A barely visible mite, the larval stage of the chigger attaches to the skin of the host by means of a hooked mouth part.

    c.   While attached, it ingests a blood meal. The mite does not burrow and releases after engorgement.

    d.   Lesions occur most frequently after contact with infested hay or grains. The mite prefers an area where it can feed undisturbed, especially under constrictions of clothing.

    e.   Macules or papules (which are very pruritic), may be up to 5 mm in size, are common after exposure. If the individual is sensitized, the eruption may vary from urticaria to a more severe granulomatous reaction. Lesions slowly regress over 1 to 2 weeks. There is potential for vector disease (see Table 3).

    f.   Wearing clothing that has been treated with DEET and is tight around the wrist and ankle offers some protection. Immediate soapy shower after exposure to infested hay

Table 3.
Potential Vector Diseases from Blood-Sucking Insects

Flea	Plague, typhus, tapeworms, and filariasis
Mosquitos	Malaria, encephalitis, dengue, and yellow fever
Chiggers	Rickettsial typhus, viral encephalitis, and Pasteurella plague
Bedbugs	Oriental sore, Chagas' disease, kala-azar, and relapsing fever (all rare occurrences)
Tick, especially deer tick	Rocky Mountain spotted fever, Lyme disease, and relapsing fever

and berry vines may reduce the number of lesions.

B. **Insecta: class of six-legged insects, many with wings, which includes bees, wasps, and ants.**
  1. Bumblebee.
     a. Largest of the Hymenoptera, found throughout the United States, is better adapted to colder regions than other bee species.
     b. The bumblebee is hairy and usually of black and yellow coloration.
     c. The bee is responsible for pollination of a wide variety of plants.
     d. Generally not aggressive, often stings when its victim disturbs it while walking in patches of clover.
     e. The bee produces one painful, stabbing defensive sting into its victim that may leave behind the barbed stinger. The surrounding skin quickly forms a red papule which becomes urticarial and edematous and may remain painful for hours.
        (1) The sting injects formic acid and proteins into its victim.
        (2) Sensitization to the protein may result in an anaphylactic reaction (see Table 4).
        (3) The venom sac is attached to the stinger and will continue to contract and inject additional venom if not removed.
        (4) The stinger should be quickly flicked off with a fingernail or blunt instrument instead of pinched with the fingers to reduce the amount of venom being injected into the victim.
        (5) A bumblebee that has lost its stinger soon dies.
     f. Caution when walking in clover or low-growing flowering plants will reduce the risk of stings. Nesting chambers with a single opening are frequently made in the abandoned nests of mice and squirrels.
  2. Honeybee.
     a. Found in all states of the United States, the honeybee is found in any area with flowers and fruits.
     b. Smaller and somewhat similar in appearance to the bumblebee.

Table 4.
Hypersensitivity Reactions

Hymenoptera: The order of insects which can cause severe hypersensitivity reactions.

The imported fire ant (IFA) bite can produce an antigen response in sensitive individuals. The local reaction is an immediate flare generally followed by a wheal of up to 10 mm. A sterile vesicle forms in the center and becomes cloudy as it fills with neutrophils. This resulting pustule is surrounded by a bright red halo. Mild nausea, malaise, and fever or even anaphylactic shock may occur over the first 24 to 48 hours. Much more severe systemic allergic reactions with urticaria, angioedema, wheezing, and syncope occur in about 1% of victims. Once identified as sensitized, the victim should seek professional advice for potential skin testing and immunotherapy. The IFA should be avoided by observing for their mounds, not walking in fields or lawns at night, and avoiding sandboxes until checked for presence of ants.

A similar generalized response may occur with the sting of other Hymenoptera such as the wasp or various species of bees. When use of an epinephrine pen is suggested, make sure the patient or parent is able to discharge the medication as instructed.

     c. Very important to pollination, the honeybee is generally not aggressive unless it perceives threat.
        (1) Since experiments in Brazil sought to cross the native honeybee with an African cousin, a much more aggressive bee has developed.
        (2) The Africanized honeybee migrated into the United States in the early 1990s.
        (3) This aggressive bee is capable of chasing a fleeing victim for up to one-quarter of a mile.
     d. If the entire hive is disturbed, a swarm of insects may attack, stinging any body surface.
     e. The sting produces an edematous red papule.
     f. Beehives should not be disturbed. If found in a dwelling, a professional beekeeper should be sought to remove the bees. This can be accomplished with the use of smoke bombs which block perception of the

chemical pheromone released with the sting that results in swarming behavior from the bees. Bright-colored, rough-textured clothing is attractive to bees.

3. Wasp.
   a. The paper wasp lives in communities while the mud dauber, potter wasp, and digger wasp are solitary.
   b. The wasp varies in color from mahogany colored to black and may be from 2 to 5 cm in length.
   c. The diet consists of other insects and vegetable matter. Some species are pollinators of crops.
   d. Like other members of the Hymenoptera, wasps sting when disturbed or threatened.
   e. Producing a similar lesion to the bee sting, the venom of all wasps contains histamine and a factor that dissolves red blood cells. Sensitization occurs across species.
   f. Children should be discouraged from knocking down wasp nests. Protective clothing and covering food at picnics reduce the chance of stings.

4. Yellow jacket.
   a. A member of the wasp family, closely related to the hornet, it is widely distributed throughout the United States.
   b. Named for its characteristic yellow markings, it is hairless and has three sets of legs and two sets of wings.
   c. The diet consists chiefly of insects and rotting fruit.
   d. Stings may be inflicted on any body part when the nest or individual yellow jacket is disturbed.
   e. Sting is similar to that of the honeybee.
   f. Nests are generally underground or close to the ground and may contain thousands of yellow jackets. Avoiding the nesting areas and placing pails of rotting fruit on the perimeter of fruit picking areas may reduce the chance of stings.

5. Hornet.
   a. A member of the wasp family, the hornet may be found in unique football-shaped nests made of papery material comprising masticated plant foliage and wood suspended from a tree limb. The hornet's habitat is more evident in the northern United States.
   b. The hornet is about 3 cm in length and is generally white-faced with black and white markings on its segments.
   c. The diet consists largely of other insects and ripe fruit.
   d. The hornet stings to protect its environment and is likely to swarm if the nest is disturbed, whether by accident or intention.
   e. The sting produces a painful edematous papule. Its sting may result in anaphylactic reaction in sensitized individuals.
   f. Only someone knowledgeable in hornet behaviors should remove the nest.

6. Ant.
   a. The wingless member of the order Hymenoptera, the imported fire ant (IFA) is the species most frequently involved in painful stings and allergic reactions. Introduced into the United States from South America, it is prevalent in most of the south.
   b. Ants are generally 2 to 5 mm long, colors varying from tan-red to black. The IFA live in large colonies often producing large mounds, especially noticeable after rains.
   c. The ant serves a useful purpose as an aerator and mixer of soil. Most species are omnivorous. The IFA can be dangerous to young or injured livestock as well as humans.
   d. Walking, gardening, and sitting in the habitat of the ant may result in one or more stings. Multiple stings, with the increased venom load, increase the risk of systemic reaction for small children and debilitated adults.
   e. See Table 4.
   f. Observing for characteristic mounds, vigilance during hand gardening, checking sandboxes prior to play sessions, and closed footwear will reduce the risk of IFA bites. Proper soil treatment to reduce ant population may be indicated.

7. Flea.
   a. A member of the order Siphonaptera, fleas can be found all over the world with cat and dog fleas causing the highest proportion of infestation in households. Human fleas are rare in the United States.
   b. Wingless, and with three pairs of legs, fleas can jump distances out of proportion to their size.
   c. Require blood meal for survival.
   d. Bites occur most frequently about the ankle of the human but may be scattered in any area as the flea attempts to hide from light.
   e. The bite produces an erythematous papule that may progress to a wheal or blister. Bites may be intensely itchy. There is potential for vector disease (see Table 3).
   f. Fleas can live for up to a year without contact with humans or pets. A thorough eradication program involves treatment of the pet, elimination of fleas and their eggs

from carpets, furniture, and flooring, and thorough treatment of the yard within the same time period.

8. Mosquito.
   a. A member of the order Diptera, the mosquito inhabits most of the globe where there is sufficient water to permit the hatching phase.
   b. A two-winged, narrow insect with long, slender legs.
   c. The male feeds on nectar but the female uses her specialized mouth parts to pierce the skin and inject saliva which inhibits clotting, permitting her to ingest blood. Infectious organisms may be transferred during feeding.
   d. The mosquito will attack any uncovered skin and is able to pierce lightweight clothing.
   e. The bite forms an urticarial papule with intense itching that may begin within 10 minutes and last for days. There is potential for vector disease (see Table 3).
   f. The use of products that contain diethyltoluamide (DEET) may serve as adequate repellants if used properly. Adding 1 to 2 teaspoons of chlorine bleach to the bath water prior to exposure may reduce natural body odors that attract the female. Eating foods high in serotonin such as bananas and peanuts also attract the female mosquito.

9. Bedbug.
   a. A member of the order Hemiptera, the bedbug is far less common than most other insects in the United States.
   b. The bedbug is 0.5 cm in length, slightly ovoid and flattened, and of reddish brown coloration.
   c. Blood meals are taken, perhaps as infrequently as twice yearly, by piercing the skin with specialized stylets, ingesting blood and dissolved epidermal tissue before releasing. The victim is rarely aware of the bite until after release.
   d. Lesions may occur on any body surface. The stylets leave behind two red marks that become pruritic papules several minutes after the bite. Depending on the sensitivity of the victim, wheals, vesicles, or hemorrhagic bullae may develop. More severe symptoms have been documented, including anaphylactic reaction.
   e. When known to be present behind baseboards, in cracks and crevices, and around beds, the bedbug can be eliminated by vacuuming and insecticide sprays.

II. ASSESSMENT

A. History and physical exam.
   1. History of exposure or potential exposure to insect.
   2. Presence of one or more lesions with characteristic appearance.
   3. Distribution of lesions consistent with biting or stinging habits of insect.
   4. Hypertension and respiratory distress noted with scorpion sting especially with presence of hypersalivation.
   5. Presence of severe muscle pain or spasms associated with black widow spider bite.
   6. Arthralgia, weakness, confusion may indicate delayed hypersensitivity reaction.
   7. Expressions of feeling of doom may indicate onset of anaphylaxis.

B. Diagnostic tests.
   1. Generally not indicated unless required to follow course of disease or with specific envenomation.
   2. Arterial blood gas may be required with anaphylaxis or with scorpion sting that may cause hypersalivation.
   3. Leukocytosis and elevated creatine phosphokinase may be present with the bite of a black widow spider.
   4. Hemoglobinemia, thrombocytopenia, and hemoglobinuria may result with envenomation of the brown recluse spider.
   5. Positive blood cultures may indicate secondary bacterial infection from any bite; often present with deep tissue necrosis of brown recluse spider bite.
   6. About 4 to 6 weeks after the bite of a tick, the enzyme-linked immunosorbent assay may be positive for the antibodies to the causative spirochete of Lyme disease. Later in the course of the disease the spirochete may be isolated in joint fluid.

III. TREATMENT MODALITIES

A. Local treatment.
   1. The bites of many insects can be rendered less painful and itching reduced by applying of cold compresses or ice packs alternated with warm compresses.
   2. Keeping the hands and skin clean and trimming nails in young children reduces the risk of secondary bacterial infection.
   3. Applying topical antihistamine lotions or systemic antihistamines may reduce the urge to scratch. Use cautiously with young children and debilitated adults.
   4. Anti-infective ointments such as bacitracin or Polysporin® may reduce secondary infection when the skin is broken.

Table 5.
Nursing Diagnoses, Outcomes, and Nursing Interventions

Nursing Diagnoses	Outcomes	Interventions
Impaired skin integrity related to bite/envenomation.	Skin healed to pre-exposure state.	Assist with wound care as required. Assess for signs of secondary infection. Offer topical measures to reduce scratching.
Risk of impaired oxygenation related to effects of venom.	Airway clear.	Support airway as required. Prepare for suctioning with diagnosis of scorpion bite. Administer bronchodilators as required with anaphylaxis.
Risk of secondary bacteria infection related to broken skin barrier.	Skin healed without further tissue damage.	Urge careful handwashing. Use comfort measures to reduce scratching. Maintain aseptic technique with dressing changes in brown recluse spider bite.
Pain and pruritus related to venom or local tissue edema.	Patient comfortable without report of pain.	Offer local measures to reduce swelling. Application of phenol-containing products may reduce pruritus. Elevate limb if indicated.

B. Treatments specific to envenomation.
1. Scorpion.
   a. Treat symptoms of severe agitation, peripheral motor jerking, and hypersalivation as needed.
   b. Be prepared to support respiration.
   c. Goat serum antivenin may be used to relieve neurologic, respiratory, and cardiovascular symptoms.
2. Black widow spider.
   a. Equine antivenin may reduce the musculoskeletal pain associated with envenomation.
   b. Parenteral calcium gluconate may be used in some centers.
3. Brown recluse spider.
   a. Dapsone® 100 mg/day (check blood for presence of G6pd; should be present before administering) for 14 days when tissue necrosis occurs.
   b. Surgical intervention is used cautiously as the toxin remains biologically active in the tissues for up to 21 days.
   c. After tissue destruction has stopped, skin flaps may be required to repair the defect.
4. Lyme disease.
   a. Doxycycline 100 mg bid or amoxicillin 250 to 500 mg tid for 21 days.
   b. With late-stage disease, parenteral antibiotics such as ceftriaxone or penicillin for 10 to 21 days are indicated.
5. Rocky mountain spotted fever.
   a. Doxycycline 100 mg bid or tetracycline hydrochloride 500 mg qid.
   b. Tetracycline should not be used during tooth development.
   c. IV chloramphenicol sodium succinate 50 to 75 mg/kg/day divided into qid dosing.

IV. COMMON NURSING DIAGNOSES, OUTCOMES, AND INTERVENTIONS (see Table 5)

Three-year-old Amy is brought to a clinic in Florida by her parents. They report that their daughter was playing in the yard near their vacation cabin yesterday morning when she began to cry and ran from the sandbox. Physical exam reveals multiple vesicles on her feet and legs with bright red halos. Amy is lethargic but attempts to scratch the lesions.

1. The source of envenomation is likely:
   a. Honeybee stings as she probably sat on their nest.
   b. Multiple bites from a scorpion in the sand.
   c. Sterile vesicles from the bites of imported fire ants nesting in the sand.
   d. Sand flea bites.

2. The cause of Amy's lethargy may be secondary to:
   a. She is sleepy because she cried so hard with the bites.
   b. Large amount of venom injected into a small individual.
   c. She is in the first stage of sleeping sickness.
   d. It is past her bedtime.

3. The physician questions the parents about previous exposure to bites from any type of wasp or bee. The reason for this is:
   a. He believes a member of the Hymenoptera family caused the stings and Amy may have been previously sensitized.
   b. He believes the bites are from a sand flea but previous exposure to bee stings can cause a severe reaction.
   c. He knows the nesting area for most bees is in sand and feels that Amy may have been stung earlier in the day.
   d. Chiggers are common in sand in Florida. Their bites cause extreme lethargy.

4. The vesicles on Amy's feet and legs contain:
   a. A coagulotoxin.
   b. A neurotoxin.
   c. Purulent material from an infection.
   d. Sterile material with many neutrophils.

Your social group is planning a summer backpacking vacation with adults and children to an area of grass and woodlands in the northeast. The group has asked you to advise them in methods to avoid insect bites and stings. You know that your trip will include some marshy areas with mosquitoes and dense brush that you know has potential for ticks.

5. Your concern is to have the group practice avoidance behaviors which may include:
   a. Wearing long-sleeved shirts and long pants tucked into socks.
   b. Use of DEET product applied to exposed skin and clothing at least every 6 hours.
   c. Keep to center of path when possible.
   d. All of the above.

6. Each evening during the trip the adults have an inspection party of all campers to remove any ticks that have managed to attach to the skin. Caution is used to gently remove any ticks without squeezing. Antiseptic is applied and hands are washed after tick removal. Two weeks after the trip a parent calls to report a strange rash behind the knee of her teenage son, Jason. She describes a large bull's eye area with clearing in the center. The rash seems asymptomatic but Jason reports flu-like symptoms about a week ago. You suspect:
   a. An isolated chigger bite which has become infected.
   b. The first presentation of Rocky Mountain spotted fever.
   c. The bite of a mosquito carrying St. Louis encephalitis.
   d. Evidence of a spirochete in her son.

7. Treatment for Jason's infection may include:
   a. Local antibiotics and steroids for the skin lesion, aspirin for the flu symptoms.
   b. Oral doxycycline or amoxicillin for at least 3 weeks. High-dose penicillin if arthritis symptoms develop.
   c. Tetracycline or intravenous chloramphenicol.
   d. Symptomatic treatment only unless infection occurs.

The local parks department has asked you to assist with their summer camp. You have access to ice, insect repellents, and a first-aid kit. You see a variety of lesions on the campers the first morning.

8. Suggestions that you might give to the parents to avoid or reduce the consequences of insect bites include all *except*:
   a. Ask the parents to spray insect repellent lightly on the child's clothes and skin, avoiding the eyes, before camp.
   b. Use RID® as a repellent, saturating socks and pants.
   c. Keep peanuts and bananas to a minimum and avoid strong perfumes and bright-colored, rough-textured clothing.
   d. Use cold compresses to reduce itching and keep nails clean and short.

Answers to Study Questions

1.	c	5.	d
2.	b	6.	d
3.	a	7.	b
4.	d	8.	b

Part II: Infestation with Ectoparasites: Scabies and Lice

OBJECTIVES

At the end of this chapter, the reader will be able to:

- Identify the causative ectoparasite in scabies and lice infestations.
- List the most common treatments and cautions for treating infestations.
- List environmental and fomite treatments which prevent re-infestation.

KEY POINTS

- All cases of very pruritic rashes with intense nighttime itching should raise the suspicion of scabies infestation.
- Calm acceptance of the patient diagnosed with scabies or lice will help the family deal with the social stigma and promote attention to treatment plans.
- Schools and institutions often require complete nit removal before a child can re-enter the school even when pediculicides are effective.
- Parent education should include methods of eradicating scabies and lice from the home environment to prevent re-infestation.

Infestation with Ectoparasites: Scabies and Lice

Marcia J. Hill, MSN, RN

SCABIES

I. OVERVIEW

The common itch mite, *Sarcoptes scabiei*, is responsible for a great deal of misery in every habitated area of the globe. It is no respecter of social or economic class, sex, gender, age, or standard of personal hygiene.

A. Ectoparasite: *Sarcoptes scabiei.*
   1. The mature female mite is about 0.5 mm in diameter.
   2. Only the female mite burrows into the skin.
   3. Mites from animals can feed on humans but do not burrow or reproduce in humans.
B. Reproduction.
   1. Reproduction takes place on the skin of the host.
   2. The female is impregnated by the male who then dies.
   3. The impregnated female penetrates the skin by producing a secretion that lyses the stratum corneum. This process takes about 45 minutes.
   4. The mature female mite lays one or two eggs each day during her 30-day lifespan.
   5. The embryo hatches in 3 to 10 days producing a six-legged larva.
   6. The larva goes through two additional shedding stages, finally producing an eight-legged nymph that matures into the adult mite.
   7. Both the larva and nymph can survive and mature outside the host.
C. Infestation.
   1. Occurs only in close physical contact with a host already infested with the mite or may be transmitted by fomites such as clothing and bed linen.
   2. The mite pushes through the corneocytes into the stratum granulosum.
   3. The motion of the mite is always forward at a rate of 0.5 to 5 mm per day producing an externally visible burrow on the skin of the host.
   4. The burrow may be 5 to 20 mm long, straight or serpentine in appearance.
D. Immune response (see Table 6).

II. ASSESSMENT

A. History and physical exam.
   1. Very pruritic eruption with increased intensity of symptoms at night.
   2. Family members and household contacts with similar rash and itching.
   3. Presence of papules, pustules, or vesicles.
   4. Presence of a thread-like linear or serpentine shaped gray-brown or pearly burrow less than 1 mm in width.
   5. Lesions tend to be concentrated in the web spaces of the fingers, around the wrists, axillae, breasts and areolae, waist, thighs, lower buttocks, and genitalia.
   6. In infants and children the lesion may be nodular and present over the back and on the head.
   7. Nodular lesions may be present in the groin or axillae in adults.
   8. Lesions in the immunocompromised patient may present with disseminated papular eruption and extensive hyperkeratotic lesions and fissuring, especially on flexor surfaces.
B. Diagnostic tests.
   1. Mineral oil prep.
      a. Scabies prep using a scalpel blade (pre-moistened with mineral oil) to scrape a

Table 6.
Immune Response

Immune response.	Caused by soluble antigen produced when the saliva, body secretions, and feces of the mite come in contact with cellular fluid.	Immune response develops over 4-6 weeks with first infestation of mite. During the latent period, the mite multiplies. When the normal allergic response begins, many mites die. Inflammatory response develops. In the immunocompromised individual, the mite continues to multiply unchecked. This super infestation is commonly called Norwegian or crusted scabies. With presence of the antigen, future infestations result in pruritus within 24 hours to several days. Past infestation does not confer future immunity.

suspected burrow and placing the material on a slide with mineral oil.

b. Examining the material under the microscope with low magnification.

c. Presence of the scabies mite, ova, or fecal pellets (scybala) are diagnostic of scabies.

2. Burrow ink test (BIT).

a. Use of a pen or nonpermanent marker to identify a suspected burrow.

b. After penetration, the excess ink is removed with an alcohol wipe.

c. A mineral oil prep is performed as above.

3. Tetracycline fluorescence technique.

a. Liquid preparation of tetracycline applied to the skin and permitted to dry.

b. After drying, the skin is wiped with an alcohol pad.

c. The skin is illuminated with a Wood's lamp and the fluorescing burrow scraped as above.

4. Biopsy.

a. Seldom used except when lesions are atypical.

b. Demonstrate extent of tunneling present in crusted scabies.

5. Blood tests.

a. IgE elevated, IgA decreased in crusted scabies.

b. Eosinophilia in crusted scabies.

C. **Differential diagnosis.**

1. Unless proved otherwise, all pruritic rashes should raise the suspicion of scabies.

2. Atopic and contact dermatitis and neurodermatitis must be ruled out.

3. Dermatitis herpetiformis, lichen planus, and psoriasis may have similar skin lesions.

III. TREATMENT MODALITIES

A. **Medication.**

1. 5% permethrin cream (Elimite®) massaged into the skin of adults and children from the neck down and washed off in the morning.

2. 5% permethrin cream (Elimite) applied from head to toe in infants over 2 months and washed off in the morning.

3. For pregnant or lactating females and infants under 2 months, 5% to 10% sulfur in petrolatum preparations.

a. Applied nightly for 3 nights and washed off in the mornings.

b. Prevent oral contact when nursing.

c. Inform your patient of objectionable odor and potential for staining of clothing and bed linen.

4. Gammabenzene hexachloride (1% lindane, Kwell®) may be used for treatment but additional cautions are warranted.

a. Treatment is often less effective than with permethrin.

b. Not for use in pregnant or lactating females.

c. Infants should be held for the 2-hour treatment time to prevent them from getting the insecticide into the mouth.

d. Application of 30 ml is sufficient for an adult.

e. Avoid retreatment unless specifically ordered by a physician to reduce chance of neurotoxicity, especially in the young.

5. Crotamiton (Eurax®) application used for 2 to 5 consecutive nights with bathing 24 hours after last application. Not for use with pregnant or lactating females.

6. Low-dose topical or systemic steroids or oral antihistamines for treating continued pruritus, secondary to presence of dead mites and ova, may be required.

7. Antibiotics may be required for secondary infections, when present.

B. **Household contacts.**

1. The most effective eradication occurs when all contacts are treated within the same time frame.

2. Include all sexual contacts in treatment.

C. **Clothing, bed linen, and environment.**

1. Change clothing and linen after overnight or recommended treatment time.

2. Launder clothing with hot water wash and dry or dry clean.

3. Vacuum all nonwashable surfaces; seal and dispose of vacuum bag.

4. Fabric articles that cannot be washed or dry-cleaned may be encased in plastic for several weeks to avoid re-infestation.

IV. COMMON NURSING DIAGNOSES, OUTCOMES, AND INTERVENTIONS (see Table 7)

V. COMPLICATIONS (see Table 8)

A. **Intense scratching in response to pruritus may result in secondary bacterial infections.**

B. **In the immunocompromised host, the lack of cell-mediated response permits the mite to multiply unchecked.**

1. Hyperkeratotic plaques may form with fissuring.

2. Normal skin flora then have a portal of entry into the bloodstream.

3. Once in the bloodstream, normal skin flora may develop into bacteremia, sepsis, and potentially death.

4. If the normal cell-mediated response does not limit the number of mites, huge numbers may tunnel in and around the fingernails promoting the spread of the mite to other body areas or caretakers.

Table 7.
Nursing Diagnoses, Outcomes, and Interventions

Nursing Diagnoses	Outcomes	Interventions
Impaired skin integrity related to infestation.	Lesions healed.	1. Medication as ordered to eradicate mites/lice. 2. Use nursing measures to reduce itch-scratch-itch response.
Risk of secondary infection related to broken skin barrier.	No evidence of secondary infection.	1. Trim fingernails to reduce abrasion of the skin. 2. Encourage frequent handwashing to reduce introduction of normal skin flora into the body. 3. Observe for development of signs and symptoms of secondary infection.
Potential alteration in body image secondary to infestation.	Able to initiate and carry through treatment for self and contacts.	1. Assure patient understands treatment plan. 2. Supportive care if evidence of delusions of parasitosis occurs. 3. Observe for evidence of overtreatment. (Lindane may cause CNS excitation or eczematous reactions secondary to irritation. Should not be used for the treatment of Norweigian scabies secondary to increased absorption; do not use in patients with a history of seizure disorder.)
Knowledge deficit related to medication use.	Able to verbalize appropriate treatment plan; understands potential for overuse.	1. Assure that patient or parent understands that the medication is an insecticide and uses with caution. 2. Provide written instructions. 3. Assure appropriate volume of product for number of treatments required to avoid over or undertreatment. 4. Assure the patient or parent has a plan for laundering of clothing and treating personal care items to avoid reinfestation.

5. The hyperkeratosis, fissuring, and numbers of mites makes eradication difficult. Appropriate treatment may include alternating Elimite and Kwell treatment at weekly intervals.
6. Overtreatment may occur when patients are not counseled about the persistence of pruritus for weeks after eradication of the mite.

VI. CONTACT CONSIDERATIONS

A. School.
   1. Skin-to-skin contact is generally required for the spread of the mite.
   2. Infestation is more common in crowded sleeping areas.
   3. Children with scabies often share a bed with an adult with scabies.
   4. Sleeping arrangements in day care centers may be a source of spread.
B. Nursing homes.
   1. The lowered immune response of the elderly may permit the mite to multiply unchecked.
   2. When huge numbers of mites are present, the potential for spread to others increases.

Table 8.
Potential Complications of Infestation and Potential Vector Diseases

Potential complications of infestation.	Keratoconjunctivitis, photophobia, secondary pyoderma, eczematization, nodular granulomas, urticaria, acarophobia, and delusions of parasitosis.
Potential vector diseases. *P. humanus* (body louse)	*Rickettsia prowazekii* Epidemic typhus fever *Borrelia recurrentis* Relapsing fever *Rickettsia quintana* Trench fever

C. Immunocompromised patient.
1. The reduced cell-medicated response does not kill off the developing mites.
2. Without the immune response, the itch-scratch-itch cycle does not occur and the individual does not come to early treatment.
3. Anyone in contact with a patient who is both HIV positive or undergoing chemotherapy and has scabies is at high risk of infestation due to the large numbers of mites present in these individuals.

PEDICULOSIS

I. OVERVIEW

There are two species of the order Anoplura which infest humans. The louse, which is visible to the naked eye, is endemic to all areas of the globe and is likely responsible for well over 10 million cases of infestation in the United States each year. Although the head louse may be found in all social and economic levels, the body louse and pubic louse are far more prevalent in those with crowded living conditions and uncertain hygiene.
A. Ectoparasite: *Pediculus humanus.*
1. Subspecies *Pediculus humanus corporis* or body louse.
2. Subspecies *Pediculus humanus capitis* or head louse.
B. Ectoparasite: *Phthirus pubis.*
1. Commonly called the crab louse.
2. Infests predominately the pubic hairs and other body hair with similar diameter.
C. Reproduction.
1. All three types of lice undergo five developmental stages.
a. The egg or oviposit which hatches in 5 to 10 days in response to body heat.
b. Three nymphal stages, which depend on blood meals for survival, develop over the next 8 or 9 days.
c. The adult louse is capable of mating within hours of reaching the adult stage.
2. The adult louse produces six to ten eggs a day and may lay up to 300 eggs during its life span.
3. All require blood meals for survival although they may live off a host for a period of 10 to 30 days if conditions of temperature and humidity are met.
D. Infestation.
1. *P. humanus capitis* attaches its oviposit or nit on scalp hair close to the skin.
2. *P. humanus corporis* attaches its oviposit on fabric fibers, particularly the seams of clothing.
3. *Phthirus pubis* attaches its oviposit on hairs at the skin line of the pubic region, the beard, eyebrows, eyelashes, and in the axillae.

E. Lesion varies by species.
1. The head louse produces pruritic red papules above the shoulders, often with dark red spots visible on the neck and shoulders from fecal droppings.
2. The body louse produces an urticarial papule. With extensive infestation, the skin may become dry and scaly with the development of hyperpigmented areas.
3. Pubic lice often produce gray-blue areas called maculae ceruleae over the trunk and thighs.
F. Immune response.
1. Develops from saliva injected into the skin when the louse prepares to feed.
2. The saliva prevents blood from clotting while feeding occurs.

II. ASSESSMENT

A. History and physical exam.
1. Presence of pruritus, often worse at night.
2. Lackluster hair and presence of cervical adenopathy and purulent dermatitis with heavy or prolonged infestation by the head louse.
3. Presence of urticarial papules, dry and scaly skin with body louse infestation.
4. Presence of macules over the thighs and trunk with infestation by the pubic louse.
5. Evidence of louse on the body or in the clothing on close inspection.
a. Presence of fecal dropping in the seams of clothing.
b. If suspicion is high and no lice are found on the clothing, question when the last change of clothing was made.
6. Presence of the nit on the hair shaft with head and pubic lice.
a. The position of the nit from the skin surface is indicative of the time since attachment, moving with the growing hair.
b. Nits spread at multiple intervals along the hair shaft indicate prolonged or repeated infestations.
c. Egg casings distant from the scalp are empty or contain killed ova.
B. Diagnostic tests.
1. Visualization of the louse on the skin or clothing, presence of oviposits.
2. Wood's light will cause fluorescence of hair infested with head lice.

III. TREATMENT MODALITIES

A. Medication for head lice.
1. 1% permethrin lotion (Elimite/Nix®) applied to hair after pretreatment shampoo, rinse, and towel drying.
a. Lotion is allowed to remain on hair for 10

minutes followed by rinse and towel drying with a clean towel.

    b. Provides protection from re-infestation for 2 weeks.

2. Gamma benzene hexachloride (GBH) (1% lindane, Kwell shampoo) may be used for treatment but additional cautions are warranted.

    a. Treatment is often less effective than with permethrin.

    b. Apply to wet hair; 15 to 30 ml for short hair, 45 ml for medium length, and up to 60 ml for very long hair.

    c. Allow to remain on the hair for 4 minutes before adding water to work up a lather.

    d. Thoroughly rinse and towel dry.

    e. To reduce chance of excess absorption, wear gloves while applying, avoid getting shampoo on other body parts, and do not apply any occlusive covering.

    f. May require one repeat treatment in 7 to 10 days.

3. Pyrethrin (RID) may be used for any type of pediculosis infestation.

    a. Available over the counter, this product is less effective than other pediculicides.

    b. Apply and wash off after 10 minutes.

    c. High potential for misuse due to lack of understanding of treatment schedule.

    d. Chemically related to chrysanthemums and may cause hypersensitivity reactions in some individuals.

B. Medications for pubic and body lice.

1. GBH 1% lotion or cream (1% lindane, Kwell) applied to dry skin after bathing, drying, and allowing skin to cool to reduce absorption of the insecticide.

    a. Lotion or cream is applied in a thin film from the neck to the soles.

    b. The application is allowed to dry and remain on the skin for 8 to 12 hours.

    c. Remove application by thorough washing; dry skin use clean towels.

    d. Dress in clothing which have already been washed in hot water or dry-cleaned.

    e. 60 ml lotion is sufficient to treat an adult; use proportionally less for children.

2. Petrolatum may be applied to eyelashes 2 to 3 times a day to aid in removing lice or nits.

3. 0.25% physostigmine ointment (Eserine®) may be used on the eyelashes. No other insecticide should be used around the eyes.

4. Pyrethrin as with scabies treatment.

5. Additional insecticides are available for special cases such as infants and pregnant and lactating females.

    a. Products generally have objectionable qualities and require multiple applications.

    b. Consult with physician, pharmacist, or drug resource.

C. Care of fomites.

1. All head coverings such as scarves and caps must be dry-cleaned or washed in hot water.

2. Combs, brushes, curlers, and hair clips and bows should be washed in hot water.

3. Clothing worn by those with heavy body louse infestation may need the additional precaution of ironing of the seams as this is the attachment area for oviposits.

IV. COMMON NURSING DIAGNOSES, OUTCOMES, AND INTERVENTIONS (see Table 7)

V. COMPLICATIONS

A. Complications rare except in debilitated individuals with secondary infections.

B. Potential for vector diseases (see Table 8).

VI. CONTACT CONSIDERATIONS

A. School.

1. The close proximity of children playing and sleeping make spread of the head louse relatively easy.

2. Children tend to share items that serve as fomites: combs, brushes, and hats.

3. All children in the same classroom or sleeping area of day care centers must be checked for possible infestation.

4. Parents must be informed to treat the infested child and all infested family members at the same time.

5. Parents must be educated about lice and appropriate treatments to reduce their anxiety and potential for hiding contacts.

6. Re-inspection should be carried out at regular intervals to reduce the possibility of re-infestation.

7. Pubic lice in young or adolescent children may indicate sexual activity.

B. Nursing homes.

1. The natural reduction in immune response that may occur in the elderly may contribute to the spread of lice without detection as the patient may not complain of itching.

2. All residents with evidence of lice must be treated at the same time.

3. The staff should develop a plan for replacing linen and clothing following treatment.

4. Families and visitors should be informed of outbreaks to reduce the potential for re-infesting the facility.

Bibliography

Billstein, S.A., & Mattaliano, V.J., Jr. (1990). The "nuisance" sexually transmitted diseases: Molluscum contagiosum, scabies, and crab lice. *Medical Clinics of North America, 74*(6), 1487-505.

Blondell, R.D. (1991). Parasites of the skin and hair. *Primary Care, 18*(1), 167-183.

Bond, G.R. (1992). Antivenim administration for Centruroides scorpion sting: Risks and benefits. *Annuals of Emergency Medicine, 21*(7), 788-9, 790-791.

Buchstein, S.R., & Gardner, P. (1991). Lyme disease. *Infectious Disease Clinics of North America, 5*(1), 103-116.

Clark, R.F., Wethern-Kestner, S., Vance, M.V., & Gerkin, R. (1992). Clinical presentation and treatment of black widow spider envenomation: A review of 163 cases. *Annals of Emergency Medicine, 21*(7), 782-787.

Elgart, M.L. (1993). Scabies: Diagnosis and treatment. *Dermatology Nursing, 5*(6), 464-467.

Hibel, J.A., & Clore, E.R. (1992). Prevention and primary care treatment of stings from imported fire ants. *Nurse Practitioner, 17*(6), 65-66, 68, 71.

Holmes, H.S. (1990). Stings and bites: Tips on coexisting comfortably with the insects. *Postgraduate Medicine, 88*(1), 75-78.

King, M.M. (1990). Lyme disease: A seasonal hazard. *Dermatology Nursing, 2*(4), 202-3.

Merck & Co, Inc (1999). *The Merck Manual of Diagnosis & Therapy.* Retrieved from: www.merck.com/pubs/ mmanual/section23/chapter 308/308d.htm.

Morgan, R.J. (1990). Bites, stings, and toxins. In W.M. Sams, Jr. & P.J. Lynch (Eds.), *Principals and practice of dermatology* (pp. 181-190). New York: Churchill Livingstone.

Morgan, R.J. (1990). Mite infestations and pediculosis. In W.M. Sams, Jr. & P.J. Lynch (Eds.), *Principals and practice of dermatology* (pp. 191-96). New York: Churchill Livingstone.

Orkin, M., & Maibach, H.I. (1999). Scabies & pediculosis. In T.B. Fitzpatrick, A. Eisen, K. Wolff, I. Freedberg, & K. Austen (Eds.), *Dermatology in general medicine.* New York: McGraw-Hill, Inc.

Pardo, R.J., & Kerdel, F.A. (1992). Parasites, arthropods, and hazardous animals of dermatological significance. In S. Moschella & J. Hurley (Eds.), *Dermatology* (pp.1957-1983). Philadelphia: W.B. Saunders Company.

Roof, G.W. (1994). Bites, stings, and infestations. In M. Hill (Ed.), *Mosby's clinical nursing series: Skin disorders* (pp. 94-115). St. Louis: Mosby.

Roenigk, H.H. Jr. (1981). Diseases due to parasites. *Office dermatology* (pp. 155-160). Baltimore: Williams and Wilkins.

Sharf, M.J., & Daly, J.S. (1999). Bites and stings of terrestrial & aquatic life. In T.B. Fitzpatrick, A. Eisen, K. Wolff, I. Freedberg, & K. Austen (Eds.), *Dermatology in general medicine.* New York: McGraw-Hill, Inc.

Spach, D.H., Liles, W.C., Campbell, G.L., Quick, R.E., Anderson, D.E., & Fritsche, T.R. (1993). Tick-borne diseases in the United States. *New England Journal of Medicine, 329*(3), 936-947.

Weber, D.J., & Walker, D.H. (1991). Rocky mountain spotted fever. *Infectious Disease Clinics of North America, 5*(1),19-35.

Wilson, D.C., Leyva, W.H., & King, L.E. (1999). Arthropod bites and stings. In T.B. Fitzpatrick, A. Eisen, K. Wolff, I. Freedberg, & K. Austen (Eds.), *Dermatology in general medicine* (pp. 2810-2826). New York: McGraw-Hill, Inc.

Mr. Garcia is a 30-year-old Hispanic male, married with no children. He comes to the office complaining of recent onset of a rash over much of his body. You note hyperkeratotic lesions on his elbows and over his knuckles. There is evidence of some fissuring on several of his fingers. He denies excessive itching, fever, chills, or any drainage from the skin. His medication history includes immunosuppressive drugs which he states he has been taking for 2 years following renal transplant.

1. In preparing for his examination by the physician, you should:
   a. Complete the history, have the patient disrobe, and await the physician.
   b. Put on gloves before conducting the examination, have the patient disrobe and place his clothes over a sheet which you have placed in a chair. Wash your hands before leaving the examination room.
   c. Put on gown, mask, and gloves. Do not permit Mr. Garcia to sit on the exam table.
   d. Treat Mr. Garcia like any other patient without need for skin barriers.

2. To help the physician prepare for diagnostic work-up, you would prepare the following equipment.
   a. A Wood's lamp.
   b. A punch biopsy kit.
   c. A number 15 blade and bottle of formalin.
   d. Mineral oil, several slides, and a number 15 scalpel.

3. After examination and diagnosis, you would expect the treatment plan for Mr. Garcia to include the following *except:*
   a. Use of 1% permethrin product and an antipruritic.
   b. Specific instructions to wash or dry-clean clothing and bed linen after treatment.
   c. Treatment of his wife.
   d. Treatment with insecticide.

4. Because of his suppressed immune system, which of the following explains why Mr. Garcia is likely to spread scabies to more casual contacts than most patients with scabies.
   a. The scabies mite multiplies faster in the immunocompetent patient.
   b. A delayed or sluggish immune response does not kill the mite, allowing it to multiply unchecked.
   c. The mite will jump off a host with suppressed immunity, seeking another host.
   d. Blood from the fissures comes in contact with other hosts.

5. A thorough understanding of the immune response to scabies in immunocompetent individuals explains which of the following signs and symptoms from Mr. Garcia's wife:
   a. Intense itching, worse at night, starting several weeks after infestation.
   b. Presence of hundreds of serpentine burrows concentrated about her hands and feet.
   c. Fever and chills which occurred 3 days after infestation.
   d. Intense itching, worse in the morning, which started several months after Mr. Garcia's transplant.

Sara Madden, age 10, has been sent home from school by the school nurse. Sara's mother is distraught and, although she has the nurse's instruction sheet on head lice, she obviously will require careful instruction.

6. All of the following beliefs about head lice which Ms. Madden is able to verbalize are true *except:*
   a. Head lice are very common among children, especially girls.
   b. Head lice are evidence of poor body hygiene.
   c. Treatment is most effective if all family members found to be infested are treated at the same time.
   d. Presence of egg casings on the hair shaft following treatment are not an indicator of treatment failure.

7. Your instruction to Ms. Madden is most effective if you include the following information.
   a. It is common for school-aged children to get head lice. Over-the-counter products for lice can be used prophylactically.
   b. All members of the family should be treated for lice at the same time. A permethrin product applied to the hair can be left on overnight before shampooing.
   c. Most pediculocides are left on the hair only 10 minutes before rinsing. Use of a nit comb will aid in removing the egg casings.
   d. Repeating the treatment for head lice 3 days in a row will assure complete eradication and provide immunity to future infestations.

8. After you calm Ms. Madden, you are able to have her participate in a plan for treatment for Sara and other family members as needed. Which of the following information is most important for Ms. Madden.
   a. Over-the-counter products are available for treating lice.
   b. All head coverings, hair ornaments, and bed linen should be washed in hot water.
   c. Permethrins and pyrethrines are effective for treatment but pyrethrines may be associated with hypersensitivity reactions in those sensitive to chrysanthemums.
   d. All of the above.

Mr. Clark arrived at your office complaining of severe itching especially over his trunk. He states that he has recently started work, has moved out of a homeless shelter into an apartment, has had no chemical exposure, and has had no recent sexual contacts.

9. Infestations are common in homeless shelters. The pattern of itching is most likely indicative of which ectoparasite.
   a. The head louse, *P. humanus capitis.*
   b. The body louse, *P. humanus corporis.*
   c. The crab or pubic louse, *Phthirus pubis.*
   d. The itch mite, *Sarcoptes scabiei.*

10. You assist with the examination of Mr. Clark. There are urticarial papules evident over much of the back, groin, and thighs. The skin is dry and scaly with hyperpigmentation prominent on the lower back. Understanding the nature of the infestation, you should expect to find:
    a. Evidence of lice in the hair of the groin with nits attached to the hair shaft.
    b. Multiple burrows, especially on the shaft of the penis, over the flexor surfaces of the wrists and in the axillae.
    c. Few or absent lice on the body, no evidence of nits.
    d. Presence of lice and nits in the pubic hair and in the axillae.

11. Because of his economic status, the following information would prove most helpful to Mr. Clark.
    a. Iron one set of underwear, shirt, and slacks tonight for use in the morning. Use prescribed treatment or over-the-counter product at bedtime. In the morning, place clothing and bed linen in a plastic bag, seal, and prepare to wash and dry them on hot cycle after work. Shower and dress in clothes that have been ironed.
    b. Iron one set of underwear, shirt, and slacks. Use product, leave on skin for 10 minutes then shower. Dress in ironed clothing. Carefully place all linen and clothing in a plastic bag and take to the laundry. Set washer and dryer on hot cycle.
    c. Use permethrin product every evening for 3 days. This eliminates the need for laundry.
    d. All clothing articles must be dry-cleaned. Use insecticide, applying as a body shampoo, and wash off after 10 minutes.

Answers to Study Questions

1.	b	5.	a	9.	b
2.	d	6.	b	10.	c
3.	a	7.	c	11.	a
4.	b	8.	d		

Chapter 16.
Bites, Stings, and Infestations

Please photocopy this test page and return.

COMPLETE THE FOLLOWING:

Name: _____

Address: _____

City: _____ State: _____ Zip: _____

Preferred telephone: (Home)_____ (Work) _____

State where licensed and license number: _____

CE application fee: DNA member $7.00
                         Nonmember $10.00

POSTTEST INSTRUCTIONS
1. To receive continuing education credit for individual study after reading the article, complete the answer/evaluation form below.
2. Photocopy and send the answer/evaluation form along with a check or money order payable to **Dermatology Nurses' Association** to: *DNA*, East Holly Avenue Box 56, Pitman, NJ 08071-0056.
3. Test returns must be postmarked by December 31, 2008. Upon completion of the answer/evaluation form, a certificate for 1.7 contact hour(s) will be awarded and sent to you.

This chapter was reviewed and formatted for contact hour credit by Marcia J. Hill, MSN, RN, Core Curriculum Editor; and Sally Russell, MN, RN,C, DNA Education Director.

ANSWER FORM

1. Name one new detail (item, issue, or phenomenon) that you learned by completing this activity.

_____

_____

_____

2. How will you apply the information from this learning activity to your practice?
   a. Patient education.
   b. Staff education.
   c. Improve my patient care.
   d. In my education course work.
   e. Other: Please describe _____

_____

_____

Evaluation

	Strongly disagree				Strongly agree
3. The offering met the stated objectives.					
a. Identify the common skin manifestations of biting and stinging insects.	1	2	3	4	5
b. List appropriate avoidance behaviors that may reduce exposure to biting and stinging insects.	1	2	3	4	5
c. Describe common therapeutic interventions used to return the skin and tissues to pre-exposure condition	1	2	3	4	5
d. Identify the causative ectoparasite in scabies and lice infestations.	1	2	3	4	5
e. List the most common treatments and cautions for treating infestations.	1	2	3	4	5
f. List environmental and fomite treatments which prevent re-infestation.	1	2	3	4	5
4. The content was current and relevant.	1	2	3	4	5
5. The content was presented clearly.	1	2	3	4	5
6. The content was covered adequately.	1	2	3	4	5
7. I am more confident of my abilities since completing this material.	1	2	3	4	5

8. The material was (check one) ☐ new, ☐ review for me.

Comments _____

_____

9. Time required to complete reading assignment: _____ minutes

This independent study is provided by the Dermatology Nurses' Association (DNA) for 1.7 contact hours. DNA is accredited as a provider of continuing education in nursing by the American Nurses Credentialing Center's Commission on Accreditation. DNA is approved as a provider of continuing education by the California Board of Registered Nursing Provider #CEP5708.

Dermatologic Considerations in Ethnic Skin

Marrise M. Phillips, BS, RN, CCRC, DNC

OBJECTIVES

At the end of this chapter, the reader will be able to:

- List normal variations in pigmentation in people of color.
- Identify skin disorders commonly occurring in ethnic individuals.
- Discuss the changes in treatment modalities necessary for skin diseases unique to the ethnic population.
- Recognize differences in the manifestation of skin disease in the ethnic population.
- Identify the psychosocial impact imposed by skin diseases unique to the ethnic population.

KEY POINTS

- The U.S. Census Bureau estimates that by the year 2050, people of ethnic skin will make up almost half of the American population. These changing demographics will change health care needs dramatically.
- For the purpose of this chapter, Asian, Black, and Hispanic skin types will be considered as representative of the ethnic population.
- Dermatology, as much as any other field, will need to expand to better serve this particular group of patients with their unique needs
- Distinguishing between normal and pathological variations in the ethnic population by the health care clinician is essential to the successful management of this group of clients.
- Social customs, traditional beliefs, mistrust, and fear influence adherence to treatment regimes.
- Post-inflammatory hyperpigmentation may persist long after the disease is cleared in darkly pigmented skin.
- Patient and family education must include precautions that will prevent disfigurement.

Dermatologic Considerations in Ethnic Skin

Marrise M. Phillips, BS, RN, CCRC, DNC

VARIANTS OF ETHNIC SKIN TYPES

I. OVERVIEW

Most skin diseases occur in all types of skin. Fitzpatrick separated skin types by photo-responsiveness; skin Types III, IV, V, and VI compose the ethnic population that is being addressed. It is important to recognize normal pigmentation variants in ethnic people in order to distinguish these variations from pathologic conditions.

A. Differences in skin type.
   1. Johnson reports pigment, follicular response, fibroblast hyperresponsivity, curly hair, and ashiness to be the major clinical differences in ethnic skin.
      a. Pigment: in black individuals, melanosomes are singly grouped and are much larger than in whites. Melanosomes in whites are grouped together, as is the case with Asians of Chinese descent. Melanosomes are distributed throughout the entire epidermis of blacks, in the lower epidermis in whites, and the distribution tends to be variable in Asians. In Hispanics, distribution is also variable and specifically related to the skin phototype.
      b. Follicular reactivity is common to many dermatologic diseases in black skin — follicular accentuation is clearly visible in darker-skinned individuals, as can be seen in pityriasis rosea, atopic dermatitis, nummular eczema, and sarcoidosis.
      c. Fibroblast hyperresponsivity, which is thought to be induced by mast cell/fibroblast interaction and prolonged by a decrease in collagenase activity, leads to another characteristic of black skin — keloid formation
      d. Curly hair: In people of African descent, hair tends to curl and spontaneously knot and break. With straight hair being stylish, reconstruction of the hair shaft performed with chemicals and heat and hot oils tend to cause hair shaft fracture and scalp scarring which can result in temporary or permanent alopecia.
      e. Ashiness: people with dark skin are ashy white when the skin is dry and scaly; although this scaling occurs in lighter skin it is not as clinically evident.

NORMAL SKIN CHANGES IN DARKER-SKINNED PATIENTS

I. DEFINITION

A. Pigmentary demarcation lines (PDLs) also described as Voigt's and Futcher's lines consist of a demarcation between darkly pigmented and lightly pigmented portions of the upper arms in blacks. For our purpose we will deal with Types A and B PDLs which are those with sharp transition.

II. ETIOLOGY

A. Unknown.
B. One theory suggests that the purpose of PDLs is protection. The dorsal skin is more heavily pigmented to provide protection from the sun.

III. INCIDENCE

A. African descent — 20% to 60%.
B. Asian descent — less frequently.
C. Japanese — 4% (more often in women than men)
D. Caucasians — rarely seen.
E. Evident at birth or is noted in childhood.

IV. ASSESSMENT

A. Physical examination.
   1. PDLs (Futcher's, Voigt's) lines are distinct lines of demarcation between darkly pigmented skin laterally and lighter skin anteromedially along the length of the arm.
   2. Lines may follow the distribution of spinal nerves.
   3. Lines are clearly seen on the skin.
   4. PDLs (Futcher's, Voigt's) lines can be present on the posteromedial aspect of the lower leg in women of African descent; and are more pronounced during pregnancy.

V. TREATMENT MODALITIES

A. PDLs have no clinical significance other than cosmetic considerations.
B. No treatment is available, but thankfully treatment is not needed.

IV. NURSING DIAGNOSES, OUTCOMES, AND INTERVENTIONS (see Table 1)

A. Alteration in body image.

Table 1.
Common Nursing Diagnoses, Outcomes, and Interventions

Nursing Diagnoses	Outcomes	Interventions
Alteration in body image related to presence of skin lesions.	Verbalization of feelings demonstrates appropriate coping with situation.	Discuss condition thoroughly with patient allowing time for questions and expression of feelings; encourage participation of family/significant other.
Alteration in comfort related to pruritus or pain.	Patient will express increased comfort level.	Decrease environmental stimuli; explain treatment and need for compliance in order to help relieve discomfort; initiate appropriate therapy (baths, soaks, humidifier, emollients) to relieve discomfort.
Increased risk for infection related to impaired integument due to scratching, rubbing, dryness, shaving.	Patient's skin will remain free of infection.	Assess skin frequently for signs of infection; educate patient about signs/symptoms of infection; emphasize importance of compliance to prescribed treatments.
Anxiety related to abnormal appearance of the skin.	Patient will verbalize confidence in ability to care for himself, and understanding of treatment or nontreatment.	Explain diagnosis thoroughly; answer all questions about any therapy planned, or if no therapy planned, explain reason.

B. Anxiety related to abnormal skin appearance.

NAIL PIGMENTATION – (Longitudinal Melanonychia)

I. DEFINITION
A. Longitudinal, linear, dark bands found in the nail plates.

II. ETIOLOGY
A. Pigmentation is due to increased melanin deposits in the nail plates.
B. May be associated with melanocytes within the nail matrix.

III. INCIDENCE
A. African descent — 50%.
B. May exceed 90% in very dark-skinned individuals.
C. Increases with age.

IV. ASSESSMENT
A. Physical examination.
    1. Longitudinal, pigmented nail stripes in the nail plates, width varying from one to several millimeters; may be single or multiple in number.

2. Distribution of nail pigment may be diffuse rather than linear.

V. DIAGNOSIS
A. Related to distribution and clinical findings.
B. Melanoma should be considered.

VI. TREATMENT MODALITIES
A. No treatment is necessary.
B. Biopsy is warranted if high suspicion of malignancy is present.

VII. NURSING DIAGNOSES, OUTCOMES, AND INTERVENTIONS (see Table 1)
A. Alteration in body image.
B. Anxiety related to abnormal skin appearance.

PALMAR AND PLANTAR PIGMENTATION

I. OVERVIEW
In dark skin, the palms and soles are usually lighter in color than the rest of the body. Palmar or plantar pigmentations frequently present in varying degrees.

II. ASSESSMENT

A. **Physical examination.**
1. Palmar pigmentation normally occurs in flexural and digital creases.
2. Small hyperkeratotic papules that evolve into discrete, conical depressions (pits) are also common; limited to palmar and digital creases.
3. Pigmented macules are commonly seen on the palms and soles of darker-skinned individuals; these lesions are usually multiple, non-erythematous, irregularly shaped with indistinct borders, varying in color from tan to dark brown.
4. Plantar pigmentation is normally present in people with dark skin; however, may be present in light skin as well.

B. **Diagnosis.**
1. Physical examination.
2. Plantar lesions also occur in secondary syphilis.
3. Possibility of melanoma should not be overlooked.

C. **Treatment modalities.**
1. None indicated.

D. **Nursing diagnoses, outcomes, and interventions (see Table 1).**
1. Alteration in body image.
2. Anxiety related to abnormal skin appearance.

COMMON DISEASES IN THE DARKER-SKINNED ADULT

I. OVERVIEW

Dermatologic diagnosis is often more difficult to reach in the darker-skinned patient because subtle changes in skin color may be hidden. Pink and light red hues may be totally missed. Dark reds and browns may appear as purple, grey, or black. Patient history, distribution of lesions, and skin surface changes become the most important diagnostic tools.

II. ATOPIC DERMATITIS

A. **Definition: an acute or subacute, usually chronic, pruritic inflammation of the epidermis and dermis.**

B. **Etiology.**
1. Hereditary predisposition.

C. **Incidence.**
1. Onset first 2 months to 12 years with 60% of patients by the first year.
2. More common in boys than girls.
3. Equal frequency in all races.

III. ASSESSMENT

A. **History and physical.**
1. Erythema, papules, scaling excoriations, and crusting.
2. Lichenification.
3. Lesions confluent and ill defined.
4. Characteristic features of atopic dermatitis in dark-skinned individuals; tendency to develop follicular lesions.
   a. Children may present with widespread follicular papules antedating the more diagnostically obvious lichenification stage.
   b. Follicular prominence may occur in many diseases of black skin, not limited to atopic dermatitis. For example:
      (1) Lichen planus.
      (2) Secondary syphilis.
      (3) Tinea versicolor.
      (4) Eczematous disorders.

B. **Diagnosis.**
1. Ancillary criteria may be necessary to diagnose atopic dermatitis in dark-skinned patients.
   a. Family history of atopy.
   b. Asthma or allergic rhinitis.
   c. Demonstrable dermographism.
   d. Biopsy confirmation of eczema.

III. COMMON TREATMENT MODALITIES (see Chapter 3)

IV. COMMON NURSING DIAGNOSES, OUTCOMES, AND INTERVENTIONS (see Table 1)

A. Alteration in body image.
B. Alteration in comfort related to pruritus or pain.
C. Increased risk for infection related to impaired integument due to scratching, rubbing, and dryness.
D. Anxiety related to abnormal skin appearance.

PITYRIASIS ROSEA

I. OVERVIEW

Self-limiting papulosquamous disorder affecting young adults.

A. **Etiology.**
1. Unknown, presumed viral.

B. **Pathophysiology.**
1. Prodromal signs are minimal or absent.
2. First sign is a herald patch 2 to 6 cm in diameter. Resembles tinea corporis.
3. From days to weeks later, a generalized eruption consisting of oval plaques develops on covered regions of the body.
4. Sites — chest, trunk, thighs, upper arms.

C. **Incidence.**
1. Occurs in all racial groups.
2. More common during the winter months.
3. Age 10 to 35.
4. Composes 2% of dermatologic outpatients.

II. ASSESSMENT

A. **History and physical.**
  1. Pruritus.
  2. Characteristic features.
     a. In light skin, lesions are salmon-pink. Color may not be seen in dark skin.
     b. In dark skin, lesions assume a dull reddish brown to deep brown or black color.
     c. The fine scale, difficult to see in light skin, is prominent in dark skin.
     d. Papular and papulovesicular variants are more commonly seen in dark skin. May resemble nummular eczema or plaques of atopic dermatitis.
     e. Lesions completely disappear in whites. Pityriasis rosea may result in persistent post-inflammatory changes in dark skin.

C. **Diagnosis.**
  1. May be difficult to distinguish from secondary syphilis, if herald patch is absent.
  2. Normal plantar macules in dark skin may be mistaken for syphilis.
  3. Pityriasis rosea does not affect the palms and soles.
  4. Examine palms and soles for stigmata of syphilis.

III. COMMON THERAPEUTIC MODALITIES

A. **Most patients require no treatment.**
B. **UVB to control pruritus.**
C. **Antipruritic lotions, emollients, antihistamines.**
D. **Topical corticosteroids in severe inflammatory cases.**

IV. NURSING DIAGNOSES, OUTCOMES, AND INTERVENTIONS (see Table 1)

A. **Alteration in body image.**
B. **Alteration in comfort related to pruritus or pain.**
C. **Increased risk for infection related to impaired integument due to scratching, rubbing, and dryness.**
D. **Anxiety related to abnormal skin appearance.**

PSORIASIS

I. OVERVIEW

Psoriasis is a visible, disfiguring disease. Clinical features and distribution in whites and dark-skinned people are the same. The presentation may be different making diagnosis difficult. It can be emotionally and mentally disturbing in the lives of patients.

A. **Definition: psoriasis is a common papulosquamous proliferation disorder.**
B. **Etiology.**

  1. Unknown, considered by some to be a hereditary disorder.
  2. Chronic disease; can resolve spontaneously in some cases.

C. **Pathology.**
  1. Typically, well-demarcated erythematous, scaly plaques of various size occurring as individual lesions or coalescing into large plaques.
  2. Scale: white and thin, resembling mica. When removed, leaves pinpoint foci of bleeding (Auspitz sign).
  3. Characteristic distribution in areas of repeated trauma (Koebner's phenomenon).

D. **Incidence.**
  1. Overall in U.S. — 1%.
  2. Affects men and women equally.
  3. Average age of onset — early 20s.
  4. Blacks of West Africa — low as 0.1%.
  5. East African black population — incidence of psoriasis equal or exceeds that in Caucasians or European descent.

II. ASSESSMENT

A. **History and physical.**
  1. Pruritus.
  2. Characteristic scaling may be absent.
  3. Lesions may appear bluish black hue due to pigment incontinence.
  4. Distribution — elbows, knees, scalp. May involve all or any part of the body, including nail beds.

B. **Diagnosis.**
  1. Aided by observing:
     a. Distribution of lesions.
     b. Ancillary physical signs:
        (1) Nail pitting.
        (2) Oil slick onycholysis.
           (a) Oil slick — discoloration around the periphery of the nails.
           (b) Onycholysis — lighter areas where nails have separated from nail bed.

III. THERAPEUTIC MODALITIES (see Chapter 3)

A. **Medical.**
  1. Depends on distribution of lesions, age, and severity of disease.
  2. Topical corticosteroids.
  3. Intralesional steroids.
  4. UVB radiation.
  5. PUVA.
  6. Systemic therapy.
  7. After therapy, post-inflammatory hyperpigmentation may persist.

IV. NURSING DIAGNOSES, OUTCOMES, AND INTERVENTIONS (see Table 1)

A. Alteration in body image.
B. Alteration in comfort related to pruritus or pain.
C. Increased risk for infection related to impaired integument due to scratching, rubbing, and dryness.
D. Anxiety related to abnormal skin appearance.

FOLLICULAR OCCLUSION TRIAD

I. OVERVIEW

The follicular occlusion triad is made up of three diseases that often occur together: hidradenitis suppurativa, acne conglobata, and dissecting cellulitis of the scalp.

A. Definition: hidradenitis suppurativa is a difficult disease to treat involving the apocrine gland-bearing skin of the axilla, groin, inflamammary area, and the anogenital region. Symptoms range from mild discomfort to debilitation. The patient with acne conglobata is affected with multiple comedomes, inflammatory nodules with pus, scarring, and sinus tracts of the back, buttocks, face, and chest. These large comedomes tend to have multiple openings. The patient with dissecting cellulitis of the scalp (also known as perifolliculitis capitis abscendens et suffodiens) is plagued by inflammatory nodules, sinus tracts, chronic drainage, crusting alopecia, and scarring.

B. Etiology.
  1. Predisposing factors.
    a. Obesity.
    b. Predisposition to acne.
    c. Obstruction of apocrine duct.
    d. Bacterial infection.

C. Pathophysiology.
  1. Apocrine duct plugged with keratinous material.
  2. Dilatation of apocrine duct and hair follicle.
  3. Severe inflammation of apocrine gland.
  4. Bacterial growth in dilated ducts.
  5. Extension of inflammation/infection secondary to ruptured duct/gland.
  6. Extension of suppuration/tissue destruction.
  7. Ulceration and fibrosis.
  8. Sinus tract formation.

D. Incidence.
  1. Onset puberty.
  2. Usually undergo a spontaneous remission with age (over 35).
  3. Men tend to be affected in anogenital area; women in axillae.

II. ASSESSMENT

A. History and physical.

1. Intermittent pain, mild to extreme tenderness.
2. Multiple inflamed erythematous nodular lesions. Abscesses are frequent and drain purulent/seropurulent material.
3. Sinus tracts form and drain pus; fibrosis, hypertrophic and keloidal scars form; contractures.
4. Open comedomes form. Double comedomes may develop even when active nodules are absent.
5. Lesions may also be found in inguinal folds, gluteal cleft, perineum, or breast and may extend over back and buttocks.
6. Obesity.
7. Severe cystic acne.

B. Diagnosis.
  1. Clinical exam and history.
  2. Bacterial cultures from drainage.
    a. *Staphylococcus aureus.*
    b. *Staphylococcus millieri.*
    c. Anaerobic streptococcus.
    d. Bacteroides species.
    e. *Pseudomonas aeruginosa.*

III. THERAPEUTIC MODALITIES

A. Medical.
  1. Antibiotics
    a. Early.
      (1) Antibiotics.
      (2) Erythromycin 250 to 500 mg qid.
      (3) Tetracycline 250 to 500 mg qid.
      (4) Minocycline 100 mg bid until lesions resolve.
      (5) Intralesional triamcinolone 3 to 5 mg/ml.
    b. Late.
      (1) Maintenance with antibiotics.
      (2) Prednisone 70 mg.
      (3) Taper over 14 days if pain and inflammation are severe.

B. Surgical.
  1. Axillary hidradenitis suppurativa responds well to removal of apocrine sweat glands.
  2. Inguinal — surgical control is more difficult and less successful.
  3. Oral 13-cis-retinoic (role not clearly established) — 2 mg/kg/day appears effective in early disease and when combined with surgical excision of individual lesions.

IV. NURSING DIAGNOSES, OUTCOMES, AND INTERVENTIONS (see Table 1)

A. Alteration in body image.
B. Alteration in comfort related to pain.
C. Increased risk for infection related to impaired integument.

KELOIDS

I. OVERVIEW

Represent bizarre exaggeration of the normal fibroblastic process involved in wound healing. Keloids are difficult to treat and recur.

A. **Definition:** shiny, hyperpigmented, thick, raised, hard, papulonodular plaques and tumors characterized by deposition of excessive amounts of collagen.

B. **Etiology.**
   1. Unknown.
   2. Usually occur following injury to skin but may appear spontaneously without skin trauma.
   3. Keloids tend to form in dark-skinned people more frequently than in people with light skin.
   4. Possible sources of keloid formation: any minor or major surgical procedure, many inflammatory or bullous skin disorders, burns, accidental traumatic events, vaccinations, and secondary infections.

C. **Pathophysiology.**
   1. Exuberant fibrous repair tissue following a cutaneous injury.
   2. Benign growths or small papules.
   3. Papules grow into large nodules and plaques, often with claw-like extensions.
   4. Growth may be slow or become large in a short time.

D. **Incidence.**
   1. Equal incidence in males and females.
   2. More common in blacks than whites.
   3. Occur more often on young adults. This enables the keloids to reach their full growth.
   4. Research indicates that keloids are also common in other groups.
      a. Chinese population in Malaysia.
      b. Light-skinned people of Finland.

II. ASSESSMENT

A. **History and physical.**
   1. Usually asymptomatic.
   2. May be pruritic or painful.
   3. Firm, smooth, hairless, shiny, and raised above the surrounding skin surface.
   4. May be red; progress to brownish red hue; become hyperpigmented or hypopigmented over time.
   5. Erythema may not be noticed in dark skin.
   6. May be linear following traumatic or surgical injury. Sometimes confused with hypertrophic scars.
      a. Keloids differ from hypertrophic scars in that keloidal tissue growth, in a traumatized site extends beyond the boundary of the injury.
      b. Tissue growth from hypertrophic scar

remains confined to the site of original injury.
      c. Hypertrophic scars tend to regress, flatten, and soften over time.
      d. Keloids may continue to expand in size for years.
      e. Hypertrophic scars are likely to form soon after injury, whereas keloids may not begin growing until months later.
   7. Spontaneous regression is rare.
   8. Common sites: ear lobes, shoulders, upper back, neck, chest, skin overlying the jaw, lateral chest (in women).

B. **Diagnosis.**
   1. Clinical examination.
   2. Biopsy not warranted; it may induce new scar.

III. THERAPEUTIC MODALITIES

A. **Medical.**
   1. Intralesional injection — triamcinolone 10 to 40 mg/ml once a month to reduce pruritus and sensitivity of lesion, reduce its volume, and flatten it.
   2. Intralesional triamcinolone plus cryotherapy may be a little more effective. The corticosteroid must be injected directly into the bulk of the keloid.
   3. Corticosteroid injections may cause temporary hypopigmentation at or around the injection site. Usually resolves within a few months.
   4. Atrophy may occur in the surrounding skin if corticosteroid inadvertently gets injected into the surrounding normal tissue.
   5. Interferon injections 0.01 to 0.1 mg three times per week for 3 consecutive weeks.
   6. Silicon gel sheeting for 12 to 24 hours daily for 8 to 12 weeks or longer may flatten keloid.

B. **Surgical.**
   1. Simple surgical excisions. Lesions may grow back larger than the original lesion.
   2. Simple surgical excisions and steroid injections followed by pressure dressing. Pressure dressing is most effective if it is maintained for at least 4 to 6 months after surgery.
   3. Laser surgery produces the best result for keloids on the earlobes or scalp.
   4. Other techniques employed — skin grafts, random pattern flaps, and radiation alone or with excision and electrosurgery.

IV. NURSING DIAGNOSES, OUTCOMES, AND INTERVENTIONS (see Table 1)

A. **Alteration in body image.**
B. **Alteration in comfort related to pruritus or pain.**
C. **Increased risk for infection related to surgical procedure.**
D. **Anxiety secondary to abnormal skin appearance.**

I. OVERVIEW

Hair and scalp disorders related to grooming practices occur more frequently in people with dark skin and curly hair. For years hot combing was the popular choice. Currently, braids and weaves are more fashionable due to easy maintenance in busy lifestyles. However, the repeated process that beautifies and makes curly hair manageable also damages the scalp and hair. Traction alopecia and hot comb alopecia are the result of using these grooming techniques extensively.

A. Definition: traction alopecia is a gradually developing patchy hair loss resulting from the cumulative effects of prolonged traction on scalp and hair. Hot comb alopecia is the traumatic hair loss caused by straightening and styling the hair with a hot comb following the application of oils or pomades.

B. Etiology: traction alopecia.
   1. Traction alopecia.
      a. Braiding: cornrowing the hair frequently and tightly; sometimes adding jewelry, beads, and synthetic hair.
      b. Weaving: cornrowing the hair, then attaching natural human or synthetic hair to the hair or gluing it to the scalp. May glue human hair strand by strand to natural hair.
   2. Hot comb alopecia.
      a. Heat from the hot comb causes the hair to break. Hot oil flows down the hair shaft damaging the fair follicles.

C. Pathophysiology.
   1. Traction alopecia.
      a. The individual's hair is braided with or without the addition of human or synthetic hair.
      b. Extensive tension is placed on the hair follicle causing follicular erythema and follicular pustules.
      c. Condition is exacerbated by oils and pomades.
      d. Follicular atrophy results in a non-inflammatory permanent alopecia.
      e. Commonly affects the frontal and temporal hairline.
   2. Hot comb alopecia.
      a. Application of oil or pomade to shampooed and dried hair.
      b. Pulling a heated metal comb from roots to end.
      c. Curling the hair with electric or marcel curling iron heated to 300 to 500 degrees F.
      d. Breakage and rearrangement of hydrogen bonds by the high temperature straightens the hair.
      e. Reverse the process by adding moisture to the hair.
      f. Burning of skin surface when hot oil flows down the hair shaft causing inflammation.
      g. Scarring causes a decrease in the number of hair follicles.
      h. Epidermal atrophy.
      i. Common site — predominantly vertex of scalp (central, frontal, and parietal areas).

D. Incidence.
   1. More common among American blacks.
   2. Black children through pre-puberty to older adults.
   3. More widespread due to fashionable acceptance of hair grooming customs.
   4. Recent studies reveal that hot comb alopecia pattern of hair loss is occurring in men who do not hot comb their hair but do use oil and pomades. The term "follicular degeneration syndrome" has been recommended to encompass the broader generalities.

II. ASSESSMENT

A. History and physical.
   1. Traction alopecia.
      a. Hair loss in frontal and temporal hairline.
      b. Inflamed and pustular follicles.
      c. Hair breakage at anchoring sites in weaves.
      d. Permanent hair loss.
      e. Headache due to scalp tension.
   2. Hot comb alopecia.

Table 2.
Interventions for Traction Alopecia

1. Do not braid hair tightly.
2. Avoid any hair style that causes prolonged tension on the scalp.
3. Professional grooming with scalp inspection once a week.
4. Remove braids after 6 to 8 weeks.
5. Change style and direction of the tension on the scalp if rebraids are desired.
6. Refit weaves every 4 to 8 weeks as natural hair grows out from the scalp.

Hot Comb Alopecia
1. Reduce heat of the hot comb to minimize damage to hair follicles.
2. Hot comb the hair on the top of the scalp out to the side, so that the hair is parallel to the ground.
3. Mild chemical relaxers: less damaging to the hair and scalp.

a. Decrease in hair and breakage in top of scalp.
b. Scarring.
c. Remaining hair may be broken, coarse, or thickened.

B. **Diagnosis.**
1. Clinical examination and history.
2. Both traction alopecia and hot comb alopecia must be distinguished from male pattern baldness (androgenetic alopecia) caused by genetic factors, age, and androgen production. Often misdiagnosed in women of color because hair loss is attributed to hot comb traction alopecia.
3. Trichogram determines the number of anagen and telogen hairs by plucking and counting the hairs of each.

III. THERAPEUTIC MODALITIES

A. Punch grafting and flap rotation techniques of hair transplantation to correct permanent traction.

IV. NURSING DIAGNOSES, OUTCOMES, AND INTERVENTIONS (see Table 2)

A. Alteration in body image.
B. Increased risk for infection related to impaired integument.
C. Anxiety related to abnormal skin appearance.

POMADE ACNE

I. OVERVIEW

The practice of grooming the hair and scalp with oils and pomades is attributed partly to traditional and cultural beliefs of blacks. Established customs in grooming the hair are difficult to break. Treatment then becomes a challenge.

A. **Definition: an eruption of closed comedomes with occasional papules and pustules.**
B. **Etiology.**
1. Prolonged habit of applying oils or greasy creams to the hair and scalp.
2. Inflammation around the hair follicle.
C. **Pathophysiology.**
1. Pomades, which are liquid or solid preparation of mineral, petrolatum, and paraffin, straighten hair by plastering it into position.
2. The heavier solid pomades tend to plug hair follicles.
3. Pustules form around the hair follicles producing an inflammatory reaction called oil folliculitis. The condition worsens as bacterial growth in the follicle increases.
4. Acne develops on the forehead and temples clinically similar to acne vulgaris but more monomorphous.

D. **Incidence.**
1. Adults and children.
2. Infantile acne secondary to pomade application to hair and scalp.

II. ASSESSMENT

A. **History and physical.**
1. Uniform open and closed comedomes.
2. Papules, pustules, and cystic nodules may be present.
3. Hair may be greasy.
4. On examination, may detect exogenous topical material.
5. Post-inflammatory hyperpigmentation may follow pomade acne.
6. Common sites — scalp, forehead, temples.
B. **Diagnosis.**
1. Clinical exam.

III. THERAPEUTIC MODALITIES

A. **Discontinue use of pomade; will resolve within a few months.**
B. **Antibiotics to treat infection.**
C. **Keratolytics (benzyl peroxide) and retinoic acid.**

IV. NURSING DIAGNOSES, OUTCOMES, AND INTERVENTIONS (see Table 1)

A. **Alteration in body image.**
B. **Alteration in comfort related to pruritus or pain.**
C. **Increased risk for infection.**
D. **Anxiety related to abnormal skin appearance.**

DISORDERS UNIQUE TO BLACKS: PSEUDOFOLLICULITIS BARBAE

I. OVERVIEW

One of the most troublesome conditions that affect black men. The simplest treatment is to stop shaving.

A. **Definition: an inflammatory disorder seen in many men of African descent who shave; also known as ingrown hairs.**
B. **Etiology.**
1. Hair follicles in many blacks grow curved or tightly coiled.
2. When the hairs emerge on the skin surface, they have a sharp point caused by shaving, turning the hair back into the skin.
C. **Pathophysiology.**
1. Many black men have tightly coiled hair.
2. After shaving, the free end may re-enter the skin and incite an inflammatory foreign body reaction.
3. Also, the top of the coiled penetrating shaft may be shaved off, leaving small pieces of hair in the skin.
4. An inflammatory reaction occurs due to

repeated hair penetrations and hair shaft remnants.
5. Common sites — chin, upper anterior neck, and mandible. May also develop on legs and axilla from shaving.

D. Incidence.
1. Occurs more frequently in black men than white men.

II. ASSESSMENT

A. History and physical.
1. Irritated papular and pustular eruption on the neck, chin, and mandible.
2. Keloids can form.
3. Over time, post-inflammatory hyperpigmentation occurs throughout the bearded area.
4. Severity: mildly bothersome to terribly traumatic eruption.

B. Diagnosis.
1. Clinical examination.
2. Bacterial culture yielding *staphylococcus albus*. The disorder is not primarily infectious.

III. THERAPEUTIC MODALITIES

A. Stop shaving.
B. If unable to stop shaving, use a new razor each time; avoid electric razors.
C. Apply hot towel to beard before shaving.
D. When possible, carefully free ingrown hairs with a sharp point.
E. Use PFB razor to shave, leaving about 6 mm of beard.
F. Brush beard gently before shaving to dislodge hairs that are attempting to re-enter the skin.
G. Use depilatory creams.
H. Limited success with topical corticosteroids, tretinoin creams, benzyl peroxide cream or gel, and glycolic cream.
I. Depilatory creams: Magic Shave®, Royal Crown® shave cream. Since Royal Crown shaving cream can be irritating, a mild steroid cream can be applied after application.
J. If secondary infection occurs, course of systemic antibiotics can be recommended.

IV. NURSING DIAGNOSES, OUTCOMES, INTERVENTIONS (see Table 1)

A. Alteration in body image.
B. Alteration in comfort related to pain (irritation).
C. Increased risk for infection related to impaired integument.
D. Anxiety related to abnormal skin appearance.

DERMATOSIS PAPULOSA NIGRA

I. OVERVIEW

Is a common entirely benign condition experienced by many black adults. It is characterized by growth on the face and neck of multiple pigmented papules. Adults who experience facial lesions also exhibit lesions on the body. Prepubescent children are rarely affected.

A. Definition: wart-like papules that may be hyperpigmented or the color of the surrounding skin. Lesions are typically 1 to 5 mm in size.
B. Etiology.
1. Nature is unclear.
2. Unknown if it is a nevoid condition, hereditary disease, eruptive tumor, or simply a variant of seborrheic keratosis.
C. Pathophysiology.
1. Histologically, epidermal tumors look like seborrheic keratosis with underlying acanthotic epidermis.
2. The keratinocytes are basaloid.
3. Horn cysts are often present.
4. Some lesions are deeply melanin pigmented.
5. They do not spontaneously regress.
D. Incidence.
1. Most unique to people of African descent; occurring in about 50% of blacks.
2. Puberty onset.
3. Women more often than men.
4. Prevalence increases with age.
5. Occurrence in other groups — Indochinese, Japanese, Mexican Indians, and sometimes in Europeans who live along the Mediterranean Sea.

II. ASSESSMENT

A. History and physical.
1. Multiple asymptomatic, hyperpigmented papules.
2. Benign lesions can be smooth, rough, or verrucous.
3. All moles look alike to patients.
4. Cosmetically unacceptable to the patient.
5. Common sites — face, neck, back, or chest.
B. Diagnosis.
1. Can be mistaken for seborrheic keratosis. The clinical appearance of multiple lesions on the face suggests a diagnosis of dermatosis papulosa nigra. It is rarely biopsied.
2. Other tumors may be hidden among the many lesions.
3. Careful physical exam to ensure no other skin tumors go undetected.

III. THERAPEUTIC MODALITIES

A. The right surgical approach is difficult to decide.

B. Light electrodesiccation is effective; may result in hyperpigmentation.

C. Cryotherapy is not a treatment of choice because of the hyperpigmentation that may be produced.

D. Scissor excision or curettage to excise lesions; causes little bleeding and no postoperative complications.

E. Chemical peels with alpha hydroxy acids will soften and flatten these lesions and seem to prevent new lesions.

IV. NURSING DIAGNOSES, OUTCOMES, AND INTERVENTIONS (see Table 1)

A. Alteration in body image.

B. Alteration in comfort related to post-procedure pain.

C. Increased risk for infection in surgical sites.

D. Anxiety related to abnormal skin appearance.

MELANOCYTIC LESIONS/CONDITIONS COMMON IN THE ASIAN PATIENT: NEVUS OF OTA

I. OVERVIEW

A macular lesion on the side of the face involving the conjunctiva and lids, as well as the adjacent facial skin, sclera, ocular muscles, and periosteum.

A. Definition: the Nevus of Ota is a facial, dermal melanocytic lesion common in the Asian patient. Nearly all lesions appear before age 30. The incidence in Japanese patients is from 0.1% to 0.2%. Females predominate.

B. Assessment.
 1. History and physical.
  a. Unilateral blue-black or brown pigment.
  b. Usually corresponds to the forehead, temple, eyelid, nose, ear, and/or scalp.
  c. Pigmentation may also be found in the sclera and oral mucosa.
  d. Cosmetically unacceptable to the patient.
  e. Bilateral occurrence is by age 30 if it happens.
  f. Pigmentation is never symmetrical.

C. Diagnosis.
 1. Histologically melanocytes are found scattered in the upper and mid dermis.
 2. Bilateral Nevus of Ota can be confused with Nevus of Ota-like macules.
  a. Pigmentation is more intense with bilateral Nevus of Ota; more subtle with bilateral Nevus of Ota-like macules.
  b. The patient is almost always an Asian or darkly pigmented woman.
  c. Bilateral Nevus of Ota-like macules never appear on the mucosa and are never

congenital whereas both congenital presentations and mucosal pigmentation often occurs with bilateral Nevus of Ota.

II. THERAPEUTIC MODALITIES

A. Camouflage is the usual approach to treatment of the condition.

III. NURSING DIAGNOSES, OUTCOMES, AND INTERVENTIONS (see Table 1)

A. Alteration in body image.

B. Anxiety related to abnormal skin appearance.

NEVUS OF ITO

I. OVERVIEW

Similar to Nevus of Ota, but the characteristic location of the former is periocular, the latter in the distribution of the posterior supraclavicular and lateral cutaneous brachial nerves

A. Definition: Nevus of Ito pigmentation of skin innervated by lateral branches of the supraclavicular nerve and the lateral cutaneous nerve of the arm.

B. Assessment.
 1. History and physical.
  a. Differentiation of epidermal nevus syndrome from hypomelanosis of Ito may be particularly difficult in children in whom there is wide variation in background pigmentation.
  b. The classic lesion has its onset at birth or childhood and shows increased pigmentation in the skin innervated by the posterior supraclavicular and lateral brachial cutaneous nerves.
  c. Usual distribution on shoulders and neck.
  d. Cosmetically unacceptable to the patient.
  e. Pigmentation is never symmetrical.

C. Diagnosis.
 1. Histologically melanocytes are found scattered in the upper and mid dermis.
 2. Lesions typically present as blue macules.

II. THERAPEUTIC MODALITIES

A. Camouflage is the usual approach to treatment of the condition.

III. NURSING DIAGNOSES, OUTCOMES, AND INTERVENTIONS (see Table 1)

A. Alteration in body image.

B. Anxiety related to abnormal skin appearance.

MONGOLIAN SPOT

I. OVERVIEW

The Mongolian spot presents as a blue-black patch on the sacrum or buttocks of a neonate. There have been suggestions to change the name to blue-gray macule of infancy to avoid using the term Mongolian. There have been many suppositions as to why these macules appear including comparing these pigmentary changes with patterns seen in young animals which camouflage them protecting them from being eaten. Why do they fade? It has been suggested that the pigmentary protection is necessary in young infants and as the skin thickens the protection is no longer necessary.

A. Definition: Mongolian spot is a poorly defined blue-to-gray area of skin discoloration present at birth, usually in the area of the buttocks and lower spine. It may also involve other areas such as the upper back, shoulders, and arms or legs; palms and soles are spared. Mongolian blue spots are flat birthmarks with wavy borders and irregular shapes, common among people of Asian, East Indian, African, and Latino heritage.

B. Assessment.
   1. History and physical.
      a. The pigmented area has large concentrations of skin cells called melanocytes, with normal skin texture. They commonly appear at birth or shortly after birth and may look like bruises.
      b. Mongolian spots may cover a large area of the back.
      c. Often appear on the base of the spine, on the buttocks, and sometimes on the ankles or wrists.

C. Diagnosis.
   1. Histologic examination of a Mongolian spot shows elongated, dendritic, melanin-containing cells scattered lightly throughout the dermis.
   2. The diagnosis of Mongolian spot is usually obvious and a biopsy is not needed. The incidence varies according to the overall depth of this birthmark.
      a. Black babies — 90%.
      b. Asian babies — 80%.
      c. Latino babies — 65%.
      d. Caucasian babies — 9.5%.
   3. The vague resemblance to a bruise has from time to time led to unfounded accusations of child abuse.

II. THERAPEUTIC MODALITIES

A. No specific treatment is required.
B. The color reaches a peak at 1 to 2 years of age and then begins to fade.
C. The majority of lesions are gone by adolescence.

D. Occasionally lesions persist to adulthood and are usually localized to the buttocks.

III. NURSING DIAGNOSES, OUTCOMES, AND INTERVENTIONS (see Table 1)

A. Alteration in perception of body image.
B. Parental anxiety related to abnormal skin appearance

Bibliography
Arndt, K.A., Laboit, P.C., Robinson, J.K., & Wintroub, B.U. (1996). *Cutaneous medicine and surgery: An integrated program in dermatology.* Philadelphia: W.B. Saunders Company.
Bigby, M.E., David, A.K., & Brown, A.E. (1994). *Recognition and management of skin diseases in people of color.* Boston: Glaxo Wellcome Inc.
Chan, H.H., Alam, M., Kono, T., & Dover, J.S. (2002). Clinical application of Lasers in Asians. *Dermatology Surgery, 28*(7), 556-63.
Fitzpatrick, T.B., Johnson, R.A., Polano, M.K., Suurmond, D., & Wolff, K. (1994). *Color atlas and synopsis of clinical dermatology common and serious disseases.* New York: McGraw-Hill Inc.
Grimes, P.E., & Davis, L.T. (1991). Cosmetics in blacks. *Dermatology Clinics in North America, 9*(1), 53-68.
Johnson, B.L., Jr., Moy, R.L., & White, G.M. (1998). *Ethnic skin: Medical and surgical.* St. Louis, MO: Mosby, Inc.
Montagna, W., Prota, G., & Kenney, J.A. Jr. (1993). *Black skin structure and function.* San Diego: Academic Press, Inc.
Rosen, T., & Martin, S. (1981). *Atlas of black dermatology.* Boston: Little, Brown and Company.

1. Mongolian spots only occur on the buttocks of African-American/Black infants.
   a. True
   b. False

2. The following diseases make up the follicular occlusion triad:
   a. Psoriasis, hidradenitis, and acne.
   b. Hidradenitis suppurativa.
   c. Acne conglobata.
   d. Dissecting cellulitis.
   e. All of the above.
   f. b, c, & d.

3. Dermatosis papulosus nigra is:
   a. Most unique to people of African descent.
   b. Is a benign condition.
   c. Typically 1 to 5 mm in length.
   d. Cosmetically acceptable to the individual.
   e. All of the above.
   f. a, b, & c.

4. Keloids are common in:
   a. Blacks or dark-skinned people.
   b. Chinese population in Malaysia.
   c. Light skinned people of Finland.
   d. A only.
   e. All of the above.

5. Mongolian spots are:
   a. Flat birthmarks with wavy borders and irregular shapes.
   b. Tend to plug hair follicles.
   c. Produce pustules and inflammation around the hair follicles.
   d. Common among people of Asian, East Indian, African, and Latino heritage.
   e. a & d.
   f. All of the above.

6. Pseudofolliculitis can best be treated by:
   a. Discontinuing shaving.
   b. Shaving with the same razor each time.
   c. Applying cold compresses before shaving.
   d. Shaving close to the skin surface.

7. Pigmentary demarcation lines:
   a. Occur in about 20% to 60% of people of African descent.
   b. May follow the distribution of spinal nerves.
   c. Are also called Voight's and Futcher's lines.
   d. Thought to provide better the skin protection from the sun.
   e. All of the above.

8. Longitudinal melanonychia:
   a. Is due to melanin deposits in the nail plates.
   b. Are stripes in the nail plates.
   c. Melanoma should be considered as a differential diagnosis.
   d. All of the above.
   e. a & c.

9. Palmar and plantar pigmentation:
   a. Presents in varying degrees.
   b. Are commonly seen on the palms and soles of darker-skinned individuals.
   c. Normally occurs in flexural and digital creases.
   d. a & c.
   e. All of the above.

10. The first sign of pityriasis rosea is the herald patch.
    a. True
    b. False

11. Clinical features and distribution of psoriasis are the same in white and dark-skinned people.
    a. True
    b. False

12. Regarding traction and hot comb alopecia:
    a. Both are related to grooming processes.
    b. Children do not experience traction alopecia.
    c. Braiding is a common cause of alopecia.
    d. Heat from the hot comb causes the hair to break.
    e. All of the above.
    f. a, c, & d.

Answers to Study Questions

1.	b	5.	e	9.	e
2.	f	6.	a	10.	a
3.	e	7.	e	11.	a
4.	e	8.	d	12.	f

Chapter 17.
Dermatologic Considerations in Ethnic Skin

Please photocopy this test page and return.

COMPLETE THE FOLLOWING:

Name: _____

Address: _____

City: _____ State: _____ Zip: _____

Preferred telephone: (Home)_____ (Work) _____

State where licensed and license number: _____

CE application fee: DNA member $10.00
                    Nonmember $13.00

POSTTEST INSTRUCTIONS
1. To receive continuing education credit for individual study after reading the article, complete the answer/evaluation form below.
2. Photocopy and send the answer/evaluation form along with a check or money order payable to **Dermatology Nurses' Association** to: **DNA**, East Holly Avenue Box 56, Pitman, NJ 08071-0056.
3. Test returns must be postmarked by December 31, 2008. Upon completion of the answer/evaluation form, a certificate for 2.4 contact hour(s) will be awarded and sent to you.

This chapter was reviewed and formatted for contact hour credit by Marcia J. Hill, MSN, RN, Core Curriculum Editor; and Sally Russell, MN, RN,C, DNA Education Director.

ANSWER FORM

1. Name one new detail (item, issue, or phenomenon) that you learned by completing this activity.

_____

_____

_____

_____

2. How will you apply the information from this learning activity to your practice?
   a. Patient education.
   b. Staff education.
   c. Improve my patient care.
   d. In my education course work.
   e. Other: Please describe _____

_____

Evaluation

	Strongly disagree				Strongly agree
3. The offering met the stated objectives.					
a. List normal variations in pigmentation in people of color.	1	2	3	4	5
b. Identify skin disorders commonly occurring in ethnic individuals.	1	2	3	4	5
c. Discuss the changes in treatment modalities necessary for skin diseases unique to the ethnic population.	1	2	3	4	5
d. Recognize differences in the manifestation of skin disease in the ethnic population.	1	2	3	4	5
e. Identify the psychosocial impact imposed by skin disease unique to the ethnic population.	1	2	3	4	5
4. The content was current and relevant.	1	2	3	4	5
5. The content was presented clearly.	1	2	3	4	5
6. The content was covered adequately.	1	2	3	4	5
7. I am more confident of my abilities since completing this material.	1	2	3	4	5

8. The material was (check one) ☐ new, ☐ review for me.

Comments _____

Time required to complete reading assignment: _____ minutes

This independent study is provided by the Dermatology Nurses' Association (DNA) for 2.4 contact hours. DNA is accredited as a provider of continuing education in nursing by the American Nurses Credentialing Center's Commission on Accreditation. DNA is approved as a provider of continuing education by the California Board of Registered Nursing Provider #CEP5708.

Hair and Nails

Kelly N. White, MS, ARNP

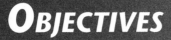

OBJECTIVES

At the end of this chapter, the reader will be able to:
- Identify normal and disease processes affecting the hair and nails.
- Discuss the treatment of hair and nail disorders.
- Define appropriate skin care and nursing management for these skin disorders.

KEY POINTS

- Hair and nails are classified as epidermal appendages.
- Hair disorders may be directly correlated with skin lesions or may develop without skin lesions.
- Nail changes can cause disfigurement and pain and may be a sign of systemic disease.

Hair and Nails

Kelly N. White, MS, ARNP

NORMAL HAIR

I. OVERVIEW

A. Hair is a keratin structure of the epidermis which serves no vital function on the human body. It does have physiologic functions including insulation, social and sexual display, camouflage, tactile perception, thermoregulation, and protection from UV light.

B. Embryonic development.
  1. First follicles form at about 9 weeks gestation, mainly in the eyebrows, upper lip, and chin. Remainder develop at 4 to 5 months gestation.
  2. Epidermal cells progressively penetrate downward into the maturing dermis, passing through "germ," "peg," and "bulbous peg" stages of development.

C. Anatomy.
  1. The hair shaft is organized into seven longitudinal regions, beginning from the epidermis (see Figure 1).
    a. Hair canal region — present only during fetal development and extends from the skin surface to the level of the epidermal-dermal junction.
    b. Infundibulum — funnel-shaped top of follicular canal. Extends to opening of the sebaceous duct.
    c. Sebaceous gland area.
    d. Isthmus — located between the entry of sebaceous duct and insertion of arrector pili muscle.
    e. Area of the bulge — site of the insertion of the arrector pili muscle.
    f. Lower follicle — extends from the area of the bulge to the top of the hair bulb.
    g. Hair bulb — is the deepest part of the hair follicle and surrounds the dermal papilla.
  2. Cross section of hair follicle reveals a series of cellular compartments (see Figure 2).
    a. A cellular basement membrane ("glassy membrane"). Surrounds entire follicle.
    b. Outer root sheath — most peripheral of cellular components.
    c. Inner root sheath — comprises three separate layers.
      (1) Henle's layer.
      (2) Huxley's layer.
      (3) Cuticle.
    d. Hair shaft — also comprises three separate layers.
      (1) Cuticle — the outside portion. Consists of overlapping cell layers arranged like shingles pointing upward. Protects the hair shaft.
      (2) Cortex — the bulk of the hair shaft. "Cigar-shaped" cells which synthesize and accumulate proteins while in the lower regions of the hair shaft.
      (3) Medulla — may not be present in all hairs. May be discontinuous.

D. Hair growth.
  1. Hair follicles undergo repeated cycles of active growth and rest (see Figure 3).
    a. Anagen — actively growing hair. Cells in dermal papilla increase in size. Germal cells show increased mitotic activity. For scalp hair, lasts 2 to 7 years.
    b. Catagen — metabolic processes associated with hair growth gradually decrease. The hair follicle regresses. Lasts approximately 2 to 3 weeks.
    c. Telogen — the resting phase. Existing hair will never grow longer. Has a club-shaped proximal end which will be shed from the follicle.
  2. Length of growth cycle varies according to body site with a general relationship of increasing hair length to a longer growth cycle.
  3. Genetic programs determine normal growth parameters for hair on different anatomical locations; for example, eyelash hairs remain short while scalp hair grows much longer.
  4. Hormones influence hair growth. Androgens influence pubic, axillary, beard, trunk, and extremity hair as well as lead to hair loss in susceptible individuals. Estrogens tend to prolong the telogen phase and delay the anagen phase.

E. Distribution of hair.
  1. Covers entire body except palms, soles, interspaces of the digits, and portions of the genitalia.
  2. Greatest density in scalp, numbering 100,000 in people with brown/black hair. Is about 10% greater in natural blondes and 10% less in redheads.
  3. Approximately 85% to 90% of hairs in anagen, 10% to 15 % in telogen, and a few percent in catagen at any given time.
  4. Normal hair shedding ranges from 50 to 100 scalp hairs per day.

F. Types of hair.
  1. Hairs are classified into four groups according to texture and length.
    a. Lanugo hairs — soft, fine lightly pigmented

Figure 1.
Anatomy of the Hair Follicle, Anagen Stage

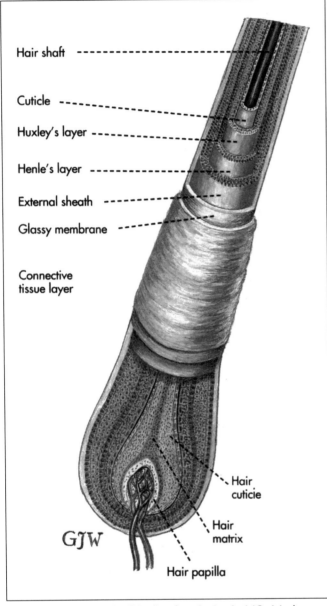

From Hill, M.J. (1994). *Skin disorders*. St. Louis, MO: Mosby.

Figure 2.
Cross Section of Hair Follicles

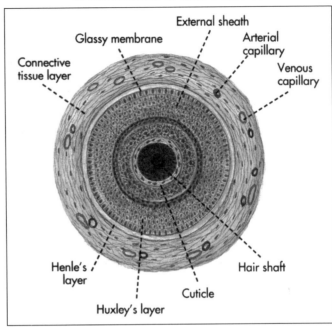

From Hill, M.J. (1994). *Skin disorders*. St. Louis, MO: Mosby.

Figure 3.
The Hair Growth Cycle

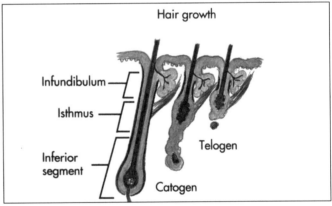

From Hill, M.J. (1994). *Skin disorders*. St. Louis, MO: Mosby.

hair. Found in utero on fetal skin.
b. Vellus hairs — fine, short hair with little pigment. Found on all parts of body except palms, soles, parts of genitalia, and periungual areas.
c. Indeterminate hairs — fall between vellus and terminal hairs in size.
d. Terminal hairs — thicker, longer, coarser hair. Frequently has central medulla and is pigmented. Found only on scalp, eyebrows, and eyelashes in children. Androgen production at puberty stimulates conversion from small to large terminal hairs in scalp, beard (males), axillary, and pubic regions.
2. Any one hair follicle can give rise to different types of hair within its lifetime; for example, during puberty former vellus hairs become terminal hairs in the beard, scalp, pubic, and axillary regions.
G. **Hair pigmentation.**
1. Melanocytes located in the matrix area of the follicle produce pigment.
2. Pigment is most prominent in the cortex of the hair shaft.
3. Any follicle can produce two types of pigment, although usually only one type at any time is found.

Dermatologic Nursing Essentials: A Core Curriculum 2nd Edition © DNA 2003

a. Eumelanin — pigment found in brown or black hairs.

b. Pheomelanin — pigment found in red or blonde hairs.

4. Generally, pigment is not found in the hair shaft during the early stages of new hair formation and in the proximal portion of telogen hairs.

5. Color intensity is generally proportional to the amount of pigment in the fiber.

6. Graying hair is a result of a decreased number of melanocytes in the hair bulb.

H. Morphology of hair.

1. Four categories: straight, spiral, helical, and wavy.

2. Caucasians are the hairiest and may contain any of these categories.

3. Asian hair is straight due to straight follicles with lower portions oriented vertically to the skin surface.

4. Hair in blacks is spiraled due to curved follicles with lower portions almost horizontal to the skin surface.

II. ASSESSMENT

A. History and physical examination.

1. Patient history — cause may be associated with a variety of other diseases which significantly affect treatment decisions. Pertinent history may include the following.

a. Disease duration, age of onset, extent of involvement including:

(1) Increase or decrease in amount of hair shedding per day.

(2) Change in color or texture.

(3) Distribution of hair normal or abnormal.

(4) Gradual or sudden onset.

(5) Symmetric or asymmetric hair loss.

b. Associated symptoms include pruritus, pain, lesions, fever, pregnancy, psychologic or physiologic stress, or presence of systemic disease.

c. Current drug therapy.

d. Exposure to environmental or occupational toxins or chemicals.

e. Nutritional status.

f. Current and past treatment and response.

2. Physical examination — inspect hair for texture, color, quality, and distribution.

B. Diagnostic tests: often the diagnosis is clinically evident. In other cases, the following tests may be indicated.

1. Hair pull and microscopic examination of the hair.

2. Biopsy.

3. KOH preparation.

4. Fungal culture.

5. Immune, endocrine, and other laboratory studies, if indicated.

6. Serologic testing, as indicated.

III. COMMON NURSING DIAGNOSES, OUTCOMES, AND INTERVENTIONS — HAIR (see Table 1)

HAIR DISORDERS: ALOPECIA AREATA

I. OVERVIEW

A. **Definition: microscopically inflammatory, usually reversible, patchy loss of hair, commonly occurring in sharply defined areas. Usually involves scalp and beard.**

B. **Etiology.**

1. Cause unknown but likely an immunologically mediated disease.

C. **Pathophysiology.**

1. Telogen and dystrophic hairs with irregular shapes and fractured ends are removed in hair pull tests.

2. Dystrophic hairs fracture forming "explanation point" hairs.

3. Lymphatic infiltrate found around affected hair bulb and lower one-third of follicle.

4. Increased number of terminal catagen and telogen hairs.

5. Normal total number of hair follicles.

6. Marked narrowing of hair shafts in severe disease.

D. **Clinical features.**

1. Classic presentation is a well-defined lesion, round or oval area of total hair loss on the scalp.

2. Paresthesia or pruritus may accompany hair loss in some patients.

3. Disease activity may be insidious or rapid.

4. Scarring is not present.

5. Nail findings may include pitting, thin or brittle fingernails and toenails, and longitudinal ridging.

E. **Incidence.**

1. Affects males and females equally.

2. Occurs in both children and adults.

II. ASSESSMENT

A. **See Normal Hair, Assessment.**

B. **Rule out drug-induced alopecia (see Tables 2a & b).**

C. **Children should undergo thyroid function testing.**

III. COMMON THERAPEUTIC MODALITIES

A. **Medical interventions.**

1. Intralesional corticosteroid injections,

Table 1.
Common Nursing Diagnoses, Outcomes, and Interventions (Hair)

Nursing Diagnoses	Outcomes	Interventions
Anxiety related to hair changes or loss.	1. The patient will demonstrate decreased anxiety, as evidenced by: • Patient's statement of ability to cope with hair changes.	1. Assess anxiety level and observe verbal and nonverbal cues. 2. Listen attentively. 3. Assist the patient to identify concerns about hair change.
Body image disturbance related to hair changes or loss.	1. Patient will demonstrate beginning adaptation to actual/perceived change in body image as evidenced by: • Statements of acceptance of self. • Active display of interest in personal appearance. • Statements of hope for future. 2. Patient will demonstrate positive social interactions.	1. Have patient describe feelings about self. 2. Assist the patient to deal with perceptions of body image. • Establish a therapeutic nurse-patient relationship. • Accept feelings of anger or hostility. • Help patient and family cope with effects of change(s). 3. Teach patient/family methods of dealing with their feelings.
Coping with hair changes or loss.	1. The patient will demonstrate effective coping skills, as evidenced by: • Statements of ability to cope. • Demonstration of positive social interactions. • Identification of own ineffective coping mechanisms.	1. Assess causative and contributing factors and the patient's premorbid responses to stress. 2. Assess for signs and symptoms that are indicative of ineffective coping (irritability, insomnia, statements of inability to cope, and fatigue). 3. Assist the patient to identify own strengths. 4. Encourage involvement of the family.
Potential social isolation related to hair changes or loss.	1. Patient will identify feelings of isolation. 2. Patient will independently engage in social activities. 3. Patient will state feelings of self-worth.	1. Encourage patient to discuss feelings of loneliness. 2. Identify available support systems to the patient. 3. Help patient identify own responsibility in resolving feelings of loneliness and isolation.
Knowledge deficit of hair changes or loss.	1. Patient will participate in the learning process. 2. Patient will state understanding of hair condition or disease and treatment.	1. Assess the patient for learning needs, readiness to learn, and factors that will influence learning. 2. Determine content to be given: • Explain disease and its course. • Teach patient about each type of treatment. • Emphasize need to comply with all provisions of treatment process. • Instruct patient in the proper application of topical medications or appropriate dosing for oral medications. Explain side effects. • Advise patient to keep followup appointments with physician. 3. Implement teaching. 4. Refer to educational resource: National Alopecia Areata Foundation (NAAF) P. O. Box 150760 San Rafael, CA 94915-0760 Web site: www.alopeciaareata.com

Dermatologic Nursing Essentials: A Core Curriculum 2nd Edition © DNA 2003

particularly on scalp or eyebrows. About 66% of patients will experience some growth.

  a. Inject involved area with dilute triamcinolone acetonide suspension up to 5 mg/ml at 1 to 2 cm intervals using a 27 or 30 gauge needle.

  b. Reinject at 4 to 6 week intervals. Discontinue after 3 months if no growth present.

  c. Thinning of regrowth may occur after 3 to 6 months and can be reinjected as necessary.

  d. Spontaneous regrowth may occur 3 to 6 months after injection.

2. Oral corticosteroids or potent topical steroid preparation. Short white or finely pigmented hairs develop within 3 to 4 months if treatment is successful.

3. Contact sensitizers such as dinitrochlorobenzene, squaric acid dibutyl ester, or diphencyprone.

  a. Patients are first sensitized to the agent using concentrations from 0.0001% to 2%.

  b. Agents are reapplied as necessary to maintain a mild erythema.

  c. Regrowth consisting of white or finely pigmented hairs develop within 3 to 4 months, if successful.

  d. If no growth in 3 to 4 months, consider another therapy.

4. Topical anthralin.

  a. Apply lowest concentration to affected area daily.

  b. If no hair growth, concentration may be increased to 1.0%. Apply to affected area 20 to 30 minutes daily.

5. Topical minoxidil, 1%, 3% or 5%, 1 mm bid.

  a. Positive results seen in only a small percentage of patients.

  b. May take up to 4 months to see regrowth.

  c. Will keep working only as long as used.

  d. New hair may be lost when drug is discontinued.

6. Psoralens, topical or systemic, with ultraviolet A. Is successful in only a small percentage of patients and treatment effectiveness currently being questioned.

B. **Surgical interventions. None.**

IV. COMMON NURSING DIAGNOSES, OUTCOMES, AND INTERVENTIONS

A. See Table 1.

B. **Identify places to obtain toupees, hair prostheses, and scarfs.**

V. HOME CARE CONSIDERATIONS

A. **Apply sunscreens (SPF>15) and wear hat/scarf** when sun exposure expected or when outside.

B. **Limit shampooing, combing, and brushing hair as much as possible.**

C. **Use cream rinse or conditioner after shampooing.**

D. **Avoid vigorous rubbing with a towel, rough combing, and brushing when hair is wet.**

E. **Use wide-toothed combs and brushes with smooth tips.**

F. **Hairstyles that pull on the hair should not be pulled tightly and should be alternated with looser hairstyles.**

ANDROGENIC ALOPECIA

I. OVERVIEW

A. **Definition: androgenic alopecia is referred to as common balding and is the most common cause of thinning hair.**

B. **Etiology.**

  1. Inherited condition from either parent.

C. **Pathophysiology.**

  1. Regression depends on androgen production with normal serum androgen levels found.

  2. Process is progressive beginning with hair shedding, followed by smaller hair shaft diameters, shortening of anagen, and lengthening of telogen growth phases.

  3. Total number of hair follicles nearly normal (about 35 per 4 mm plug).

  4. Reduced ratio of terminal and indeterminate hairs.

  5. Increased number of vellus and indeterminate hairs.

  6. Fibrous "streamers" found in fat which is evidence of hair miniaturization.

  7. Increased telogen count when compared with uninvolved scalp.

D. **Clinical features.**

  1. Occurs most commonly in late adolescence or in early 20s.

  2. Patterns of male androgenic alopecia.

    a. Hamilton's classification system (see Table 3, Figure 4).

    b. Norwood's classification system (see Figure 5).

  3. Ludwig's classification system used to describe female androgenic alopecia (see Table 4, Figure 6).

II. ASSESSMENT

A. **See Normal Hair, Assessment.**

III. COMMON THERAPEUTIC MODALITIES

A. **Medical interventions.**

  1. Topical minoxidil 2% or 5%, 1 ml. Apply to

Table 2a.
Causes of Hair Loss

Type of Loss	Possible Causes
Telogen effluvium-loss of resting hair	Acute blood loss Childbirth Crash diets Drugs (coumarins, heparin, propranolol, vitamin A) High fever Physical/psychological stress Hypothyroidism
Anagen effluvium-abrupt loss of hair growing phase	Chemotherapy Thallium/arsenic poisoning Radiation
Generalized patchy loss	Secondary syphilis

Adapted from Habif, T.P. (1990). *Clinical dermatology: A color guide to diagnosis and treatment* (p. 601). St. Louis, MO: C.V. Mosby.

Table 2b.
Drugs and Chemicals Reported to Cause or Possibly Cause Telogen Hair Loss

Allopurinol
Androgens (danazol)
Angiotensin-converting enzyme inhibitors (captropril, enalapril)
Anticholesterolemic drugs (clofibrate)
Anticoagulants (warfarin, dextran, heparinoids)
Antimitotic agents (colchicine, methotrexate)
Antithyroid medications (carbimazole, methylthiouracil, propylthiouracil)
Benzimidazoles (albendazole, mebendazole)
Beta blockers (systemic: metroprolol, propranolol; topical ophthalmic: betazalol, levobunolol, timolol)
Bromocriptine
Cimetidine
Gold
Immunoglobulin

Interferon (alpha, gamma)
Levodopa
Methysergide
Minoxidil
Oral contraceptives
Proguanil
Psychotropic medications (amphetamines, desipramine, dixyrazine, fluoxetine, imipramine, lithium, tranylcypromine, valproic acid)
Pyridostigmine bromide
Retinoids
Sulfasalazine
Vitamin A

From Olsen, E.A. (1994). *Disorders of hair growth, diagnosis and treatment.* New York: McGraw Hill, Inc.

scalp bid.
a. May take 4 months to begin to work.
b. Will keep working only as long as it is used.
c. New hair is lost when drug is stopped.
2. Finasteride (Propecia®) 1 mg taken daily, acts as a specific competitive inhibitor of steroid type II5 alpha-redoctase.

3. Topical, intralesional, and oral anti-androgens currently under study.
B. **Surgical interventions.**
1. Hair transplant.
2. Scalp reduction.

Dermatologic Nursing Essentials: A Core Curriculum 2nd Edition © DNA 2003

Table 3.
Hamilton's Classification of Male Androgenic Alopecia

Type	Clinical Features
I	Normal frontoparietal hairline.
II	Symmetrical triangular areas of recession in the frontoparietal regions.
III	Borderline cases.
IV	Deep frontotemporal recession in association with hair loss along the midfrontal border of the scalp.
V	Extensive frontoparietal and frontal recession in association with sparse hair growth on the vertex.
VI	Vertex region of alopecia is separated from the anterior area of hair loss by a region of sparse scalp hair density.
VII	Area dividing the crown region with the anterior area of hair loss begins to disappear.
VIII	Complete baldness.

From Hordinsky, M.K. (1996). Hair. In Sams, W.M., & Lynch, P.J. (Eds), *Principles and practice of dermatology* (pp. 779 -800). New York: Churchill Livingstone.

IV. COMMON NURSING DIAGNOSES, OUTCOMES, AND INTERVENTIONS

A. See Table 1.
B. Identify places to obtain toupees, hair prostheses, and scarfs.

V. HOME CARE CONSIDERATIONS

A. Apply sunscreens (SPF>15) and wear hat/scarf when sun exposure expected or when outside.
B. Limit shampooing, combing, and brushing hair as much as possible.
C. Use creme rinse or conditioner after shampooing.
D. Avoid vigorous rubbing with a towel, rough combing, and brushing when hair is wet.
E. Use wide-toothed combs and brushes with smooth tips.
F. Hairstyles that pull on the hair should not be pulled tightly and should be alternated with looser hairstyles.

HIRSUTISM

I. OVERVIEW

A. Definition: growth of coarse terminal hairs on the face or body of a woman in a pattern more typical of that seen in men.
B. Etiology.
   1. Ovarian and adrenal diseases causing increased production of ovarian and/or adrenal androgens.
   2. Abnormal regulation of androgen production by the pituitary gland.
   3. Sex hormone-binding proteins depressed despite normal levels of total androgen.
   4. Increase in end-organ sensitivity with normal free androgen levels.
   5. Genetic factors.
   6. Elevated prolactin.
   7. Acromegaly.
   8. Oral contraceptives or androgen-containing drugs.
C. Pathophysiology.
   1. Coarse, terminal hairs on androgen-dependent areas of the body, such as the chin, periauricular area, chest, abdomen, and anterior thighs.
D. Clinical features.
   1. Pubic and axillary hairs are not affected.
   2. Major racial and ethnic variations occur with hair growth, so what is normal in one may be hirsutism in another.
   3. Onset rapid at puberty with increases noted into the 3rd decade.
   4. May only involve one area of the body such as breasts or mustache region.
   5. Onset gradual.
   6. Balding usually does not occur.
   7. A low hair line and heavy eyebrows usually present.
E. Incidence.
   1. Occurs only in women.

Figure 4.
Hamilton's Classification of Male Androgenic Alopecia

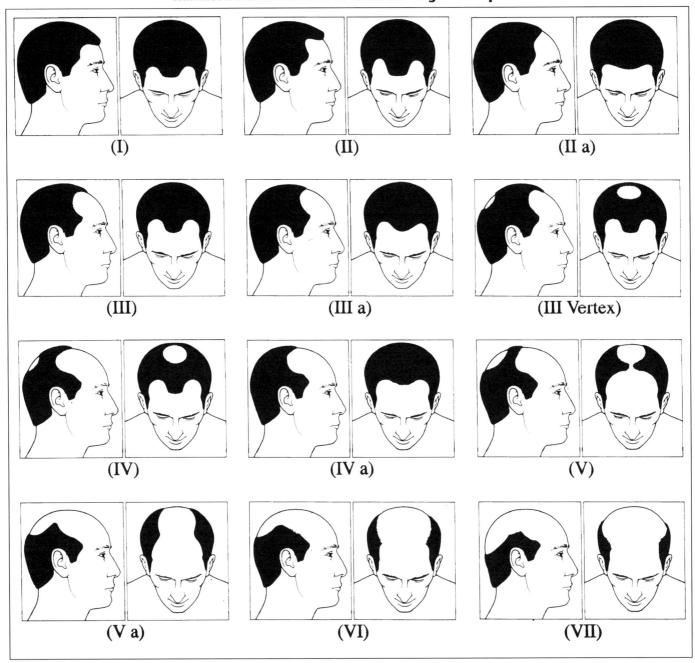

(I)   (II)   (II a)

(III)   (III a)   (III Vertex)

(IV)   (IV a)   (V)

(V a)   (VI)   (VII)

From Olsen, E.A. (1994). *Disorders of hair growth, diagnosis and treatment.* New York: McGraw Hill, Inc.

II. ASSESSMENT

A. See Normal Hair, Assessment.
B. Review current medication regimen to determine presence of drugs reported to cause hirsutism (see Table 5).
C. Obtain laboratory tests for free and total testosterone levels, dehydroepiandrosterone sulfate (DHEAS), the luteinizing hormone/follicle stimulating hormone ratio (LH/FSH), and prolactin. Repeat to confirm diagnosis.
D. Normal menstrual history is consistent with nonendrocrine cause.
E. Ultrasound and computed tomography (CT) if screening suggests underlying disease.

Figure 5.
Norwood's Classification of Male Androgenic Alopecia

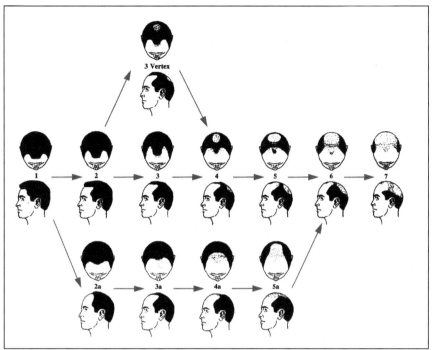

Olsen, E.A. (1994). *Disorders of hair growth, diagnosis and treatment.* New York: McGraw Hill, Inc.

III. COMMON THERAPEUTIC MODALITIES

A. Medical interventions.
1. Estrogen to suppress gonadotrophic production. Dose 1.25 to 2.5 mg conjugated estrogens daily with 5 days of medroxyprogesterone acetate each month.
2. Prednisone, 5 mg/day or dexamethasone, 0.5 mg/day to suppress pituitary-adrenals if indicated.
3. Cyproterone acetate, 50 to 100 mg/day with ethinyl estradiol, 0.05 mg daily. Leads to decreased hair growth in 60% to 90% women in 3 months.
4. Anti-androgens such as spironolactone, 50 mg to 200 mg/day.
5. Bromocriptine to decrease prolactin, if indicated.
B. Surgical interventions.
1. Laparoscopy may be necessary to visualize the ovaries and obtain a biopsy for diagnostic purposes.

IV. COMMON NURSING DIAGNOSES, OUTCOMES, AND INTERVENTIONS (see Table 1)

V. HOME CARE CONSIDERATIONS

A. Physical methods such as plucking, waxing, chemical depilation, and shaving produce temporary removal of unwanted hair.
B. Bleaching with hydrogen peroxide will make unwanted hair less obvious.
C. Electrolysis can produce permanent removal of hair.

TRICHOTILLOMANIA

I. OVERVIEW

A. Definition: a form of alopecia resulting from repetitive pulling, plucking, and breaking of one's own hair.
B. Etiology.
1. Attributed to a variety of psychodynamic conflicts.
2. Ultimate cause unclear.
C. Pathophysiology.
1. Total number of hairs, both terminal and vellus normal.
2. Presence of distorted intrafollicular portions of anagen hairs.
3. Many empty distorted follicles, often with melanin casts.
4. No significant peribulbular inflammation.
D. Clinical features.
1. May involve single or multiple areas of the scalp, particularly the frontal, parietal, or

Table 4.
Ludwig's Classification of Female Androgenic Alopecia.

Type	Clinical Features
I	Mild decrease in hair density on the crown; hairs in this area become thinner, shorter, and less pigmented; frontal hairline is retained.
II	Moderate decrease in hair density on the crown; frontal hairline is still retained.
III	Extensive decrease in hair density on the crown; sparse frontal hairline.

occipital regions, with remainder of scalp normal.

2. Involvement of eyebrows and eyelashes may be seen in 25% of affected patients.
3. Alopecia patches are often unilateral, occurring on the same side at the patient's dominant hand, are variable in size and usually irregular, oval, or asymmetrical.
4. Telogen hairs missing and anagen hairs twisted and broken at various lengths in involved sites.
5. Texture and color of broken hairs unaffected.
6. Pruritus uncommon although some patients may complain of itching and may have excoriations.
7. Teenage and adult patients with more severe disease usually deny touching their hair and rarely admit to the self-induced nature of their hair loss.

E. Incidence.
   1. Two-thirds of affected patients are children, adolescents, and young adults.
   2. Boys outnumber girls by 3 to 2, but females predominate in the older age groups.

II. ASSESSMENT

A. See Normal Hair, Assessment.
B. Biopsy from involved area reveals:
   1. Decreased number of telogen follicles and an increased number of catagen follicles.
   2. Normal follicles found among involuted, damaged, or empty follicles.
   3. Presence of pigmented casts, usually in the isthmus or infundibular area, representing clumps of melanin and keratinaceous debris.

III. COMMON THERAPEUTIC MODALITIES

A. Medical interventions.
   1. Discuss the problem frankly with patient and/or parents of an affected child.
   2. Perform "hair window" by occluding a clipped area in a location that the patient cannot see. Removal of the occlusion in 1 to 3 weeks

Figure 6.
Patterns of Female Androgenic Alopecia

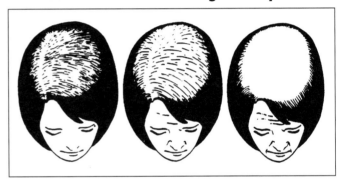

Ludwig, 1977

Table 5.
Drugs Reported to Cause Hirsutism

Acetazolamide	Levonorgestrel
ACTH (Adrenocorticotropic Hormone)	Mestranol + Norethindrone
	Methylprednisone
Buserelin	Methyltestosterone
Calusterone	Metyrapone
Chlorotrianisene	Minoxidil
Clonazepam	Nandrolone
Cortisone	Oxandrolone
Cyclosporine	Oxymetholone
Danazol	Paramethasone
Deflazacort	Penicillamine
Dexamethasone	Phenytoin
Diazoxide	Prednisolone
Dionestrol	Prednisone
Diethylstilbestrol	Quinestrol
Estrogens	Spironolactone
Ethosuximide	Stanozolol
Etretinate	Tacrolimus
Fluocortolone	Testosterone
Fluoxetine	Thioridazine
Fluoxymesterone	Triamcinalone
Lamotrigine	

Dermatologic Nursing Essentials: A Core Curriculum 2nd Edition © DNA 2003

should show proportional 1 cm per month hair growth.

3. Arrange psychiatric consultation for psychotherapy, behavior modification therapy, and antidepressant medication including desipramine, clomipramine, or fluoxetine.

B. Surgical interventions. None.

IV. COMMON NURSING DIAGNOSES, OUTCOMES, AND INTERVENTIONS (see Table 1)

V. HOME CARE CONSIDERATIONS

A. Identify and avoid factors that provoke emotional trauma, stress, anxiety, and fear.

NORMAL NAILS

I. OVERVIEW

A. Definition: the nail covers the upper surface of each finger and toe and acts as a protective covering to the end of each digit. Nails serve as scratching organs and have an increasingly important esthetic and cosmetic purpose.

B. Embryonic development.
1. 9 weeks: proximal lateral and distal groves of the nail field first appear.
2. 12 weeks: future nail bed has both granular and horny layers. Vessel formation present.
3. 18 weeks: nail bed loses granular zone.
4. 20 weeks: matrix cells exhibit adult keratinization.

C. Anatomy: the nail unit consists of components which form, ensheathe, support, anchor, and frame the nail plate (see Figure 7).
1. Nail matrix.
   a. Most proximal portion, extending 5.0 mm beneath proximal nail fold.
   b. Bordered proximally by proximal nail fold and distally by nail bed.
   c. Major function is to produce the nail plate. Basal cells flatten, nuclei fragment, and cytoplasm condense to form horny, keratinized cells that adhere strongly to each other.
2. Nail plate.
   a. Major visible part of the nail arising from matrix.
   b. Usually flat and rectangular in shape.
   c. Approximately 0.5 mm thick in females, 0.6 mm thick in males.
   d. Distal plate thickness can be ranked thumb, index, middle, ring, little finger.
   e. Length of matrix determines thickness of nail plate.
3. Proximal nail fold.
   a. An extension of the skin of surface fingers

and toes. Becomes a fold and lies superficial to matrix.
   b. Contains two layers.
      (1) Cuticle or superficial layer.
         (a) Adheres and moves a short distance on the surface of nail plate before being shed normally.
         (b) Can be seen from the exterior.
      (2) Ventral or deep layer is continuous with the matrix epithelium.
4. Lunula.
   a. White, crescent-shaped area extending from under the proximal nail fold.
   b. Is the most distal and visible portion of matrix.
   c. Determines shape of free edge of nail plate.
   d. White color due to effect of light scattered by nucleated matrix cells and the thick layer of epithelial cells in the matrix.
   e. Marks the end of nail matrix and is the site of mitosis and nail growth.
5. Nail bed.
   a. Supports entire nail plate.
   b. Extends from lunula to hyponychium.
   c. Has longitudinal ridges that fit in a tongue and groove fashion with dermal ridges which are responsible for striations observed on surface of nail plate.
   d. Normal pink color due to enriched vascular network and transparency of nail plate.
   e. Is continuous with matrix and comprises a highly vascular dermis.
6. Dermis.
   a. Is limited by the underlying phalanx with no subcutaneous tissue.
   b. Dermal ridges fit into the parallel and longitudinal groves of epidermal layers and contain the fine capillaries of the nail bed.
7. Hyponychium.
   a. Is the area where the nail plate lifts off the nail bed.
   b. Normally not seen but can be observed in fingers of nail biter.

D. Nail growth.
1. Rate.
   a. Controlled by turnover rate of cells in nail matrix.
   b. Fingernail rate 0.1 to 0.12 mm/day; toenail rate 1/2 to 1/3 fingernail rate.
   c. Growth greater in 2nd and 3rd decades with a slight decline thereafter.
   d. Growth rate factors (see Table 6).
   e. Factors that decrease growth rate (see Table 7).
2. Thickness.
   a. Determined by size of basal cell population in nail matrix.
   b. An increase in matrix length leads to an increase in the thickness of nail.

Table 6.
Factors that Increase Nail Growth Rate

- Summer
- Pregnancy
- Nail biting
- Regrowth after avulsion
- Dominant hand
- Male sex
- Psoriasis/Onycholysis

Table 7.
Factors that Decrease Nail Growth Rate

- Lactation
- Ischemia
- Immobilization/Paralysis
- Cold climates
- Starvation
- Serious systemic illness
- Night
- Antimitotic drugs
- Yellow nail syndrome

II. ASSESSMENT

A. **History and physical examination.**
   1. Patient history.
      a. Detailed history important and should include attention to the evolution of the problem, topical substance exposure, medical, family, and drug histories.
      b. Determine whether underlying systemic disease, recent physical or psychological stress, physical trauma, or exposure to topical agents is a factor.
      c. Explore any relationship to exposure to drugs, environmental hazards, chemicals or toxins, or prolonged immersion in water.
   2. Physical examination.
      a. Remove polish or lacquer when present.
      b. Always inspect all 20 nails as multiple nails are usually involved.
      c. Examine with digits relaxed and not pressed against any surface.
      d. Adequate lighting is essential.
      e. Usually fingernails provide more subtle information that toenails.
      f. Assess color, shape, adherence to nail bed, and presence of lesions.
      g. Note whether nails are soft, hard, brittle, peeling, pitted, or splitting.
      h. Examine skin, hair, and mucous membranes for additional evidence of disease.
      i. Perform a complete physical examination as indicated.
B. **Diagnostic tests: often the diagnosis is clinically evident. In other cases the following tests may be indicated.**
   1. KOH preparation.
   2. Fungal cultures.
   3. Bacterial cultures.
   4. Nail biopsy.
   5. X-ray.

Figure 7.
Structures of the Normal Nail

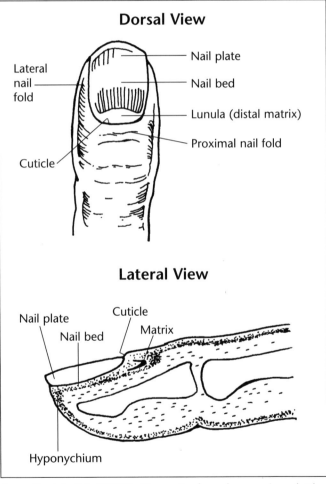

From Daniel, C.R. (1996). *Diagnosis of onychomycosis and other nail disorders.* Marceline, MO: Walsworth Publishing Co.

Dermatologic Nursing Essentials: A Core Curriculum 2nd Edition © DNA 2003

Table 8.
Common Nursing Diagnoses, Outcomes, and Interventions (Nails)

Nursing Diagnoses	Outcomes	Interventions
Anxiety related to nail changes.	1. The patient will demonstrate decreased anxiety, as evidenced by: • Patient's statement of ability to cope with changes.	1. Assess level and observe verbal and nonverbal cues. 2. Listen attentively. 3. Assist the patient to identify concerns about nail changes.
Body image disturbance related to nail changes.	1. Patient will demonstrate beginning adaptation to actual/perceived change in body image as evidenced by: • Statements of acceptance of self. • Active display of interest in personal appearance. • Statements of hope for the future.	1. Have patient describe feelings about self. 2. Implement measures to assist the patient to deal with perceptions of body image. • Establish a therapeutic nurse-patient relationship. • Accept feelings of anger or hostility. • Assist the patient and family in coping with effects of change(s). 3. Teach patient/family methods of dealing with their feelings.
Knowledge deficit related to nail changes.	1. Patient will participate in the learning process. 2. Patient will state understanding of nail condition or disease and treatment.	1. Assess the patient for learning needs, readiness to learn, and factors that will influence learning. 2. Determine the content to be given. • Explain disease and its course. • Teach the patient about each type of treatment. • Emphasize need to comply with all provisions of the treatment process. • Instruct the patient in the proper application of topical medications or appropriate dosing for oral medications. Explain side effects. 3. Implement teaching. 4. Evaluate the patient's success.

6. Fluorescence with black light.
7. Exfoliative cytology.
8. Nail composition studies.

III. COMMON NURSING DIAGNOSES, OUTCOMES, AND INTERVENTIONS (NAILS) (see Table 8)

NAIL DISORDERS: ONYCHOMYCOSIS

I. OVERVIEW

A. **Definition: one of the most common fungal infections of the nail unit. Heat, moisture, trauma, tinea pedis, diabetes mellitus, inheritance, aging, and altered immunologic status are predisposing factors.**

B. **Etiology.**
   1. Approximately 90% to 95% caused by dermatophytes.

C. Pathophysiology.
   1. Fungus penetrates the hyponychium or lateral nail fold region.

D. Clinical features.
   1. More common in toenails than fingernails.
   2. Distal subungual onychomycosis most common.
   3. Predisposing factors include years of trauma, decreased peripheral circulation, nail plate dystrophy, malalignment of nail folds, and immunosuppression.
   4. Early stages associated with yellowish or whitish discoloration of nail.
   5. Nails become thickened, lusterless with subungual debris. Nail plate may crumble.
   6. Splinter hemorrhages, onycholysis, and isolated white or yellow islands on nail plate may also be present.

E. Incidence.
   1. Rare to see in prepubertal child.

Figure 8.
Nails, Unexpected Findings

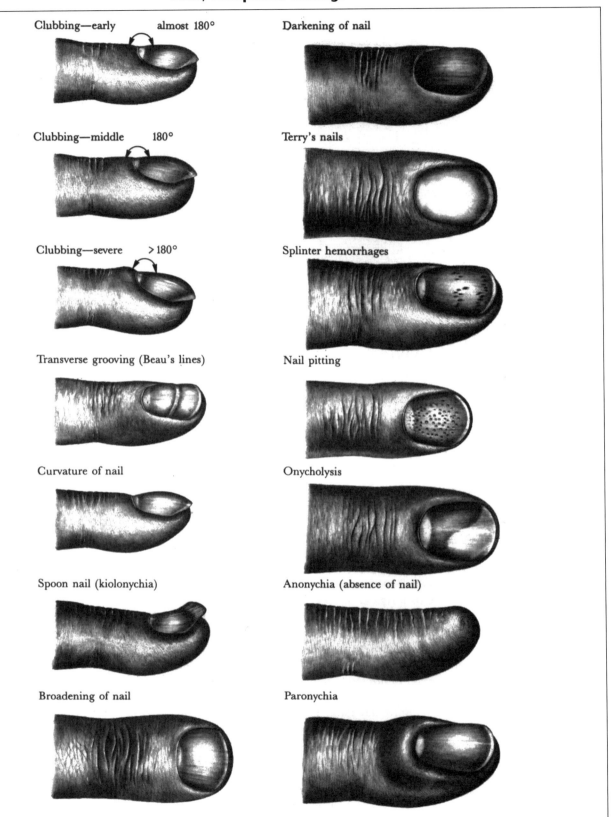

Clubbing—early   almost 180°

Clubbing—middle   180°

Clubbing—severe   >180°

Transverse grooving (Beau's lines)

Curvature of nail

Spoon nail (kiolonychia)

Broadening of nail

Darkening of nail

Terry's nails

Splinter hemorrhages

Nail pitting

Onycholysis

Anonychia (absence of nail)

Paronychia

From Hill, M.J. (1994). *Skin disorders*. St. Louis, MO: Mosby.

Table 9.
Common Nursing Diagnoses, Outcomes, and Interventions (Pain)

Nursing Diagnoses	Outcomes	Interventions
Pain related to infection.	1. Patient will demonstrate diminished pain as evidenced by: • Statement of diminished or absent pain. • Need for analgesics is decreased or nonexistent.	1. Initiate nursing measures to relieve pain. • Warm soaks. • Apply topical antibiotics. • Administer oral antibiotics and analgesics as necessary. 2. Teach patient or family about: • Signs and symptoms of infection. • Transmission and recurrence of infection. • How to avoid aggravating factors, for example, tight clothing, excess moisture.

II. ASSESSMENT

A. See Normal Nails, Assessment.
B. Correct diagnosis by KOH, culture, or biopsy extremely important before beginning therapy.

III. COMMON THERAPEUTIC MODALITIES

A. Medical interventions.
1. Clip abnormal nail and curette underlying nail bed.
2. Terbinafine (Lamisil®), 250 mg qd for 6 weeks for fingernails and 12 weeks for toenails. Itraconazole (Sporanox®) 200 mg bid for 1 week of each month (pulse therapy). Two pulses for fingernails and three pulses for toenails. Liver functions tests midway through therapy for both drugs.
3. Topical solutions of sulconazole (Exelderm®), clotrimazole (Lotrimin®), mycelex or miconazole lotion (Monistat® Derm) may be used in combination with oral therapy.
4. Chemical avulsion using various combinations of urea, salicylic acid, or potassium iodide.
B. Surgical interventions.
1. Nail avulsion, although infrequent.

IV. COMMON NURSING DIAGNOSES, OUTCOMES, AND INTERVENTIONS (see Table 8)

V. HOME CARE CONSIDERATIONS

A. Dry nails and between digits thoroughly after bathing.
B. Apply talcum powder or antifungal powder at least daily.
C. Shoes should fit well and be nonocclusive. Leather shoes or sandals best.
D. Avoid wearing plastic footwear or sneakers.
E. Wear absorbent cotton socks.
F. Avoid stockings with wool or synthetic fibers.
G. Change hand and bath towels frequently and launder in hot water.

PARONYCHIA

I. OVERVIEW

A. Definition: common condition characterized by redness, swelling, and pain of the nail folds. May be acute or chronic, infectious or noninfectious (see Figure 8).
B. Etiology.
1. Exogenous factors such as trauma most likely.
C. Pathophysiology.
1. *S. aureus,* streptococci, and pseudomonas are most common causative organism in acute conditions.
2. Candida and low-grade bacterial infection commonly present in chronic conditions.
D. Clinical features.
1. Predisposing factors such as heat, moisture, trauma to nail folds, local dermatitis, local irritants, diabetes mellitus frequently present.
2. Once a primary infection has occurred in a nail fold, the area is often predisposed to chronic paronychia.
3. Number of fingers involved is associated with chronicity.
4. May be infectious or noninfectious.
E. Incidence.
1. More common in women.

II. ASSESSMENT

A. See Normal Nails, Assessment.
B. Important to inquire about the nature of the patient's occupation, household activities, and hobbies.

III. COMMON THERAPEUTIC MODALITIES

A. Medical interventions.
1. Warm saline or Betadine® soaks, 15 to 20 minutes bid for 5 to 7 days.
2. Topical or oral antibiotics.
B. Surgical interventions.
1. Possible incision and drainage.
2. Possible debridement.

IV. COMMON NURSING DIAGNOSES, OUTCOMES, AND INTERVENTIONS

A. See Table 8.
B. See pain information (Table 9).

V. HOME CARE CONSIDERATIONS

A. All wet work must be stopped.
B. Limit exposure to predisposing factors (trauma and irritants).
C. Wear gloves to protect hands.
D. Avoid nail cosmetics while disorder is healing.
E. Avoid touching the cuticle.
F. Use proper nail care, cutting toe nails straight.

NAIL INVOLVEMENT ASSOCIATED WITH PSORIASIS

I. OVERVIEW

A. Definition: psoriasis is one of many dermatologic disorders that involve the nails. Nail changes can involve any part of the nail unit and cause a variety of clinical and pathological changes.
B. Etiology: strong genetic component. Approximately one out of three people with family history of psoriasis also have the condition.
C. Pathophysiology.
1. Mild to severe hyperkeratosis.
D. Clinical features.
1. Nail pitting due to small psoriatic lesions in the nail matrix.
2. Salmon patch or "the oil drop change" caused by the exudation of a serum glycoprotein which "weeps" onto the nail bed. Causes yellowish color. Resembles a spot of oil.
3. Onycholysis and separation of the distal and lateral edges of nail plate due to psoriatic lesion in the hyponychium and distal nail bed.
4. Subungual thickening due to psoriatic lesions in the hyponychium and distal nail bed for longer duration than onycholysis.
5. Uplifting of nail plate due to extensive cornification.
6. Nail plate that crumbles easily.
7. Subungual splinter hemorrhages.
8. Nail psoriasis without psoriasis on other parts of the body is rare.
9. Severity of nail involvement does not correlate with the severity of cutaneous disease.
E. Incidence.
1. Varies from 10% to 50% of individuals affected with psoriasis.
2. Fingernails affected more often than toenails.

II. ASSESSMENT

A. See Normal Nails, Assessment.
B. Lesions commonly seen are pits (see Figure 8), discoloration, distal or lateral onycholysis (see Figure 8), subungual thickening, and crumbling and grooving of the nail plate.

III. COMMON THERAPEUTIC MODALITIES

A. Medical interventions.
1. No consistently effective treatment.
2. Intralesional steroids involving triamcinolone acetonide 2.5 mg/ml to 5 mg/ml injections into proximal nail fold every 3 to 4 weeks.
3. High-potency topical steroids under occlusion after gently removing the onycholytic nail. Use for only 2 weeks. Do not use in children under 12. Mildly useful.
4. Topical 5-fluorouracil solution gently massaged into fold areas bid for 4 to 6 months. Useful in matrix disease.
5. PUVA or localized psoralen and long-wave ultraviolet light treatments.
6. Methotrexate.
7. Oral etretinate (Tegison®), 0.5 mg to 1 mg/kg/day.
B. Surgical interventions. None.

IV. COMMON NURSING DIAGNOSES, OUTCOMES, AND INTERVENTIONS (see Table 8)

V. HOME CARE INSTRUCTIONS

A. Avoid nail irritants.
B. Keep nails short.
C. Treat psoriasis elsewhere on body.

Bibliography

Arndt, K.A. (1991). *Manual of dermatologic therapeutics* (4th ed.). Boston/Toronto: Little, Brown and Company.

Balden, H.P., & Kvedar, J.C. (1971). Nails. In T.B. Fitzpatrick, A.Z. Eisen, K. Wolf, I.M. Freedberg, & K.F. Austen (Eds.), *Dermatology in general medicine* (pp. 696-709). New York: McGraw-Hill.

Balden, H.P., & Kvedar, J.C. (1971). Biology of nails. In T.B. Fitzpatrick, A.Z. Eisen, K. Wolf, I.M. Freedberg, & K.F. Austen (Eds.). *Dermatology in general medicine* (pp. 294-297). New York: Mc Graw-Hill.

Bertolino, A.P., & Freedberg, I.M. (1971). Disorders of epidermal appendages and related disorders. In T.B. Fitzpatrick, A.Z. Eisen, K. Wolf, I.M. Freedberg, & K.F. Austen (Eds.), *Dermatology in general medicine* (pp. 671-694). New York: Mc Graw-Hill.

Bertolino, A.P., Klein, L.M., & Freedberg, I.M. (1971). Biology of hair follicles. In T.B. Fitzpatrick, A.Z. Eisen, K. Wolf, I.M. Freedberg, & K.F. Austen (Eds.), *Dermatology in general medicine* (pp. 289-293). New York: McGraw-Hill.

Burrell, L.O. (1992). *Adult nursing in hospital and community settings.* Nowalk, CT: Appleton & Lange.

Daniel, C.R. (1996). *Diagnosis of onychomycosis and other nail disorders.* Marceline, MO: Walsworth Publishing Co.

Danial, C.R., & Scher, R.K. (1996). The nail. In W.M Sams, & P.J. Lynch (Eds.), *Principles and practice of dermatology* (pp. 767-777). New York: Churchill Livingstone.

Goldstein, A.M., & Wintroub, B.W. (1994). *Adverse cutaneous reactions to medication — A physician's guide.* New York: CoMedica Inc.

Hamilton, J.B. (1942). Male hormone stimulation is a prerequisite and an incitant in common baldness. *American Journal of Anatomy, 71,* 451-480.

Hill, M.J. (1994). *Skin disorders.* St. Louis, MO: Mosby.

Hordinsky, M.K. (1996). Hair. In W.M Sams, & P.J. Lynch (Eds.), *Principles and practice of dermatology* (pp. 779-800). New York: Churchill Livingstone.

Ludwig, E. (1977). Classification of the types of androgenic alopecia (common baldness) arising in the female sex. *British Journal of Dermatology, 97,* 249-253.

Norwood, O.T. (1975). Male pattern baldness: Classification and incidence. *Southern Medical Journal, 68,* 1359-1365.

Olsen, E.A. (1994). *Disorders of hair growth, diagnosis and treatment.* New York: McGraw Hill.

Scher, R.K., & Daniel, C.R. (1990). *Nails: Therapy, diagnosis, surgery.* Philadelphia: W.B. Saunders Company.

Spindler, J.R., & Data, J.L. (1992). Female androgenic alopecia: A review. *Dermatology Nursing, 4*(2), 93-100.

Hair

1. A club hair is in which growth phase of the hair follicle?
   a. Anagen.
   b. Catagen.
   c. Telogen.
   d. Terminal.

2. What is the active growth phase of the hair follicle?
   a. Anagen.
   b. Catagen.
   c. Telogen.
   d. Vellus.

3. In the normal scalp, what is the percentage of hair follicles in the resting phase of the growth cycle at any time?
   a. 1%.
   b. 5%.
   c. 10%.
   d. 20%.

4. Testosterone is necessary for converting small terminal hairs to large terminal hairs in both males and females.
   a. True.
   b. False.

5. If androgenic alopecia is manifested in young women, an endocrinologic evaluation is also indicated if there is significant:
   a. Acne.
   b. Hirsutism.
   c. Trichotillomania.
   d. All of the above.
   e. None of the above.

6. Nail changes that may occur with alopecia areata include:
   a. Pitting.
   b. Longitudinal ridging.
   c. Beau's lines.
   d. Onychomycosis.
   e. b & c.
   f. a & b.
   g. c & d.

7. Hirsutism may occur:
   a. When there is increased production of ovarian and/or adrenal androgens.
   b. When there is increased end-organ sensitivity with normal free androgen levels.
   c. When sex hormone binding proteins are depressed despite normal levels of total androgen.
   d. All of the above.

Nails

1. The nail component responsible for the shape of the free edge of the nail is:
   a. Matrix.
   b. Hyponychium.
   c. Cuticle.
   d. Lunula.

2. A factor that decreases the growth of the nails includes:
   a. Psoriasis.
   b. Lactation.
   c. Summer.
   d. Immobilization.

3. The thick portion of the nail bed beneath the proximal nail fold from which the nail develops is called:
   a. Nail unit.
   b. Nail matrix.
   c. Lunula.
   d. Ventral Layer.

4. Pitting is a specific finding in psoriasis of the nail plate.
   a. True.
   b. False.

5. What common nail disorder is characterized by redness, swelling, and pain of the nail folds?
   a. Onycholysis.
   b. Onychomycosis.
   c. Pitting.
   d. Paronychia.

6. Onychomycosis may be caused by:
   a. Heat and moisture.
   b. Thyroid dysfunction.
   c. Contact allergy to nail lacquers and hardeners.
   d. *Candida albicans.*

7. Treatment options of nail psoriasis include:
   a. Pulsed-dye laser therapy.
   b. Electrocautery.
   c. Tretinoin formulations.
   d. Cryotherapy.

Answers to Study Questions

Hair		Nails	
1.	c	1.	d
2.	a	2.	d
3.	c	3.	b
4.	a	4.	a
5.	b	5.	d
6.	f	6.	d
7.	d	7.	c

Chapter 18.
Hair and Nails

Please photocopy this test page and return.

COMPLETE THE FOLLOWING:

Name: _____

Address: _____

City: _____ State: _____ Zip: _____

Preferred telephone: (Home)_____ (Work) _____

State where licensed and license number: _____

CE application fee: DNA member $7.00
                       Nonmember $10.00

POSTTEST INSTRUCTIONS
1. To receive continuing education credit for individual study after reading the article, complete the answer/evaluation form below.
2. Photocopy and send the answer/evaluation form along with a check or money order payable to **Dermatology Nurses' Association** to: **DNA**, East Holly Avenue Box 56, Pitman, NJ 08071-0056.
3. Test returns must be postmarked by December 31, 2008. Upon completion of the answer/evaluation form, a certificate for 1.0 contact hour(s) will be awarded and sent to you.

This chapter was reviewed and formatted for contact hour credit by Marcia J. Hill, MSN, RN, Core Curriculum Editor; and Sally Russell, MN, RN,C, DNA Education Director.

ANSWER FORM

1. Name one new detail (item, issue, or phenomenon) that you learned by completing this activity.

_____

_____

_____

_____

2. How will you apply the information from this learning activity to your practice?
   a. Patient education.
   b. Staff education.
   c. Improve my patient care.
   d. In my education course work.
   e. Other: Please describe _____

_____

Evaluation

	Strongly disagree				Strongly agree
3. The offering met the stated objectives.					
a. Identify normal and disease processes affecting the hair and nails.	1	2	3	4	5
b. Discuss the treatment of hair and nail disorders.	1	2	3	4	5
c. Define appropriate skin care and nursing management for these skin disorders.	1	2	3	4	5
4. The content was current and relevant.	1	2	3	4	5
5. The content was presented clearly.	1	2	3	4	5
6. The content was covered adequately.	1	2	3	4	5
7. I am more confident of my abilities since completing this material.	1	2	3	4	5

8. The material was (check one) ☐ new, ☐ review for me.

Comments _____

9. Time required to complete reading assignment: _____ minutes

This independent study is provided by the Dermatology Nurses' Association (DNA) for 1.0 contact hour. DNA is accredited as a provider of continuing education in nursing by the American Nurses Credentialing Center's Commission on Accreditation. DNA is approved as a provider of continuing education by the California Board of Registered Nursing Provider #CEP5708.

Cutaneous Manifestations of HIV

Margaret Sabatini, MS, BSN, RN

OBJECTIVES

At the end of this chapter, the reader will be able to:

- Identify the disease process of the human immunodeficiency virus (HIV).
- Identify the risk factors of HIV.
- Recognize common cutaneous manifestations of HIV.
- List the common cutaneous disorders associated with HIV.

KEY POINTS

- Cutaneous manifestations of HIV can be indicators in diagnosis.
- Universal precautions should be followed with all patients.
- Continued nursing and patient education are essential in patient care.
- Chemoprophylaxis after occupational exposure to HIV may be recommended.
- Patients with HIV often develop common skin disorders with an atypical appearance and/or cases which are severe and explosive.

Cutaneous Manifestations of HIV

Margaret Sabatini, MS, BSN, RN

HIV

I. OVERVIEW (see Figure 1)

HIV compromises the immune system rendering the body more susceptible to illnesses and infections. Early symptomology includes fatigue, fever, diarrhea, lymphadenopathy, weight loss, oral candidiasis, and night sweats. Cutaneous manifestations of HIV include skin cancer, viral, bacterial, and fungal infections, and other cutaneous disorders.

A. Definition: HIV (human immunodeficiency virus) is the virus that causes AIDS (acquired immune deficiency syndrome), the syndrome of opportunistic infections that occur in the final stage of HIV infection. HIV/AIDS is a transmissible blood-borne infectious process.

B. Etiology.
   1. HIV is transmitted through sexual contact and exposure to infected blood or blood products.
   2. Transmission may also occur perinatally from mother to neonate.

   3. Epidemiologic evidence has implicated blood, semen, vaginal secretions, and breast milk as modes of transmission.

C. Pathophysiology.
   1. HIV is transmitted across the mucocutaneous barrier with extension to regional lymph tissue presumably by dendritic cells (days).
   2. Massive viremia with extensive involvement of the lymph tissue (days to weeks).
   3. Immune response with partial control (ascribed to cytotoxic T-cell response, humoral response, and cytokines) (weeks to months).
   4. Persistent HIV replication with relatively constant levels of HIV RNA viremia and gradual CD4 cell depletion over a mean of 8 to 10 years.
   5. Massive destruction of the immune system with susceptibility to opportunistic pathogens and opportunistic tumors when the CD4 cell count reaches <200/mm^3.

D. Risk factors.
   1. Sexual transmission through:
      a. Receptive anal intercourse is considered

Figure 1.
Indicator Conditions in Case Definition of AIDS (1987-1992, Adults)
(Centers for Disease Control, 1992)

Candidiasis of esophagus, trachea, bronchi, or lungs
Cervical cancer, invasive[c,d]
Coccidioidomycosis, extrapulmonary[c]
Crytococcosis, extrapulmonary
Cryptosporidiosis with diarrhea > 1 month
Cytomegalovirus of any organ other than liver, spleen, or lymph nodes
Herpes simplex with mucocutaneous ulcer > 1 month or bronchitis, pneumonitis, esophagitis
Histoplasmosis, extrapulmonary[c]
HIV-associated dementia[c]: disabling cognitive and/or motor dysfunction interfering with occupation or activities of daily living
HIV-associated wasting[c]: involuntary weight loss > 10% of baseline plus chronic diarrhea
   (> 2 loose stools/day > 30 days) or chronic weakness and documented enigmatic fever > 30 days
Isosporosis with diarrhea > 1 month[c]
Kaposi sarcoma in patient under 60 yr (or over 60 yr)[c]
Lymphoma of brain in patient under 60 yr (or over 60 yr)[c]
Lymphoma, non-Hogkins of B cell or unknown immunological phenotype and histology showing small, noncleaved lymphoma or
   immunoblastic sarcoma
Mycobacterium avium or M. kansasii, disseminated
Mycobacterium tuberculosis, disseminated[c]
Mycobacterium tuberculosis, pulmonary[c,d]
Nocardiosisc
Pneumocystis carinii pneumonia
Pneumonia, recurrent-bacterial[c,d]
Progressive multifocal leukoencephalopathy
Salmonella septicemia (nontyphoid), recurrent[c]
Strongyloidosis, extraintestinal
Toxoplasmosis of internal organ

[c]Requires positive HIV serology.
[d]Added in the revised case definition, 1993.

Table 1.
Common Lesions of the HIV Patient

Pseudomembranous candidiasis (thrush)
Erythematous candidiasis
Hyperplastic candidiasis
Hairy leukoplakia
Angular cheilitis
Kaposi's sarcoma
HIV gingivitis
HIV periodonitis

    high risk.
  b. Unprotected and/or unsafe sexual activity with an HIV-infected individual.
  c. Unprotected sexual intercourse with multiple partners.
 2. Intravenous/needle transmission by:
  a. Sharing needles to inject drugs and/or steroids.
  b. Needlestick injuries in health care workers.
 3. Maternal transmission via:
  a. Neonatal transmission in utero or during birth from HIV-infected mother.
  b. Breastfeeding is also a route of transmission from HIV-infected mother.
 4. Other risk factors include:
  a. History of blood transfusion of blood products prior to April 1994.
  b. Occupational exposure in health care workers.

E. Incidence.
 1. According to the CDC and United Nations Programme on HIV/AIDS (UNAIDS) (2000) the following are current HIV/AIDS incidence data:
  a. It is estimated that 800,000 to 900,000 persons in the United States are living with HIV infection, one-third of whom are unaware of their infection.
  b. In the United States approximately 40,000 new HIV infections occur each year of which 70% are men and 30% are women.
  c. Half of all new HIV infections occur in people younger than 25 years of age.
  d. Of new infections among men in the United States, approximately 50% are black, 30% are white, 20% are Hispanic, and a small percentage are members of other racial/ethnic groups.
  e. Of new infections among women in the United States, approximately 64% are black, 18% are white, 18% Hispanic, and a small percentage are members of other racial/ethnic groups.
  f. AIDS is the fifth leading cause of death in the United States among people aged 25 to 44, and is the leading cause of death for

black men in this age group.
  g. Worldwide, approximately 1 in every 100 adults aged 15 to 49 is HIV infected.
  h. Approximately 47% of the 36.1 million adults living with HIV/AIDS are women.
  i. In 2000 alone, HIV/AIDS-associated illnesses caused the deaths of approximately 3 million people worldwide, including an estimated 500,000 children younger that 15 years.

II. **CUTANEOUS ASSESSMENT**

A. **History and physical exam.**
 1. Total body skin exam including oral and genito/anal exam should be conducted (see Table 1).
 2. A complete medical history including sexual history should be obtained.
 3. HIV disease should be considered in the following:
  a. Patient categorized in high-risk group:
   (1) Homosexual/bisexual male.
   (2) History of intravenous drug use (IVDU) or sharing needles to inject drugs or steroids.
   (3) History of sexually transmitted diseases.
   (4) History of recipient of blood or blood products.
   (5) History of unprotected and/or multiple sexual partners.
  b. Insidious onset of skin disorder with:
   (1) Primary or secondary diagnosis of cutaneous manifestation of HIV disease.
   (2) Clinical presentation of skin disorder.
   (3) Patient demographic information, including age.

B. **Diagnostic tests.**
 1. Biopsy if indicated for clinical diagnosis.
 2. KOH and/or fungal or tissue culture per differential diagnosis.
 3. Tzanck test if indicated.
 4. HIV counseling and testing should be encouraged at visit.
 5. Other appropriate blood tests per clinical and differential diagnosis.

III. **CUTANEOUS NEOPLASM**

A. **Kaposi's sarcoma (see Figure 19-1, page 242).**
 1. An opportunistic cancer of the skin and blood vessels included in the AIDS defining group of pathogens and opportunistic infections.
 2. Most common skin manifestation of HIV disease (CD4 200-500) (see Table 1).
 3. Individual lesions of Kaposi's sarcoma (KS) vary in color from pink > dark red > purple > brown macules, plaques, and/or nodules.
 4. Size of the lesions may vary from a few

millimeters to 1.0 centimeter.
5. Lesions can appear anywhere on the skin, mucosa (oral and anal involvement is common) and may also involve the lymphatic system, and internal organs: spleen, liver, stomach, bowel, and lungs.
6. Soles of the feet and buccal mucosa are common sites of involvement.
7. Biopsy of lesion(s) needed to confirm diagnosis.
8. Although treatment response is poor, treatment modalities may include:
   a. Liquid nitrogen therapy.
   b. Chemotherapy.
   c. Chemical destruction.
   d. Intralesional injections with various chemotherapeutic drugs.
   e. Surgical excision.

IV. VIRAL INFECTIONS

A. **Herpes simplex (see Figure 19-2, page 242).**
   1. Very common, contagious viral infection of the skin (primarily mucocutaneous involvement) consisting of herpes simplex virus type 1 (HSV-1) and herpes simplex virus type 2 (HSV-2) with a normal course of 10 days to 2 weeks.
   2. Involves the skin, mucous membrane, mouth, eyes, nose, rectal, and genital areas.
   3. Primary infection of the HSV is more severe and remains dormant until reactivation.
   4. Recurrent herpes simplex infection produces a milder and shorter duration than primary HSV.
   5. Site of involvement becomes erythematous with the development of vesicular lesions in a herpetiform distribution.
   6. Prodrome includes pain, burning, and itching at site of involvement.
   7. In immune-suppressed patients the herpes simplex virus may lead to dissemination causing the following symptoms:
      a. Increased temperature.
      b. Mental confusion.
      c. Weakness.
      d. Headache.
   8. In immune-suppressed patients lesions may present as:
      a. Persistent erosions and ulcerations.
      b. Intractable perirectal ulcerations.
      c. Other infections.
   9. Diagnostic testing includes:
      a. Viral culture; most reliable in obtaining an accurate diagnosis.
      b. Flourescent antibody blood testing.
      c. Tzanck test preparation to obtain immediate diagnosis includes:
         (1) Obtaining smear of cells at base of herpetic lesion.
         (2) Smear cells on a glass slide.
         (3) Stain slide with Wright's or Giemsa's stain.
         (4) Microscopic exam demonstrates multinucleated giant cells.
   10. Treatment modality includes the following:
      a. Famicyclovir (Famvir®, 250 mg 3 times a day) or valcyclovir (Valtrex®, 100 mg twice a day). Both have higher bioavailability and require less frequent dosing.
      b. Acyclovir prophylaxis for recurrent infection (400 mg BID).
      c. Hospitalization and intravenous acyclovir indicated for disseminated HSV.

B. **Herpes zoster (shingles).**
   1. Infectious viral infection (varicella-zoster virus) of the skin.
   2. Development of herpes zoster may be the first sign of HIV infection in young patients (CD4 200 to 500).
   3. Prodrome includes mild to moderate to severe pain at dermatome of involvement, erythema, and a cluster of vesicular lesions in a zosteriform distribution.
   4. Most distinctive feature of herpes zoster is the unilateral distribution of lesions.
   5. Severe pain is caused by inflammation of the nerve endings.
   6. Post neuralgic pain may continue for months after resolution of dermal involvement.
   7. Involvement of the nasociliary branches commonly causes ocular complications including:
      a. Unilateral conjunctivitis.
      b. Acute keratitis.
      c. Optic neuritis.
      d. Corneal ulceration.
      e. Secondary glaucoma.
   8. Trigeminal nerve involvement may be evidenced by lesions present on the tip and side of the nose.
   9. Diagnosis obtained clinically and by obtaining viral culture.
   10. Treatment of herpes zoster includes the following:
      a. Famicyclovir (Famvir®, 250 mg 3 times a day) or valcyclovir (Valtrex®, 100 mg twice a day). Both have higher bioavailability and require less frequent dosing.
      b. Acyclovir orally, 800 mg 5 times daily x 10 days.
      c. Pain control medication as indicated.
      d. Referral to ophthalmologist if ocular involvement is suspected.
      e. Patient avoidance of individuals with suppressed immune systems and individuals, including young children with no history of chickenpox (varicella virus).
      f. Hospitalization/isolation as indicated.

C. **Molluscum contagiosum.**
1. Common cutaneous viral infection seen in patients in late and advanced stages of HIV infection (CD4 < 100).
2. Skin lesions present as translucent papules with central umbilication varying in size from 1 mm up to 1 cm and may be clustered.
3. Site of involvement is common on upper trunk, neck, face, and genital/anal areas although lesions may appear anywhere.
4. Treatment should be instituted when first lesions appear for most effective results.
5. Treatment modalities include the following:
   a. Destructive techniques:
      (1) Liquid nitrogen (LN2) application.
      (2) Curettage.
      (3) Electrodesiccation and curettage.
   b. Topical therapy:
      (1) Retinoic acid 0.05% or 0.1% qd-bid.
      (2) Salicylic acid preparations.

D. **Verruca vulgaris (warts).**
1. Common papilloma virus of the skin.
2. Lesions are verrucous, keratotic growths appearing anywhere on the body but more prominent in genital/anal areas of immune-compromised individuals.
3. Multiple lesions are common in HIV infection and are more resistant to therapy.
4. Most common verrucous lesions include the following:
   a. Common warts (verruca vulgaris).
      (1) Scaly, papular, and/or nodular and flat (flat warts) lesions.
      (2) Mostly found on the hands, although can appear anywhere on skin surface.
   b. Plantar warts.
      (1) Located on the plantar aspect of the feet.
      (2) Hyperkeratotic, painful lesions with dermal vessels present.
   c. Genital warts (penile warts/condyloma acuminata, anogenital).
      (1) Singular or multiple verrucous lesions that may appear on the penile shaft, perianally, perineum to labia majora.
      (2) Lesions may vary in size from 1 to 3 mm to large, crusted "cauliflower" growths.
5. Diagnostic procedures include:
   a. Biopsy is indicated in clinically suspicious lesions.
6. Treatment modalities depending on size, location, and type of wart include the following:
   a. Liquid nitrogen application.
   b. Caustic and acid preparations; salicylic, lactic, bichloraectic acids.
   c. Electrodesiccation and curettage.
   d. Surgical intervention.

E. **Oral hairy leukoplakia.**
1. HIV-associated disorder of the oral mucosa believed to be caused by Epstein-Barr virus.
2. Presents as white plaque-like lesions commonly found on the lateral aspects of the tongue.
3. Lesions may extensively involve the oral and buccal mucosa.
4. Plaque-like lesions may also have a verrucous appearance that are not removable.
5. Diagnostic tests include:
   a. Clinical diagnosis
   b. Biopsy as indicated
6. Treatment modality includes:
   a. Intravenous or oral acyclovir as indicated.
   b. Spontaneous resolution may occur.

V. BACTERIAL INFECTION

A. **Impetigo.**
1. Most commonly seen bacterial infection in HIV-infected individuals.
2. Skin manifestations characterized by multiple, oozing, vesicular lesions developing a honey yellow crust.
3. Lesions ulcerate and crust.
4. Diagnostic testing includes:
   a. Bacterial cultures and sensitivity of vesicular lesion obtained to:
      (1) Identify specific causative agent.
      (2) Initiate appropriate antibiotic therapy.
5. Treatment of impetigo consists of the following:
   a. Antibiotic therapy per culture and sensitivity results.
   b. Antibacterial wash to area bid.
   c. May also include topical antibacterial/anti-biotic therapy.

VI. FUNGAL INFECTIONS

A. **Oral candidiasis (thrush)(see Figure 19-3, page 242).**
1. Most common yeast infection associated with HIV-infected individuals.
2. Oral lesions present as white, curd-like patches/plaques on the tongue and buccal mucosa.
3. Symptoms associated with candidiasis of the mouth (thrush) include the following:
   a. Soreness of the mouth and throat.
   b. Difficulty swallowing.
   c. Loss of taste.
4. Oral candidiasis can spread to the esophagus causing symptoms of pain and burning upon swallowing.
5. Diagnostic tests include:
   a. Clinical diagnosis is usual.
   b. KOH demonstrates budding yeast and hyphae.
   c. Scraping and culture of lesion.

6. Treatment modalities may include the following:
   a. Nystatin gargles.
   b. Clotrimazole troches.
   c. Fluconazole p.o.
B. **Tinea unguium (onychomycosis) (see Figure 19-4, page 242).**
   1. Fungal infection of the fingernails and/or toenails is common in HIV patients.
   2. Nails present as thickened and white with proximal subungual debris.
   3. Development of proximal white subungual onychomycosis in both fingernails and toenails is commonly seen in patients with HIV disease.
   4. Most proximal or superficial white onychomycosis in HIV patients is caused by *T. rubrum.*
   5. Candida is the primary pathogen of the nail bed and plate causing dystrophy to the nail in HIV patients (CD4 < 100).
   6. Diagnostic tests include:
      a. KOH preparation and microscopic exam.
      b. Fungal culture.
   7. Treatment modalities include:
      a. Oral medication and dosage as indicated may include:
         (1) Griseofulvin.
         (2) Ketoconazole.
         (3) Itraconazole.
      b. Topical treatment:
         (1) Miconazole.
         (2) Clotrimazole.
C. **Tinea manum.**
   1. Fungal infection of the palm(s) of the hand often seen with proximal subungual onychomycosis (tinea unguium) in HIV-infected patients.
   2. Presents as fine white scale on the palmer aspect of the hand.
   3. Usually present on one hand, but may also involve both.
   4. Diagnostic tests include:
      a. KOH preparation with microscopic exam.
      b. Fungal culture.
   5. Treatment modalities include:
      a. Oral medication and dosage per indications:
         (1) Griseofulvin.
         (2) Ketoconazole.
         (3) Itraconazole.
      b. Topical treatment as indicated:
         (1) Miconazole.
         (2) Clotrimazole.
D. **Other fungal infections.**
   1. Tinea pedis.
      a. Fungal infection of the feet.
      b. Presents with dryness and scale on plantar aspect of the feet.

c. Maceration of toe webs is common.
      d. Vesicular and/or pustular lesions may also be present.
   2. Tinea cruris.
      a. Fungal infection of the groin.
      b. Often called "jock itch."
      c. Pruritic erythematous rash with scaling extending to upper anterior thighs.
      d. May also present with well-defined elevated border.
   3. Diagnostic tests include:
      a. KOH preparation with microscopic exam that demonstrates branching hyphae.
      b. Fungal culture if indicated.
   4. Treatment of fungal infection may include:
      a. Oral medication as indicated.
      b. Topical antifungal creams.
      c. Recurrent fungal infections of the skin is common in HIV-infected patients.

VII. OTHER CUTANEOUS DISORDERS

A. **Dry skin.**
   1. Common cutaneous disorder seen in HIV-infected individuals.
   2. May present as mild, moderate, or severe.
   3. Dry, flaky skin can also result in pruritus.
   4. Diagnostic tests may include:
      a. Usually a clinical presentation diagnosis.
      b. KOH preparation and microscopic exam to rule out dermatophyte infection and/or scabies.
   5. Plan of treatment includes:
      a. Decreased water temperature when bathing.
      b. Use of mild soaps.
      c. Moisturizing skin regularly, especially after bathing when skin is wet.
      d. Topical 1% hydrocortisone if indicated.
      e. Oral antihistamines for pruritus if indicated.
B. **Seborrheic dermatitis.**
   1. Common cutaneous skin disorder in HIV-infected individuals.
   2. Presents as red, dry flaky skin condition involving the nasolabial folds bilaterally, forehead, eyebrows, and ears; may be severe and extensive.
   3. Seborrhea of the scalp is also commonly known as dandruff.
   4. Other areas of skin that may be involved are the chest and groin.
   5. Diagnostic tests include:
      a. Usually clinical diagnosis per presentation
      b. KOH preparation and microscopic exam to rule out dermatophyte infection
   6. Treatment modality includes:
      a. Topical 1% hydrocortisone cream.
      b. In severe cases, the use of stronger topical

therapy may be indicated.
c. Anti-seborrheic shampoos indicated for scalp involvement.
d. Oral ketoconazole or topical cream.

C. **Psoriasis.**
1. Cutaneous skin disorder presenting with erythematous to pink-salmon plaques with overlying white scale.
2. Plaques are commonly seen anywhere on the cutaneous surface but most often on the surface of the elbows, knees, and umbilicus.
3. Involvement of the scalp is common and may be severe.
4. HIV-infected individuals with a past history of psoriasis often develop worsening of this skin condition.
5. Total body psoriasis with erythema and scaling and accompanying intense pruritus can also be seen in the immune-compromised individual.
6. The development of pustular lesions on the palms and soles (pustular psoriasis) may also be present.
7. Diagnostic tests include:
   a. KOH preparation and microscopic exam to rule out dermatophyte infection.
   b. Biopsy of plaque(s) may be indicated to confirm diagnosis and rule out other cutaneous disorders.
8. Treatment consists of the following:
   a. Topical cortisone creams or ointments and/or tar preparations.
   b. Skin care instruction including bathing techniques.
   c. Moisturization with emollient creams and/or ointments.
   d. Ultraviolet light therapy may be indicated.
   e. Oral antihistamines may be indicated for extreme pruritus.
   f. Other oral medications such as methotrexate and advanced therapy may be contraindicated rendering further suppression of the immune system in the HIV-infected individual.

D. **Eosinophilic pustular folliculitis.**
1. Common cutaneous disorder presenting with follicular pustules and erythematous papules which may be asymptomatic to pruritic.
2. May present as widespread acneiform eruption.
3. Common areas of involvement include:
   a. Face and scalp.
   b. Chest and/or trunk.
   c. Buttocks and lower extremities.
4. Secondary impetigination and infection may occur as the result of pruritic pustules and papules and/or self-manipulation.
5. Diagnostic tests include:
   a. Usually a clinical presentation diagnosis.
   b. Culture and sensitivity of pustular lesions

indicated in suspected cases of secondary infection.
6. Treatment modalities include:
   a. Topical steroids.
   b. Oral antihistamines may be indicated for pruritus.
   c. Oral antibiotics are indicated in cases with secondary infection.
   d. Ultraviolet light treatment may be indicated.

VIII. NURSING CONSIDERATIONS (see Table 2)

A. **The nursing assessment of the patient is critical for managing and providing optimal patient care. The role of the nurse includes:**
1. Education.
   a. Providing patient education in overview of the disease process.
   b. Providing educational tools to the patient; pamphlets, resource materials, etc.
   c. Providing instruction and application of use of medications indicated for patient care.
   d. Provide education to family members and significant others as indicated.
   e. Providing HIV counseling as indicated.
2. Resource.
   a. The nurse provides resource information to the patient in the following areas:
      (1) Support group information.
      (2) Educational materials.
      (3) Drug trials.
      (4) Medical care and support information.
3. Medical care.
   a. Provides skilled nursing care in assisting surgical procedures.
   b. Provides skilled nursing care in wound and dressing care.
   c. Provides skilled nursing care in sterile techniques.
   d. Provides skilled nursing care in dermatologic procedures.
   e. Provides skilled nursing care in universal precautions.

IX. UNIVERSAL PRECAUTIONS (see Table 3)

A. **Universal precautions should be practiced with ALL patients.**
1. Universal precautions include:
   a. The use of barrier precautions.
      (1) To avoid skin or mucous membrane exposure.
   b. Routine and regular handwashing.
      (1) To avoid contamination with blood and/or body fluids.
   c. Sharps and needlestick protection.
      (1) Do not recap needles.
      (2) Dispose sharps, blades, needles, and

Table 2.
Nursing Diagnoses, Interventions, and Outcomes in Cutaneous Manifestations of HIV

Nursing Diagnoses	Interventions	Outcomes
Anxiety related to: HIV/AIDS disease.	Reduce anxiety. Better understanding of HIV disease. Resource information available in the community to ensure patient has available support systems. Referral to appropriate provider or resources.	Patient education of HIV/AIDS, including physiology, risk factors, transmission, common skin disorders and resources. Provide HIV counseling as indicated.
Skin disorders.	Better understanding of common skin disorders and the cutaneous manifestations of HIV. Patient verbalization and increased level of comfort.	Provide patient with educational materials. Provide patient with overview of disorder. Encourage questions and concerns.
Surgical procedures.	Reduce anxiety and stress. Increased level of patient comfort.	Discuss and explain surgical procedures with the patient. Encourage questions and concerns.
Altered physical discomfort: pain and pruritus related to skin disorder and/or surgical procedures. Pain	Identify level of patient discomfort. Patient verbalization and increased level of comfort. Increase the level of patient comfort. Decrease or alleviate pain.	Assess level of pain and patient discomfort. Encourage questions, concerns, and feelings. Discuss the use of prescribed pain medication and/or the use of analgesics and anti-inflammatory drugs to decrease pain.
Pruritus and dry skin.	Pruritus alleviated or subsided. Well hydrated skin. Decreased or alleviated patient discomfort. Patient verbalizes level of comfort.	Discuss the use of anti-pruritics, including dosage, adherence, and safety. Educate patient in methods of moisturization and choices of moisturizers. Discuss medication and/or moisturization application techniques. Assess level of patient comfort and concerns.

Table 2. (continued)
Nursing Diagnoses, Interventions, and Outcomes in Cutaneous Manifestations of HIV

Nursing Diagnoses	Interventions	Outcomes
Decreased self-esteem related to body image and skin manifestations.	Patient will verbalize concerns, fears, and feelings. Increased self-esteem.	Encourage patient to verbalize concerns, fears, and feelings. Acknowledge medical interventions and response to treatments. Discuss cosmetic interventions when applicable.
Potential side effects to medications.	Patient demonstrates understanding of medications. Patient understanding of common side effects. Increased patient understanding to treatment. Demonstrates adherence to medication regimen and positive outcomes. Participates in continued care, followup and needed interventions.	Discuss oral and/or topical medications. Inform patient of potential side effects. Discuss how and when to take oral medications. Educate patient on topical medication application techniques. Acknowledge the importance of adherence to treatment. Instruct patient to report on treatment modalities and any questions and concerns. Instruct patient on followup appointment.

syringes in a puncture-resistant container.
d. The use of resuscitation devices.
(1) Mouthpieces and/or ventilation devices should be used in resuscitation.
e. Caregivers at risk.
(1) Presence of dermatitis.

X. POST EXPOSURE PROPHYLAXIS (see Table 4)

A. U.S. Centers for Disease Control and Prevention guidelines on post HIV exposure prophylaxis and recommendations for chemoprophylaxis of HIV infection in health care workers exposed to the virus include:
1. Type of exposure includes:
   a. Percutaneous exposure.
   b. Mucous membrane exposure.
   c. Skin, increased risk.

2. Source.
   a. Blood.
   b. Fluid containing blood.
   c. Infectious fluid/body fluid.
   d. Tissue.
3. Antiretroviral prophylaxis.
4. Regimen of chemoprophylaxis includes the following for combination therapy:
   a. AZT, zidovudine (Retrovir®).
   b. 3TC, lamivudine (Epivir®).
   c. IDV, indinavir sulfate (Crixivan®).

Dermatologic Nursing Essentials: A Core Curriculum 2nd Edition © DNA 2003

Table 3.
Universal Precautions to Prevent Transmission of HIV

1. All healthcare workers should routinely use appropriate barrier precautions to prevent skin and mucous membrane exposure when contact with blood or other body fluids of any patient anticipated. Gloves should be worn for touching blood and body fluids, mucous membranes, or non-intact skin of all patients, for handling items or surfaces soiled with blood or body fluids, and for performing venipuncture and other vascular access procedures. Gloves should be changed after contact with each patient. Masks and protective eyewear or face shields should be worn during procedures that are likely to generate droplets of blood or other body fluids to prevent exposure of mucous membranes of the mouth, nose and eyes. Gowns or aprons should be worn during procedures that are likely to generate splashes of blood or other body fluids.

2. Hands and other skin surfaces should be washed immediately and thoroughly if contaminated with blood or other body fluids. Hands should be washed immediately after gloves are removed.

3. All healthcare workers should take precautions to prevent injuries caused by needles, scalpels, and other sharp instruments or devices during procedures; when cleaning used instruments; during disposal of used needles; and when handling sharp instrument after procedures. To prevent needlestick injuries, needles should not be recapped, purposely bent or broken by hand, removed from disposable syringes, or otherwise manipulated by hand. After they are used, disposable syringes and needles, scalpel blades, and other sharp items should be placed in puncture-resistant containers for disposal; the puncture-resistant containers should be located as close as practical to the use area. Large-bore reusable needles should be placed in a puncture-resistant container for transport to the reprocessing area.

4. Although saliva has not been implicated in HIV transmission, to minimize the need for emergency mouth-to-mouth resuscitation, mouthpieces, resuscitation bags, or other ventilation devices should be available for use in areas in which the need for resuscitation is predictable.

5. Healthcare workers who have exudative lesions or weeping dermatitis should refrain from all direct patient care and from handling patient-care equipment until the condition resolves.

6. Pregnant healthcare workers are not known to be at greater risk of contracting HIV infection than healthcare workers who are not pregnant; however, if a healthcare worker develops HIV infection during pregnancy, the infant is at risk of infection resulting from perinatal transmission. Because of this risk, pregnant healthcare workers should be especially familiar with and strictly adhere to precautions to minimize the risk of HIV transmission.

Centers for Disease Control (1987)

Bibliography
Bartlett, J.G. (1996). *The John Hopkins Hospital 1996 guide to medical care of patients with HIV infection*. Baltimore, MD: Williams and Wilkins.
Centers for Disease Control and Prevention Public Health Image Library (2002). Retrieved June 21, 2002 from http://phil.cdc.gov/phil/search_page.asp
Centers for Disease Control and Prevention. (1995). *HIV/AIDS surveillance report, 7*(2), 1-5.
Centers for Disease Control and Prevention. (1992). Indicator conditions in case definition of AIDS (1987-1992, adults). *MMWR, 41*, 1-9.
Centers for Disease Control and Prevention. (1996). Recommendations for chemoprophylaxis after occupational exposure to HIV. *MMWR, 45*(22), 468-472.
Centers for Disease Control and Prevention. (1987). Recommendations for prevention of HIV transmission in healthcare settings. *MMWR, 36*(2S), 1S-18S.

Daniel, C.R. (1996). *Diagnosis of onychomycosis and other nail disorders*. New York: Springer.
Elmets, C. (1993). Management of common superficial fungal infections in patients with AIDS. *Journal of the American Academy of Dermatology, 31*, S60-S63.
Fitzpatrick, T.B., Eisen, A.Z., Wolff, K., Freedberg, I.M., & Austen, K.F. (1987). *Dermatology in general medicine*. New York: McGraw-Hill.
National Institute of Health. (2002). *AIDS history*. Retrieved June 21, 2002 from http://aidshistory.nih.gov/imgarchive/index.html#HIV
Pantaleo, G., Graziosi, C., & Fauci, S. (1993). The immunopathogenesis of human immunodeficiency virus infection. *New England Journal of Medicine, 328*(5), 327-335.
UNAIDS. (2000, December). *Report on the global HIV/AIDS epidemic*.

Table 4.
Provisional Public Health Service Recommendations for Chemoprophylaxis After Occupational Exposure to HIV, by Type of Exposure and Source Material - 1996

Type of Exposure	Source Material*	Antiretroviral Prophylaxis[†]	Antiretroviral Regimen[§]
Percutaneous	Blood[¶] Highest risk Increased risk No increased risk Fluid containing visible blood, other potentially infectious fluid[††], or tissue. Other body fluid (for example, urine)	Recommended Recommended Offer Offer Not Offer	ZDV plus 3TC plus IDV ZDU plus 3TC, + IDV** ZDU plus 3TC ZDU plus 3TC
Mucous Membrane	Blood Fluid containing visible blood, other potentially infectious fluid[††], or tissue. Other body fluid (for example, urine)	Offer Offer Not Offer	ZDU plus 3TC, + IDV** ZDU + 3TC
Skin Increased Risk[§§]	Blood Fluid containing visible blood, other potentially infectious fluid, or tissue. Other body fluid (for example, urine)	Offer Offer Not Offer	ZDU plus 3TC, + IDV** ZDU, + 3TC

Key: ZDU, zidovudine (Retrovir®); 3TC, lamivudine (Epivir®); IDV, indinavir sulfate (Crixivan®).

* Any exposure to concentrated HIV (e.g., in a research laboratory or production facility) is treated as percutaneous exposure to blood with highest risk.

† Recommend—Postexposure prophylaxis (PEP) should be recommended to the exposed worker with counseling (see text). Offer—PEP should be offered to the exposed worker with counseling (see text). Not offer—PEP should not be offered because these are not occupational exposures to HIV.

§ Regimens: Zidovudine (ZDV), 200 mg 3 times a day; lamivudine (3TC), 150 mg 2 times a day; indinavir (IDV), 800 mg 3 times a day (if IDV is not available, saquinavir may be used, 600 mg 3 times a day). Prophylaxis is given for 4 weeks. For full prescribing information, see package inserts.

¶ Highest risk—BOTH larger volume of blood (e.g., deep injury with large diameter hollow needle previously in source patient's vein or artery, especially involving an injection of source-patient's blood) AND blood containing a high titer of HIV (e.g., source with acute retroviral illness or end-stage AIDS; viral load measurement may be considered, but its use in relation to PEP has not been evaluated). Increased risk—EITHER exposure to larger volume of blood OR blood with a high titer of HIV. No increased risk — NEITHER exposure to larger volume of blood NOR blood with a high titer of HIV (e.g., solid suture needle injury from source patient with asymptomatic HIV infection).

** Possible toxicity of additional drug may not be warranted (see text).

†† Includes semen; vaginal secretions; cerebrospinal, synovial, pleural, peritoneal, pericardial, and amniotic fluids.

§§ For skin, risk is increased for exposures involving a high titer of HIV, prolonged contact, an extensive area, or an area in which skin integrity is visibly compromised. For skin exposures without increased risk, the risk for drug toxicity outweighs the benefit of PEP.

Source: Update: Provisional Public Health Service recommendations for chemoprophylaxis after occupational exposure to HIV. MMWR 1996; *45* (22), 468-472.

1. According to the Centers for Disease Control, the estimated number of people living with HIV infection in the United States is:
   a. 40,000.
   b. 500,000.
   c. 800,000 to 900,000.
   d. 10 million.
   e. 36.1 million.

2. AIDS is the fifth leading cause of death in the United States among people aged 25 to 44 and is the leading cause of death in this age group among:
   a. Hispanic women.
   b. Black women.
   c. Hispanic men.
   d. Black men.
   e. None of the above.

3. According to the CDC, indicator conditions in the case definition of AIDS include the following *except*:
   a. Cervical cancer, noninvasive.
   b. Pneumocystis carinii pneumonia.
   c. Cryptococcosis with diarrhea > 1 month.
   d. *Mycobacterium avium.*
   e. Progressive multifocal leukoencephalopathy.

4. In the patient with HIV, a common lesion(s) include:
   a. Hairy leukoplakia.
   b. Erythematous candidiasis.
   c. Angular cheilitis.
   d. HIV gingivitis.
   e. All of the above.

5. Ocular complications associated with herpes zoster resulting from involvement of the nasociliary branches include:
   a. Acute keratitis.
   b. Optic neuritis.
   c. Bilateral conjunctivitis.
   d. a & b.
   e. a, b, & c.

6. A very common, contagious viral infection of the skin with a normal course of 10 days to 2 weeks is:
   a. Molluscum contagiosum.
   b. Herpes zoster.
   c. Herpes simplex virus.
   d. Kaposi's sarcoma.
   e. Disseminated herpes simplex.

7. Eosinophilic pustular folliculitis is a common cutaneous disorder that:
   a. Presents as an isolated lesion.
   b. Involves the buccal mucosa.
   c. Treatment modality includes cryotherapy.
   d. Surgical intervention may be indicated.
   e. None of the above.

8. The HIV-associated viral infection believed to be caused by the Epstein-Barr virus is:
   a. Herpes simplex.
   b. Oral hairy leukoplakia.
   c. Molluscum contagiosum.
   d. Verruca vulgaris.
   e. Herpes zoster.

9. Symptoms associated with oral candidiasis (thrush) include:
   a. Soreness of the mouth and throat.
   b. Difficulty swallowing.
   c. Loss of taste.
   d. Loss of smell.
   e. a, b, & c.

10. A Tzanck test preparation for microscopic exam is used for the diagnostic testing of the following cutaneous lesion(s):
    a. Kaposi's sarcoma.
    b. Herpes simplex.
    c. Verruca vulgaris.
    d. Oral hairy leukoplakia.
    e. All of the above.

11. Universal precautions to prevent transmission of HIV should be practiced with all patients and include:
    a. The use of barrier precautions.
    b. Routine and regular handwashing.
    c. Sharps and needlestick protection.
    d. Use of resuscitation devices.
    e. All of the above.

Answers to Study Questions

1.	c	5.	d	9.	e
2.	d	6.	c	10.	b
3.	a	7.	e	11.	e
4.	e	8.	b		

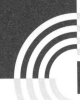
Chapter 19.
Cutaneous Manifestations of HIV

Please photocopy this test page and return.

COMPLETE THE FOLLOWING:

Name: _____

Address: _____

City: _____ State: _____ Zip: _____

Preferred telephone: (Home)_____ (Work) _____

State where licensed and license number: _____

CE application fee: DNA member $10.00
                        Nonmember $13.00

POSTTEST INSTRUCTIONS

1. To receive continuing education credit for individual study after reading the article, complete the answer/evaluation form below.

2. Photocopy and send the answer/evaluation form along with a check or money order payable to **Dermatology Nurses' Association** to: **DNA**, East Holly Avenue Box 56, Pitman, NJ 08071-0056.

3. Test returns must be postmarked by December 31, 2008. Upon completion of the answer/evaluation form, a certificate for 2.4 contact hour(s) will be awarded and sent to you.

This chapter was reviewed and formatted for contact hour credit by Marcia J. Hill, MSN, RN, Core Curriculum Editor; and Sally Russell, MN, RN,C, DNA Education Director.

ANSWER FORM

1. Name one new detail (item, issue, or phenomenon) that you learned by completing this activity.

   _____

   _____

   _____

   _____

2. How will you apply the information from this learning activity to your practice?

   a. Patient education.
   b. Staff education.
   c. Improve my patient care.
   d. In my education course work.
   e. Other: Please describe _____

   _____

   _____

Evaluation

	Strongly disagree				Strongly agree
3. The offering met the stated objectives.					
a. Identify the disease process of the human immunodeficiency virus (HIV).	1	2	3	4	5
b. Identify the risk factors of HIV.	1	2	3	4	5
c. Recognize common cutaneous manifestations of HIV.	1	2	3	4	5
d. List the common cutaneous disorders associated with HIV.	1	2	3	4	5
4. The content was current and relevant.	1	2	3	4	5
5. The content was presented clearly.	1	2	3	4	5
6. The content was covered adequately.	1	2	3	4	5
7. I am more confident of my abilities since completing this material.	1	2	3	4	5

8. The material was (check one) ☐ new, ☐ review for me.

Comments _____

9. Time required to complete reading assignment: _____ minutes

This independent study is provided by the Dermatology Nurses' Association (DNA) for 2.4 contact hours. DNA is accredited as a provider of continuing education in nursing by the American Nurses Credentialing Center's Commission on Accreditation. DNA is approved as a provider of continuing education by the California Board of Registered Nursing Provider #CEP5708.

CHAPTER TWENTY

Wound Healing

Janice Zeigler Cuzzell, MA, RN

OBJECTIVES

At the end of this chapter, the reader will be able to:
- Describe the phases of wound healing.
- Differentiate between healing by tissue regeneration versus healing by scarring and wound contraction.
- List three factors that delay the wound healing process.
- Distinguish between intrinsic and extrinsic factors that affect wound healing.
- Identify various wound dressings and how to use them to optimize healing.

KEY POINTS

- Wound healing comprises a naturally occurring series of events (cascade) that are dependent on specialized cells.
- Delayed healing or failure to obtain wound closure is usually due to a disruption in the normal cascade of healing.
- The host's status must be optimized to adequately support tissue repair.
- Choosing an appropriate treatment depends on accurate wound assessment and identification of the phase of healing.
- Knowledge of dressing materials and their appropriate use is essential in choosing products.

Wound Healing

Janice Zeigler Cuzzell, MA, RN

Author's Note: A wound is defined as any disruption in the integrity and/or function of the skin that incites normal or abnormal repair responses (Eaglestein et al., 1990). Normal wound healing is an orderly process that occurs as a cascade of biocellular events mediated by the actions of specialized cells. These events begin at the moment of wounding and, if not interfered with, will proceed to a predictable end point — a healed wound.

I. PHYSIOLOGY OF WOUND HEALING

A. Definition: the wound healing process is a series of events, or cascade (see Table 1), that is dependent on specialized cells and cellular functions that lead to a healed wound. Wounds heal by one of two methods — regeneration or scar formation. The depth of damage will determine the type of healing that a wound will undergo. Epithelial regeneration (re-epithelialization) is limited to wounds that involve the epidermis and upper layers of the dermis. Scar formation is the wound healing process that is required for repair of deeper wounds with more extensive tissue destruction.

B. Phase I — Inflammation: the body's immediate response to wounding is "defensive;" this begins with hemostasis followed immediately by inflammation. The goal of this phase is to control bleeding, defend the body against invasion by harmful agents in the environment, and to initiate tissue repair. The clinical characteristics of this phase are the classic signs of inflammation: erythema, edema, warmth, and pain.

1. Hemostasis — the clotting process is initiated at wounding with the disruption of cellular and vascular components; blood is exposed to collagen initiating the release of clotting factors, platelet aggregation, and fibrin deposition.

2. Vascular/cellular response — vasodilatation and increased vascular permeability lead to leakage of protein-rich fluid into the wound space causing edema, erythema, and warmth; leukocytes (PMNs) migrate into the wounded area and begin to digest debris and bacteria; macrophages gradually replace leukocytes as "scavengers" in the wound space; macrophages also mediate the release of growth factors and chemoattractants that are critical to initiating the proliferative phase of healing.

C. Phase II — Proliferative phase: this phase overlaps the inflammatory phase beginning about the 4th day post wounding and lasts for approximately 15 to 16 days. The goal of the proliferative phase of healing is to repair damaged tissue and restore the barrier function of the skin. The clinical characteristics of this phase are re-epithelialization, granulation, and tissue contraction.

1. Granulation — the formation of new connective (scar) tissue which provides a structural matrix for migration of epithelial cells; involves two processes, neoangiogenesis and collagen synthesis; these processes occur simultaneously and are co-dependent; wound contraction occurs concurrently with granulation.

   a. Neoangiogenesis — the process of new blood vessel formation is stimulated by hypoxia resulting from vascular disruption at the time of wounding.

Table 1.
Wound Healing Cascade

Inflammatory Phase (Defense)
- Begins with hemostasis and release of growth factors at the time of wounding — platelets are the primary mediator in this phase.
- Phagocytosis (breakdown of necrotic material) — polymorphonuclear leukocytes and macrophages are the primary mediators in this phase.

Proliferation Phase
- Formation of granulation tissue; wound contraction and epithelialization occur in this phase.
- Fibroblasts, endothelial cells, and keratinocytes are the primary mediators in this phase.

Maturation Phase
- Remodeling of scar tissue through collagen synthesis and collagen breakdown.
- Macrophages and fibroblasts are the primary mediators in this phase.

b. Collagen synthesis — a complex process that involves the formation of connective tissue substances combined with the synthesis of new collagen fibers; collagen synthesis is initiated by fibroblasts, specialized cells controlled by macrophage-mediated growth factors; this process requires oxygen and nutrients, therefore the vascular and nutritional status of the patient are crucial to normal tissue repair.

2. Epithelialization — resurfacing of the wound which begins at the wound edges and from undamaged skin appendages; in deep dermal wounds epithelialization occurs in conjunction with collagen synthesis; in more extensive wounds, epithelialization does not occur until granulation tissue is present.

3. Contraction: pulling together of the tissue and skin surrounding the wound in the direction of least resistance, gradually reducing the size of the defect.

D. Phase III — Maturation phase: overlaps with the proliferative phase and continues for up to a year or longer after the wound has closed; in full-thickness wounds collagen is remodeled. Disorganized collagen is broken down (lysed) and redeposited in a more organized fashion. The goal of the maturation phase is to maximize the tensile strength of the wound and protect the scar from rupture due to mechanical stress. The tensile strength of a healed wound is always less than that of uninjured tissue. This phase is characterized clinically by raised erythematous scar tissue that gradually flattens and no longer blanches when pressure is applied.

Note: Superficial wounds do not scar; deep dermal wounds will scar.

II. FUNCTION OF CELLS IN WOUND HEALING

The cells involved in the wound healing process include platelets, leukocytes, macrophages, fibroblasts, myofibroblasts, and epithelial cells (keratinocytes).

A. Platelets: the smallest cell in the blood is essential for coagulation of blood and maintenance of hemostasis; becomes active in clot formation when blood becomes exposed to collagen after tissue injury; platelets release growth factors that assist in wound repair.

B. Leukocytes: polymorphonuclear leukocytes (PMNs) migrate into the wound space immediately after injury; PMNs are attracted to the wound by chemoattractants produced by platelets, activated clotting factors, and fibrin; the function of these early, short-lived (approximately 4 days) cells is to provide protection from infection.

C. Macrophages: the most significant cells in wound healing; phagocytic cell that gradually replaces leukocytes beginning approximately 4 days after wounding; the macrophage aggressively ingests bacteria and necrotic tissue, produces chemoattractants and growth factors, converts macromolecules into amino acids and sugars necessary for wound healing, and secretes lactate to stimulate collagen synthesis.

D. Fibroblasts: undifferentiated cell in connective tissue responsible for the synthesis of collagen and other connective tissue substances during wound repair; chemoattractants and growth factors released by platelets and macrophages stimulate fibroblasts to migrate to the wound bed beginning at the end of the inflammatory phase; lactate and ascorbate stimulate fibroblasts to synthesize collagen.

E. Myofibroblasts: fibroblasts with characteristics similar to those of smooth muscle cells; myofibroblasts stimulate wound contraction as they migrate within the wound space.

F. Epithelial cells: keratinocytes; proliferate and migrate from wound edges and intact skin appendages to re-establish epidermal barrier; in partial-thickness (superficial) wounds epidermal resurfacing begins within 24 hours; in deeper (full-thickness) wounds dermal repair must take place before epithelial cells can begin to migrate.

III. WOUND CLOSURE

There are three types of wound healing — primary intention, secondary intention, and tertiary or delayed primary intention.

A. Primary intention: a surgically closed wound; approximation of wound edges minimizes tissue defect and potential for infection; wounds heal quickly with minimal scar formation.

B. Secondary intention: wound is left open and allowed to heal by production of connective tissue (scar); requires a longer healing time for connective tissue to fill the defect; higher risk for infection due to absence of protective barrier; examples of wounds that heal by secondary intention are pressure ulcers and abdominal wounds left open to fascia.

C. Tertiary intention: describes the process when there is an intentional delay between injury and closure; requires more connective tissue formation (scar) than wounds closed by primary intention, less than those that heal by secondary intention. Example of a wound that heals by tertiary intention — contaminated abdominal wound left open to drain following surgery and later approximated when the wound is granulating and free of infection.

IV. ACUTE WOUNDS

Defined as those wounds caused intentionally (surgery) or by trauma (scrape, burn, cut); vasculature is disrupted, hemostasis occurs; in a healthy host healing proceeds in a timely manner.
A. Etiology.
   1. Mechanical — stab wound, laceration, abrasion, blister, surgical.
   2. Thermal — burns including sunburn, frostbite and thermal.
   3. Chemical — A wound intentionally made through the use of a chemical agent (such as a chemical peel) or unintentionally by exposure to a caustic substance; heal primarily by secondary intention/regeneration.

V. CHRONIC WOUNDS

A result of a failure of the normal healing process to proceed in an orderly and timely manner; can be a result of many factors including vascular insufficiency or an underlying medical condition; examples of chronic wounds include vascular ulcers and pressure ulcers.

VI. PATHOPHYSIOLOGY OF WOUND HEALING

Delayed healing or nonhealing is usually due to some disruption in the normal cascade of healing. Many factors can impair healing. It is imperative that these factors be recognized and addressed to augment the body's natural ability to heal.
A. Negative factors affecting wound healing.
   1. Intrinsic factors (related to patient's general physical or mental condition).
      a. Age — normal skin changes seen with aging affect the skin's function and healing response through decreased wound contraction, decreased tensile strength, and increased metabolic response. Age-related alterations that increase the potential for injury and impair healing include:
        (1) Decreased collagen density.
        (2) Increased capillary fragility.
        (3) Decreased sensory reception.
        (4) Decreased amount/distribution of subcutaneous fat.
        (5) Reduced inflammatory response.
        (6) Slower rate of neoangiogenesis and wound contraction.
        (7) Fewer fibroblasts.
        (8) Fragmentation of elastin fibers.
        (9) Insufficient tensile strength (increased potential for wound dehiscence).
        (10) Decreased tissue perfusion secondary to vascular disease.

b. Nutrition — plays a vital role in tissue regeneration.
   (1) Protein — provides the structural component for tissue repair; deficiency results in decreased fibroblast proliferation, reduced collagen synthesis, decreased angiogenesis, and disrupted maturation; slow gain in tensile strength and increased incidence of wound healing abnormalities are associated with protein-calorie malnutrition.
   (2) Vitamins — A affects collagen cross-linkage, supports epithelial proliferation and migration, and enhances immune system; B affects enzyme activity, collagen cross-linkage, and immune response; C necessary for collagen synthesis; D instrumental in the uptake of calcium and phosphorus from the GI tract; E plays a protective role in antioxidant defense.
   (3) Carbohydrates — provide energy needed for wound repair; insufficient carbohydrate intake initiates body protein catabolism and increases potential for infection.
   (4) Trace elements — zinc stabilizes membrane structure and function, acts as a co-factor in enzyme systems, affects immune response, and inhibits bacterial growth; copper aids in collagen linkage; iron corrects iron-deficiency anemia and affects collagen synthesis.
c. Medical condition — underlying disease states alter the body's normal response to healing:
   (1) Diabetes — altered leukocyte function increases risk of infection; neuropathy contributes to wound deterioration and recurrence.
   (2) Hypotension — vasoconstriction promotes tissue ischemia.
   (3) Peripheral vascular disease — tissue perfusion is decreased resulting in hypoxia.
   (4) Renal disease — uremia disrupts collagen deposition and interferes with granulation tissue formation.
   (5) Hematopoietic abnormalities — inadequate numbers of RBCs impair oxygen transport; inadequate platelets delay the healing cascade.
   (6) Gastrointestinal disease — inhibits absorption and compromises nutritional status.
   (7) Cardiopulmonary disease — PaO_2 is decreased contributing to tissue hypoxia.

(8) Cancer and HIV positive — immune response is altered; risk of infection is increased.

d. Infection — defined as bacterial concentrations greater than 105 organisms per gram of tissue; highly virulent organisms can cause infection at lower concentrations; important to distinguish between infection and colonization.

(1) Signs of local and regional infection (suppressed in immunocompromised patients):
  (a) Erythema.
  (b) Edema.
  (c) Induration.
  (d) Pain.
  (e) Purulent or foul-smelling drainage.
  (f) Crepitance.
  (g) Lympadenopathy.

(2) Signs of systemic infection:
  (a) Fever/chills.
  (b) Elevation of white blood cell (neutrophil) count; increase in number of bands/segs (shift to the left).
  (c) Positive blood cultures.
  (d) Hypotension.
  (e) Decreased urine output.

e. Drugs — particularly important to evaluate patient's medicines when a chronic, nonhealing wound is present; examples of drugs which may impair healing:

(1) Corticosteroids — systemic steroids inhibit fibroblast formation and collagen synthesis; topical steroids may have varying effects on epidermal resurfacing and dermal collagen synthesis.

(2) Anticoagulants — implied effect on healing by preventing hemostasis.

(3) Nonsteroidal anti-inflammatory drugs (NSAIDS) — may inhibit inflammatory phase of healing.

(4) Corticosteroids —inhibit the inflammatory phase of healing; interfere with fibroblast formation and collagen synthesis.

(5) Immunosuppressives — azathioprine and prednisone are associated with significant reduction in tensile strength.

(6) Chemotherapeutic agents — affect on wound healing depends on the specific drug, dose, and time of administration; increased risk of infection (due to decreased WBCs), acts on any rapidly dividing cells; alters the function of fibroblasts and myofibroblasts; impairs collagen synthesis and re-epithelialization.

f. Hypoxia — poor tissue oxygenation slows or completely inhibits healing; this is seen in patients with cardiopulmonary disease (decreased PaO_2), peripheral vascular disease, and diabetes; sustained tissue pressure compromises circulation leading to tissue ischemia, hypoxia, and cell death.

g. Stress — impairs healing by altering normal physiologic response; psychological stress, pain, and noise stimulate the sympathetic nervous system releasing vasoactive substances that promote vasoconstriction and alter tissue perfusion.

2. Extrinsic factors.

a. Topical antimicrobials/cleansers — inappropriate use of disinfectants and antiseptics (povidone-iodine, hydrogen peroxide, acetic acid, chlorhexidine, and hypochlorites) impair healing by having cytotoxic effects on fibroblasts; "never put in a clean wound what you wouldn't put in your eye."

(1) Liquid detergents — may retard healing by changing the pH of the wound bed or by cytotoxic action on fibroblasts.

(2) Antiseptic cleansers (acetic acid, Dakin's® solution, Hibiclens®, povidone iodine/Betadine®, hydrogen peroxide) — cytotoxic to fibroblasts.

b. Necrotic tissue — prolongs the inflammatory phase of healing; supports microbial growth; delays epithelial cell migration; provides a physical obstacle to wound contraction.

c. Continued tissue trauma — unrelieved pressure and edema leads to progressive tissue hypoxia and cell death; friction destroys epidermal cells and alters the barrier function of the skin; shearing forces angulate blood vessels, causing localized tissue hypoxia and chronic inflammation; excessive moisture leads to tissue maceration and promotes the growth of microorganisms; wound desiccation prolongs inflammation, retards epithelial cell migration, and impairs collagen synthesis.

d. Radiation therapy — dose, frequency, and location of irradiated area in relation to wound site will have implications for therapy; residual effects of radiation are permanent; irradiated tissue is easily damaged and slower to heal; impairs healing through:
  (1) Injury to fibroblasts.
  (2) Injury to endothelial cells.
  (3) Decrease in collagen production.
  (4) Destruction of cells in mitosis.

(5) Vascular damage.

(6) Increased risk of infection.

VII. WOUND CLASSIFICATION

A. National Pressure Ulcer Advisory Panel (NPUAP) criteria for staging pressure ulcer: NPUAP classification system is for pressure ulcers only; do not use to classify leg ulcers or other chronic wounds; the stage of a pressure ulcer represents the initial depth of tissue destruction and remains constant; a wound cannot be staged if necrotic tissue is present.

1. Stage I — nonblanchable erythema of intact skin; the heralding lesion of skin ulceration.

2. Stage II — partial-thickness skin loss involving epidermis and/or dermis; presents clinically as an abrasion, blister, or shallow crater (usually painful due to exposed dermal nerve endings).

3. Stage III — full-thickness skin loss involving damage or necrosis of subcutaneous tissue that may extend down to, but not through, underlying fascia; presents clinically as a deep crater with or without undermining of adjacent tissue.

4. Stage IV — full-thickness skin loss with extensive destruction, tissue necrosis, or damage to muscle, bone, or supporting structures; undermining and sinus tracts may also be associated with Stage IV pressure ulcers.

B. Classification of wound by tissue depth.

1. Superficial partial thickness — involves epidermis and upper layers of dermis; heals primarily by re-epithelialization; painful due to exposed nerve endings; examples include superficial abrasion, scald burn, chemical peel, skin tear.

2. Deep partial thickness – damage extends to the lower layers of the dermis but does not penetrate the dermis; heals by epithelialization in conjunction with varying degrees of collagen synthesis; examples include grease burn, dermal biopsy.

3. Full thickness — damage extends through the epidermis and dermis into deeper structures (subcutaneous tissue and possible fascia); healing occurs primarily by collagen synthesis and soft tissue contraction; examples include Stage III or IV pressure ulcer, open abdominal wound.

VIII. WOUND ASSESSMENT (see Tables 2 & 3; Figures 1-4; Figures 20-1 to 20-8, pages 243-244).

A. Anatomic location: Provides information about wound etiology and healing potential, for example pressure ulcers commonly occur over bony prominences and lower-extremity wounds take longer to heal.

B. Size: wound measurement is a basic parameter of assessment; a healing wound decreases in size over time; interventions should promote a gradual decrease in wound size, except following debridement when wound size can be expected to increase; assessment of size is a way to effectively evaluate efficacy of treatment.

1. Two or three-dimensional measurement (two dimensional measurement does not provide information regarding depth of the wound).

a. Linear measurements — greatest length, width and depth in cm or mm; gently insert cotton-tipped applicator into deepest area of wound to obtain depth measurement; patient should be in same position each time for accurate measurement of full-thickness wounds (soft tissue displacement can alter linear measures).

b. Wound tracings — useful when wound margins are irregular or poorly demarcated and linear measurement is difficult; use double layer transparent acetate and permanent marking pen to trace configuration; label clean tracing with date; mark direction of head and foot on tracing for subsequent comparisons.

c. Wound photography — gold standard of wound documentation; use in conjunction with linear measurement and other assessment parameters; provides visual data to verify change or lack of change in linear dimensions — color of tissue, the amount of exudate, and the condition of the surrounding skin.

2. Volume measurement.

a. Wound molds — use to assess the volume of open wounds; biocompatible molding material is poured into open wound and allowed to harden; change in size/weight of mold over time indicates progress; not practical in most clinical settings.

b. Fluid instillation — instill a known quantity of solution into the wound cavity, filling it to the perimeter; extract fluid with a syringe or suction and record the amount; requires serial measurements; use is limited to deep full-thickness wounds; not practical in most clinical settings.

C. Undermining, tracts, or tunneling: evaluate full-thickness (Stage III or IV pressure ulcers) wounds carefully for undermining/tracts; undermining most often occurs in wounds as a result of shear (pressure ulcers); sinus tracts occur generally as a result of dehiscence, infection, or a combination of neuropathy and arterial insufficiency; soft tissue tunneling is common in deep granulating wounds; use a

Figure 1.

PRESSURE ULCER PROTOCOL

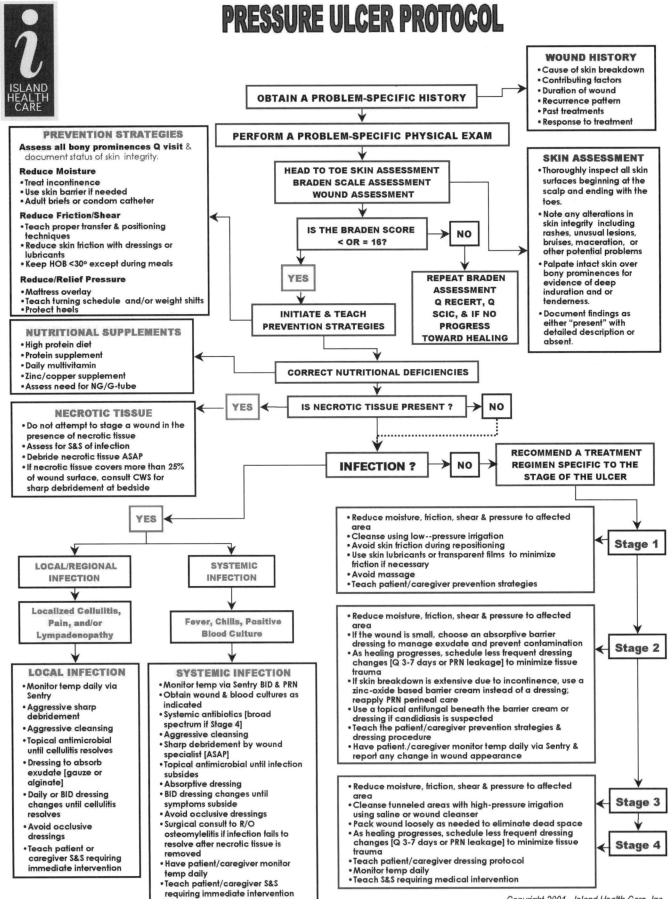

Copyright 2001 - Island Health Care, Inc.

Dermatologic Nursing Essentials: A Core Curriculum 2nd Edition © DNA 2003

Figure 2.

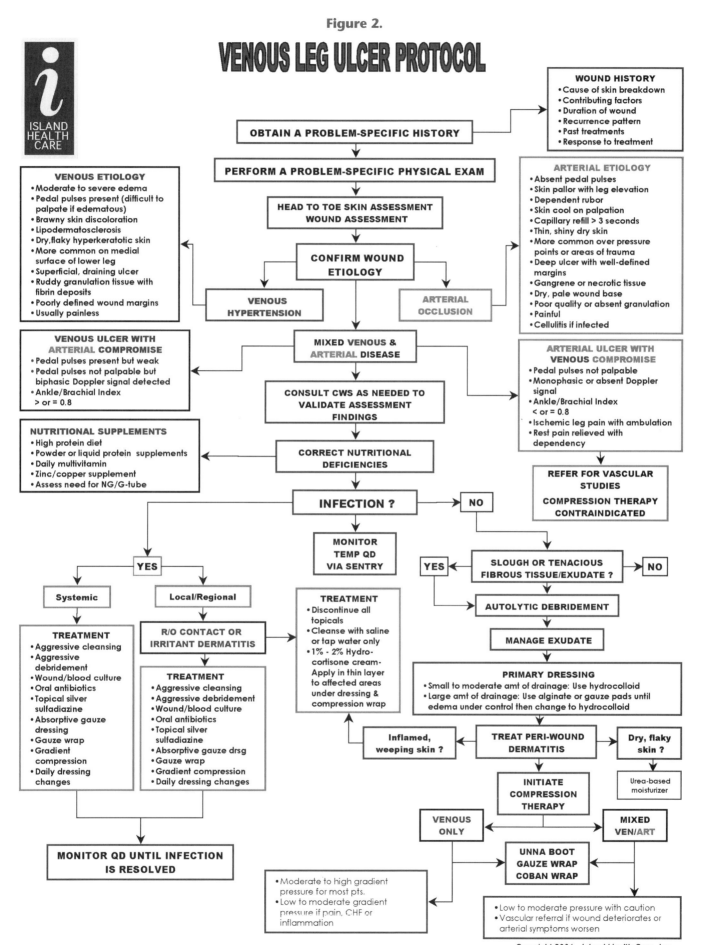

VENOUS LEG ULCER PROTOCOL

Figure 3.

DIABETIC ULCER PROTOCOL

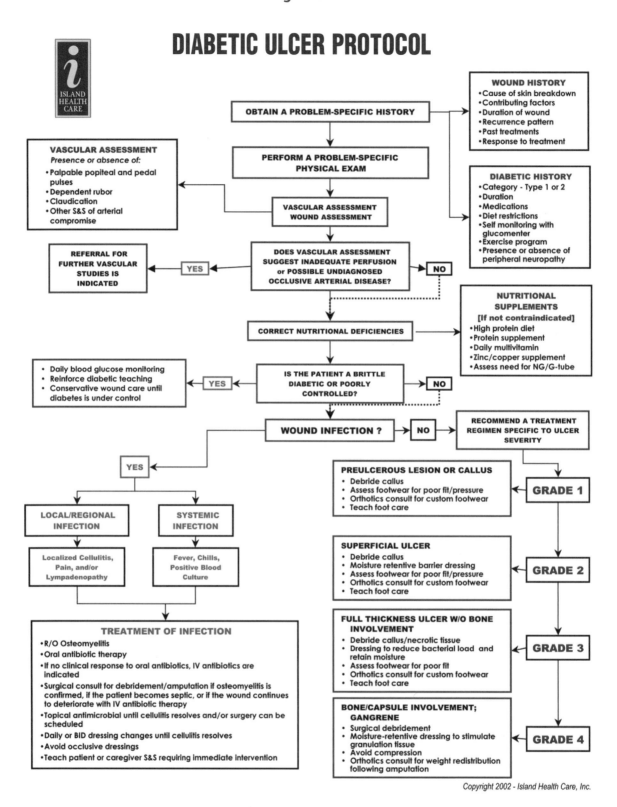

Copyright 2002 - Island Health Care, Inc.

Dermatologic Nursing Essentials: A Core Curriculum 2nd Edition © DNA 2003

Figure 4.

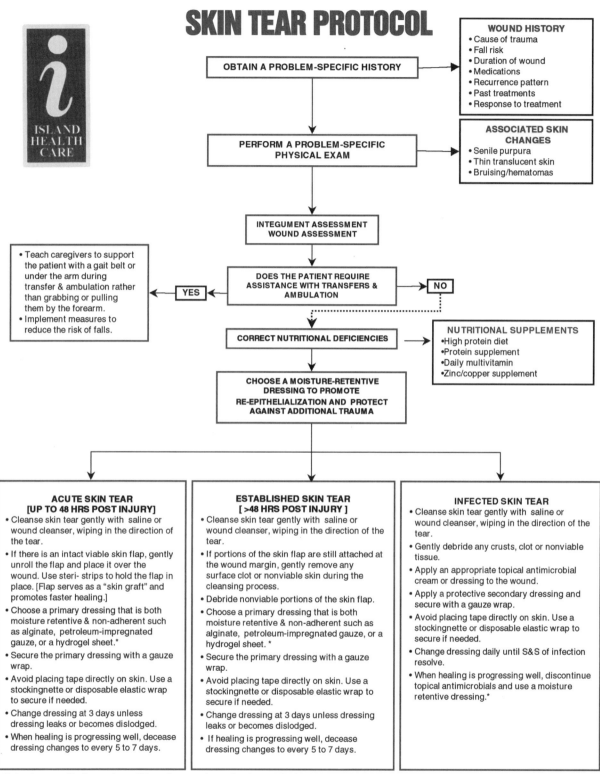

SKIN TEAR PROTOCOL

ISLAND HEALTH CARE

OBTAIN A PROBLEM-SPECIFIC HISTORY

WOUND HISTORY
- Cause of trauma
- Fall risk
- Duration of wound
- Medications
- Recurrence pattern
- Past treatments
- Response to treatment

PERFORM A PROBLEM-SPECIFIC PHYSICAL EXAM

ASSOCIATED SKIN CHANGES
- Senile purpura
- Thin translucent skin
- Bruising/hematomas

INTEGUMENT ASSESSMENT WOUND ASSESSMENT

DOES THE PATIENT REQUIRE ASSISTANCE WITH TRANSFERS & AMBULATION   YES   NO

- Teach caregivers to support the patient with a gait belt or under the arm during transfer & ambulation rather than grabbing or pulling them by the forearm.
- Implement measures to reduce the risk of falls.

CORRECT NUTRITIONAL DEFICIENCIES

NUTRITIONAL SUPPLEMENTS
- High protein diet
- Protein supplement
- Daily multivitamin
- Zinc/copper supplement

CHOOSE A MOISTURE-RETENTIVE DRESSING TO PROMOTE RE-EPITHELIALIZATION AND PROTECT AGAINST ADDITIONAL TRAUMA

ACUTE SKIN TEAR [UP TO 48 HRS POST INJURY]
- Cleanse skin tear gently with saline or wound cleanser, wiping in the direction of the tear.
- If there is an intact viable skin flap, gently unroll the flap and place it over the wound. Use steri- strips to hold the flap in place. [Flap serves as a "skin graft" and promotes faster healing.]
- Choose a primary dressing that is both moisture retentive & non-adherent such as alginate, petroleum-impregnated gauze, or a hydrogel sheet.*
- Secure the primary dressing with a gauze wrap.
- Avoid placing tape directly on skin. Use a stockingnette or disposable elastic wrap to secure if needed.
- Change dressing at 3 days unless dressing leaks or becomes dislodged.
- When healing is progressing well, decease dressing changes to every 5 to 7 days.

ESTABLISHED SKIN TEAR [>48 HRS POST INJURY]
- Cleanse skin tear gently with saline or wound cleanser, wiping in the direction of the tear.
- If portions of the skin flap are still attached at the wound margin, gently remove any surface clot or nonviable skin during the cleansing process.
- Debride nonviable portions of the skin flap.
- Choose a primary dressing that is both moisture retentive & non-adherent such as alginate, petroleum-impregnated gauze, or a hydrogel sheet. *
- Secure the primary dressing with a gauze wrap.
- Avoid placing tape directly on skin. Use a stockingnette or disposable elastic wrap to secure if needed.
- Change dressing at 3 days unless dressing leaks or becomes dislodged.
- If healing is progressing well, decease dressing changes to every 5 to 7 days.

INFECTED SKIN TEAR
- Cleanse skin tear gently with saline or wound cleanser, wiping in the direction of the tear.
- Gently debride any crusts, clot or nonviable tissue.
- Apply an appropriate topical antimicrobial cream or dressing to the wound.
- Apply a protective secondary dressing and secure with a gauze wrap.
- Avoid placing tape directly on skin. Use a stockingnette or disposable elastic wrap to secure if needed.
- Change dressing daily until S&S of infection resolve.
- When healing is progressing well, discontinue topical antimicrobials and use a moisture retentive dressing.*

Note: Some patients may benefit from the use of an adhesive product [transparent film, thin hydrocolloid, adhesive foam] to maintain dressing integrity. Adhesive dressings can cause reinjury and should be used with caution.

Table 2.
Characteristics of Common Problem Wounds

	Arterial Ulcer	Venous Ulcer	Diabetic Ulcer	Pressure Ulcer	Skin Tear
Predisposing Factors	• Arteriosclerosis • Peripheral vascular disease (PVD) • Diabetes mellitus • Advanced age	• History of: ➡ Deep vein thrombosis ➡ Thrombophlebitis ➡ Leg fracture or trauma • Incompetent valves in perforating veins • Calf pump failure • History of venous ulcers or family history of ulcers • Obesity • Pregnancy (in women with a family history of venous ulcers) • Advanced age	• Diabetes • Peripheral neuropathy • Peripheral vascular disease	• Multiple medical diagnoses • Advanced age • Impaired mobility • Loss of sensation • Altered mental status • Poor nutritional status • Sedation • Incontinence • Impaired circulation	• Advance age • Solar damaged skin • Chronic steroid therapy
Location	• Usually distal to impaired arterial supply • At sites subjected to trauma or rubbing of footwear: ➡ Phalangeal heads ➡ Lateral malleolus ➡ Tips of toes ➡ Interdigital spaces	• Can occur anywhere between the knee and ankle • Medial malleolus is most common site	• Any sites on the foot and lower limb subjected to repetitive pressure, friction, shear, or trauma: • Plantar surface over metatarsal heads (especially first and fifth) • Great toe • Calcaneus	• Can occur over any bony prominence subjected to pressure, friction, or shearing forces • Sacrum, heels, elbows, and trochanter are most common sites in bedridden patients • Occurs over ischial tuberosity with prolonged sitting	• Forearms • Pretibial surface • Skin areas subject to friction or shearing forces
Depth	• Can be shallow but usually deep, crater-like wound • Exposed tendons common	• Usually shallow	• Usually deep, but may be shallow depending on disease severity • May have tracking and/or undermining • Exposed tendons are common	• Ranges in depth from circulatory compromise (Stage 1) to deep tissue destruction involving underlying structures such as bone and tendon (Stage 4)	• Shallow (partial thickness to deep partial thickness)
Wound Appearance	• Thick, dry, leathery eschar often present • Digits may appear gangrenous • Pale, gray, or yellow wound base following debridement • Absent or poor quality granulation tissue • Cellulitis may be present and usually indicates advanced infection.	• Ruddy, "beefy" red granulation tissue • Superficial fibrin deposits (looks like a gelatinous film) may occur suddenly on top of healthy appearing granulation tissue	• Almost always accompanied by thick, leathery eschar that requires sharp debridement • Following debridement, base may appear dry and fibrotic • Wound granulates slowly, especially if PVD is present • Cellulitis or osteomyelitis is common, particularly with neuropathic ulcers	• Stage 1 - Non-blanchable erythema over a pressure point indicating prolonged tissue ischemia • Stage 2 - Superficial skin loss with exposure of pink, moist dermal tissue • Stage 3 - Full-thickness crater with eschar formation; heals primarily by granulation and contraction • Stage 4 - Extensive tissue necrosis down to and involving bone. Undermining, sinus tracts, or soft tissue tunneling may be present • Stage 3 or 4 may present as a "silent" ulcer - clinical characteristics are similar to a Stage 1, but with deep tissue induration on palpation indicating necrosis beneath the epidermal lesion	• Superficial or deep partial thickness skin flap (often partially attached at wound margin) • Commonly occur over areas of purpura • Pink to red moist dermal base • Hematoma may be present
Exudate/Drainage	• Minimal exudate • Dry, fibrous wound base	• Moderate to heavy exudate • Exudate decreases with treatment of venous hypertension	• Small to moderate amounts of exudate • Infected ulcers usually have purulent drainage • Excessive drainage usually indicates underlying osteomyelitis	• Amount of drainage varies with stage of ulcer and whether or not the wound is infected	• Small to moderate amounts of exudate

Dermatologic Nursing Essentials: A Core Curriculum 2nd Edition © DNA 2003

Table 2. (continued)
Characteristics of Common Problem Wounds

	Arterial Ulcer	Venous Ulcer	Diabetic Ulcer	Pressure Ulcer	Skin Tear
Wound Shape & Margins	• Sharp, well-defined margins that conform to the type of skin trauma • "Punched out" appearance	• Irregular, poorly-defined margins that make measurement difficult	• Sharp, well-defined margins • Wound may be small at the surface with a large subcutaneous abscess beneath • Callus around the ulcer in areas caused by ill-fitting shoes • Edges often undermined	• Usually uniform in shape with well-defined margins • Large ulcers caused by shearing forces may have irregular margins and extensive undermining	• Shape of wound is consistent with a traumatic tear caused by skin friction or tissue shearing
Surrounding Skin	• Pale or cyanotic color • Dependent rubor • Skin is thin, shiny and cool to the touch • Hair loss over dorsal skin surfaces • Minimal to no edema	• Brawny, hyperpigmented skin in gaiter (sock) area • Moderate to severe edema • Lipodermatosclerosis • Localized areas of maceration from excessive drainage • Dry, flaky skin (hyperkeratosis)	• Dry, thin, frequently callused • Periwound hyperkeratosis is common and indicates repeated pressure or trauma • Infection may be difficult to assess due to microcirculatory compromise	• Skin may be macerated or have secondary yeast infection if patient is incontinent • Clinical infection is indicated by localized redness, warmth, and induration	• Paper-thin, fragile skin • Senile purpura (bruising)
Pain Response	• Often accompanied by severe pain at rest (claudication), numbness, and parasthesias • Pain often increases with leg elevation • Pain may increase with ambulation (time of onset depends on severity of disease)	• Pain varies unpredictably • Small, deep ulcers around malleoli are typically the most painful • May complain of a throbbing pain if leg edema is severe and not being adequately treated • Pain often improves with leg elevation and edema control	• Varies from no pain to constant or intermittent numbness or burning • Neuropathic ulcers are almost always accompanied by numbness and parasthesias	• Varies from mild to severe (Pressure ulcers are less common in patients that have sensation and can communicate discomfort). • Many patients experience pain but are unable to express it due to altered consciousness	• Pain response varies • Usually mild to moderate pain during cleansing, but subsides once wound is covered
Expected Outcome	• Rate of healing depends primarily on disease severity and adequacy of tissue perfusion • The presence of necrotic tissue will delay healing significantly • Open wounds will either not heal or will recur if ostomyelitis is inadequately treated • If perfusion is poor and revascularization isn't an option, the outcome of a healed wound is very unlikely	• Outcome depends directly on patient compliance with edema control measures • Epithelialization often fails despite good granulation • Average time to healing depends on: ➡ Disease severity ➡ Extent of lipoder-matosclerosis ➡ Presence of cardiovascular disease ➡ Successful reversal of venous hypertension and edema control	• Patient must comply with diet, glucose regulation, exercise, and foot care in order for healing to occur • Achieving a healed wound may require aggressive revascularization or appropriate antibiotic therapy • Open wounds will either not heal or will recur if osteomyelitis is inadequately treated • Custom or specialized shoes will reduce pressure and help prevent ulcer recurrence	• Must eliminate or significantly reduce pressure, shear, and friction in order to achieve a healed wound • Prevention measures and appropriate skin care are critical to maintaining intact skin once healing is achieved	• Must prevent continued or recurrent skin trauma in order to achieve healing • Adequate education of patient and caregivers should reduce recurrence rate

clock face to describe the direction of undermining, tracts and tunnels; obtain linear measurements when possible.

D. Tissue type: accurate assessment of the wound bed leads to appropriate treatment and decreased morbidity. [Note: Viable subcutaneous tissue, fascia, muscle, tendon, and bone may also be visible at the base of deep wounds, especially after surgical debridement.]

1. Epithelial tissue — regrowth of skin from wound edges or skin appendages; initially one cell layer thick, then stratifies; presents clinically as pearly pink wound margins (full-thickness wounds) or fleshy budding of the hair follicles (partial-thickness wounds).

2. Granulation tissue — combination of newly formed blood vessels and collagen deposited into the wound space during the proliferative

Table 3.
Wound Documentation Guidelines

Goal	Assessment Guidelines	What to Document	Documentation Tools
Wound Location will remain unchanged.	■ The location of the wound provides information about the possible cause of skin/tissue breakdown.	**On Admission** ■ Anatomical location of the wound(s). ■ Distribution or percent body surface area involved if large wound (burn), rash, or multiple sites. ■ Proximity of the wound to a bony prominence.	■ Body line drawing. ■ Photograph
Wound Size will decrease with healing at a rate dependent upon the amount of necrotic tissue present and the patient's overall condition.	■ Wound size increases as necrotic tissue is debrided. ■ Wound size decreases as infection is controlled and healing occurs by re-epithelialization and contraction. ■ The wound changes in shape as healing occurs. ■ Large superficial wounds may become multiple smaller wounds as new skin growth occurs.	**Every 2 Weeks and PRN Changes in Wound Status** ■ Length in cm (largest dimension from head to toe). ■ Width in cm (largest dimension from hip to hip). ■ Extent of undermining at wound margins in cm (circumferentially). **Daily** ■ Changes in plan of care.	■ Disposable measuring device. ■ Plastic "baggie" and marker (for tracing irregularly shaped wounds). ■ Polaroid or digital camera. ■ Cotton-tipped applicator stick (to measure undermining).
Wound Depth will decrease with healing at a rate dependent upon the amount of necrotic tissue present and the patient's overall condition.	■ Wound depth increases as necrotic tissue is removed. ■ Wound depth decreases as granulation tissue forms. ■ The amount of packing material needed to fill deep wounds decreases as healing progresses. ■ Tissue color changes from black to yellow to red as healing progresses.	**On Admission** ■ Stage of pressure ulcer (if wound base visible). ■ Partial or full-thickness designation (if wound is not pressure related or if unable to stage necrotic tissue). **Every 2 Weeks and PRN Changes in Wound Status** ■ Depth in cm at deepest portion of wound. ■ Depth and direction of soft tissue tunneling. ■ Amount of packing material needed to loosely pack deep wound cavities. **Daily** ■ Changes in plan of care.	■ Cotton-tipped applicator stick. ■ Gloved finger to gently probe wound if deep tunneling is present. ■ Wound drawing using a clock-face to describe the direction of soft tissue tunneling.
Tissue Type will progress from no healing (necrosis, infection) to partially granulating to fully granulating.	■ Tissue color changes from black to yellow to red as healing progresses. ■ The percentage of black necrotic tissue, yellow slough, and incidence of infection decreases with appropriate treatment. ■ The percentage of granulation and new epithelial tissue increases with appropriate treatment.	**Every 2 Weeks and PRN Changes in Wound Status** ■ Percent of black tissue. ■ Percent of yellow slough. ■ Percent of granulation tissue. **Daily** ■ Changes in plan of care.	■ Good light source. ■ Photograph Q 2 weeks.
Wound Exudate will decrease in amount once necrotic tissue is removed and infection is controlled.	■ Amount of serosanguinous exudate increases suddenly prior to surgical wound dehiscence. ■ Exudate increases in amount and viscosity with autolytic debridement of necrotic tissue using occlusive dressings. ■ Exudate decreases in amount once necrotic tissue is removed and the wound is granulating. ■ Exudate increases in amount and viscosity if wound becomes infected. ■ Exudate increases in amount with venous leg ulcers if compression is not adequate or patient is noncompliant with measures to reverse venous hypertension.	**Every 2 Weeks and PRN Changes in Wound Status** ■ Amount of drainage as quantified by: ➡ Small, moderate, and large. ➡ Frequency of dressing changes to control drainage. ➡ Number of gauze pads saturated with drainage at each dressing change. **Daily** ■ Changes in plan of care.	■ Patient reports of drainage on linens, etc.

Dermatologic Nursing Essentials: A Core Curriculum 2nd Edition © DNA 2003

Table 3. (continued)
Wound Documentation Guidelines

Goal	Assessment Guidelines	What to Document	Documentation Tools
Surrounding Skin will remain intact and free of signs and symptoms of infection.	■ Skin around the wound becomes macerated and colonized with yeast if drainage is excessive and not controlled by use of an absorptive dressing. ■ A pruritic "burn-like" skin reaction that has well-defined borders usually indicates an allergic reaction to the dressing material. ■ Cellulitis and tenderness extending more than 2 cm beyond the wound margins indicates possible infection. ■ Local signs and symptoms of wound infection may be masked in immunocompromised patients.	**Every 2 Weeks and PRN Changes in Wound Status** ■ Condition of surrounding skin (intact or not intact). ■ Description of skin changes if present (including associated symptoms). **Daily (if infected)** ■ Extent of cellulitis (measurement in cm). ■ Amount and type of wound drainage. ■ Presence or absence of wound odor. ■ Presence or absence of induration. ■ Presence or absence of tenderness ■ Presence or absence of systemic symptoms (fever, lymphadenopathy, etc.) **Daily** ■ Changes in plan of care.	■ Good light source. ■ Palpation ■ Patient reports of discomfort (increased tenderness, pruritus, etc.). ■ Photograph.

phase of healing; presents clinically as fleshy granular projections of tissue; healthy granulation is moist, pink to beefy-red, and has a spongy texture.

3. Eschar — necrotic epidermis and dermis (full-thickness wounds only); delays wound healing by slowing epithelial cell migration and serving as a physical obstacle to wound contraction; presents clinically as thick, dry leathery necrotic tissue attached to the wound surface (for example, dry gangrene); usually black in color.

4. Slough — soft, stringy necrotic tissue that may appear black, gray, yellow, or tan in color; often associated with thick drainage and increased numbers of bacteria.

E. **Exudate: the amount, viscosity, and color of exudate will vary with the phase of healing, amount and type of necrotic tissue present, and wound dressing.**

1. Volume — volume of exudate should decrease as inflammation subsides, necrotic tissue is removed and infection is controlled; volume of exudate increases with use of moisture-retentive dressings for autolytic debridement, osteomyelitis, or spontaneous drainage of a soft tissue abscess; a sudden increase in the volume of exudate may signal impending wound dehiscence in primarily closed wounds; quantify volume of exudate as scant, moderate, or large.

2. Color — the color of exudate changes as tissue repair progresses through the various phases of healing; inflammatory wound transudate is initially yellow-tinged and watery (serous) as protein-rich transudate leaks from dilated blood vessels; may be blood-tinged (serosanguinous)

or show evidence of fresh bleeding (sanguineous); chronic wound exudate changes color (cream, brown, gray, green) with increased proliferation of microorganisms.

3. Consistency — the viscosity of wound exudate changes from a watery consistency (inflammatory transudate) in acute wounds to a purulent consistency in chronic or infected wounds; change in consistency caused by accumulation of blood cells and living or dead organisms.

F. **Odor: colonization or infection with certain microorganisms gives the wound a distinct odor (Pseudomonas); a pungent, strong, foul, fecal, or musty odor together with increased erythema, tenderness, and volume of exudate usually suggests infection; some moisture-retentive dressings are also associated with an unpleasant odor in the absence of infection.**

G. **Condition of periwound skin.**

1. Color — assess for erythema, hypo/hyperpigmentation, cyanosis, etc.; color changes are more difficult to assess in individuals with darker skin.

2. Texture – assess for blistering, maceration, dryness/cracking, rashes, etc.

3. Signs of active infection — a ring of redness or halo of erythema extending for several centimeters, deep induration of periwound skin.

H. **Pain response: assess and document the presence of severe pain or tenderness within or around the wound; may indicate infection, underlying tissue destruction, or vascular insufficiency; absence of pain may indicate nerve**

Table 4.
Treatment Goals

Full-Thickness Wounds with Necrosis
- Debride
- Cover
- Protect
- Hydrate
- Insulate
- Absorb
- Cleanse
- Prevent infection
- Promote granulation

Full-Thickness Wounds with Exudate of Dead Space
- Absorb
- Obliterate dead space
- Cover
- Protect
- Hydrate
- Insulate
- Cleanse
- Prevent infection
- Promote granulation

Clean and Proliferating Full-Thickness Wounds
- Cover
- Protect
- Hydrate
- Insulate
- Prevent infection
- Promote granulation

destruction.
I. **Previous treatment: always question the patient about previous treatment modalities; some treatments may alter wound appearance clinically or retard the healing process.**
J. **Infection: bacterial infection negatively affects wound healing; it may either delay the wound healing process, or lead to severe morbidity or death; accurate evaluation of bacterial load in a wound is important to treatment planning.**
K. **General health assessment: assess the host — wounds do not exist in a vacuum. It is imperative to assess the status of the host and to correct/optimize any conditions recognized.**
 1. Age — with normal aging there is a decrease in the inflammatory response, delayed angiogenesis, decreased collagen synthesis and degradation, slowed epithelialization and decreased functioning of sebaceous glands; older patients are at higher risk for slow or nonhealing wounds.
 2. Chronic illness — assess for concomitant medical problems associated with delayed healing: diabetes, COPD, hypertension, etc.
 3. Medications — assess for medications known to slow/inhibit healing: systemic corticosteroids,

anticoagulants, NSAIDs, immunosuppressives, chemotherapeutic agents.
 4. Nutritional status — healing may require an increase in calorie intake, vitamins, and trace elements; if a patient is in a state of hypoproteinemia, then healing will be negatively affected.
 5. Infection — assess systemic conditions that may increase potential for infection; immune incompetence (interferes with mitosis, protein synthesis and increases risk of infection).
 6. Psychosocial — assess patient's ability/willingness to be compliant with treatment; assess hygiene; assess support systems/resources available to patient.

IX. TREATMENT (see Table 4)

A. **Debridement: the removal of dirt, foreign objects, damaged tissue, and cellular debris from the wound surface. The primary objectives of wound debridement are to promote timely progress along the healing continuum from inflammation to proliferation, prevent infection by removing food source for microorganisms, and correct abnormal wound repair.**
 1. Nonselective debridement — removes devitalized tissue from the wound but may also damage healthy tissue.
  a. Wet-to-dry dressings — uses saline and gauze; wet gauze is placed directly onto wound base and allowed to dry before removal; removal mechanically pulls debris from the wound surface; painful to the patient and nonselective (can injure viable tissue); limit use to wounds that contain a large amount of soft necrotic slough or when insoluble debris is not easily removed by rinsing or cleansing.
  b. Irrigation — uses water or saline to flush the wound and remove superficial nonattached cellular debris; irrigation technique may be forceful (high pressure) or gentle (low pressure); high-pressure irrigation can damage healthy tissue and is not indicated for clean, noninfected wounds, granulating wounds, or superficial wounds.
  c. Hydrotherapy (whirlpool) — indicated for debridement of large wounds with loosely adherent necrotic tissue and yellow fibrinous or gelatinous exudate, to soak off adherent dressings, to cleanse wounds of dirt and foreign contaminants; facilitates softening and separation of eschar and desiccated tissues; limit to Stage III and IV wounds with extensive amounts (>50%) of necrotic tissue; addition of antibacterial agents to the whirlpool may by cytotoxic to healing tissue and should be done with

Dermatologic Nursing Essentials: A Core Curriculum 2nd Edition © DNA 2003

caution.

d. Surgical debridement — use of a scalpel or other instrumentation to dissect and remove necrotic tissue; technique of choice when time is a factor (infected wound that may lead to increased morbidity or even mortality); prepares open wounds for closure; extensive surgical debridement may involve the sacrifice of viable tissue.

e. Topical agents — Dakin (sodium hypochlorite) solution chemically loosens/removes cellular debris; may be toxic to healthy cells and a chemical irritant to intact skin; not indicated for use on clean superficial wounds.

2. Selective debridement — selectively removes devitalized tissue from the wound without disruption or damage to healthy tissue.

a. Non-ionic wound cleansers, surfactants, and sterile normal saline — Indicated for cleansing wounds with minimal-to-moderate amounts of slough or when wounds are edematous

b. Conservative sharp debridement (minor) — requires no anesthesia; can be done on an outpatient basis or at home using forceps and scissors; only devitalized tissue is removed.

3. Enzymatic debridement — enzyme preparations applied topically to necrotic tissue to break down targeted substrates (necrotic protein, fibrin, or collagen); products require moisture for activation; active in limited pH range (<6.0 to 8.0); inactivated in wounds with pH of <5.0 or when exposed to heavy metal ions such as mercury or silver (present in some antiseptics); debris should be flushed from the wound before application (if granulation tissue present, flush with either surfactants or normal saline).

a. Fibrinolytic and proteolytic enzymes — combination products containing proteolytic enzymes, fibrinolysin and deoxyribonuclease; used to debride denatured proteins as well as fibrin clots and fibrinous exudates.
   (1) Glassy, edematous wounds.
   (2) Edematous wounds.
   (3) Venous insufficiency ulcers with fibrinous exudates.

b. Proteinases — used to debride eschar and denatured proteins found more superficially in the wound bed.

c. Collagenases — hydrolyzes adherent denatured collagen usually found at the base of the wound.

4. Autolytic debridement — naturally occurring enzymes produced by bacteria and macrophages in wound fluid are used to promote liquefaction of necrotic tissue; autolysis (self-digestion) is promoted by the use of moisture-retentive dressings which trap fluid next to the wound surface.

a. Indicated in wounds with manageable amounts of necrotic tissue.

b. Contraindicated in infected wounds.

c. Use contraindicated for more than 2 weeks without objective indications of progress toward healing.

d. Use with caution in wounds with poor perfusion, diabetic and immunocompromised patients.

X. CHOOSING THE APPROPRIATE TREATMENT OPTION (see Table 5)

Base choice of product on the wound/host assessment, expected outcome of intervention, and cost of treatment.

A. Principles of wound management.
   1. Reduce/eliminate causative factors.
   2. Provide systemic support.
   3. Remove foreign bodies/necrotic tissue.
   4. Choose appropriate topical therapy.
   5. Control bacterial proliferation.
   6. Control drainage.

B. Goal of wound cleansing/debridement — to remove surface bacteria and other microorganisms; to hasten the removal of devitalized tissue.

C. Goals of topical therapy.
   1. Create an optimum wound environment.
   2. Manage exudate.
   3. Obliterate dead space.
   4. Provide insulation.
   5. Protect from trauma.

Note: Wounds with red, granulating base DO NOT REQUIRE CLEANSING UNLESS INFECTED.

D. Dressing options.
   1. Semipermeable film dressing — acronyms include moisture vapor-permeable (MVP) dressings, vapor-permeable (VPM), transparent film dressings (TFDs), synthetic adhesive moisture vapor-permeable (SAM) dressings, and polyurethane films (PUFs); hydrates wounds with minimal exudate without macerating periwound skin; waterproof; permits oxygen and water vapor to cross the barrier; impermeable to bacteria and contaminants; maintains moist environment; promotes autolysis of necrotic tissue; provides insulation; allows for visualization of the wound; adhesive products may injure new epithelium on removal; indications include:
   a. Superficial, partial thickness wounds.
   b. Wounds with minimal necrosis or slough.

Table 5.
Wound Dressing Categories

Category	Description	Indications	Side Effects	Examples
Absorptive Filler	✓ A variety of product types including absorptive powders, pastes, and beads ✓ *Highly* absorptive ✓ Oxygen permeable ✓ Moisture retentive ✓ Secondary cover dressing required	• Absorption in full-thickness wounds with moderate to heavy exudate • Autolytic debridement of yellow slough in deep wounds with dead space • Odor control • Hydrophilic cleansing action and reduction of surface bacteria	• Will desiccate wound and cause further damage if exudate is minimal • Some products may be difficult to remove if wound is deep with tunneling	Bard Absorption Dressing Chronicure Comfeel Powder DuoDERM Paste HydraGran Iodosorb Gel Multidex
Alginate	✓ Nonwoven mass of calcium-sodium alginate fibers that form a moisture-retentive gel on contact with wound fluid ✓ Moisture retentive ✓ Nonocclusive ✓ Varying levels of absorbency ✓ Nonadhesive ✓ Available in pads and ropes for packing dead space ✓ Secondary cover dressing required	• Absorption of heavy to moderate wound exudate in superficial and deep wounds • Autolytic debridement of yellow slough • Infected wounds (after debridement of necrotic tissue, appropriate antibiotic therapy, and with close monitoring of wound progress) • "Filler" for deep or tunneling wounds (rope form) • Promotes hemostasis • Insulates wound	• May contribute to wound desiccation if wound exudate is minimal and gel dries (moisten with saline if dressing adheres to surface) • Contraindicated for use on third-degree burns • Limited hemostatic properties	CURASORB Kaltostat Sorbsan
Foam	✓ Semipermeable polyurethane foam dressings that have varying barrier properties ✓ Moisture retentive ✓ Conformable ✓ Available in pads and pillows for filling wound cavities ✓ Available in adhesive and nonadhesive forms ✓ Some products require tape or a secondary cover dressing to secure	• Absorption of moderate to heavy exudate in superficial and deep wounds • Protection of friable peri-wound skin (nonadhesive pads) • Insulates wound • Infected wounds (after appropriate intervention and with close monitoring of wound progress) • Autolytic debridement of yellow slough • Padding of tracheostomy sites • Padding and protection of high-risk areas from repeated trauma (pretibial area, forearms, etc.)	• May promote wound dehydration and desiccation if exudate is minimal • Contraindicated for sinus tracts	Allevyn CURAFOAM Flexzan LyoFoam MitraFlex
Gauze (Woven)	✓ Absorbent, 100% meshed cotton fabric woven into squares, rolls and packing strips ✓ Available in sterile and nonsterile packaging	• Protection of surgical wounds • Mechanical debridement of yellow slough (wet-to-dry gauze) • Autolytic debridement (saline-moistened gauze) • Absorption of minimal to heavy exudate in superficial and deep wounds • "Filler" for packing dead space in large, deep wound cavities • Moisten or impregnate with antimicrobials for infection	• May adhere to healthy tissue and cause injury in removal • Some products may shed, leaving lint in wound	Curity Gauze Sponges KERLIX Super Sponge KLING Gauze Rolls NUGAUZE Packing Strips
Hydrocolloid	✓ Conformable material made of gelatin, pectin and carboxymethlcellulose particles suspended in an adhesive base ✓ Moisture retentive ✓ Highly occlusive ✓ Wafers are available in a regular and extra-thin forms and in a variety of shapes ✓ Some products have borders to prevent rolling of edges	• Autolytic debridement of minimal to moderate amounts of yellow slough • Protection of high-friction areas • Protection from exogenous contamination (excellent barrier function) • Absorption of minimal to moderate exudate in superficial and shallow full-thickness wounds • Fibrinolytic activity (venous leg ulcers) • Can be used in combination with other wound fillers (alginates, pastes, etc.)	• Occlusive properties can promote infection in high-risk patients • Contraindicated for third-degree burns • May promote hypertrophic granulation tissue • Some products leave residue in wound on removal • Some products have an unpleasant odor on dressing removal	Comfeel Cutinova DuoDERM Restore Tegasorb
Hydrogel	✓ Semipermeable hydrophilic polymers composed primarily of water or glycerin ✓ Available in both sheet and gel forms ✓ Hydrate wound and are moisture retentive ✓ Secondary cover dressing required	• Absorption of minimal to moderate exudate in superficial and deep wounds • Autolytic debridement of yellow slough and softening of black eschar • Pain relief in radiation-damaged tissue and superficial burns (store dressing in refrigerator to cool) • Ultrasound treatments • Liquid and gel forms can be used as filler for deep wounds	• Not indicated for heavily exuding wounds • May contribute to peri-wound maceration • May promote growth of yeast	Carrington Gel Geliperm IntraSite Gel Nu-Gel Vigilon CURAGEL Elasto-Gel

Dermatologic Nursing Essentials: A Core Curriculum 2nd Edition © DNA 2003

Table 5. (continued)
Wound Dressing Categories

Category	Description	Indications	Side Effects	Examples
Transparent Film	✓ Transparent polyurethane and polyethylene films coated with adhesive ✓ Semipermeable ✓ Moisture vapor transmission rates vary with product type ✓ Impermeable to microorganisms ✓ Moisture retentive ✓ Nonabsorptive	• Protection of high-friction areas (heels, beneath restraints, Stage I, etc,) • Superficial wounds with minimal exudate • Autolytic debridement of yellow slough in shallow wounds • Protection of IV sites • Waterproof cover dressing for fillers and other, more absorptive dressing materials	• Not recommended as primary dressing for wounds with moderate or heavy exudate • May cause skin tears or adhesive stripping of peri-wound skin • Contributes to peri-wound maceration and yeast colonization if exudate collects beneath dressing • Contraindicated in sinus tracts and infected wounds	Bioclusive Tegaderm OpSite Polyskin II

c. Wounds with little or no exudate.

d. Use as a secondary (cover) dressing.

2. Hydrocolloid dressing — pastes, powders, or occlusive adhesive wafers composed of pectin-like material; provides moist environment; promotes autolysis and granulation; insulates wound; impermeable to bacteria and other contaminants; atraumatic removal; provides moderate absorption; may use with compression stockings/pumps, wraps, or Unna's boot for:
   a. Partial-thickness wounds.
   b. Shallow full-thickness wounds.
   c. Granulating full-thickness with minimal-to-moderate exudate.

3. Foam dressing — wound contact surface is semipermeable or hydrophilic; outer dressing surface is hydrophobic; nonadherent; maintains moist wound environment; promotes autolytic debridement; minimal-to-moderate absorption; protects from trauma; insulates; atraumatic removal; indications include:
   a. Partial-thickness wounds with minimal-to-moderate drainage.
   b. Full-thickness wounds with depth or dead space; use packing to fill cavity; may use under compression.
   c. A primary dressing to provide absorption or insulation.
   d. Secondary dressing for wounds with packing.
   e. To absorb drainage around tubes (trach sites, chest tubes, gastrostomy tubes, etc.).

4. Absorption dressing — includes various preparations composed of dextranomer beads and co-polymer starches; absorbs large amounts of exudate; conforms to the wound surface and eliminates dead space; maintains moist wound environment; promotes autolytic debridement; use for:
   a. Full-thickness wounds with moderate-to-heavy exudate.
   b. Wounds with sinus tracts, undermining and soft tissue tunneling.
   c. Wounds with moderate to small amounts of necrotic tissue.

5. Calcium alginate dressing — derived from brown seaweed; highly absorbent (can absorb 20 times its weight in wound exudate); conforms to the shape of the wound; indications include:
   a. Partial and full-thickness wounds with moderate-to-heavy exudate.
   b. Wounds with tunneling or sinus tracts.
   c. Wounds with moderate-to-small amounts of necrotic tissue.
   d. Infected and noninfected wounds.

6. Biosynthetic/biologic dressing — composed of tissue derived from animal or human sources; indicated for treatment of grafts, donor sites, and burns; limited application in conservative chronic wound care.

7. Hydrogel dressing — water or glycerin-based amorphous gel, impregnated gauze, or sheet; promotes autolytic debridement; maintains moist environment; limited absorption of exudate; atraumatic removal; refrigerated product provides some pain relief; indications include:
   a. Partial or full-thickness wounds.
   b. Deep wounds with minimal exudate.
   c. Wounds with varying amounts of necrosis

or slough.

    d. Burns or tissue damaged by radiation.

8. Composite dressings — combination of two or more dressing materials, moisture-retentive properties; absorptive; provides a bacterial barrier; indications include:

    a. Partial-thickness or full-thickness wounds.

    b. Wounds with moderate-to-heavy exudate.

    c. Granulating, necrotic, or mixed wounds.

9. Gauze dressings — available in many forms — impregnated, nonimpregnated, nonadherent, nonwoven. Indications include:

    a. Mechanical debridement of necrotic tissue and debris (wet-to-dry dressings).

    b. Exudating wounds (to wick drainage away from the wound).

    c. To fill dead space.

    d. To deliver topical medications to the wound bed.

    e. To promote a moist environment for healing.

10. Vaccum-assisted closure (V.A.C.) — wound dressing device that applies uniform negative pressure to the wound surface to increase perfusion and facilitate removal of surface bacteria and debris.

    a. Sterile foam dressing is cut to fit geometry of wound. Foam is attached to fenestrated evacuation tube, which is in turn connected to a vacuum source.

    b. Foam and tubing are sealed with adhesive occlusive film.

    c. Continuous or intermittent vacuum is applied to the closed system.

    d. Indications include:

        (1) Acute, traumatic, and sub-acute wounds.

        (2) Grafts and flaps.

        (3) Nonhealing chronic wounds that have not responded to conventional treatments.

        (4) Acceleration of granulation tissue formation in poorly perfused wounds.

        (5) To draw wound edges together (large open wounds healing by secondary intention).

        (6) Relieve fluid pressure and exudate control in heavily draining wounds.

        (7) Reduce periwound tissue edema.

    e. Contraindications include:

        (1) Malignant wounds.

        (2) Active bleeding.

        (3) Anticoagulant therapy.

        (4) Wounds with necrotic tissue.

        (5) Untreated osteomyelitis.

        (6) Sinus tracts or fistulas connecting to organs or body cavities.

        (7) Placement directly over exposed veins or arteries.

Note: It is extremely important that wound assessment, interventions, and evaluation of response to treatment are documented accurately to allow the clinician to appropriately monitor progress toward healing.

XI. VASCULAR ULCERS

A. Venous ulcers.

1. Definition: ulcerations resulting from chronic venous insufficiency.

2. Etiology/Pathophysiology.

    a. Dysfunction of the deep venous system (femoral, popliteal, and tibial veins), perforating, or superficial veins causing increased hydrostatic pressure; venous hypertension causes stretching of the vessel walls with leakage of plasma and fibrin into the extravascular space. Fibrin cuffs form around capillaries, preventing diffusion of oxygen and nutrients needed for normal cellular function. Predisposing factors include:

        (1) Deep vein thrombosis (DVT).

        (2) Valvular incompetence of deep venous system.

        (3) Postphlebitic syndrome.

        (4) Congestive heart failure.

        (5) Obesity.

        (6) Pregnancy.

        (7) Superficial vein regurgitation.

        (8) Muscle weakness secondary to paralysis.

        (9) Previous bone fracture.

3. Events related to venous disease.

    a. Increased hydrostatic pressure.

    b. Venous hypertension.

    c. Edema.

    d. Dermal ulceration.

4. Contributing factors.

    a. Malnutrition.

    b. Hypoalbuminemia.

    c. Immobility.

    d. Trauma.

5. Clinical characteristics.

    a. Stasis dermatitis — brown discoloration and scaling of the skin in the gaitor (sock) area of the lower extremities. Increased venous hypertension leads to chronic edema and rupture of dermal capillaries with deposition of hemosiderin, an iron-containing pigment, in the dermis.

    b. Ulcerations have a predilection for area proximal to the medial malleolus.

    c. Lipodermatosclerosis — induration of skin and subcutaneous tissue.

    d. Pitting edema.

    e. Dull, constant pain which improves on elevation.

Dermatologic Nursing Essentials: A Core Curriculum 2nd Edition © DNA 2003

f.   Ulcers may have sharply demarcated or poorly defined borders and may be deep or superficial.

g.   Pedal pulses usually palpable.

h.   With removal of crust, a moist, granulating base will be revealed.

6.   Incidence.

a.   Affects 1% of the general population and 3.5% of persons over 65.

b.   Recurrence rate approaches 70%.

c.   Women affected three times more often than men.

7.   Assessment.

a.   History and physical examination.

b.   Complete review of medical history.

(1)   Previous pregnancies.

(2)   Leg trauma.

(3)   Cardiac disease.

(4)   Nutritional status.

(5)   History of deep vein thrombosis.

(6)   Previous lower extremity surgery.

c.   Physical exam.

(1)   Varicose veins.

(2)   Lipodermatosclerosis and edema of the lower extremity usually present.

(3)   Stasis dermatitis — induration, erythematous hyperpigmentation, hemosiderin deposition, scaling and weeping; may be pruritic.

(3)   Ankle flare sign — a collection of small venular channels inferior to the medial malleolus extending onto the medial foot.

(4)   Trendelenburg test is generally positive.

(a)   Place patient in supine position with leg elevated for 5 to 10 minutes.

(b)   Place a tourniquet above the knee to occlude venous circulation and prevent retrograde flow.

(c)   Have patient stand and note manner in which veins refill.

(d)   If superficial veins fill rapidly with the tourniquet in place, the perforator valves are incompetent.

(e)   Remove tourniquet and if sudden additional filling occurs, the valves of the saphenous vein are incompetent.

8.   Diagnostic tests.

a.   Doppler ultrasonography — noninvasive assessment of deep venous system.

b.   Photoplethysmography (PPG) — measures vascular volume with infrared light giving an index of valvular incompetence.

c.   Duplex scanning with color-flow imaging — locates venous reflux in the superficial, deep, and perforator systems.

d.   Radionuclide venography (RV) — invasive procedure to assess the venous system.

e.   Contrast venography — invasive procedure utilizing radiopaque dye.

f.   Laboratory.

(1)   Visceral protein — to assess nutritional status of patient and ability to heal.

(2)   Glucose.

(3)   CBC.

9.   Treatment.

a.   Treat underlying cause of venous dysfunction.

b.   Compression and elevation to enhance venous return.

c.   Appropriate dressing for the wound based on assessment.

d.   Avoid restrictive garments.

10.   Nursing considerations (see Table 6).

B.   **Arterial ulcers.**

1.   Definition: ischemic ulcerations secondary to arterial insufficiency (PVD) with acute (for example, thrombosis) or chronic (for example, arteriosclerosis obliterans) presentation.

2.   Etiology/Pathophysiology.

a.   Peripheral vascular disease (PVD).

b.   Arteriosclerosis — thickening and decreased elasticity of arterial walls due to deposition of plaque, lipids, fibrin, platelets, and other cellular debris.

c.   Involves bilateral lower extremities.

d.   Contributing factors.

(1)   Smoking.

(2)   Diabetes mellitus.

(3)   Hyperlipidemia.

(4)   Hypertension.

e.   Signs and symptoms of ischemic disease.

(1)   Progressive pain; usually increases with leg elevation.

(a)   Pain with exercise; relieved with rest (intermittent claudication).

(b)   Nocturnal pain; usually precedes rest pain (ischemic neuritis).

(c)   Pain at rest; demonstrates very advanced disease.

(2)   Impaired circulation — seen prior to ulceration.

(a)   Decreased pulses.

(b)   Change in skin temperature.

(c)   Delayed capillary and venous filling.

(d)   Pallor on elevation.

(e)   Dependent rubor.

(f)   Development of gangrene.

(3)   Ischemic skin changes.

(a)   Smooth, shiny, thin epidermis.

(b)   Absence of hair on lower extremities and feet.

(c)   Slow nail growth.

(4)   Generally affects vessels below the knee (tibial and peroneal arteries) in diabetics.

(5)   Generally affects femoral, iliac, and

Table 6.
Nursing Considerations for Wounds

Nursing Diagnoses	Outcomes	Interventions
Impaired skin integrity.	Skin integrity will improve evidenced by decrease in size of wound, decrease in drainage, and presence of granulation tissue.	Accurately assess the wound; cleanse wound as indicated; implement appropriate topical therapy using principles of wound care.
High risk for infection.	Patient will be monitored closely for the development or progression of any infection; patient will be free of infection.	Continually assess wound and periwound skin for signs of infection; use appropriate dressings to provide protection from infection.
Pain	Pain will be reduced or eradicated through appropriate interventions.	Use both topical and parenteral methods to reduce/relieve any pain associated with wounds.
Altered nutritional status leading to decrease healing.	Nutritional status will be optimized leading to enhanced healing.	Assess patient's nutritional status; employ dietary supplements as indicated to improve patient's nutritional status.
Body image alteration secondary to the presence of wounds.	Positive body image will be evident.	Assess patient's perceptions and feelings regarding the presence of open wounds; allow patient to express feelings.
Impaired mobility secondary to the presence of wounds.	Maximum mobility is attained.	Assess limitations and institute appropriate measures to enhance mobility.
Knowledge deficit.	Patient will have knowledge regarding causative or exacerbating factors and comply with treatment regimen.	Assess knowledge or understanding of causative or exacerbating factors related to wound formation.
Ineffective coping mechanisms (for patients with factitial ulcers).	Patient will develop healthier coping mechanisms.	Assess patient's psychosocial needs and implement appropriate measures to assist patient in correcting problems.

aortic vessels in common population.
3. Clinical presentation.
   a. Punched-out appearance.
   b. Well-demarcated borders.
   c. Location — areas exposed to traumatic injury.
      (1) Over toes.
      (2) Interdigital spaces.
      (3) Dorsum of the foot.
      (4) Lateral malleolus.
   d. May be deep, exposing tendon.
   e. Base of ulcer generally necrotic and pale, lacking granulation tissue.
   f. Gangrenous skin may be seen adjacent to or surrounding the ulcer.
4. Incidence of PVD.

   a. More common in diabetics.
   b. More common at earlier age in diabetics.
   c. Male/female ratio 2:1 in diabetics, 30:1 in nondiabetics.
   d. Diabetics generally have bilateral lower-extremity involvement.
   e. Nondiabetics generally have unilateral involvement.
5. Assessment.
   a. History.
      (1) Ask about events/symptoms specific to arterial insufficiency.
         (a) Pain.
         (b) Impaired circulation.
         (c) Ischemic skin changes.
      (2) Evaluate history of the ulcer.

Dermatologic Nursing Essentials: A Core Curriculum 2nd Edition © DNA 2003

(a) Length of time ulcer present.
(b) Any traumatic event that may have initiated the ulcer.
(c) Topical treatments used for treatment.
(d) History of diabetes, surgery, vascular problems.
(e) History of smoking.
(f) Presence of co-existing systemic conditions (anemia, sickle cell disease, arthritis, or venous insufficiency).

6. Physical examination.
   a. Inspection.
      (1) Ischemic skin changes.
      (2) Evidence of gangrene.
      (3) Pallor with delayed capillary filling.
      (4) Wound bed — desiccated; dry leathery eschar or pale granulation.
      (5) Drainage — scant to minimal.
   b. Palpation.
      (1) Decreased or absent pulses (femoral, popliteal, posterior tibial, and dorsalis pedis).
      (2) Mild (1+) to severe (3+) edema.
      (3) Temperature of skin is cool in the presence of arterial disease.
      (4) Wound bed.
         (a) Palpate, probe wound bed to identify presence of tunnels and sinus tracts.
         (b) Palpate necrotic bed; if boggy/spongy, suspect liquefaction of necrotic tissue or infection.

7. Diagnostic tests.
   a. Noninvasive.
      (1) Doppler ultrasonography — assesses competency of deep arterial system; also measures ankle-brachial index (ABI).
      (2) Transcutaneous oxygen tension.
   b. Invasive.
      (1) Angiography.
   c. Laboratory.
      (1) Visceral protein — to assess nutritional status of patient and ability to heal.
      (2) Glucose.
      (3) CBC.
      (4) Culture (if infection suspected).

8. Treatment.
   a. Avoid compression.
   b. Legs to be kept neutral or slightly dependent position (no elevation).
   c. Avoid restrictive garments.
   d. Eliminate causative factors — enhance arterial profusion either through surgery or pharmacotherapy.
   e. Optimize microenvironment — debridement; eradication of infection.

   f. Optimize the host — enhance nutritional status; control edema; control underlying medical conditions; control smoking.
   g. Appropriate wound dressing.
9. Nursing considerations (see Table 6).

C. **Neuropathic (Diabetic) ulcers.**
   1. Definition: skin ulcers secondary to peripheral neuropathy that commonly accompany diabetes mellitus; ulcer also referred to as malperforans or neurotrophic.
   2. Etiology/Pathophysiology.
      a. Sensory neuropathy — decreased protective sensation places the patient at risk for mechanical, chemical, and thermal trauma, which leads to development of neurotrophic ulcers.
      b. Motor neuropathy — muscular atrophy of the foot.
         (1) Changes patient's gait.
         (2) Causes claw toes.
         (3) Repetitive stress on metatarsal head (callus buildup first sign of increased pressure) — leads to ulceration.
      c. Autonomic neuropathy— generally leads to infection/gangrene.
         (1) Distal anhydrosis.
         (2) Xerosis.
         (3) Cracks/fissures.
   3. Clinical presentation.
      a. Usually isolated lesions on the plantar surface of the foot (correlate with areas of increased weight loading).
      b. Round, dry, punched-out lesion (well-defined edges).
      c. Elevated hyperkeratotic rim.
      d. Foot warm, pink, with pedal pulses present.
      e. Xerosis and fissuring may be present.
      f. Eschar/necrotic debris uncommon unless accompanied by vascular disease, cellulitis, or osteomyelitis.
      g. Absence of normal skin sensation.
   4. Incidence.
      a. Estimated to be between 10% to 20% of diabetics.
      b. Three times more patients with diabetes are admitted to a hospital for foot ulcers secondary to neuropathy than ischemic pain.
   5. Assessment.
      a. History.
         (1) Complete medical history similar to that for ischemic ulcers.
         (2) Previous trauma.
         (3) Compliance with diabetic foot care.
         (4) Types of shoes/orthotics being worn (examine for worn areas).
         (5) Pain relieved by walking.
         (6) Paresthesias or insensate areas.

Table 7.
Characteristics of Ulcers

	Venous	Arterial	Neurotrophic (Diabetes)
Wound base	Red/ruddy. Yellow fibrin. May have granulation.	Pale. Necrotic tissue common. Little or no granulation. Tendons may be exposed.	Granular/red (unless arterial disease present). Deep. Hyperkeratotic rim.
Edges	Irregular/jagged.	Well defined. "Punched-out" appearance.	Even. Well-defined.
Exudate	Moderate-to-heavy (secondary to edema).	Minimal to no exudate.	Low-to-moderate.
Pain	Minimal unless infected or desiccated.	Severe.	Insensate.
Skin changes	Stasis dermatitis.	Dry, cracked. Thickened toenails. Cool to touch at site and distal of ulcer. Indurated wound edges. Shiny, taut, atrophic. Hair loss.	Cellulitis. Decreased or absent sensation. Warm to touch.
Pulses	Difficult to palpate (generally due to edema).	Decreased or absent.	Palpable (unless arterial disease present).

b. Physical examination — always distinguish between traumatic ulcers secondary to peripheral neuropathy and those secondary to arterial insufficiency.
    (1) Diminished or absent sensation in feet.
    (2) Deep, circular lesions.
    (3) Indolent lesions.
    (4) Pedal pulses generally present.
    (5) Skin changes — xerosis, fissures.
    (6) Foot deformities.
    (7) Foot usually warm.
c. Diagnostic tests.
    (1) Doppler ultrasonography and/or angiography to rule out macrovascular disease (PVD).
    (2) Toe pressures or transcutaneous oxygen measurements.
    (3) Ankle-brachial index (ABI) usually inaccurate due to microvascular calcification.
d. Laboratory.
    (1) Visceral proteins.
    (2) CBC.
    (3) Glucose.
    (4) Culture if infection suspected.
6. Treatment.
    a. Avoid trauma — chemical, thermal, or mechanical.
    b. Inspect feet daily — look specifically for corns/calluses that can cause pressure and

between toes for maceration/fissures.
c. Wash feet daily with mild soap and dry completely.
d. Moisturize skin; avoid interdigital spaces.
e. Wear properly fitting shoes.
f. Have podiatrist trim nails, corns/calluses when necessary; avoid OTC corn/callus removers.
g. Orthotics.
h. Prevent mechanical trauma.
i. Redistribute weight of foot.
j. Total contact casting.
    (1) Temporary intervention.
    (2) Increases the surface area of contact when ulcer present.
    (3) Leave in cast for 3 to 7 days.
7. Nursing considerations (see Table 6).
Note: Table 7 shows characteristics of venous, arterial, and neurotrophic ulcers.
D. Pressure ulcers.
1. Definition: tissue destruction as a result of compression of soft tissue, usually between a bone and an external surface; leads to progressive tissue ischemia.
2. Etiology: unrelieved pressure.
3. Contributing factors.
    a. Poor nutritional status.
    b. Shear, friction.
    c. Excessive moisture and maceration (for example, incontinence).

Dermatologic Nursing Essentials: A Core Curriculum 2nd Edition © DNA 2003

d. Immobility.

e. Diminished pain sensation.

f. Oversedation.

4. Pathophysiology.

  a. Pressure — amount of force exerted on a given area.

    (1) Normal capillary filling pressure is approximately 32 mmHg at arteriolar end; 12 mmHg at venous end.

    (2) Pressure greater than 32 mmHg restricts blood flow.

    (3) Increased pressure collapses capillaries leading to thrombosis, ischemia and eventual cell death.

    (4) Decreased oxygen and nutrition reaches tissues.

    (5) Pressure increases as body surface area decreases.

  b. Shear — a mechanical force that is parallel rather than perpendicular to a body area; combination of gravity and friction.

    (1) Main effect is on deep tissue (sacral, coccygeal, trochanteric, ischial areas).

    (2) Blood vessels become angulated, obstructed, torn, and/or stretched.

    (3) Shearing decreases the time that tissues can tolerate pressure forces.

    (4) Shear produces triangular-shaped sacral ulcers.

    (5) Undermining or tunneling commonly occur as a result of shear.

  c. Friction — created by the forces of two surfaces moving across one another.

    (1) Wound resembles an abrasion.

    (2) Alters skin integrity, increasing potential for deeper tissue damage.

  d. Excessive moisture — usually due to incontinence.

    (1) Macerates epidermis.

    (2) Causes epidermal sloughing.

    (3) Predisposes to secondary yeast infection.

5. Incidence.

  a. Prevalence rates vary due to variances in methodology of collection and interpretation of data.

  b. 11.1% to 29.5% of patients in acute care are estimated to have pressure ulcers.

  c. 2.4% to 23% of patients in long-term care are estimated to have pressure ulcers.

6. Assessment (see AHCPR Guidelines, Figures 5 to 8).

7. Treatment (see AHCPR Guidelines, Figures 9 to 11 and Table 8 for classification of support surfaces).

8. Nursing considerations (see Table 6).

E. Factitial ulcers (factitial dermatitis).

1. Definition: a self-inflicted lesion created or perpetuated by manipulation of the skin and is

Figure 5.
Management of Pressure Ulcers: Overview

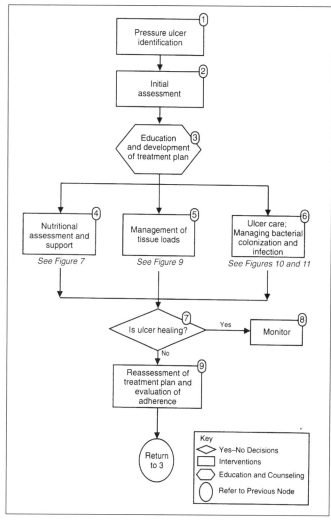

AHCPR Clinical practice guidelines: Pressure ulcer treatment: Quick reference guide for clinicians. (1995). *Dermatology Nursing, 7*(2), 87-101.

generally secondary to underlying emotional factors.

2. Etiology: unknown whether emotional factors precede the skin manifestations or vice versa

3. Pathophysiology.

  a. Dermatologic features.

    (1) Blisters.

    (2) Ulcers.

    (3) Burns.

    (4) Bizarre patterns.

      (a) Unilateral.

      (b) Sharply demarcated.

      (c) Angular wound margins.

      (d) Unusual sites or large areas of destroyed skin in a few locations.

    (5) Sudden appearance of lesions.

  b. Psychiatric features.

Figure 6.
Sample Pressure Ulcer Assessment Guide

Patient Name: _____ Date: _____ Time: _____

<u>Ulcer 1:</u>
Site _____
Stage^a _____
Size (cm)
  Length _____
  Width _____
  Depth _____

<u>Ulcer 2:</u>
Site _____
Stage^a _____
Size (cm)
  Length _____
  Width _____
  Depth _____

Ulcer 1	No	Yes	Ulcer 2	No	Yes
Sinus Tract	☐	☐	Sinus Tract	☐	☐
Tunneling	☐	☐	Tunneling	☐	☐
Undermining	☐	☐	Undermining	☐	☐
Necrotic Tissue	☐	☐	Necrotic Tissue	☐	☐
Slough	☐	☐	Slough	☐	☐
Eschar	☐	☐	Eschar	☐	☐
Exudate	☐	☐	Exudate	☐	☐
Serous	☐	☐	Serous	☐	☐
Serosanguineous	☐	☐	Serosanguineous	☐	☐
Purulent	☐	☐	Purulent	☐	☐
Granulation	☐	☐	Granulation	☐	☐
Epithelialization	☐	☐	Epithelialization	☐	☐
Pain	☐	☐	Pain	☐	☐

<u>Surrounding Skin:</u>					
Erythema	☐	☐	Erythema	☐	☐
Maceration	☐	☐	Maceration	☐	☐
Induration	☐	☐	Induration	☐	☐

Description of Ulcer(s):

_____

_____

Indicate Ulcer Sites:

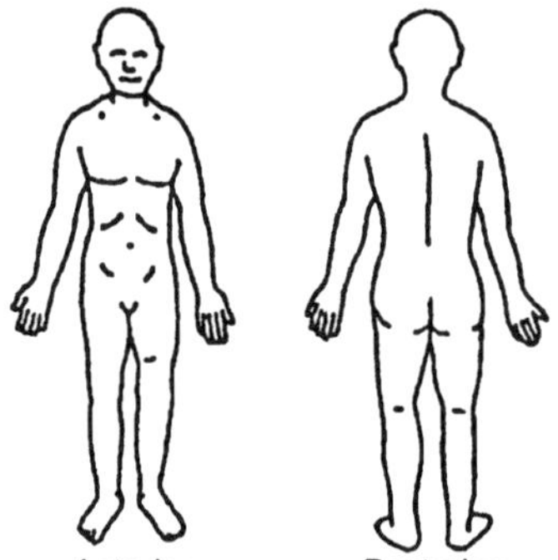

Anterior   Posterior

(Attach a color photo of the pressure ulcer[s] [Optional])

^aClassification of pressure ulcers:
Stage I: Nonblanchable erythema of intact skin, the heralding lesion of skin ulceration. In individuals with darker skin, discoloration of the skin, warmth, edema, induration, or hardness may also be indicators.
Stage II: Partial thickness skin loss involving epidermis, dermis, or both.
Stage III: Full thickness skin loss involving damage to or necrosis of subcutaneous tissue that may extend down to, but not through, underlying fascia. The ulcer presents clinically as a deep crater with or without undermining adjacent tissue.
Stage IV: Full thickness skin loss with extensive destruction, tissue necrosis, or damage to muscle, bone, or supporting structures (e.g., tendon or joint capsule).

AHCPR Clinical practice guidelines: Pressure ulcer treatment: Quick reference guide for clinicians. (1995). *Dermatology Nursing, 7*(2), 87-101.

Table 8.
Selected Characteristics for Classes of Support Surfaces

Performance Characteristics	Air-Fluidized	Low-Air-Loss	Alternating Air	Static Flotation (air or water)	Foam	Standard Mattress
Increased support area	Yes	Yes	Yes	Yes	Yes	No
Low moisture retention	Yes	Yes	No	No	No	No
Reduced heat accumulation	Yes	Yes	No	No	No	No
Shear reduction	Yes	?	Yes	Yes	No	No
Pressure reduction	Yes	Yes	Yes	Yes	Yes	No
Dynamic	Yes	Yes	Yes	No	No	No
Cost per day	High	High	Moderate	Low	Low	Low

AHCPR Clinical practice guidelines: Pressure ulcer treatment: Quick reference guide for clinicians. (1995). *Dermatology Nursing, 7*(2), 87-101.

Figure 7.
Nutritional Assessment of Patient with Pressure Ulcer(s)

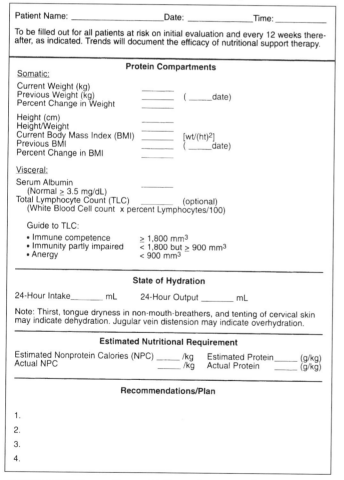

AHCPR Clinical practice guidelines: Pressure ulcer treatment: Quick reference guide for clinicians. (1995). *Dermatology Nursing, 7*(2), 87-101.

Figure 8.
Nutritional Assessment and Support

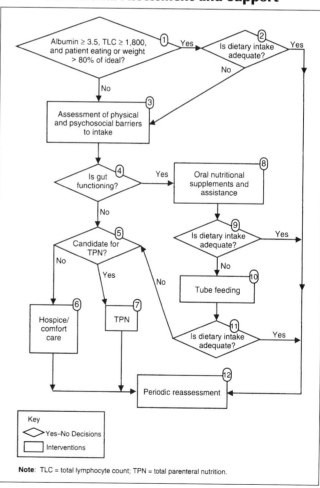

AHCPR Clinical practice guidelines: Pressure ulcer treatment: Quick reference guide for clinicians. (1995). *Dermatology Nursing, 7*(2), 87-101.

Figure 9.
Ulcer Care

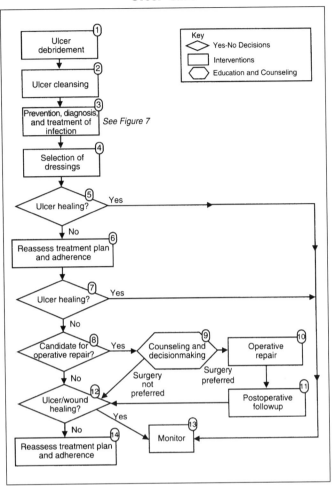

AHCPR Clinical practice guidelines: Pressure ulcer treatment: Quick reference guide for clinicians. (1995). *Dermatology Nursing, 7*(2), 87-101.

Figure 10.
Managing Bacterial Colonization and Infection

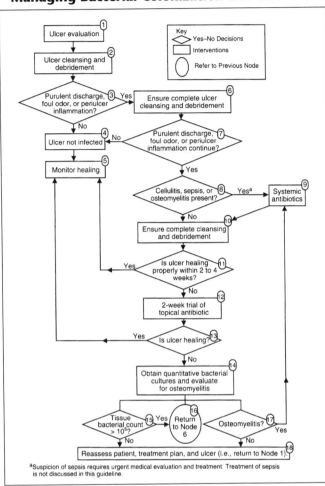

AHCPR Clinical practice guidelines: Pressure ulcer treatment: Quick reference guide for clinicians. (1995). *Dermatology Nursing, 7*(2), 87-101.

(1) Immature personality.
(2) Lesions signal an "appeal for help."
(3) Suicide uncommon.
4. Incidence.
   a. Ratio of female to males is 4:1.
   b. "Hollow history" — patient cannot describe how lesions evolved.
5. Assessment.
   a. History.
     (1) Complete medical history to rule out physiologic etiology.
     (2) Ascertain evolution of lesion(s).
     (3) Social and psychological assessment.
   b. Physical examination.
     (1) Evaluate pattern of lesion(s).
     (2) Evaluate location of lesion(s).
6. Treatment.
   a. Psychological.
     (1) Supportive, empathetic approach.
     (2) Family involvement.
     (3) Environmental manipulation as indicated

FIVE P's OF ACUTE ARTERIAL ISCHEMIA

Pain

Paresthesia

Paralysis

Pallor

Pulselessness

Ulceration is the result of chronic ischemia

(reduce stressful situations, etc).
     (4) Psychological counseling or psychiatric care.
   b. Physical.
     (1) Occlusive dressings/casts to reduce manipulation.
     (2) Removal of trigger factors — heat, dryness, humidity, sweating, pruritus, irritating topical preparations.

Figure 11.
Management of Tissue Loads

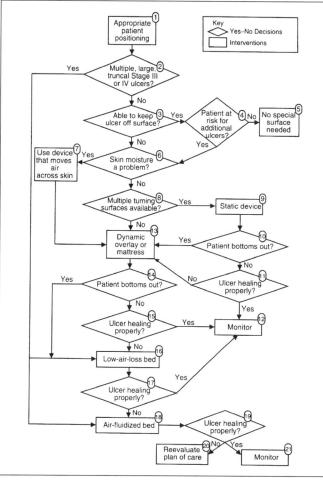

AHCPR Clinical practice guidelines: Pressure ulcer treatment: Quick reference guide for clinicians. (1995). *Dermatology Nursing, 7*(2), 87-101.

 (3) Topical steroids as indicated to reduce symptomology.

 (4) Sedatives/tranquilizers — in acute situations.

 7. Nursing considerations (see Table 6).

Bibliography

AHCPR clinical practice guidelines: Pressure ulcers in adults: Prediction and prevention. (1993). *Dermatology Nursing, 5*(1), 17-31.

AHCPR clinical practice guidelines: Pressure ulcer treatment: Quick reference guide for clinicians. (1995). *Dermatology Nursing, 7*(2), 87-101.

Ayello, E.A., & Braden, B. (2002). How and why to do pressure ulcer risk assessment. *Skin & Wound Care, 15*(3), 125-133.

Bolton, L., & van Ryswijk, L. (1991). Wound dressings: Meeting clinical and biological needs. *Dermatology Nursing, 3*(3), 146-161.

Bowker, J.H., & Pfeifer, M.A. (2000). *Levin and O'Neal's the diabetic foot.* St. Louis, MO: Mosby Year Book.

Bryant, R.A. (2000). *Acute and chronic wounds: Nursing management* (2nd ed.). St. Louis, MO: Mosby Year Book.

Chang, H., Wind, S., & Kerstein, M.D. (1996). Moist wound healing. *Dermatology Nursing, 8*(3),174-204.

Cuzzell, J.Z. (1988, October). The new RYB color code. *American Journal of Nursing,* 1342-1346.

Cuzzell, J. (2002). Wound healing: Translating theory into clinical practice. *Dermatology Nursing, 14*(4), 257-261.

Cuzzell, J. (2002). Wound dressings: Confusion or choice? *Dermatology Nursing, 14*(3), 187-188.

Cuzzell, J. (2002). Wound documentation guidelines. *Dermatology Nursing, 14*(4), 265-266.

Dolynchuk, K., Keast, D., Campbell, K., et al. (2000). Best practices for the prevention and treatment of pressure ulcers. *Ostomy/Wound Management, 46*(11), 38-54.

Eaglestein, W.H., Baxter, C., Mertz, P.M., Oot-Giromini, B., Rodeheaver, G., Rudolph, R., Shannon, M.S., & Silane, M. (1990). *New directions in wound healing.* Princeton, NJ: E.R. Squibb and Sons, Inc.

Goldsmith, S.P. (1996). Wound care: Combining three classification systems to select dressing. *Home Health Care Management & Practice, 8*(6), 17-26.

Haas, A.F. (1995). Wound healing. *Dermatology Nursing, 7*(1), 28-34.

Hess, C.T. (1995). *Nurse's clinical guide: Wound care.* Springhouse, PA: Springhouse Corporation.

Ierardi, R.P., Wind, S., & Kerstein, M.D. (1995). Neuropathic wounds. *Dermatology Nursing, 7*(4), 223-225.

Inlow, S., Orstead, H., & Sibbald, R.G. (2000). Best practices for the prevention, diagnosis, and treatment of diabetic foot ulcers. *Ostomy/Wound Management, 46*(11), 55-68.

Koblenzer, C.S. (1993). Psychologic aspects of skin disease. In T.B. Fitzpatrick, A.Z. Eisen, K. Wolff, I.M. Freedberg, & K.F. Austen, (Eds.), *Dermatology in general medicine* (4th ed.). New York: McGraw Hill.

Krasner, D., & Kane, D.(Eds.) (1997). *Chronic wound care: A clinical source book for healthcare professionals* (2nd ed.). Wayne, PA: Health Management Publications.

Krasner, D., Kennedy, K.L., Rolstad, B.S., & Roma, A.W. (1993). The ABCs of wound care dressings. *Ostomy/Wound Management, 39*(8), 66-86.

Kunimoto, B.T. (2001). Management and prevention of venous leg ulcers: A literature-guided approach. *Ostomy/Wound Management, 47*(6), 36-49.

Maklebust, J., & Sieggreen, M. (1996). *Pressure ulcers guidelines for prevention and nursing management.* West Dundee, IL: S-N Publications.

Margolis, D., & Nguyen, T.V. (1993). Diagnosis of lower-extremity ulcers. *Dermatology Nursing, 5*(1), 46- 48.

Phillips, T.J. (1996). Leg ulcer management. *Dermatology Nursing, 8*(5), 333-340.

Sibbald, R.G., Williamson, M.B., Orsted, H., et al. (2000). Preparing the wound bed-Debridement, bacterial balance, and moisture balance. *Ostomy/Wound Management, 46*(11), 14-35.

Torrence, B.P., Hovanec, R., Bartunek, C., & Brodell, R.T. (1993). Stasis dermatitis: Practical pearls for the dermatologic nurse. *Dermatology Nursing, 5*(3), 186-192.

STUDY QUESTIONS

1. The proliferative phase of healing is characterized by all of the following *except:*
   a. Formation of new blood vessels.
   b. Hemostasis.
   c. Collagen deposition.
   d. Collagen lysis.
   e. Wound contraction.

2. An example of a wound that heals by primary intention is:
   a. Diabetic foot ulcer.
   b. Venous leg ulcer.
   c. Open abdominal wound.
   d. Sutured laceration.
   e. Skin tear.

3. Intrinsic factors that can delay healing include all of the following *except:*
   a. Unrelieved pressure.
   b. Protein malnutrition.
   c. Increased capillary fragility.
   d. Pre-existing cardiac disease.

4. The best example of a full thickness wound is a:
   a. Skin tear.
   b. Basal cell excision.
   c. Shave biopsy.
   d. Dermabrasion.
   e. Stage 2 pressure ulcer.

5. Of the following, the best clinical indicator of progress toward healing is:
   a. Decrease in wound dimensions.
   b. Decrease in wound volume.
   c. Increase in percent of granulation tissue.
   d. a & c.
   e. b & c.

6. An example of nonselective wound debridement is removal of necrotic tissue using:
   a. Dakin's solution.
   b. High pressure saline irrigation.
   c. Wet-to-dry dressings.
   d. None of the above.
   e. All of the above.

7. Dressings that promote autolytic debridement include all of the following *except:*
   a. Hydrocolloid dressings.
   b. Alginate packing.
   c. Wet-to-dry saline dressings.
   d. Semipermeable film dressings.
   e. Absorption dressings.

8. Clinical signs of inadequate wound perfusion include:
   a. Dry, fibrotic wound surface.
   b. Nocturnal pain.
   c. Pale granulation tissue.
   d. Well-demarcated wound borders.
   e. a & c.
   f. All of the above.

9. Appropriate treatment of neuropathic ulcers includes all of the following *except:*
   a. Liberal moisturization of feet and interdigit spaces.
   b. Avoiding over-the-counter corn and callus removers.
   c. Redistributing body weight to minimize pedal pressure points.
   d. Avoiding the use of heating pads when feet are cold.

10. The dressing material that is least likely to impair new epithelial growth is a:
    a. Transparent film dressing.
    b. Wet-to-dry saline dressing.
    c. Betadine gauze packing.
    d. Hydrogel dressing.

11. One contraindication to use of enzymatic debriding agents is:
    a. Significant edema of the peri-wound tissue.
    b. The presence of a thick leathery eschar.
    c. Use of antimicrobial solutions containing mercury.
    d. The presence of healthy granulation tissue.
    e. None of the above.

12. A deep diabetic foot ulcer with exposed tendon at the base should be classified as a:
    a. Deep partial thickness ulcer.
    b. Stage IV ulcer.
    c. Stage III ulcer.
    d. Full-thickness ulcer.

Answers to Study Questions

1.	c	5.	e	9.	a
2.	d	6.	e	10.	d
3.	a	7.	c	11.	c
4.	b	8.	f	12.	d

Dermatologic Nursing Essentials: A Core Curriculum 2nd Edition © DNA 2003

DNAP320

CE Answer/Evaluation Form

Chapter 20.
Wound Healing

Please photocopy this test page and return.

COMPLETE THE FOLLOWING:

Name: _____

Address: _____

City: _____ State: _____ Zip: _____

Preferred telephone: (Home)_____ (Work) _____

State where licensed and license number: _____

CE application fee: DNA member $13.00
                        Nonmember $16.00

POSTTEST INSTRUCTIONS
1. To receive continuing education credit for individual study after reading the article, complete the answer/evaluation form below.
2. Photocopy and send the answer/evaluation form along with a check or money order payable to **Dermatology Nurses' Association** to: **DNA**, East Holly Avenue Box 56, Pitman, NJ 08071-0056.
3. Test returns must be postmarked by December 31, 2008. Upon completion of the answer/evaluation form, a certificate for 3.9 contact hour(s) will be awarded and sent to you.

This chapter was reviewed and formatted for contact hour credit by Marcia J. Hill, MSN, RN, Core Curriculum Editor; and Sally Russell, MN, RN,C, DNA Education Director.

ANSWER FORM

1. Name one new detail (item, issue, or phenomenon) that you learned by completing this activity.

   _____

   _____

   _____

2. How will you apply the information from this learning activity to your practice?
   a. Patient education.
   b. Staff education.
   c. Improve my patient care.
   d. In my education course work.
   e. Other: Please describe _____

   _____

   _____

Evaluation	Strongly disagree				Strongly agree
3. The offering met the stated objectives.					
a. Describe the phases of wound healing.	1	2	3	4	5
b. Differentiate between healing by tissue regeneration versus healing by scarring and wound contraction.	1	2	3	4	5
c. List three factors that delay the wound healing process.	1	2	3	4	5
d. Distinguish between intrinsic and extrinsic factors that affect wound healing.	1	2	3	4	5
e. Identify various wound dressings and how to use them to optimize healing.	1	2	3	4	5
4. The content was current and relevant.	1	2	3	4	5
5. The content was presented clearly.	1	2	3	4	5
6. The content was covered adequately.	1	2	3	4	5
7. I am more confident of my abilities since completing this material.	1	2	3	4	5

8. The material was (check one) ☐ new, ☐ review for me.

Comments _____

9. Time required to complete reading assignment: _____ minutes

This independent study is provided by the Dermatology Nurses' Association (DNA) for 3.9 contact hours. DNA is accredited as a provider of continuing education in nursing by the American Nurses Credentialing Center's Commission on Accreditation. DNA is approved as a provider of continuing education by the California Board of Registered Nursing Provider #CEP5708.

Dermatologic Emergencies

Bonita Weyrauch, RN, CWS, CCT

OBJECTIVES

At the end of this chapter, the reader will be able to:
- Identify dermatologic disease processes which may progress to become life threatening, and require emergency or acute care interventions.
- Recognize patients who are at risk of severe, acute disease.
- Describe therapeutic interventions used to promote healing and prevent complications.

KEY POINTS

- Rapid assessment of the extent and progression of the disease will allow for implementation of measures to reduce complications and tissue damage.
- Information and education for the patient and family must include avoidance of the causative agent, if known, and interventions for possible recurrent episodes.
- Nursing care for the acute phases of disease includes consideration of maintenance of fluid balance, prevention of secondary infections and complications, pain management, wound care, and psychosocial support.

Dermatologic Emergencies

Bonita Weyrauch, RN, CWS, CCT

Bacterial Infections:
STAPHYLOCOCCAL SCALDED SKIN SYNDROME

I. OVERVIEW

Staphylococcal scalded skin syndrome (SSSS) is a severe cutaneous reaction to toxin from certain strains of gram-positive cocci.

A. Definition: a generalized cutaneous bullous and exfoliative process caused by a toxin produced by *Staphylococcus aureus*, phage groups 1, 2, and 3.

B. Etiology.
1. SSSS is usually associated with relatively mild staphylococcal infection of the eyes, ears, nose, throat, anus, wound, or skin. Bacteremia is not detected in children even when SSSS is severe.
2. A milder form of SSSS, staphylococcal scarlet fever, presents with an erythematous rash, followed by mild to moderate desquamation and is distinguished from streptococcal scarlet fever by lacking the pharyngeal involvement and strawberry tongue typical of streptococcal scarlet fever.
3. Only a few phage types of *S.aureus* produce the exfoliative toxin which is responsible for the severe form of the disease.

C. Pathophysiology.
1. *S. aureus,* phage groups 1, 2, and 3, may produce exfoliative endotoxin which causes a split in the granular layer of the skin, and results in vesicle formation beneath the stratum corneum.
2. Initially an erythematous, blanchable, macular rash with a sandpaper texture begins around the mouth and in the body folds and spreads to cover the body within 24 hours.
3. Vesicles enlarge to form fragile bullae, which extend and rupture with friction, leaving large areas of erosion and denudation.
4. Mucous membranes are spared, although crusting around orifices may be present.

D. Incidence.
1. SSSS is usually seen in association with poor renal clearance of toxin or a compromised immune system.
2. Successful antibody production by the patient against the exfoliative toxin limits the disease.
3. Adults with immunosuppression due to tumors, alcoholism, steroids, bone marrow transplantation, and AIDS have developed SSSS and may have a 50% mortality rate.

E. Considerations across the life span.
1. Infants and children under 5 years, due to a lower renal clearance rate, are at risk.
2. A compromised immune system in children and adults contributes to the development of SSSS.
3. Adults with SSSS usually have renal insufficiency, immunosuppression, or sepsis. Skin changes are similar to those of children, but bacteremia is detected and bullae are culture positive.

II. ASSESSMENT

A. History and physical examination.
1. A child or infant with superficial infection of eyes, ears, orifices, or skin, or an adult with reduced renal function or immunosuppression presents with an erythematous rash or bullae.
2. The erythema spreads over the body within 24 hours and the skin becomes tender, with the texture of sandpaper, then wrinkled and bullous.
3. The bullae may appear in the skin folds of the body, and spread to any skin surface.
4. Friction will cause extension and rupture of the bullae to reveal raw, wet erosions.
5. Pain is severe from the denuded areas of the skin surface.
6. Nikolsky's sign is positive.
7. In contrast to toxic epidermal necrolysis, which appears similar on the skin surface and is more common in adults, the mucous membranes, including the conjunctiva, are not affected.

Note: Nikolsky's sign — horizontal pressure across the skin, with the fingertip, will cause separation of the epidermis and result in bullae formation or a torn skin surface.

B. Diagnostic tests.
1. Skin biopsy of the lesions shows a split in the granular layer beneath the stratum corneum.
2. Tissue frozen sections or cells from the exfoliated tissue of Nikolsky positive areas and Tzank preparation show flattened nucleated squamous cells with a "fried egg" appearance.
3. Culture of sites colonized by staphylococci is positive for *S. aureus* phage groups 1, 2, and 3.

III. COMMON THERAPEUTIC MODALITIES

A. Medical interventions.
1. Intravenous antibiotics such as oxacillin, nafcillin, first-generation cephalosporins or vancomycin, if SSSS is suspected.
2. Topical preparations such as Vaseline® gauze, silver sulfadiazine, or mafenide acetate to prevent fluid loss and super infection of lesions,

Table 1.
Common Nursing Diagnosis, Outcomes, and Interventions: SSSS

Nursing Diagnoses	Outcomes	Interventions
Impaired skin integrity related to inflammatory process.	Skin integrity has been improved or maintained.	Wet compresses, barriers, and topical medications applied to denuded area of skin. Observe for signs of healing.
At risk for infection related to lack of skin barrier function.	Patient will remain free from infection.	Observe for signs of infection in skin lesions and other organs.
Fluid volume deficit related to impaired skin integrity.	Patient will maintain normal fluid balance.	Monitor fluid intake and output.
Pain related to skin lesions.	Patient's pain will be relieved.	Maintain adequate pain control, based on the patient's report of pain. Give pain medication prior to painful procedures.

except on infants less than 2 months old due to the risk of kernicterus. Observe for signs of metabolic acidosis (mafenide acetate), bone marrow suppression, hemolytic anemia related to use of topical medications. Avoid silver sulfadiazine and mafenide acetate if patient has had an adverse reaction to sulfonamides.
3. Maintenance of fluid and electrolyte balance.
4. Contact isolation precautions especially for neonates. ICU or burn unit care depending on the extent of denudation.
B. Surgical interventions.
   1. None.

IV. COMMON NURSING DIAGNOSES, OUTCOMES, AND INTERVENTIONS (see Table 1).

V. HOME CARE CONSIDERATIONS

A. Due to rapid re-epithelialization, recovery without scarring may occur within 7 to 14 days.
B. Topical dressing may be discontinued once the intact epidermis develops.

TOXIC SHOCK SYNDROME

I. OVERVIEW

Toxic shock syndrome (TSS) is an acute illness, presenting with fever, rash, and hypotension, progressing to widespread organ dysfunction. *S. aureus* toxin may be responsible, as in SSSS.
A. Definition: a condition characterized by fever (39.9° C), rash, desquamation, hypotension, and multi-system involvement.
B. Etiology.

1. Colonization with *S. aureus* phage group 1 results in toxin production.
2. The condition has been associated with menstruating women who use tampons and may also have cervical-vaginal ulceration, but non-menstruating adults have also been affected.
3. Other contributing factors to TSS are childbirth, surgical wound infection, nasal packing, and non-surgical cutaneous or subcutaneous infections such as abscesses and insect bites.
4. Healthy people can be carriers of the *S. aureus* strain.
C. Pathophysiology.
   1. Phage group 1 *S. aureus* produces a toxin labeled toxic shock syndrome toxin 1 (TST-1) which may be the cause of hypotension and skin desquamation.
   2. Other *S. aureus* strains produce toxins which cause similar systemic effects.
   3. An adequate immune response to the toxin seems to protect from developing the syndrome.
D. Incidence.
   1. Colonization or infection with phage group 1 *S. aureus* may give rise to TSS in menstruating women, non-menstruating adults, and also children.
   2. Healthy people may be carriers, with a 22% carrier rate in people under 20 years.
E. Considerations across the life span.
   1. Young adults, particularly women and children, are at risk of TSS.

Table 2.
Common Nursing Diagnoses, Outcomes, and Interventions: TSS

Nursing Diagnoses	Outcomes	Interventions
Impaired skin integrity related to inflammatory process.	Skin integrity will be restored.	Cleanse infected sites. Monitor for skin breakdown.
At risk for fluid volume deficit related to skin lesions, renal function, and fluid loss.	Patient will maintain normal fluid balance.	Encourage oral intake. Maintain intravenous access. Monitor fluid intake and output.
At risk for hemodynamic instability related to infection.	Patient will maintain normal vital signs.	Monitor vital signs, cardiac electrical activity, and urine output.
At risk for impaired gas exchange related to disease process.	Patient will maintain normal oxygenation.	Monitor respiratory function.

II. ASSESSMENT

A. **History and physical examination.**
   1. Onset of TSS may be 24 hours to several weeks after surgery.
   2. Women may give a history of using tampons.
   3. Primary features of TSS are fever, chills, myalgia, nausea, vomiting and diarrhea, rash, and hypotension.
   4. The rash appears as a nonpruritic macular erythroderma, with a sandpaper texture, especially in the skin folds. It may be widespread or limited to the trunk, extremities, perineum, or vaginal area.
   5. Edema of the hands, face, and feet may be present.
   6. Mucous membranes are tender and conjunctivitis, strawberry tongue, oral ulcerations, and pharyngitis are also present.
   7. Muscle tenderness on the trunk and upper parts of the limbs; arthritis is common.
   8. Orthostatic hypotension, dizziness, or hypotensive shock are evidence of cardiovascular involvement.
   9. Leakage of fluid through capillaries, vasodilatation, cardiomyopathy, and diarrhea lead to shock.
   10. Complications due to renal failure, liver damage, toxic encephalopathy, adult respiratory distress syndrome (ARDS), and myocardial irritability may result in death.
   11. While recovering from TSS, peeling desquamation of the hands and feet is common.

B. **Diagnostic tests.**
   1. Negative cultures except for blood which may be positive for *S. aureus*.
   2. Platelets less than or equal to 100,000/mm, leukocytosis.
   3. Nikolsky's sign is negative.

III. COMMON THERAPEUTIC MODALITIES

A. **Medical interventions.**
   1. Because of the possible risk of going into shock, blood pressure monitoring will help to determine the need for vasopressor agents and intravenous fluids.
   2. If the characteristic fever, rash, and hypotension are present, the patient should be in ICU.
   3. Continuous monitoring of cardiac electrical activity, heart rate, blood pressure, respiratory rate, and urine output.
   4. Laboratory tests for liver function, complete blood count, electrolytes, blood urea nitrogen, creatinine, calcium, phosphorus, albumen, prothrombin time, and partial thromboplastin time.
   5. A chest x-ray.
   6. Cultures from orifices and wounds will verify the diagnosis.
   7. Cleansing of purulent sites, removal of tampons and surgical packing will reduce the bacterial load.
   8. Intravenous antibiotics may reduce the morbidity and mortality.
   9. Shock is treated with intravenous normal saline or Ringer's lactate to maintain circulation volume, with vasopressors as necessary.
   10. Oxygen by nasal cannula unless ARDS develops, when mechanical ventilation will be necessary.
   11. Recovery is evident when there is hemodynamic stability, reduced erythroderma, and mucosal inflammation.

IV. COMMON NURSING DIAGNOSES, OUTCOMES, AND INTERVENTIONS (see Table 2)

V. HOME CARE CONSIDERATIONS

A. Affected women should avoid tampon use and watch for signs and symptoms with menses in the future.

B. Renal status may require followup visits.

C. Five to 12 days after the erythematous rash resolves, desquamation of the hands and feet occur. There may be reversible hair and nail loss and fatigue.

**Viral Infections:
ECZEMA HERPETICUM
(Kaposi's Varicelliform Eruption)**

I. OVERVIEW

Herpes viruses are enveloped, double-stranded DNA viruses, which replicate in the nuclei of affected cells and can remain latent for long periods. Herpes simplex virus-I is the most common cause of eczema herpeticum in patients with pre-existing disease such as atopic dermatitis.

A. Definition: a generalized eruption caused by herpes simplex virus in patients with pre-existing skin disease or immunosuppression.

B. Etiology.

1. Herpes simplex is a human virus found worldwide. Various strains predominantly affect the lips (HSV-I) and genitalia (HSV-II) as recurrent infections.

2. The virus remains latent in the sensory nerve ganglia after the primary infection and can be reactivated and infective when triggered by sun exposure, local trauma, hormonal changes, or stress.

3. The viruses can become life threatening when immune competence decreases in the host or they may spread to a person with established skin disease.

4. Transmission is by close person-to-person contact when virus-laden secretions penetrate mucocutaneous layers. Contact isolation measures should be instituted for patients with disseminated cutaneous systemic involvement and close observation in an ICU or burn unit may be needed.

5. Eczema herpeticum due to primary HSV infection or recurrent disease occurs in people with atopic dermatitis, neurodermatitis, Darier's disease, seborrheic dermatitis, pemphigus vulgaris, congenital ichthyosiform erythroderma, mycosis fungoides, and severe burns.

6. Patients with pre-existing skin diseases can be protected from HSV infection by avoiding contact with health care providers with active, moist HSV lesions and not being roomed with patients with active herpes virus diseases.

C. Pathophysiology.

1. Primary lesions of eczema herpeticum are 1 to 3 mm vesicles over areas of previous dermatitis and on normal skin. A cluster may disseminate over larger areas. Vesicles are discrete with peripheral enlargement and central umbilication, and progress to pustular, then crusted stages over several days.

2. Secondary infection with staphylococci or streptococci causes purulent exudates and crusting.

3. Vesicles appear in crops over 2 to 6 weeks or all at the same time.

4. Fever, with dehydration, electrolyte imbalance, localized or generalized lymphadenopathy in predisposed patients identifies the condition of eczema herpeticum.

D. Incidence.

1. Infants, children, and adults with deficient cellular immunity are at greatest risk for severe disease. Otherwise, the disease may be limited to 2 to 3 weeks.

2. Antiviral therapy and good supportive care have reduced the mortality rate from 50% to 10% for the severe form of the disease.

E. Considerations across the life span.

1. Antibodies to HSV-I and to HSV-II can be detected in children after puberty.

2. Infants born to infected mothers may be infected during birth.

3. Children under 5 years are at risk of developing eczema herpeticum on primary exposure to HSV.

II. ASSESSMENT

A. History and physical examination.

1. A history of pre-existing skin disease.

2. An underlying compromised immune system.

3. Age of the patient: at risk groups are infants, children, and young adults.

4. Primary or recurrent signs of HSV-I on lips, in the oropharynx, in the eyes.

5. Primary herpes genitalis infection in young adults, caused by HSV-II.

6. Primary lesions on areas of dermatitis or on normal skin.

   a. Lesions are vesicles, often in clusters, which disseminate and coalesce.

   b. Initially discrete, with peripheral enlargement and some central indentation, they progress to pustular, then crusted forms.

   c. Fissures, erosions, superficial ulceration,

Table 3.
Common Nursing Diagnoses, Interventions, and Outcomes: Eczema Herpeticum

Nursing Diagnoses	Outcomes	Interventions
Impaired skin integrity related to infection.	Patient's skin will be free from lesions.	Apply Burrow's solution soaks as ordered.
High risk for infection related to lesions.	Patient will remain free from infection.	Observe for signs of infection.
Pain related to lesions.	Patient's pain will be relieved.	Analgesics as needed. Topical applications and comfort measures.
Altered nutrition related to disease process.	Patient will maintain or improve nutritional status.	Assess nutritional needs. Obtain soft or liquid diet, and supplements. Initiate oral care regimen.
Altered body image related to disease process.	Patient will maintain positive body image.	Allow patient to discuss perceptions and feelings.

pus, and a hemorrhagic appearance are secondary changes.

7. Fever.
8. Dehydration and electrolyte imbalance.
9. Localized or generalized lymph node enlargement.

B. Diagnostic tests.
   1. Tzanck smear taken from the base of the vesicle — large multinucleated giant cells.
   2. Direct fluorescent antibody.
   3. Culture of vesicle fluid.
   4. Skin biopsy.
   5. Serology — HSV antibody level.

III. COMMON THERAPEUTIC MODALITIES

A. Medical interventions.
   1. Antivirals — intravenous acyclovir decreases the duration of disease and vesicle formation. Oral acyclovir for patients who are not acutely ill.
   2. Topical therapy.
      a. Burrow's solution soaks for 15 minutes, 4 times a day, for antibacterial action and resolution of vesicles.
      b. Observe for exacerbation of eczematous areas due to the drying effect of Burrow's solution.
      c. Discontinue soaks when vesicles have crusted.
   3. Intravenous antibiotics if dissemination is extensive and secondary bacterial infection possible.
   4. Monitor blood pressure and mental status for signs of encephalitis.

B. Surgical interventions.
   1. None.

IV. COMMON NURSING DIAGNOSES, INTERVENTIONS, AND OUTCOMES (see Table 3)

V. HOME CARE CONSIDERATIONS

A. Recurrence of the disease is likely, especially with pre-existing disease, although it may be less severe.
B. The patient should be aware that triggers like sun exposure, local trauma, hormonal changes, or stress may reactivate the virus.
C. Patients with pre-existing skin disease should avoid contact with lesions of HSV-I or II.

Varicella-Zoster

I. OVERVIEW

The varicella-zoster virus (VZV) produces a primary infection, chicken pox or varicella, and a latent form which reappears as shingles or herpes zoster. It is the most communicable of the herpes viruses.

A. Definition: VZV causes infectious disease in a primary attack as chicken pox, and a recurrent form as shingles, or as disseminated disease of varicella or zoster in immunocompromised patients.
B. Etiology.
   1. Varicella is common in temperate climates, with epidemics in winter and spring.
   2. Transmission is by airborne and then contacts routes after vesicles form on the skin.
   3. Patients are infectious 1 to 2 days before the rash appears until 4 to 5 days after, or when all the lesions are crusted.
   4. Adults who contract a primary infection (chicken pox) have a 25% death rate.

5. Immunocompromised patients with primary or reactivated infection have a longer infectious period, and have a higher risk of dissemination and complications like pneumonitis and encephalitis.

C. **Pathophysiology.**
1. The incubation period for varicella is 9 to 21 days with a median of 14 days.
2. The lesions are pruritic, and start to appear over the scalp, face, and trunk. Vesicles are thin-walled, 2 to 3 mm diameter with an erythematous base ("dewdrop on a rose petal").
3. Vesicles appear in crops, spreading from the trunk to the extremities, with excoriations, and crusting usually complete by day 6.
4. Mucous membranes, GI tract, and conjunctiva may also be involved.
5. Fever, chills, malaise, headache, anorexia, and sore throat may be present before the rash appears and also concurrently.
6. Generalized vesicular eruption and illness in the elderly, immunocompromised, or pregnant patient may be prolonged and more severe with systemic complications.
   a. Pneumonitis: cough, tachypnea, dyspnea, fever, pleuritic chest pain, cyanosis, and hemoptysis.
   b. Encephalitis: ataxia, headache, nausea and vomiting, cerebral rigidity, altered mental status. Seizures (in adults) indicate higher mortality.
   c. Cutaneous: super infection leading to cellulitis, purpura fulminans.
7. Although not life threatening, zoster can cause blindness, especially when the ophthalmic branch of the trigeminal nerve is affected and vesicles appear on the tip of the nose.

D. **Incidence.**
1. Although it is a self-limiting disease in immunocompetent patients, varicella and zoster can cause increased morbidity and mortality in patients with malignancy, organ transplant, congenital or acquired immunodeficiency, severe malnutrition, severe burns, severe dermatitis, immunosuppressive therapy, collagen vascular disorder, rheumatic fever, or psoriasis.
2. Zoster is triggered by surgery, trauma, irradiation, immunosuppressive agents, arsenic, or diseases which are normally contained by cell-mediated immunity, like tuberculosis.

II. ASSESSMENT

A. **History and physical examination.**
1. Primary infection (varicella, chicken pox) — fever to 102° F, chills, malaise, arthralgia,

headache, anorexia, sore throat, rash in which discrete vesicles appear in crops.
2. Disseminated varicella — presents with a higher fever and appearance of new lesions after a week of rash, indicating further circulation of virus has occurred. Vesicles are deeper and umbilicated, found on the palms and soles. Also abdominal pain and back pain are significant.
3. Secondary disease — zoster.
   a. Localized eruption in dermatomes of spinal or cranial nerves, most commonly thoracic (50%), cranial usually trigeminal (15%), and cervical and lumbar (10%).
   b. Erythematous plaque develops into papules, then clusters of clear vesicles which may become confluent within the dermatome.
   c. After 8 days vesicles become pustular then crusted.
   d. Fever, malaise, headache, severe pain, or burning in the area for 1 to 4 days.
4. Disseminated zoster — vesicles outside the dermatome indicate cutaneous viral spread. Herpes zoster ophthalmicus is more likely to spread internally although virus from any dermatome can spread to lungs, brain, liver, pancreas, or eye.

B. **Diagnostic tests.**
1. Varicella.
   a. Inoculation of vesicle fluid into tissue culture; 7 to 10 days to identify.
   b. Skin biopsy.
   c. Tzanck smear identifies herpes simplex as well as varicella zoster.
   d. Direct immunofluorescence differentiates herpes simplex and herpes zoster.
2. Zoster.
   a. Tzanck stain.
   b. Skin biopsy.
   c. Direct immunofluorescence.
   d. Culture of super infected sites.

III. COMMON THERAPEUTIC MODALITIES

A. **Medical interventions.**
1. Those at risk of dissemination must be monitored for pulmonary and central nervous system (CNS) involvement.
2. Monitor for disseminated intravascular coagulation (varicella).
3. Non-aspirin antipyretics.
4. Antipruritics.
5. Analgesics.
6. Antibiotics for secondary infection.
7. Burrow's solution or cool water compresses to vesicles 4 times a day.
8. Antivirals — intravenous acyclovir for

immunosuppressed patients, varicella in neonates, varicella pneumonia, disseminated zoster. It is also given for CNS and ophthalmic zoster in patients with normal immunity. Monitor for renal toxicity. Oral acyclovir, famciclovir, or valacyclovir is used for patients with herpes zoster.

9. Vidarabine and alpha interferon may be used but have high toxicity.

10. Varicella-zoster immunoglobulin has been effective in susceptible patients with household contacts and the immunosuppressed if administered within 96 hours of exposure. It also reduces complications. It is not routinely used with patients with typical chicken pox or shingles.

11. Zoster in association with lymphoma may have especially severe complications and residual damage.

B. Surgical interventions. None.

IV. COMMON NURSING DIAGNOSES, OUTCOMES, AND INTERVENTIONS (see Eczema herpeticum) (see Table 3)

V. HOME CARE CONSIDERATIONS

A. Children with varicella should be separated from newborn infants, during the infectious stage.

B. People who are immunosuppressed should stay away from children who may have had contact with varicella and those with open lesions of zoster.

C. Pregnant women who have not had varicella should also avoid contact with people with infectious stages of varicella and zoster.

Hypersensitivity Reactions: ERYTHEMA MULTIFORME, STEVENS-JOHNSON SYNDROME, and TOXIC EPIDERMAL NECROLYSIS

I. OVERVIEW

Erythema multiforme (EM) is a group of self-limiting, acute inflammatory conditions, which include EM minor, EM major, bullous EM, Stevens-Johnson syndrome (SJS), and toxic epidermal necrolysis (TEN). The rash is characterized as a slightly pruritic erythema, with target and iris lesions, and may also occur as extensive blisters or bullae on any mucosal surface and the skin, resulting in life-threatening epidermal loss. The causes of the reactions may include herpes simplex, mycoplasma, and many other infectious agents, numerous chemicals and drugs, radiation therapy, and disease processes in a delayed immune response in the skin and mucous membranes.

A. Definition.

1. Erythema multiforme is a self-limiting episodic acute inflammatory disorder, lasting less than 4 weeks, characterized by a distinctive rash, mucousal erosions, and epidermal loss of varying degrees of severity.

B. Etiology.

1. Erythema multiforme minor may follow a recurrent infection of HSV type I or II as seen in papules, target, and iris lesions and blisters on the skin.

2. Respiratory infection by *Mycoplasma pneumoniae,* especially in children and young adults, may be followed by erosions on the mucosa and bullous skin lesions diagnosed as SJS or bullous EM.

3. Drugs like sulfonamides (topical and systemic), penicillins, anticonvulsants, and non-steroidal anti-inflammatory agents and many other drugs have been associated with extensive mucosal erosions, large bullae, confluent erythema, and epidermal loss several weeks after initiating therapy. This serious reaction, usually termed SJS or TEN, does not recur unless the drug or a cross-reacting drug is administered again. Other factors may also cause this severe form of EM.

4. For about half the cases, the causative agent may not be identified.

C. Pathophysiology.

1. Skin lesions are dull red to pink papules, slightly pruritic or tender, distributed symmetrically on the extremities.

2. Some lesions will have concentric rings of pink and white, with the center becoming white or gray as fluid accumulates. These "target" and "iris" lesions may not always be present. In EM minor, these lesions resolve spontaneously with minor desquamation and minimal hyper pigmentation.

3. In EM major, the lesions form blisters and bullae, involving the mucous membranes, particularly the mouth, pharynx, and eyes (SJS). More extensive epidermal desquamation and mucosal damage is known as bullous EM or TEN.

4. At the cellular level, an inflammatory infiltrate of lymphocytes is seen around the upper dermal vessels initially, followed by complement (C3) and IgM antibody deposition along the basement membrane.

D. Incidence.

1. EM may occur in 1/10,000 of the population per year but cases requiring hospitalization may be less than 1/100,000.

2. One-third of the EM cases are recurrent.

3. There may be genetically determined characteristics of a person's immune response

Table 4.
Common Nursing Diagnoses, Outcomes, and Interventions: Hypersensitivity Reactions

Nursing Diagnoses	Outcomes	Interventions
Impaired skin integrity.	Skin integrity and barrier function will be restored.	Wet dressings and topical medications. Remove loose necrotic tissue. Apply wet dressings of Burrow's solution, Vaseline gauze, synthetic membranes.
Body image disturbance.	Patient will show a positive body image.	Discuss patient's feelings about disease process and healing.
Ineffective thermoregulation.	Patient's body temperature will remain within normal range and patient will be comfortable.	Adjust room temperature. Light clothing and covers as needed. Warm wet wraps.
Oral mucous membranes, altered.	Patient's oral mucosa will be intact.	Establish oral care regimen.
Altered nutrition, less than body requirements (TEN).	Patient will remain at normal body weight.	Maintain fluid and feedings by nasogastric route.
Pain	Patient will achieve maximum comfort.	Monitor patient's report of pain level and give medications until acceptable level of pain control is achieved. Encourage nonpharmacologic pain control measures: distraction, relaxation, imagery.
Altered vision.	Patient's vision will remain normal.	Apply medications. Monitor condition of lesions, reaction to light.
Impaired gas exchange.	Patient will maintain adequate pulmonary function.	Monitor respiratory status (TEN).
Infection, at risk for.	Patient will remain free from secondary infection.	Monitor for fever, sepsis. Avoid invasive accesses, if possible, or remove as soon as possible. Observe for development of oral candidiasis. Culture skin, mucosa, urine.

which increases the likelihood of developing EM.

E. **Considerations across the life span.**
   1. EM typically affects otherwise healthy young adults but can occur in any age group, in both sexes and all races.

II. ASSESSMENT

A. **History and physical examination.**
   1. Prodromal symptoms of fever, headache, sore throat, cough, and malaise may precede the development of cutaneous lesions.
   2. The mucosal lesions are erythematous maculopapules which have a burning sensation.
   3. If the lesions are bullous, the condition is known as SJS.
   4. Any mucosal surface may be involved, including the lips, pharynx, esophagus, anus, genitalia, respiratory system, and conjunctiva.

5. The bullae rupture and cause erosions which develop pseudomembranous or hemorrhagic, crusted surfaces.
6. The conjunctiva may have a purulent discharge.
7. A diffuse erythema which becomes painful in a few hours will evolve into blisters, bullae, and eroded skin.
8. A positive Nikolsky's sign can be demonstrated when the skin surface separates with minimal friction.
9. If the lesions in the skin and mucosa become confluent, the condition is labeled TEN.
10. Respiratory failure may result from erosion of the pulmonary mucosa.
11. Septicemia and secondary infection are likely complications.
12. Fluid and electrolyte imbalance due to skin desquamation and inability to maintain fluid intake orally will be detected.

13. Visual impairment or blindness may result from scarring in the eye.
14. Renal damage is seen in TEN, by the presence of proteinuria, hematuria, and elevated creatinine.
15. Severe pain is experienced by the patient.
B. Diagnostic tests.
   1. Skin biopsy shows complement C3 and IgM antibodies along the basement membrane.
   2. Complete blood count — leukopenia.
   3. Urinalysis — protein, hematuria.
   4. Serum creatinine: may be elevated.

III. COMMON THERAPEUTIC MODALITIES

A. Medical interventions.
   1. Discontinue medications known to cause SJS or which have been implicated in mild or severe skin desquamation.
   2. Prophylactic acyclovir for EM induced by HSV.
   3. For SJS and TEN, systemic corticosteroid until no new lesions are seen or until healing has started. Extended use may allow infections to progress and other complications to develop.
   4. Antihistamines for pruritus.
   5. Systemic antibiotics to reduce secondary infections by bacteria and fungi.
   6. Oral fluid, as able, using viscous xylocaine for oral lesions and antacids for GI involvement especially if corticosteroids are administered.
   7. Intravenous fluid and maintenance of electrolyte balance.
   8. Ophthalmology consultation.
      a. Saline eye irrigation.
      b. Topical steroids.
      c. Antibiotics.
   9. Topical dressings, wet compresses to exudative lesions.
   10. Observation for hypothermia.
   11. Other management.
      a. Nursing patient in ICU or burn unit.
      b. Porcine or cadaver grafts to denuded skin as soon as possible, to reduce pain, fluid and protein loss, risk of infection, and to assist re-epithelialization in patients with TEN.
      c. Plasmapheresis has been effective in some cases of drug-induced TEN.
      d. Hyperbaric oxygen to enhance skin healing.
      e. Pre-existing disease like diabetes, congestive heart failure must be monitored.
B. Surgical interventions.
   1. Repair of conjunctival scars to improve vision.
   2. Repair of scars and complications caused by extensive disease.

IV. COMMON NURSING DIAGNOSES, OUTCOMES, AND INTERVENTIONS (see Table 4)

V. HOME CARE CONSIDERATIONS

A. In uncomplicated cases, skin heals in 14 days.
B. Hyper/hypopigmentation of lesions.
C. Transient loss of fingernails and toenails (TEN).
D. Hair loss will be temporary.
E. Eye problems will need followup.
F. Avoid precipitating drug, agent, and sunlight.

DRUG ERUPTIONS

I. OVERVIEW

Cutaneous eruptions due to drugs and other agents often resolve uneventfully once the cause of the reaction is removed. However, some reactions can be life-threatening, because of the rapid progression to severe symptoms and respiratory and cardiovascular collapse.
A. Gel and Coombs classification of immune reactions.
   1. Type I (immediate hypersensitivity) mediated by IgE antibody specific for the drug or drug-carrying complex (hapten). Drug and antibody combine with the mast cells to allow release of histamine, leukotrienes, and prostaglandins from the cells. This affects the skin as urticaria and angioedema, which may progress to anaphylaxis. Penicillin and insulin can cause this reaction.
   2. Type II (cytotoxic antibody reactions) result from antigen combining with normal tissue and stimulating formation of antibodies to the tissue affected, which results in damage to the tissue. Thus, quinine and sulfonamides can cause hemolytic anemia or thrombocytopenia.
   3. Type III (immune complex mediated) occurs when the drug combines with IgM or IgG to make a complex which is deposited in blood vessels and organs. Complement fixation occurs, which stimulates further damage as other immune responses are initiated at the sites. This occurs in serum sickness, vasculitis, and urticaria. The reaction may be 7 to 12 days after exposure to antigen and resolve in 3 to 4 days but will develop in a day if the host has been previously sensitized. Penicillins, sulfonamides, and phenytoin are examples of drugs which may stimulate this reaction.
   4. Type IV (delayed hypersensitivity) is associated with topical contact, giving either an irritant dermatitis which is dose related and is found in 70% of contact dermatitis, or allergic contact dermatitis which is not dose related and affects a few who have a genetic basis.

Table 5.
Common Nursing Diagnoses, Outcomes, and Interventions: Drug Eruptions

Nursing Diagnoses	Outcomes	Interventions
At risk for decreased cardiac output related to response to allergen.	Patient's pulse and blood pressure will remain normal.	Monitor pulse and blood pressure. Reduce vasodilatation by controlling environmental and skin temperature.
At risk for altered breathing pattern related to swelling.	Patient's respirations will remain normal.	Observe for swelling of the lips, oropharynx.

B. **Types of cutaneous adverse reactions.**
   1. Immune mediated.
      a. Urticaria/angioedema/anaphylaxis.
      b. Serum sickness.
      c. Purpura secondary to drug-induced thrombocytopenia.
      d. Contact dermatitis (allergic).
   2. Immune-like reactions (cause is non-immune or uncertain).
      a. Erythema multiforme/Stevens-Johnson syndrome.
      b. Morbilliform (measles like).
      c. Toxic epidermal necrolysis.
      d. Anaphylactoid reactions.
      e. Contact dermatitis (irritant).

II. URTICARIA

A. **Definition: urticaria is a pruritic, erythematous eruption of papules and reddish plaques which appear rapidly in response to mast cell stimulation and subsequent histamine release. The reaction may occur within days of contact with the agent or within minutes if the patient has been sensitized by previous contact. It can progress rapidly to angioedema and/or anaphylaxis where the patient becomes unresponsive and cardiovascular collapse ensues.**

B. **Etiology.**
   1. Type I: exposure to drugs in the groups of penicillins, cephalosporins, vaccines, insulin (polypeptide hormones).
   2. Type III: sulphonamides, phenytoin, streptomycin, thiouracil, and many other agents.
   3. Other agents cause urticaria such as food, chemicals, infections, stings, internal diseases, psychogenic factors, and physical factors.

C. **Pathophysiology.**
   1. Acute urticaria results from a type I IgE-mediated reaction, when the drug attached to a protein forms a hapten which combines with a specific antibody. The complex attaches to mast cells which release histamine, prostaglandin. Fluid leaks from capillaries into tissue.
   2. Type III reactions are stimulated by combination of the drug with IgG or IgM antibodies and complement in blood vessels, which produces inflammation of the vessels, surrounding edema, and increased white cells.
   3. Some reactions are direct effects of the drug on the mast cells as seen with radiocontrast media, opiates, bacterial toxins, vancomycin, and others.
   4. Desensitization can be attempted if the patient needs the offending drug, such as insulin or penicillin.
   5. Angioedema is similar to urticaria in origin but involves deeper dermal and subcutaneous tissue, with little pruritus. Areas of loose tissue like eyelids and lips swell in this reaction. A rare condition, hereditary angioedema carries a mortality rate of 30% due to airway obstruction.
   6. A generalized drug eruption most commonly is seen as a maculopapular rash, with numerous pruritic, erythematous macules and papules, which spread to become confluent. Symmetrical distribution over the trunk may progress to cover the whole body, sometimes the hands and feet. The bright red lesions become brownish and dull as they fade, to be followed by a fine dry desquamation.
   7. Erythroderma can be severe if it occurs in patients with pre-existing cardiovascular disease, with excessive shunting of blood to the skin. If generalized confluent erythema develops there is a risk of it progressing to TEN.

D. **Incidence.**
   1. Adverse reactions related to hypersensitivity to drugs and other agents are seen in 2% to 3% of hospitalized patients.
   2. Reactions are more likely to drugs given intramuscularly, intravenously, or orally than by other routes.

3. Many reactions resolve rapidly once the agent is identified and removed.
4. AIDS patients have a higher rate of cutaneous reactions to trimethoprim-sulfamethoxazole.

E. Considerations across the life span.
  1. Any age group is at risk of hypersensitivity reactions to drugs.

III. ASSESSMENT

A. History and physical examination.
  1. History of use of medications known to cause urticarial reactions.
  2. Well-demarcated erythematous, edematous, papules and plaques of various sizes which are pruritic.
  3. Lesions resolve in 24 hours once the agent has been removed.
  4. If the patient response is rapid, respiratory or cardiovascular changes may occur within hours of contact with the agent. Emergency, intensive care may be needed as the patient becomes unresponsive.

B. Diagnostic tests.
  1. Skin biopsy to exclude urticarial vasculitis if lesions persist longer than 24 hours.

IV. COMMON THERAPEUTIC MODALITIES

A. Medical interventions.
  1. Antihistamines.
  2. Topical antipruritics
  3. Bland emollients.
  4. Prednisone if the eruption is severe.
  5. For anaphylaxis:
     a. Subcutaneous epinephrine 0.3 to 0.5 ml 1:1000 should be given every 15 minutes until the patient becomes responsive. Children: 0.01 ml/kg subcutaneously or intramuscularly. Epinephrine can also be given intravenously 1:10,000, slowly.
     b. Cardiac monitoring.
     c. Systemic corticosteroids which will take affect 4 to 6 hours later.
     d. H1 and H2 antihistamines.
     e. Intravenous fluids and vasopressors may be required to maintain blood pressure.
     f. Aminophylline for respiratory symptoms.
  6. For erythroderma:
     a. Monitor fluid balance.
     b. Apply open wet dressings with lukewarm water which may encourage vasoconstriction.
     c. Monitor for hypoalbuminemia and anemia.

B. Surgical interventions.
  1. None.

V. COMMON NURSING DIAGNOSES, OUTCOMES, AND INTERVENTIONS (see Table 5)

VI. HOME CARE CONSIDERATIONS

A. For the patient at risk for an anaphylactic reaction, epinephrine should be made available at all times.
B. The patient should avoid contact with any known allergen.
C. The patient should be aware of signs of an impending reaction and of the need for emergency medical assistance.

EXFOLIATIVE DERMATITIS (Erythroderma)

I. OVERVIEW

Exfoliative dermatitis (ED) is a skin manifestation of other disorders, in which large areas of the body are covered with scaly, erythematous dermatitis.

A. Definition: a scaling, erythematous dermatitis often progressing to desquamation of skin and mucous membranes, usually associated with an underlying disorder.
B. Etiology.
  1. People with pre-existing psoriasis, atopic, or seborrhea dermatitis are at risk of developing ED.
  2. Chemicals which act as toxins or which suppress normal immune processes may be involved in development of ED.
  3. Drug eruptions, scabies infestation, and lymphoma can progress to ED.
C. Pathophysiology.
  1. IgE antibodies have been identified in cases associated with atopic dermatitis.
  2. Desquamation which follows the erythema may affect conjunctiva, mucous membranes of the upper respiratory tract, and result in hair loss.
D. Incidence.
  1. Variable, depending on the predisposing factors.
E. Considerations across the life span.
  1. Infants with atopic dermatitis may develop severe disease.
  2. Children and older adults with pre-existing disease are at risk.

II. ASSESSMENT

A. History and physical examination.
  1. History of atopic dermatitis or psoriasis.
  2. ED may have an acute or gradual onset.
  3. Erythematous scaling plaques and papules develop over much of the body.
  4. Pruritus is severe and excoriations usually visible.
  5. Fever, chills, malaise, fatigue, skin tightness

Table 6.
Common Nursing Diagnoses, Outcomes, and Interventions: Exfoliative Dermatitis

Nursing Diagnoses	Outcomes	Interventions
Impaired skin integrity related to pathologic process and mechanical factors.	Skin is well hydrated and inflammation is reduced.	Cleanse crusted lesions. Apply occlusive dressings. Instruct patient in hygiene and handwashing procedures.
High risk for impaired skin integrity (pruritus) related to inflammatory process.	Pruritus has been relieved.	Apply cool compresses for wet skin and oil compresses for dry skin. Instruct patient in use of antipruritics.
High risk for secondary infection related to skin excoriation.	Patient is free from infection.	Observe for signs of infection on excoriated areas.
Hypothermia related to altered skin integrity.	Patient maintains normal body temperature.	Maintain warm environment (70° F). Prevent drafts. Use layers of clothes and covers. Use light, nonirritating materials.

(edema) are present.

6. People with underlying cardiac problems, respiratory disease, or edema may develop exacerbated disease due to the blood flow being shunted to the skin.

B. Diagnostic tests.
1. Serum IgE — elevated (in severe atopic dermatitis).
2. Skin biopsy — usually inconclusive in atopic dermatitis and psoriasis.
3. Skin prick test — immediate wheal skin test response to common allergens like food.
4. Patch test — may help identify contact allergies and prevent future episodes.

III. COMMON THERAPEUTIC INTERVENTIONS

A. Medical interventions.
1. Topical corticosteroids applied to affected areas under occlusive dressings or wet wraps, to reduce inflammation and pruritus.
2. Sedative antihistamines to alleviate pruritus, anxiety, and allow sleep.
3. Systemic antibiotics for secondary bacterial skin infections.
4. Underlying disease may need to be controlled with systemic corticosteroids.
5. Emollients will soothe the skin and provide a temporary barrier.
6. Ultraviolet light treatment (PUVA or UVB) for widespread disease not responsive to steroids.

B. Surgical interventions.
1. None.

IV. COMMON NURSING DIAGNOSES, OUTCOMES, AND INTERVENTIONS (see Table 6)

V. HOME CARE CONSIDERATIONS

A. Daily soaks in a warm bath for 15 to 20 minutes will hydrate the skin, followed immediately by applying an emollient while the skin is still damp, will reduce dryness and itching.
B. Use of super-fatted soaps.
C. Use of appropriate occlusive topical emollients will reduce xerosis.
D. Medicated topical agents may be prescribed and correct application technique must be demonstrated.
E. Patient must observe skin for signs of infection.
F. External irritants can be reduced by using well-rinsed laundry, loose-fitting clothes, showering after swimming.
G. Use of sunscreens reduces irritation by sun.
H. Maintaining a comfortable environmental temperature reduces blood shunting to the skin.

Bullous Eruptions: PEMPHIGUS

I. OVERVIEW

Pemphigus and pemphigoid encompass a group of bullous diseases, more often seen in middle-aged and older adults, caused by an autoimmune process in the skin and mucous membranes. Flaccid bullae rupture to produce large denuded areas from which protein is lost.

A. Definition: pemphigus is characterized by widespread blister and bulla formation with rupture, and crusting of the resulting erosions,

Table 7.
Common Nursing Diagnoses, Outcomes, and Interventions: Pemphigus

Nursing Diagnoses	Outcome	Interventions
Impaired skin integrity related to skin lesions.	Skin's barrier function is restored.	Provide temporary barrier with topical medications and dressings.
Pain (pruritus) related to skin lesions.	Patient will remain free from pruritus and pain.	Antipruritics as needed for comfort. Cool moist dressings and medicated baths.
Risk for infection related to skin lesions.	Patient will be free from infection.	Observe for signs of infection.
Altered nutrition, less than body requirements.	Patient's nutritional status has been maintained or improved.	Offer mouthwashes before eating. Maintain good oral hygiene. Offer bland food, non-acidic liquids with protein, milkshakes.

due to autoimmune reactions to components in the epidermis.
B. Etiology.
1. Until the use of corticosteroids and other immunosuppressive agents, the condition was often fatal.
2. Some races and ethnic groups may have a genetic predisposition to develop this disease.
C. Pathophysiology.
1. Pemphigus vulgaris plaques and pemphigus vegetans blisters form just above the level of the stratum basalis causing acantholysis or breakdown of the keratinocytes.
2. Inflammatory infiltrate is absent.
3. IgG auto antibodies are bound to the epidermal cell membranes, with tissue-bound complement C3.
4. In pemphigus foliaceous the epidermal reaction occurs just below the level of the stratum granulosum, giving rise to more shallow lesions.
5. Pemphigus erythematosus is similar in reaction to pemphigus foliaceous except for a band-like pattern also seen in lupus patients.
D. Incidence.
1. Higher incidence in South America, especially Brazil.
E. Considerations across the life span.
1. Adults older than the 4th decade are more prone to develop pemphigus.
2. Occasionally children may contract the disease.

II. ASSESSMENT

A. History and physical examination.
1. Extensive generalized blistering often starts on the head, trunk, oral mucous membranes, and intertriginous areas.
2. Nikolsky's sign is positive.
3. The skin is fragile and forms flaccid, 1 cm or

greater blisters, which rupture easily, releasing a malodorous protein fluid.
4. Erosions form where the blisters burst, crust over and heal, often with hyperpigmentation.
5. Oral lesions can be extensive and interfere with food and fluid intake.
6. Pruritus, burning, and pain are felt at the sites where bullae develop.
7. Sometimes ocular or genito-urinary erosions occur.
8. With widespread damage, there may be significant loss of fluid and protein, also electrolyte imbalance. With prolonged disease, malnutrition and proteinemia can contribute to death.
9. Secondary bacterial infections can also be fatal.
10. Pain and discomfort in the oropharynx and areas of denuded skin.
B. Diagnostic tests.
1. Skin biopsy — intra-epidermal bullae, acantholysis.
2. Tzanck test — scraping of the base of bullae reveals acantholysis.
3. Immunofluorescent microscopic examination for tissue-bound and/or circulating anti-intracellular substance (IgG) antibodies.
4. CBC — progressive anemia, leukocytosis, eosinophilia.
5. Electrolytes — sodium, chloride, and calcium decreases; potassium increases as disease progresses.
6. Serum protein electrolytes — decreased albumin, increased alpha 1 and alpha 2 globins.

III. COMMON THERAPEUTIC MODALITIES

A. Medical interventions.
1. Localized forms of pemphigus are treated with topical or intralesional corticosteriods and wet

Table 8.
Common Nursing Diagnoses, Outcomes, and Interventions: Dermatomyositis

Nursing Diagnoses	Outcomes	Interventions
Impaired mobility related to proximal muscle weakness.	Patient maintains maximum mobility.	Assess joint function, mobility. Plan rest periods, ROM, exercise, ambulation. Bedrest during exacerbation.
Impaired swallowing related to involvement of pharyngeal muscles.	Patient maintains adequate nutrition status with few episodes of aspiration.	Assist with feeding, nutrition supplements. Position patient to avoid aspiration.
Increased risk of respiratory infection.	Patient remains free from respiratory infection.	Monitor respiratory status. Observe for signs of infection.
Increased risk of high cardiac output failure related to diffuse erythema.	Cardiac status is maintained.	Monitor blood pressure, cardiac status during erythrodermic states.
Body image disturbance related to appearance change and decreased mobility.	Patient exhibits adequate coping mechanisms.	Allow patient's expression of concern about effects of disease on body and self-esteem.
Impaired skin integrity.	Skin's barrier function is protected during episodes of skin breakdown.	Assess for erythroderma and open skin lesions.

compresses.

2. High-dose corticosteroids orally or intravenously in severe cases may be required to suppress widespread involvement.
3. Steroid-sparing immunosuppressants such as methotrexate, azathioprine, or cyclophosphamide are used additionally.
4. Antimalarials like chloroquine and sulfones like dapsone have also been used.
5. Plasmapheresis may reduce autoantibody rebound in severe cases.
B. Surgical interventions.
1. None.

IV. COMMON NURSING DIAGNOSES, OUTCOMES, AND INTERVENTIONS (see Table 7)

V. HOME CARE CONSIDERATIONS

A. Wound care for lesions, to promote healing and prevent secondary infections.
B. High-protein nutritional supplement and suggestions on food and fluid intake.
C. If taking immunosuppressive therapy or systemic steroids, information on the medications and followup visits to monitor for GI bleeding, diabetes.

DERMATOMYOSITIS

I. OVERVIEW

Dermatomyositis and polymyositis are inflammatory conditions with skin involvement, which may also be associated with connective tissue disease. Childhood dermatomyositis is a distinct disease in which calcinosis and vasculopathy are more apparent.

A. Definition: dermatomyositis and polymyositis are inflammatory diseases affecting striated muscle. Muscle weakness, pain, and edema are associated with polymyositis, while additionally, erythema of the face (reddish purple on the eyelids) and knuckles, periungual erythema and cuticle fragmentation indicate dermatomyositis. Internal involvement occurs in the cardiac, pulmonary, and gastrointestinal systems.

B. Etiology.
1. The cause is unknown but an association with malignancy (breast and lung) has been identified.
2. Both humoral and cellular immunity may be involved in the disease process.

C. Pathophysiology.
1. Striated muscle tissue of the proximal muscles is abnormal, with an inflammatory reaction and necrosis evident in the biopsy.

2. Muscle enzymes are elevated and the electromyogram is abnormal.
3. Biopsy of skin lesions is not diagnostic and may be similar to lupus erythematosus.

D. Incidence.
1. Women are more often affected than men.
2. Children have a somewhat different disease with calcinosis and vasculopathy in addition to muscle weakness.
3. Acute, subacute, chronic, or cyclic forms of the disease develop, with spontaneous remission in some cases.
4. A 10% mortality rate in children and 10% to 25% in adults especially if the heart and lungs become involved.

E. Considerations across the life span.
1. In children, dermatomyositis has more calcinosis and vasculopathy which progresses over time to ulceration, scarring on the skin, in the gastrointestinal tract, and in the muscles.
2. Children may have more disability from contractures, joint damage, and calcifications.

II. ASSESSMENT

A. History and physical examination.
1. Violaceous eruption on the face, especially on the eyelids, often prior to other symptoms.
2. Edema of the eyelids.
3. Violaceous papular eruption of the neck, upper trunk, and extensor surfaces of the elbows, and knees.
4. Raised flat-topped violaceous papules over knuckles (Gottron's papules).
5. Photosensitivity.
6. Periungual erythema, telangiectasia, and fragmentation of cuticles.
7. Poikiloderma, with atrophy and ulceration.
8. Especially in children, calcification and ulcerative lesions due to vasculopathy.
9. Internal organ involvement.
   a. Proximal muscle weakness and pain.
   b. Cardiomyopathy.
   c. Pulmonary fibrosis.
   d. Esophageal dysmotility.
   e. Vasculopathy of gastrointestinal tract.
   f. Malignancies.

B. Diagnostic tests.
1. Serum creatine phosphokinase, aldolase, SGOT — elevated.
2. Electromyography abnormal.
3. Biopsy — segmental necrosis, atrophy of muscle fibers, lymphocytic infiltrate.
4. Histopathology of skin lesions — non-diagnostic or similar to acute cutaneous lupus erythematosus.

III. COMMON THERAPEUTIC MODALITIES

A. Medical interventions.
1. Systemic steroids used at high doses and tapered very slowly, depending on the recovery rate of muscle strength.
2. Cytotoxic drugs like methotrexate, azathioprine.
3. Physical rest initially and physical therapy later.
4. Sun protection, sunscreens.
5. Antimalarial drugs.
6. Screening for malignancy.

B. Surgical interventions.
1. None.

IV. COMMON NURSING DIAGNOSES, OUTCOMES, AND INTERVENTIONS (see Table 8)

V. HOME CARE CONSIDERATIONS

A. Physical therapy and exercise at home.
B. Patient and caregivers' awareness of signs and symptoms of respiratory infection, breathing difficulties, or cardiac problems.
C. Explain the disease process and possible exacerbation, when to seek help.

Bibliography
White, G., & Cox, N. (2000). *Diseases of the skin: A color atlas & text.* St. Louis: Mosby.
Eisen D., & Lynch D.P. (1998). *The mouth: Diagnosis & treatment.* London: Mosby.
Hawk J.L.M. (1998). Cutaneous photobiology. In R.H. Champion, J.L. Burton, D.A. Durns, S.M. Breathnack (Eds.), *Textbook of dermatology* (6th ed.). Oxford: Blackwell Science.
Jung, M., Kippes W., & Messner G. (1999). Increased risk of bullous pemphigoid in male & very old patients. A population-based study on incidence. *Journal of the American Academy of Dermatology, 41,* 266-8.
Berkow, R. (1992). *The Merck manual of diagnosis and therapy.* Rahway, NJ: Merck & Co.
Hill, M.J. (1994). *Skin disorders.* St. Louis, MO: Mosby-YearBook.
Rasmussen, J.E. (1995). Erythema multiforme, Stevens-Johnson syndrome and toxic epidermal necrolysis. *Dermatology Nursing, 7*(1), 37-43.
Sams, W.M., & Lynch, P.J. (1996). *Principles and practice of dermatology.* New York: Churchill Livingstone.
Sivak, E.D., Higgins, T.L., & Seiver, A., (1995). *The high risk patient: Management of the critically ill.* Media, PA: Williams & Wilkins.

A 46-year-old factory worker comes to the emergency department with a fever of 103° F, bullous lesions on the soles of his feet, on the outer aspects of his arms, and an extensive erythematous maculopapular rash over his face and neck. He has oropharyngeal lesions and conjunctivitis. He is diagnosed with Stevens-Johnson syndrome. In taking his history, he tells you he has taken medications for his heart for 5 years and recently started taking allopurinol for gout.

1. The possible cause for his SJS is:
   a. Bacterial infection.
   b. Viral infection.
   c. Cardiac medications.
   d. Allopurinol.

2. The most urgent nursing diagnosis and interventions will address:
   a. His understanding of the diagnosis.
   b. The need to avoid precipitating factors for SJS.
   c. Protection of his eyes and vision.
   d. Protecting his skin from secondary infection.

3. He complains of pain at the sites of the lesions. You would:
   a. Administer intramuscular analgesic.
   b. Apply warm wet dressings to the painful sites.
   c. Assess his ability to swallow oral analgesic.
   d. Explain pain management techniques like imagery.

4. His oral lesions prevent him from taking adequate food and fluid. You plan to:
   a. Establish an oral care regimen.
   b. Encourage him to swallow fluids only.
   c. Ask his family to bring him his favorite food.
   d. Allow the lesions to heal without intervention since he is on antibiotic.

5. The patient's temperature has been normal for 48 hours but rises rapidly to 101.5° F. He has chills and a cough. He may be developing:
   a. Secondary infection of skin lesions.
   b. Pneumonia, caused by mucosal lesions and secondary infection.
   c. Viral infection.
   d. Septicemia.

6. A 65-year-old female with a history of pemphigus reports increased discomfort and an increase in the number of lesions on her skin. On assessment her oral mucosa has extensive erosions also. She will need teaching about the corticosteroids she has been ordered and also teaching about:
   a. Her need for exercise.
   b. Improvements in her hygiene.
   c. A balanced diet and protein supplements.
   d. The prognosis for this disease.

7. When teaching her about preventing or reducing possible infection, you advise her to:
   a. Follow all the components of the ordered treatment.
   b. Continue with her part-time job at a day-care center.
   c. Continue her exercise routine with the swimming club.
   d. Stay in the sun for a short time each day.

8. A 25-year-old female patient tells you she has developed a very painful rash with blisters on her lower abdomen. On assessment you find erythema, with vesicles in clusters, some pustules and crusted erosions. She has fever and enlarged lymph nodes in her groin. She reports she tested positive for HIV 18 months ago but did not want to have any medical care. She is at risk for:
   a. Cellulitis.
   b. Varicella-zoster.
   c. Eczema herpeticum.
   d. Stevens-Johnson syndrome.

9. Even if the patient had not told you she was HIV positive, to assess the site you would:
   a. Wear gloves because of the moist lesions.
   b. Use skin cleanser as a barrier on your hands.
   c. Avoid touching her clothing and skin.
   d. Wash your hands thoroughly instead of wearing gloves.

10. You advise her that she needs treatment as soon as possible because:
    a. The infection spreads by the airborne route.
    b. It may cause permanent damage to her skin.
    c. The virus can be cured with acyclovir.
    d. She is at risk of herpes infection spreading all over her body due to her HIV status.

Answers to Study Questions

1.	d	5.	b	9.	a
2.	c	6.	c	10.	d
3.	b	7.	a		
4.	a	8.	c		

Dermatologic Nursing Essentials: A Core Curriculum 2nd Edition © DNA 2003

Chapter 21.
Dermatologic Emergencies

Please photocopy this test page and return.

COMPLETE THE FOLLOWING:

Name: _____

Address: _____

City: _____ State: _____ Zip: _____

Preferred telephone: (Home)_____ (Work) _____

State where licensed and license number: _____

CE application fee: DNA member $13.00
                        Nonmember $16.00

POSTTEST INSTRUCTIONS
1. To receive continuing education credit for individual study after reading the article, complete the answer/evaluation form below.
2. Photocopy and send the answer/evaluation form along with a check or money order payable to **Dermatology Nurses' Association** to: **DNA**, East Holly Avenue Box 56, Pitman, NJ 08071-0056.
3. Test returns must be postmarked by December 31, 2008. Upon completion of the answer/evaluation form, a certificate for 3.5 contact hour(s) will be awarded and sent to you.

This chapter was reviewed and formatted for contact hour credit by Marcia J. Hill, MSN, RN, Core Curriculum Editor; and Sally Russell, MN, RN,C, DNA Education Director.

ANSWER FORM

1. Name one new detail (item, issue, or phenomenon) that you learned by completing this activity.

   _____

   _____

   _____

   _____

2. How will you apply the information from this learning activity to your practice?
   a. Patient education.
   b. Staff education.
   c. Improve my patient care.
   d. In my education course work.
   e. Other: Please describe _____

   _____

Evaluation	Strongly disagree				Strongly agree
3. The offering met the stated objectives.					
a. Identify dermatologic disease processes which may progress to become life-threatening, and require emergency or acute care interventions.	1	2	3	4	5
b. Recognize patients who are at risk of severe, acute disease.	1	2	3	4	5
c. Describe therapeutic interventions used to promote healing and prevent complications.	1	2	3	4	5
4. The content was current and relevant.	1	2	3	4	5
5. The content was presented clearly.	1	2	3	4	5
6. The content was covered adequately.	1	2	3	4	5
7. I am more confident of my abilities since completing this material.	1	2	3	4	5

8. The material was (check one) ☐ new, ☐ review for me.

Comments _____

9. Time required to complete reading assignment: _____ minutes

This independent study is provided by the Dermatology Nurses' Association (DNA) for 3.5 contact hours. DNA is accredited as a provider of continuing education in nursing by the American Nurses Credentialing Center's Commission on Accreditation. DNA is approved as a provider of continuing education by the California Board of Registered Nursing Provider #CEP5708.

CHAPTER TWENTY-TWO   22

Psychosocial Effects of Dermatologic Disease and Psychodermatoses

Marcia J. Hill, MSN, RN

OBJECTIVES

At the end of this chapter, the reader will be able to:

- Identify the psychic functions of the skin.
- Describe the psychosocial effects of dermatologic disease.
- Discuss the concept of body image and its relationship to dermatologic disease.
- Explain factors influencing body image.
- Discuss methods to assist the dermatology patient in adapting successfully to body image alterations.
- Describe psychosocial assessment and implementation strategies for patients with dermatologic disease.
- Define psychodermatoses.
- List the disease classifications and treatment of psychodermatoses.
- Discuss the nursing interventions for psychocutaneous disease.

KEY POINTS

- The skin is the physical boundary and psychic organ of contact between the individual and the environment.
- Many patients with dermatologic diseases find themselves physically uncomfortable and psychosocially disadvantaged due to the stigmatism attached to an abnormal skin appearance.
- Skin diseases cause alterations in appearance and thereby affect body image.
- Individuals experiencing alterations in their body image will experience the stages of the grief process.
- Psychodermatoses or psychocutaneous diseases are skin diseases with a psychologic origin.
- Patients presenting with dermatologic symptoms that appear psychogenic in origin must first be thoroughly assessed and evaluated for any underlying systemic or dermatologic disease.

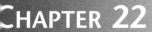

Psychosocial Effects of Dermatologic Disease and Psychodermatoses

Marcia J. Hill, MSN, RN

INTRODUCTION

This chapter is divided into two sections, both dealing with the psychosocial issues of dermatologic disease. The first section discusses the normal or expected psychologic effects of dermatologic disease and how to assist the patient in coping with the skin condition or disease. The second section describes the various diseases that are classified as psychodermatoses — conditions in which diseases of the skin overlap diseases of the mind.

EFFECTS OF DERMATOLOGIC DISEASE

I. PSYCHIC FUNCTIONS OF THE SKIN

A. The skin is the physical boundary and psychic organ of contact between the individual and the environment.
  1. Ego formation of the individual with skin disease is influenced by the visual effect leading to the formation of abnormal interpersonal relationships.
  2. Rejection by others frequently occurs.
  3. Interpretation of outside stimuli is adversely affected.
  4. Expression of enjoyment from outside stimulation is adversely affected.
    a. Sensory pleasure is adversely affected.

B. The skin affects the psyche.
  1. The epidermis has the same embryologic origin as the nervous system.
  2. The skin acts as a sense organ for touch, cold, heat, pain, and an erogenous organ.
  3. The skin acts as the shelter which protects us.
  4. The skin separates us from the outside world.
    a. The skin may be a source of anxiety.
    b. Early cutaneous tactile experience has a long-reaching effect on growth, physical and emotional development.

C. The psyche affects the skin.
  1. The skin acts as a facade which displays us.
  2. The skin involuntarily communicates to others some of our emotional states.
  3. The skin acts as an intermediary between the individual's inner-self and the outside world.
  4. The skin is an organ of emotional expression.
  5. The skin conveys temperature differences, pain, affection, tenderness, and sexual stimulation.

D. The skin is one of the most important psychosomatic organs.
  1. The impression an individual makes depends on the skin's condition.

  2. Unsightly skin provokes negative feelings in the observer.
  3. Unsightly skin triggers feelings of revulsion, shame, and inferiority.

II. PSYCHOSOCIAL EFFECTS OF DERMATOLOGIC DISEASE

A. Patients who present with symptoms of dermatologic conditions and diseases, and those undergoing dermatologic treatments often experience uncomfortable and unsightly skin. While these conditions present physical problems, they elicit emotional reactions as well.

B. Treatment for dermatologic diseases often requires time-consuming, expensive, and unpleasant topical medications. With many conditions, treatment and healing are slow. With some, the disease is intractable.

C. Significant others and the public most often do not understand skin diseases and are repulsed at the site of their appearance. They fear the diseases are contagious and communicate their thoughts and feelings, both verbally and nonverbally, to the individuals with the diseases. The public also interprets skin lesions as a sign of poor personal hygiene.

D. Many patients with dermatologic diseases find themselves physically uncomfortable and psychosocially disadvantaged due to the stigmatism attached to an abnormal skin appearance. They experience humiliation, self-disgust, and anxiety. Some fear going out in public and socially isolate themselves. The effects of skin disease can lead to difficulties in coping with an altered body image and diminished self-esteem.

III. BODY IMAGE

A. Given the visibility of the skin and the potential effects of skin disease on individuals and their psychologic functioning, it is important for the dermatology nurse to understand the concept of body image and how changes in physical appearance affect it.

B. Body image.
  1. The mental picture of how individuals view their bodies.
  2. Includes a perception of how the body looks and the feelings, attitudes, and emotions toward it.
    a. Is the means by which individuals interact with the environment.

b. If cutaneous perceptions from the environment are not favorable, body image may be unstable or fragmented which may lead to an individual becoming obsessional about skin appearance; this made lead to misperceptions of delusional proportion.

c. Fragmentation and blurring of boundaries may result in factitious disease in order for the individual to maintain dependency.

C. **Self-image is a perspective of self that includes:**
1. Role.
2. Status.
3. Goals.
4. Value systems.
5. Strengths and weaknesses.

D. **Self-concept consists of emotional expression of self-perception and persona.**

E. **Self-esteem is an evaluation of self, positive or negative, and includes personal, social, and family characteristics.**

F. **Body boundary is an understanding of the partition that distinguishes an individual's body boundary; indicates the safety the person feels in the world.**

IV. CONCEPTS IN BODY IMAGE

A. **Development of body image begins in infancy and continues through all phases of the life cycle.**
1. Children develop their body image and self-esteem by the actions of their primary caregiver. Warm, nurturing caregivers reinforce positive behaviors, help the children feel loved, and contribute to children feeling good about themselves. This creates a basis for a positive self-esteem and body image.
2. The adolescent body image is influenced by the surge of hormones and is in a constant state of change.

B. **Body image is a dynamic state of change, depending on the individual's life experiences and feedback from others.**

C. **Body image is a part of self-concept. Its importance varies with the values and emotions invested in it.**

D. **Human interaction begins and ends with the appearance and disappearance of the person's body or its parts. The body is the vehicle for psychologic interaction, both verbal and nonverbal.**

E. **Body image delineates the body's boundaries.**
1. Establishes where the body begins and ends.
2. Determines one's own space; intruding on this buffer zone creates discomfort.

F. **The face is the focal point for body image.**
1. It is the center for vision, hearing, and speech.
2. Facial appearance often leads others to

conclusions about a person's intelligence or personality.
3. Alterations in the face or its functions can significantly influence a person's psychologic equilibrium.
4. When people look "different," the world reacts to them differently. The affected individuals find coping with others' reactions difficult because they feel essentially the same as before the changes in their appearance.

V. INFLUENCES ON BODY IMAGE

A. **Developmental.**
1. Developmental tasks must be completed before an individual can move to the next task.
2. Normal growth and development may be influenced by physical appearance.
3. Social stereotypes may interfere with an individual's development (for example, individuals with skin disease are "dirty").

B. **Sociocultural.**
1. Individuals with dermatologic disease may experience difficulty coping with body image changes due to a deviation from present day accepted societal norms of perfect skin.
   a. Leads to anxiety and depression due to their perception of disfigurement.
2. Physical fitness and a suitable body appearance are valued.
3. Fashion trends emphasize greater body exposure.
4. Advertising reinforces fashion climate.
5. Stereotypical responses to disfigurement can adversely affect a person's mental health and potential for success in life.

C. **Intrapersonal.**
1. Changing health status.
2. Intelligence, social status, profession.

D. **Interpersonal.**
1. Opinions and reactions of significant others, both verbal and nonverbal, are often incorporated into an individual's concept of body image.
2. An illness may benefit the person as the overindulgent focus of the family.
3. The family dynamics of an individual with chronic skin disease may play a part in the course of a disease.
   a. The family unit may be or may become dysfunctional.
4. An individual's appearance will influence others' responses to him/her. These responses influence how the individual feels about himself/herself.
5. Sexual function and sexuality may also be considered.

E. **Other.**
1. The use of covering, clothing, wigs, and

makeup are incorporated into body image.
2. Pain, chronic or acute, affects the body image.
3. Drugs may influence body image through altered sensory input (for example, local anesthesia, sedation).

VI. BODY IMAGE ALTERATIONS

A. Skin diseases cause alterations in appearance and thereby affect body image. Examples include the following.
   1. Abnormal skin texture such as xerosis and psoriasis.
   2. Abnormal odor such as hidradenitis suppurativa and pemphigus vegetans.
   3. Disfiguring lesions such as acne vulgaris and vitiligo.
   4. Abnormal nails such as paronychia and tinea unguium.
   5. Abnormal hair such as alopecia areata and alopecia universalis.
   6. Physical limitations and abnormal appearance such as psoriatic arthritis.

VII. ADAPTATIONS TO BODY IMAGE ALTERATIONS

A. Adaptation to changes in the physical body is a complicated process that occurs over time. Adaptation depends on several factors.
   1. The nature of the change and how the individual perceives it.
   2. The importance of the body area affected.
   3. The individual's coping behaviors.
   4. The response of others to the body changes.
   5. The support available.
B. Individuals experiencing alterations in their body image will experience the stages of the grief process (shock, denial, anger, bargaining, depression, acceptance).
C. The individual's ability to look at, touch, and care for the affected body area is a positive step in the adaptation process. Involving supportive significant others can also promote a positive adaptation.
D. The patient's attitude toward his/her body image changes is affected significantly by the reactions of significant others. Nurses and other health care providers are often included among those significant others, especially during the treatment phase. Patients are sensitive to the nurse's feelings and attitudes as evidenced by the way the nurse touches the patient and handles the affected body area, and the willingness to listen and discuss the patient's feelings and concerns.
E. Body image distortion.
   1. The discrepancy between the actual physical body and the way the person views it.
   2. A degree of distortion is normal as everyone

experiences it to some extent.
   3. Body changes, even those that are strongly desired, may be followed by a lengthy adjustment period. Patients may worry about their mental state during this adjustment period.
F. Body image disturbance.
   1. Occurs when the individual has difficulty accepting body changes and adapting to them.
   2. This is an actual state of crisis in which normal patterns of responses and coping mechanisms are inadequate. Extra resources from within the patient, significant others, and the health care team are necessary.
   3. The degree of anxiety interferes with the person's physical and/or psychologic functioning.
G. Body image reintegration.
   1. During the reintegration period, patients begin to reorganize their psychologic defenses and incorporate the changed physical appearance into their body image.
   2. Incorporating a change in appearance into the body image takes time; in some, it may take 6 weeks to 6 months.
   3. Some patients may never accept their changes in appearance. They may resort to other health care providers, other treatment methodologies, or psychiatric intervention.

VIII. COMMON NURSING DIAGNOSES, OUTCOMES, AND INTERVENTIONS (see Table 1)

PSYCHODERMATOSES

I. DEFINITION AND BACKGROUND

A. Psychodermatoses or psychocutaneous diseases are defined as skin diseases that are psychologic in origin.
B. Several factors precipitate psychodermatologic diseases.
   1. Stress.
   2. Impact of mood and anxiety disorders.
   3. Influence, importance, and presence/absence of social support.
   4. Role of specific psychologic or personality disorders such as hostility, low self-esteem, perfectionism.
C. Patients presenting with dermatologic symptoms that appear psychogenic in origin must first be thoroughly assessed and evaluated for any underlying systemic or dermatologic disease. A careful history can be very helpful in determining psychologic wellness or disease.

Table 1.
Nursing Diagnoses, Outcomes, and Interventions
Psychosocial Effects of Dermatologic Disease

Nursing Diagnoses	Outcomes	Interventions
Alteration in body image related to actual and and perceived change in appearance.	Patient will progress toward a positive integration of physical changes into his/her body image.	**Assessment:** A psychosocial assessment is important to understand the patients' ability to cope successfully with the effects of the disease and function socially. Listed below are four broad areas for psychosocial evaluation. In each category, several questions are identified which can be used to explore the effects of the disease process on patients. 1. Assess their perception of the disease. • What do they know about the disease? • How do they feel it affects their appearance? • How do they feel it affects the texture of their skin? • How do they feel it affects their personal odor? 2. Assess the psychosocial effect of the disease process on patients. • How is the disease process affecting their daily lives? • Is the disease process affecting their lifestyle? • Are they anxious or depressed? • Do they cry easily? • Can they do the things they want to do? • Can they manage life's daily problems? • Do they seek assistance from others? • Do they have a positive focus? • Do they obtain and follow through with treatments as recommended? 3. Assess the "family unit." • Are they supportive of the individual? • Do they have a positive focus? • Are there stressors in the relationships? • What do they know about the disease? • What does it mean to them? 4. Assess patients' ability to function in society. • How is it affecting their relationships with others? • Have they ever worked and, if so, are they able to continue working? • Have they developed effective coping mechanisms? **Implementation:** Individuals with dermatologic diseases need assistance in coping with the physical appearance of their disease and adapting to an altered body image. The dermatology nurse can provide the following interventions: • Establish a trusting nurse/patient relationship. • Explain to the patient and significant other what to expect with the disease and its treatment. Discuss routines and procedures. Allow opportunities to address questions and concerns. • Demonstrate a positive and nonjudgmental attitude. • Listen actively and be aware of nonverbal messages. • Provide consistent emotional support in a nonthreatening and supportive manner. • Honestly discuss treatment progress, reinforce behaviors that contribute to healing, and focus on the progress that has been made toward the desired outcome. • Show sensitivity to the patient's experience and be aware of any specific needs. • Assist the individual in understanding his/her feelings and reactions to altered body image. Explain the stages of the grief process and reinforce that these stages are a normal part of coping and are temporary. Empathize with the individual's feelings in a positive and accepting manner. • Reinforce positive coping behaviors and assist in changing maladaptive responses by providing coping suggestions and mobilizing support systems.

Table 1. (continued)
Nursing Diagnoses, Outcomes, and Interventions
Psychosocial Effects of Dermatologic Disease

		Interventions
		• Encourage the individual to look at, touch, and care for the affected body area. Involve supportive significant others. • Explore with the patient how others are reacting to his/her skin condition and how the patient is responding to others. Provide reinforcement and helpful suggestions. • Assist patients in coping with temporary distortions in appearance due to the effects of treatment (for example, redness, dryness, edema). • With a child, encourage the normal growth and development skills consistent with age. • Provide ways of enhancing appearance such as cleanliness and cosmetics. • Assist significant others in understanding the disease, treatment, and reactions to altered changes in body image. Provide support and assist significant others in developing strategies to help the patient with his/her care and in psychologically coping with the disease. • Emphasize that the distortions from treatment (redness, dryness, edema) are temporary and a normal part of treatment and healing. • Observe significant others' reactions to the patient, the diseased area, and treatment modalities. Encourage expression of feelings, questions, and concerns. • Refer to an appropriate support group or other health care professional as indicated.

II. DISEASE CLASSIFICATIONS

A. **Psychiatric disorders expressed in the skin.**
   1. Dermatoses primarily emotional in origin.
      a. Hallucinations — auditory, visual, olfactory, or tactile (chronic cutaneous dysesthesia syndrome).
      b. Delusions and hallucinations — if consistent in content and persistent are pathognomonic of psychosis.
         (1) Delusional parasitosis — Infestation by bugs, mites, or worms; a false perception of disordered cutaneous structure or function (dysmorphic delusion).
         (2) Evaluation and treatment are uniform regardless of ideational content.
   2. Factitious syndromes.
      a. Dermatitis artefacta, factitious dermatitis (lesions of the skin that are self-inflicted).
      b. Cutaneous compulsions — neurotic excoriations, trichotillomania.
      c. Malingering — lesions created for secondary gain.
      d. Cutaneous hypochondriasis — dysmorphophobia.
      e. Vulvodynia and the perineal syndrome.
      f. Psychogenic purpura.
   3. Dermatoses aggravated or perpetuated by self-inflicted trauma.
      a. Lichen simplex.
      b. Acne excoriee.
      c. Prurigo.
      d. Auto-erythrocyte sensitization.
   4. Dermatoses due to accentuated physiological responses.
      a. Hyperhidrosis.
      b. Blushing.
   5. Phobic states.
      a. Syphilophobia.
      b. Erythrophobia.
      c. Acarophobia, etc.
   6. Dermatoses in which emotional precipitating or perpetuating factors may be important.
      a. Vesicular eczema of palms and soles.
      b. Atopic dermatitis in the adult.
      c. Seborrheic dermatitis.

B. **Dermatologic disorders with a psychophysiologic component.**
   1. Psychogenic pruritus.
   2. Chronic urticaria.
   3. Psychogenic purpura syndromes.
   4. Alopecia areata.
   5. Telogen effluvium.
   6. Typical pain syndromes.
   7. Chronic inflammatory dermatoses.

C. Somatopsychic reactions.
D. Other factors.
1. Age, sex, life experiences, and social circumstances.
2. Psychologic source.
3. Environmental catalysts such as stress.

III. ETIOLOGY/CLINICAL PRESENTATION

A. Dysmorphic delusions and hallucinations.
1. Etiology.
   a. Phenomenologically resemble delusions of parasitosis.
   b. Share ideational content.
   c. Obsessional worry about abnormal cutaneous structure or function.
B. Delusions of parasitosis (Ekbom's disease).
1. Etiology.
   a. Pruritus or paresthesias from environmental or somatic sources (senile xerosis, static electricity, systemic disease, previously treated infestation).
   b. Social isolation, visual or auditory impairment, and recent psychosocial stress may be contributory factors.
2. Clinical presentation.
   a. Anxiety and profound preoccupation with delusional belief.
   b. Difficulty engaging patients; has a obsessively recount in minutest detail of the morphology, life cycle, and idiosyncratic habits of their personal personalities along with all the "treatments" they have done to rid themselves of the parasites.
   c. Patients bring "specimens" (usually pieces of lint, debris, parts of insects) to prove the existence of the parasites.
   d. Paranoid rage may be cleverly controlled.
   e. Cutaneous lesions — excoriations, scratch papules, or gouges may or may not be present; irritant dermatitis may predominate due to use of caustics, abrasives, or insecticides to get rid of the parasites.
C. Factitious syndromes.
1. Etiology.
   a. Part of general spectrum of factitious disease.
   b. Personality disorders in adults characterized by infantile, dependent, manipulative behavior and poor impulse control.
   c. In childhood, the mother-child relationship is dysfunctional to varying degrees, may include physical or emotional abuse.
2. Clinical presentation.
   a. Single or multiple, bilateral or symmetrical, or within easy reach of the dominant hand; self-mutilations.

   b. Morphology is bizarre — often angulated or geometric with surface necrosis or linear streaks that do not resemble any other dermatosis.
   c. Patients give a "hollow history."
   d. Denial and noncompliance are parts of the syndrome.
   e. Depression is common.
   f. Ritualized picking.
D. Body dysmorphic disorder (obsessional concerns).
1. Etiology.
   a. Affects both body image and self-esteem.
   b. There is a suggestive relationship to obsessive-compulsive disorder and mood disorder.
   c. Characteristic of dysfunctional family constellation.
2. Clinical presentation.
   a. Spectrum of severity but clinical picture consistent.
   b. Patient obsessed with perceived abnormality — constantly checking appearance; may engage in excessive grooming.
   c. Suffering is intense; patient's life is disrupted; shame is common; social phobia present; relationships impaired; occupational performance impaired.
   d. Suicidal ideation and completed suicides.
E. Psychiatric aspects of dermatologic disease (pruritus, chronic urticaria, psychogenic purpura syndromes, alopecia areata, telogen effluvium, atypical pain syndromes, chronic inflammatory skin disease).
1. Etiology.
   a. Stress.
   b. Depression.
2. Clinical presentation.
   a. Severe pruritus either generalized or localized.
   b. May trigger urticaria.
   c. Clinical presentation of psychogenic purpura remarkably consistent; severe pain, malaise, chills, nausea, and vomiting followed by dysthesia.
F. Somatopsychic effect — affects the sufferer emotionally, socially, and occupationally.

IV. DIFFERENTIAL DIAGNOSES

A. True parasitic infestation.
B. Somatic disease.
1. Toxic psychosis (alcohol, amphetamines, cocaine).
2. Drugs (glucocorticoids, methylphenidate).
3. Organic brain syndromes.
4. Renal disease.

5. Diabetes.
6. Hepatic disease.
7. Lymphoma.
8. Pellagra.
9. Vitamin B12 deficiency.
10. Folate deficiency.
C. **Obsessional fears.**
D. **True delusional belief.**
   1. Monosymptomatic hypochondriacal psychosis.
   2. Paranoid schizophrenia.
   3. Bipolar affective disorder.
   4. Major depressive disorder.
   5. Induced psychosis.

V. TREATMENT

A. **Actual systemic or dermatologic disease must first be ruled out. Often these patients have been seen previously by more than one practitioner. They have been treated conventionally for various diseases with no response. After ruling out disease, a diagnosis and treatment plan for psychodermatoses can be developed.**

B. **Treatment takes skill and patience. Time must be taken to establish a positive and trusting relationship.**

C. **Initial treatment begins with the appropriate medication to treat the symptoms. Medications may include tricyclic antidepressants, MAO inhibitors, and MAO inhibitors in combination with neuroleptics. There are varying degrees of success reported with these drugs.**

D. **Psychiatric referral, although difficult to accomplish due to rejection by the patient, is the preferred method of treatment especially in cases which do not respond to medication.**

IV. COMMON NURSING DIAGNOSES, OUTCOMES, AND INTERVENTIONS (see Table 1)

Bibliography
Arndt, K.A., et al. (1997). *Primary care dermatology.* Philadelphia: W.B. Saunders Co.
Arndt, K.A., et al. (1996). *Cutaneous medicine and surgery — an integrated program in dermatology.* Philadelphia: W.B. Saunders Co.
Brahler, E. (Ed.). (1988). *Body experience — the subjective dimension of psyche and soma* (pp. 62-73). New York: Springer-Verlag.
Cotterill, J.A. (1989, November). Psychiatry and the skin. *British Journal of Hospital Medicine, 42,* 401-404.
De Korte, J., et al. (1986). *Family dynamics in psychodermatology.* Proceedings of the 15th European Conference on psychosomatic research (pp. 287-289).
Eller, J. (1974). Skin disorders and psyche. *Cutis, 13,* 395-416.
Gieler, U. (1988). The skin as mirror of the soul. In E. Brahler (Ed.), *Body experience — the subjective dimension of psyche and soma.* New York: Springer-Verlag.
Gould, W.M., & Gragg, T.M. (1976). Delusions of parasitosis: An approach to the problem. *Archives in Dermatology, 112,*669.

Hardy, G.E. (1983). Body image: The psyche and the skin. *Seminars in Dermatology, 2*(3), 207- 211.
Jobling, R.G. (1976). Psoriasis — a preliminary questionnaire study of sufferer's subjective experience. *Clinical and experimental dermatology, 1,* pp. 233-236.
Koblenzer, C.S. (1999). Psychological aspects of skin disease. In T.B. Fitzpatrick, et al. (Eds.), *Dermatology in general medicine.* New York: McGraw-Hill.
Koblenzer, C.S. (1994). Managing the "difficult" patient in the dermatology office. *Dermatology Nursing, 6*(3), 203-206, 220.
Koblenzer, C.S. (1987). *Psychocutaneous disease.* Orlando: Grune & Stratton.
Koblenzer, C.S. (1983, June). Psychosomatic concepts in dermatology. *Archives of Dermatology, 119,* 501-512.
Musaph, H. (1977). Skin, sex, and touch. In J. Money, & H. Musaph, H. (Eds.), *The handbook of sexology* (pp. 1157-1165).
Olbricht, S., Bigby, M.E., & Arndt, K.A. (1992). *Manual of clinical problems in dermatology.* Boston/London/Toronto: Little, Brown and Co.
Rankin, M., & Mayers, P. (1996). Psychosocial care of the plastic surgical patient. In T. Goodman (Ed.), *Core curriculum for plastic and reconstructive surgical nursing* (pp. 81-95). Pitman, NJ: ASPRSN.
Rook, R., Wilkinson, D.S., Ebling, F.J.G., Champion, R.H., & Burton, J.L. (Eds.). (1986). *Textbook of dermatology* (4th ed). Oxford, London: Blackwell Scientific Publications.
Sands, G.E. (1996). Three monosymptomatic hypochondriacal syndromes in dermatology. *Dermatology Nursing, 8*(6), 420-425.
Shuster, S., et al. (1975). The effects of skin disease on self image. *British Jouranl of Dermatology,* 18-19.
Sneddon, J. (1983). Patients who do not want to get better. *Seminars in Dermatology, 2*(3), 183-187.
Updike, J. (1985, September 2). At war with my skin. *The New Yorker,* 39-57.
Updike, J. (1976, July 19). From the journal of a leper. *The New Yorker,* 28-33.
Wittkower, E. (1952). Skin and psyche. *The Urologic and Cutaneous Review, 56,* 95-98.

1. The epidermis has the same embryologic origin as which of the following systems?
   a. Cardiovascular.
   b. Nervous.
   c. Pulmonary.
   d. Gastrointestinal.

2. Which of the following is one of the most important psychosomatic organs?
   a. Heart.
   b. Brain.
   c. Lungs.
   d. Skin.

3. Jesse, a 13-year-old male, presents in the dermatology office for evaluation of an obvious skin problem. His mother reports difficulties in school, difficulties making friends, and that he is generally rebellious and uncooperative. Jesse is exhibiting:
   a. Typical teenage behavior.
   b. Schizophrenic behavior.
   c. Emotional reaction to a dermatologic condition.
   d. Neurotic reaction to a dermatologic condition.

4. Dermatologic conditions often heal:
   a. Readily and easily.
   b. Slowly with careful treatment.
   c. Rapidly with the correct treatment.
   d. Completely without relapse.

5. The public often interprets skin lesions as a sign of which of the following?
   a. Poor personal hygiene.
   b. Good personal hygiene.
   c. A neurotic condition.
   d. A psychotic condition.

6. Body image is defined as how individuals:
   a. View bodies of others.
   b. View their own bodies.
   c. Display their bodies in pictures.
   d. Present their bodies to the public.

7. The development of body image begins during which phase of the life cycle?
   a. Infancy.
   b. Toddlerhood.
   c. Puberty.
   d. Adulthood.

8. Individuals experiencing alterations in their body image will experience stages of which of the following processes?
   a. Development.
   b. Grief.
   c. Growth.
   d. Maturation.

9. Often persons with dermatologic conditions experience which body image alteration?
   a. Recognition.
   b. Psychosis.
   c. Neurosis.
   d. Distortion.

10. Psychodermatoses are conditions that primarily have which of the following origins?
    a. Physiologic.
    b. Sociologic.
    c. Psychologic.
    d. Biologic.

Answers to Study Questions

1.	b	5.	a	9.	d
2.	d	6.	b	10.	c
3.	c	7.	a		
4.	b	8.	b		

CE Answer/Evaluation Form

Chapter 22.
Psychosocial Effects of Dermatologic Disease and Psychodermatoses

Please photocopy this test page and return.

COMPLETE THE FOLLOWING:

Name: _____

Address: _____

City: _____ State: _____ Zip: _____

Preferred telephone: (Home)_____ (Work) _____

State where licensed and license number: _____

CE application fee: DNA member $7.00
                       Nonmember $10.00

POSTTEST INSTRUCTIONS
1. To receive continuing education credit for individual study after reading the article, complete the answer/evaluation form below.
2. Photocopy and send the answer/evaluation form along with a check or money order payable to **Dermatology Nurses' Association** to: **DNA**, East Holly Avenue Box 56, Pitman, NJ 08071-0056.
3. Test returns must be postmarked by December 31, 2008. Upon completion of the answer/evaluation form, a certificate for 1.4 contact hour(s) will be awarded and sent to you.

This chapter was reviewed and formatted for contact hour credit by Marcia J. Hill, MSN, RN, Core Curriculum Editor; and Sally Russell, MN, RN,C, DNA Education Director.

ANSWER FORM

1. Name one new detail (item, issue, or phenomenon) that you learned by completing this activity.

   _____

   _____

   _____

   _____

2. How will you apply the information from this learning activity to your practice?

   a. Patient education.
   b. Staff education.
   c. Improve my patient care.
   d. In my education course work.
   e. Other: Please describe _____

   _____

Evaluation

	Strongly disagree				Strongly agree
3. The offering met the stated objectives.					
a. Identify the psychic functions of the skin.	1	2	3	4	5
b. Describe the psychosocial effects of dermatologic disease.	1	2	3	4	5
c. Discuss the concept of body image and its relationship to dermatologic disease.	1	2	3	4	5
d. Explain factors influencing body image.	1	2	3	4	5
e. Discuss methods to assist the dermatology patient in adapting successfully to body image alterations.	1	2	3	4	5
f. Describe psychosocial assessment and implementation strategies for patients with dermatologic disease.	1	2	3	4	5
g. Define psychodermatoses.	1	2	3	4	5
h. List the disease classifications and treatment of psychodermatoses.	1	2	3	4	5
i. Discuss the nursing interventions for psychocutaneous disease.	1	2	3	4	5
4. The content was current and relevant.	1	2	3	4	5
5. The content was presented clearly.	1	2	3	4	5
6. The content was covered adequately.	1	2	3	4	5
7. I am more confident of my abilities since completing this material.	1	2	3	4	5

8. The material was (check one) ☐ new, ☐ review for me.

Comments _____

9. Time required to complete reading assignment: _____ minutes

This independent study is provided by the Dermatology Nurses' Association (DNA) for 1.4 contact hours. DNA is accredited as a provider of continuing education in nursing by the American Nurses Credentialing Center's Commission on Accreditation. DNA is approved as a provider of continuing education by the California Board of Registered Nursing Provider #CEP5708.

Regulatory Guidelines

Maryann Forgach, BSN, RN

OBJECTIVES

At the end of this chapter, the reader will be able to:

- Identify major federal agencies responsible for regulatory issues that affect both the patient and the health care worker.
- Identify agencies used for obtaining appropriate facility accreditation.
- Define OSHA regulations pertinent to bloodborne pathogens.
- Describe specific regulatory issues and be able to locate resources for additional information.

KEY POINTS

- Surveillance, prevention, and control of hazards provides for a safe environment.
- Both patients and workers are protected by government standards.
- Federal agencies make and enforce laws that influence both the delivery and receipt of health care.
- Agencies providing accreditation inspect facilities for compliance to federal law.

Regulatory Guidelines

Maryann Forgach, BSN, RN

I. OVERVIEW

A regulation is defined as a law, rule, or other order prescribed by authority, especially to regulate conduct. There are numerous issues of conduct within the hospital and health care industry that pertain to both the caregiver and those receiving their care. This chapter will present an overview of some of the more frequently encountered regulations and supporting guidelines that are relevant to dermatology. Included are issues related to bloodborne pathogens and biological hazards, materials handling, lazer hazards, and clinical laboratories. There are many other important issues that are *not* included due to the broad scope of this topic. These issues include, but are *not* limited to: hazards of sterilization, X-ray hazards, drug exposures, ergonomic hazards from lifting and repetitive tasks, chemical exposure, mechanical maintenance, medical equipment maintenance, laundry, etc.

II. FEDERAL AGENCIES

There are two primary federal agencies that establish pertinent regulations and guidelines for protecting health and safety. The U.S. Department of Labor, whose focus is employee safety, and the U.S. Department of Health and Human Resources, whose focus is the health and safety of everyone they serve (see Table 1).

III. ACCREDITATION AGENCIES

Accreditation by an agency approved by The Centers for Medicare and Medicaid (CMS) (formerly HCFA) assures that a facility has been inspected to meet required standards and that it uses appropriate quality control and quality assurance procedures to benefit the patients it serves. Examples of two approved, independent, accreditation agencies are JCAHO (Joint Commission for the Accreditation of Health Organizations) and CAP (College of American Pathologists) (see Table 2).

IV. OSHA STANDARD 29CFR 1910.1030 BLOODBORNE PATHOGENS

A. Selective definitions.
1. Bloodborne pathogen — pathologic microorganisms that are present in human blood and can cause disease in humans. These pathogens include, but are not limited to, hepatitis B virus (HBV) and human immunodeficiency virus (HIV).
2. Clinical laboratory – means a workplace where diagnostic or other screening procedures are performed on blood or other potentially infectious materials.
3. Blood — human blood, human blood components, and products made from human blood.
4. Contaminated — the presence or the reasonably anticipated presence of blood or other potentially infectious materials on an item or surface.
5. Contaminated laundry — laundry which has been soiled with blood or other potentially infectious materials or may contain sharps.
6. Contaminated sharps — any contaminated object that can penetrate the skin including, but not limited to, needles, scalpels, broken glass.
7. Decontamination — the use of physical or chemical means to remove, inactivate, or destroy bloodborne pathogens on a surface or item to the point where they are no longer capable of transmitting infectious particles and the surface or item is rendered safe for handling, use, or disposal.
8. Engineering controls — means controls (for example, sharps disposal containers, self-sheathing needles, safer medical devices, such as sharps with engineered sharps injury protections and needleless systems) that isolate or remove the bloodborne pathogens from the workplace.
9. Exposure incident — a specific eye, mouth, other mucous membrane, non-intact skin, or parenteral contact with blood or other potentially infectious materials that results from the performance of an employee's duties.
10. Handwashing facilities — a facility providing an adequate supply of running potable water, soap, and single-use towels or hot air drying machines.
11. Needleless systems — means a device that does not use needles for:
    a. The collection of bodily fluids or withdrawal of body fluids after initial venous or arterial access is established.
    b. The administration of medication or fluids.
    c. Any other procedure involving the potential for occupational exposure to bloodborne pathogens due to percutaneous injuries from contaminated sharps.
12. Occupational exposure — means reasonably anticipated skin, eye, mucous membrane, or

Table 1.
Federal Agencies

Federal Department	Agency	Mission	Regulations/Guidelines	Resource
Department of Labor	**OSHA** (Occupational Safety and Health Administration) Created in 1971 under the Occupational Safety and Health Act of 1970 (Federal Code of Regulations (CFR) title 29	Responsible for creating and enforcing workplace safety and health regulations.	-**Bloodborne Pathogens** 29CFR 1910.1030 -**Needlestick Prevention** 29CFR 1910.1030 29CFR 1910.1904 -**Exposure Control Plans** 29CFR 1910.1030 -**Hazard Communication** (MSDS) 29CFR 1910.1200 -**Chemical Hygiene Plan** CFR 1910.1410(non mandatory) -**Laser/Electrosurgery Plume** No specific standard. Hazards can be addressed under: a. General Duty Clause 5(a)(1) b. Respiratory Protection 29CFR 1910.134 c. Bloodborne Pathogens 29CFR 1910.1030	www.osha.gov
Department of Health and Human Resources	**CDC** (Center for Disease Control and Prevention)	Responsible for protecting the health and safety of the people of the U.S. by developing and applying disease prevention and control, environmental health, and health promotion and educational activities.	- CDC is responsible for the CLIA studies and proving scientific and technical support/consultation to DHHS/CMS.	www.cdc.gov
	NIOSH (National Institute for Occupational Safety and Health) The Institute is part of the CDC and was established under the OSA of 1970.	Responsible for conducting research and making recommendations for the prevention of work related disease and injury.	- Investigates potentially hazardous working conditions when requested. - Makes recommendations and disseminates information on preventing workplace disease, injury, and disability.	www.cdc.gov/niosh
	CMS (Centers for Medicare and Medicaid Services) formerly HCFA	Responsible for strengthening the health care services and information available to Medicare and Medicaid beneficiaries and the health care providers who serve them.	- CMS is charged with the implementation of CLIA.	www.cms.hhs.gov
	CLIA (Clinical Laboratory Improvement Amendments) 1988 CFR,Title42,Part 493	Established quality standards for all laboratory testing to ensure the accuracy, reliability, and timeliness of patient test results regardless of where the test is performed. Sets standards designed to improve quality in all laboratory testing and includes specifications for quality control, quality assurance, patient test management, personnel and proficiency testing. CLIA applies to any facility which performs laboratory testing on specimens derived from humans for the purpose of providing information for the diagnosis, prevention, treatment of disease, or impairment of or assessment of health. (This applies to Mohs Micrographic Labs)	-Test categorization under CLIA. -MDR (Medical Device Reporting) Regulation 21 CFR Part 803 Determines when an event involving needlesticks and blood exposure is reportable as a serious injury and when it is reportable as a malfunction.	www.cms.hhs.gov/clia
	FDA (Food and Drug Administration)	Assures the safety of foods and cosmetics, and the safety and efficacy and pharmaceuticals, biological products and medical devices.	- FDA is responsible for the test categorization.	www.fda.gov

parenteral contact with blood or other potentially infectious materials that may result from the performance of an employee's duties.

13. Other potentially infectious materials include:
    a. The following human body fluids: any body fluid that is visibly contaminated with blood, and all body fluids in situations where it is difficult or impossible to differentiate between body fluids.
    b. Any unfixed tissue or organ (other than intact skin) from a human.
    c. HIV-containing cell or tissue.

14. Personal protection equipment is specialized clothing or equipment worn by an employee for protection against a hazard. General work clothes (for example, uniforms, pants, shirts, or blouses) not intended to function as protection against a hazard are not considered to be personal protective equipment.

15. Regulated waste — means liquid or semi-liquid blood or other potentially infectious materials; contaminated items that would release blood or other potentially infectious materials in a liquid or semi-liquid state if compressed; items that are caked with dried blood or other potentially infectious materials and capable of releasing these materials during handling; contaminated sharps; and pathological and microbiological wastes containing blood or other potentially infectious materials.

16. Sharps with engineered sharps injury protection — means a non-needle sharp or a needle device used for withdrawing body fluids, accessing a vein or artery, or administering medications or other fluids, with a built-in safety feature or mechanism that effectively reduces the risk of an exposure incident.

17. Source Individual — means any individual, living or dead, whose blood or other potentially infectious materials may be a source of occupational exposure to the employee.

18. Sterilize — means the use of a physical or chemical procedure to destroy all microbial life including highly resistant bacterial endospores.

19. Universal Precautions — is an approach to infection control. According to the concept of Universal Precautions, all human blood and certain human body fluids are treated as if known to be infectious for HIV, HBV, and other bloodborne pathogens.

20. Work practice controls — means controls that reduce the likelihood of exposure by altering the manner in which a task is performed (e.g., prohibiting recapping of needles by a two-handed technique).

B. **Synopsis of OSHA regulation 29CFR 1910.1030. Bloodborne Pathogens.**
    1. Each employer having an employee(s) with

occupational exposure shall establish a written exposure control plan. This exposure control plan should minimally contain:
    a. Exposure determination.
    b. Schedule and method of implementation for methods of compliance (for example, Universal Precautions; engineering and work practice controls; handwashing facilities; contaminated needles/sharps; food and drink in potentially hazardous places; specimen collection, handling, processing, storage, transport, or shipping; personal protective equipment (PPE); housekeeping; regulated waste containment; laundry.
    c. Hepatitis B vaccination and post-exposure evaluation followup.
    d. Communication of hazards to employees (labels, red bags).
    e. Recordkeeping of the plan as well as the procedure for evaluating the circumstances surrounding exposure incidents.

2. Universal Precautions shall be observed.

3. Engineering and work practice controls shall be used to eliminate or minimize employee exposure. Where occupational exposure remains after instituting these controls, PPE shall be used. PPE shall be provided by the employer at no cost to the employee. PPE includes, but is not limited to, gloves, gowns, laboratory coats, face shields or masks and eye protection, mouthpieces, resuscitation bags, pocket masks, or other ventilation devices. PPE will be considered appropriate only if it does not permit blood or other potentially infectious materials to pass through to or reach the employee's work clothes, street clothes, undergarments, skin, eyes, or other mucous membranes under normal conditions of use and for the duration of time it will be used. All PPE must be removed prior to leaving the work area.

4. Handwashing facilities shall be readily accessible.

5. Contaminated needles and other contaminated sharps shall not be bent, recapped, or removed, unless no alternative is feasible or such action is required by a specific medical procedure. (In this situation bending, removal, or recapping must be accomplished through the use of a mechanical device or one-handed technique).

Note: The Needlestick Safety and Prevention Act (HR 5178) became effective April 18, 2001. It mandated revision of 29CFR 1910.1030 Bloodborne Pathogens to strengthen the requirements related to safety engineered sharp devices. Synopsis of law:
    a. Exposure control plans must be reviewed

Table 2.
Independent Accreditation Agencies

Agency	Mission	Sites Accredited	Resource
JCAHO Joint Commission on Accreditation of Healthcare Organizations	To continuously improve the safety and quality of care provided to the public through the provision of health care accreditation and related services that support performance improvement in health care organizations.	- Hospitals - Ambulatory care providers - Outpatient surgery facilities - Group practices - Clinical laboratories	www.jcaho.org
CAP College of American Pathologists	Represent the interests of patients, the public, and pathologists by fostering excellence in the practice of pathology and laboratory medicine. Inspectors are pathologists and other laboratory professionals who combine knowledge of pathology with proper quality assurance procedures to determine whether a lab meets the standard for accreditation.	Mohs micrographic labs	www.cap.org

Figure 1.
Universal Biohazard Symbol

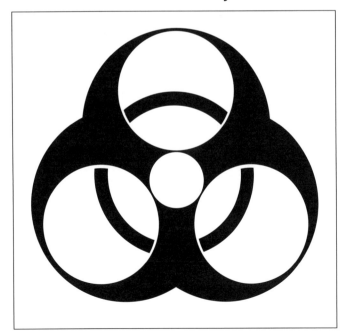

and updated annually to reflect changes in sharps safety technology.

b. Requires employers to document in their plans that they have evaluated and implemented safety-engineered sharp devices and needleless systems.

c. Requires employers to solicit input from nonmanagerial (frontline) health care workers when selecting safety engineered devices, and document this in their exposure control plan.

d. Requires a sharps injury log to be maintained with detailed information concerning injury, type and brand of device involved, how and where incident occurred.

e. Expands definition of "engineering controls" to include devices with engineered sharps injury protection.
The new law does not recommend specific devices but requires all employers to evaluate what's available and implement appropriate devices promptly.

f. Contaminated sharps shall be placed in containers that are labeled appropriately, puncture resistant, and leak proof.

g. Eating, drinking, smoking, applying

Dermatologic Nursing Essentials: A Core Curriculum 2nd Edition © DNA 2003

cosmetics or lip balm, and handling contact lenses are prohibited in areas of possible occupational exposure.

h. Food and drink cannot be kept where blood or other potentially infectious materials are kept (for example, refrigerators, shelves, cabinets, countertops).

i. All equipment, environmental, and work surfaces shall be cleaned and decontaminated after contact with potentially infectious materials.

j. Appropriate training, vaccinations, post exposure evaluation, and followup pertinent to HBV and HIV shall be available to all employees with occupational exposure, at no cost to the employee.

k. Appropriate signs and labels shall be affixed to containers used for potentially infectious materials (see Figure 1).

l. All employees with potential occupational exposure shall participate in a training program, provided by the employer at no cost to the employee:

(1) Upon assignment to tasks with possible exposure.

(2) Within 90 days of the effective date of a standard.

(3) At least annually thereafter

V. OSHA STANDARD 29CFR 1910.1200 HAZARD COMMUNICATION

Requires employers to maintain in the workplace copies of the required MSDS (Material Safety Data Sheets) for each hazardous chemical. These shall be readily accessible during each work shift to employees when they are in their workplace.

MSDS list the *hazardous* ingredients of a product, its physical and chemical characteristics (for example, flammability, explosive properties), its effect on human health, the chemicals with which it can adversely react, handling precautions, the types of measures that can be used to control exposure, emergency and first aid procedures, and the methods to contain a spill. Examples of some potentially hazardous chemicals include: acetic acid, hydrogen peroxide, acetone, isopropyl alcohol, formaldehyde, and TCA (trichloroacetic acid).

VI. LASERS

A. Plume — present there is no specific standard related to laser or electrosurgery plume. Safety from such hazards can be addressed from the:

1. OSH Act of 1970, General Duty Clause 5 (a)(1).

2. OSHA Standard 1910.134 Respiratory Protection.

3. OSHA Standard 1910.1030 Bloodborne Pathogens

B. **General hazards.**

1. The only OSHA standard that applies to general lazer hazards is: OSHA Standard 1926.54 Nonionizing Radiation. OSHA, however, has written a directive and technical manual that contains information that will assist in the recognition and evaluation of lazer hazards. (Information available at www.osha.gov.) In addition, OSHA confers with ANSI (American National Standards Institute) a private, non-profit organization that administers and coordinates the U.S. voluntary standardization and conformity system. Their publication ANSI Z136.3-1996, entitled "Safe Use of Lazers in Health Care Facilities," provides reasonable and adequate guidelines for the safe use of lazers and lazer systems in health care facilities.

VII. RESOURCES (see Table 3)

Table 3.
Resources

Resource	Location	Web Site
ANSI	1819 L Street, NW Suite 600 Washington, DC	www.ansi.org
CAP	325 Wakegan Road Northfield, IL 60093 FAX 1-847-832-8006 Phone 1-800-323-4040	www.cap.org
Department of Health and Human Resources	200 Independence Avenue, SW Washington, DC 20201 Phone 1-877-696-6775	www.cms.hhs.gov
CMS	7500 Security Boulevard Baltimore, MD 21244-1850 Phone 1-410-786-3000	
CDC	1600 Clifton Road Atlanta, GA 30333 Phone 1-404-639-3534 1-800-311-3435	
FDA	5600 Fishers Lane Rockville, MD 20857-0001 Phone 1-888-INFO-FDA 1-888-463-6332	
NIOSH	200 Independence Avenue, SW Washington, DC 20201 Phone 1-800-35-NIOSH 1-800-232-3299 Fax 1-888-232-3299	
Department of Labor OSHA	200 Constitution Avenue, NW Washington, DC 20210 Phone 1-800-321-OSHA	www.osha.gov
JCAHO	601 13th Street, NW Suite 1150N Washington, DC 20005 Phone 1-202-783-6655 Fax 1-202-783-6888	www.jcaho.org

STUDY QUESTIONS

1. The federal agency responsible for OSHA is:
   a. NIOSH.
   b. CDC.
   c. Department of Labor.
   d. Department of Health and Human Resources.

2. Only hospitals are required to follow government regulations concerning health care?
   a. True
   b. False

3. Which of the following protect the health and safety of workers?
   a. CMS.
   b. OSHA and NIOSH.
   c. CLIA and CMS.
   d. CLIA.

4. Which of the following protect the patient's rights and safety?
   a. NIOSH and OSHA.
   b. OSHA and CLIA.
   c. CMS and CLIA.
   d. CMS and NIOSH.

5. All clinical settings are required by law to have a written exposure control plan?
   a. True
   b. False

6. The Needlestick Safety and Prevention Act of 2001:
   a. Requires health care employers to document in their exposure control plan that they have evaluated and implemented regarding safety-engineered sharp devices and needleless systems.
   b. Requires that exposure control plans be reviewed and updated at least annually to reflect changes in sharps safety technology.
   c. Requires each health care facility to maintain a sharps injury log with detailed information on percutaneuos injuries.
   d. Requires employers to solicit input from nonmanagerial health care workers when identifying, evaluating, and selecting safety-engineered sharp devices.
   e. All of the above.

7. The Needlestick Safety and Prevention Act of 2001 allows devices to be chosen on a facility's specific needs and does not mandate particular devices?
   a. True
   b. False

8. The Needlestick Safety and Prevention Act of 2001:
   a. Becomes effective after an employer uses up old devices and orders new ones.
   b. Became effective on April 18, 2001.
   c. Becomes effective when all new safety devices become available through manufacturers.
   d. Becomes effective based on individual facility needs.

9. Accreditation agencies play an important role in protecting patients' rights and reimbursement issues?
   a. True
   b. False

Answers to Study Questions

1. c	5. a	9. a
2. b	6. e	
3. b	7. a	
4. c	8. b	

Chapter 23.
Regulatory Guidelines

Please photocopy this test page and return.

COMPLETE THE FOLLOWING:

Name: _____

Address: _____

City: _____ State: _____ Zip: _____

Preferred telephone: (Home)_____ (Work) _____

State where licensed and license number: _____

CE application fee: DNA member $7.00
                        Nonmember $10.00

POSTTEST INSTRUCTIONS

1. To receive continuing education credit for individual study after reading the article, complete the answer/evaluation form below.

2. Photocopy and send the answer/evaluation form along with a check or money order payable to **Dermatology Nurses' Association** to: *DNA*, East Holly Avenue Box 56, Pitman, NJ 08071-0056.

3. Test returns must be postmarked by December 31, 2008. Upon completion of the answer/evaluation form, a certificate for 1.4 contact hour(s) will be awarded and sent to you.

This chapter was reviewed and formatted for contact hour credit by Marcia J. Hill, MSN, RN, Core Curriculum Editor; and Sally Russell, MN, RN,C, DNA Education Director.

ANSWER FORM

1. Name one new detail (item, issue, or phenomenon) that you learned by completing this activity.

    _____

    _____

    _____

    _____

2. How will you apply the information from this learning activity to your practice?

    a. Patient education.
    b. Staff education.
    c. Improve my patient care.
    d. In my education course work.
    e. Other: Please describe _____

    _____

Evaluation

	Strongly disagree				Strongly agree
3. The offering met the stated objectives.					
a. Identify major federal agencies responsible for regulatory issues that affect both the patient and the health care worker.	1	2	3	4	5
b. Identify agencies used for obtaining appropriate facility accreditation.	1	2	3	4	5
c. Define OSHA regulations pertinent to bloodborne pathogens.	1	2	3	4	5
d. Describe specific regulatory issues and be able to locate resources for additional information.	1	2	3	4	5
4. The content was current and relevant.	1	2	3	4	5
5. The content was presented clearly.	1	2	3	4	5
6. The content was covered adequately.	1	2	3	4	5
7. I am more confident of my abilities since completing this material.	1	2	3	4	5

8. The material was (check one) ☐ new, ☐ review for me.

Comments _____

9. Time required to complete reading assignment: _____ minutes

This independent study is provided by the Dermatology Nurses' Association (DNA) for 1.4 contact hours. DNA is accredited as a provider of continuing education in nursing by the American Nurses Credentialing Center's Commission on Accreditation. DNA is approved as a provider of continuing education by the California Board of Registered Nursing Provider #CEP5708.

Disorders of Glands

Elizabeth Bevan (Betty) Kasper, MS, ARNP-C

OBJECTIVES

At the end of this chapter, the reader will be able to:

- Identify common dermatology disorders of the sebaceous, apocrine, and eccrine glands.
- Recognize the epidemiology, etiology and pathogenesis, diagnostic hallmarks, course and prognosis, clinical presentation, and differential diagnosis for each disease state.
- Describe common therapeutic modalities for each disease state.
- Specify common nursing diagnoses, outcomes, and interventions for each disease state.
- List home-care considerations for each disease state.

KEY POINTS

- Distribution of lesions, presence of true comedones, and degree of erythema all aid in differentiation of acne from acne-like lesions.
- Rosacea, unrelated yet often co-existing with acne, does not present with comedones.
- Hidradenitis suppurativa, a chronic, suppurative, scarring disease of apocrine gland-bearing skin, is sometimes associated with severe nodulocystic acne, but whereas acne comedones are found singularly, this disorder is characterized by paired comedones.
- Primary hyperhidrosis has no known cause but may be brought on by anxiety. Secondary hyperhidrosis has an underlying cause that needs to be found and treated.
- Miliaria crystallina (self-limited), miliaria rubra (common prickly heat), and miliaria profunda (found in patients who have had several bouts of miliaria rubra) are all sweat-retention diseases related to heat exposure.

Disorders of Glands

Elizabeth Bevan (Betty) Kasper, MS, ARNP-C

I. OVERVIEW

A. The pilosebaceous unit comprises the hair follicle and one or more sebaceous glands attached to it. Sebaceous glands are found in greater numbers on the face, scalp, chest, and anogenital regions. Sebaceous glands are small at birth, enlarge between 8 and 10 years of age with maturation continuing through adolescence, and remain unchanged until later years. They decrease in menopause in females and after the 70th decade in males. As people age, sebum secretion decreases even though the size of sebaceous glands increases. Development of sebaceous glands and sebogenesis are hormone-dependent (testosterone, androstenedione, dehydroepiandrosterone).

B. Apocrine gland ducts usually open into the hair follicle above the entrance of the sebaceous glands but some ducts open directly upon the surface of the skin. Apocrine glands are found in the axillae, around the areolae, the periumbilical, perineal, circumanal areas, prepuce, scrotum, mons pubis, labia minora, external ear canal, and eyelids. Like sebaceous glands, the activity of the apocrine glands is hormone dependent, but also stimulated by epinephrine and norepinephrine. The apocrine gland secretion is modified by the action of bacteria in the follicular infidibulum causing production of short-chain fatty acids, ammonia, and other odiferous substances.

C. Eccrine sweat glands are not associated with hair follicles and are found everywhere on the body except for mucocutaneous junctions. They are found in the greatest concentration on the palms, soles, axillae, and forehead. Eccrine sweat glands function to help regulate the body's temperature. This is accomplished by the production of eccrine sweat that flows to the skin surface and cools by evaporation. Eccrine sweat is an odorless, colorless, hypotonic solution and is excreted during periods of stress and heat. Axillary eccrine sweat glands contribute to the odor-producing secretion of the apocrine glands by providing a moist environment that is conducive to bacterial proliferation.

SEBACEOUS GLAND DISORDERS: ACNE VULGARIS
(Pearl: think obstruction & inflammation)

I. OVERVIEW

A. Definition: Pilosebaceous (hair follicle/sebaceous gland) inflammation occurs secondary to the plugging of the unit with open and closed comedones and pustules. In severe acne, cysts or nodules may develop.

B. Epidemiology.
1. Age: affects all ages, with higher incidence (approximately 85%) between ages of 12 to 25.
2. Sex: more severe in males than in females. In males, usually subsides by mid 20s. In females, may occur at any age.
3. Race: lower incidence in Asians and darkly pigmented individuals.
4. Genetic aspects: genetic influence of sebum excretion.
5. Other factors:
   a. Emotional stress, exacerbates.
   b. Occlusion and pressure on skin, exacerbate.
   c. Certain cosmetics, exacerbate.
   d. Diet, little or no effect.
   e. Systemic steroids, exacerbate.

C. Etiology and pathogenesis.
1. Basic cause thought to be multifactoral, complex interaction between androgen hormone and bacteria colonization in pilosebaceous units.
2. Increased sebum production secondary to stimulation by androgenic hormones.
3. Abnormal follicular keratinization.
4. Bacterial colonization with *Proprionibacterium acnes* (*P. acnes*), an anaerobic bacterium.
5. Inflammation.

D. Diagnostic hallmarks.
1. Distribution: face (which is usually oily), forehead and chin (first areas to be noticed) neck, upper arms, trunk, and buttocks.
2. Lesions: comedones (pathognomonic lesions), papules, pustules, and inflammatory nodules and cysts.

E. Course and prognosis.
1. Hormonal factors greatly affect development and course of acne; use of anabolic steroids likely to worsen.
2. Cystic lesions and severe acne more common in men.
3. In women, activity may peak during week prior to menses; may clear up or substantially worsen

during pregnancy.
4. Presence of cysts and family history of scarring acne are prognostic signs for predicting future severity.
5. Postinflammatory hyperpigmentation or hypopigmentation may persist for months.

II. ASSESSMENT

A. History.
1. Duration of lesions: weeks to years.
2. Season: may be worse in the fall and winter and better in the summer.
3. Symptoms: lesions may be painful, especially nodulocystic type.

B. Clinical presentation (Pearl: stretching the skin aids in detecting comedones.)
1. Open comedones (blackheads) — incompletely blocked pores; no scarring.
2. Closed comedones (skin-colored) — completely blocked pores; no scarring.
3. Pustules — plugged duct ruptures with extrusion of keratin plug into surrounding dermis causing inflammatory response; no scarring.
4. Nodules — plugged duct ruptures at level too deep to result in a visible pustule; no scarring.
5. Cysts — plugged duct ruptures at level of the sebaceous gland itself; heals with scar formation.

C. Atypical findings.
1. Acne conglobata — scarring severe cystic acne with more involvement of the trunk rather than the face (genetically malformed sebaceous follicles present; or rarely seen in XYY genotype of tall males who are slightly mentally retarded with aggressive behavior; or in polycystic ovary syndrome).
2. Acne excoriee — individuals neurotically pick at their lesions.
3. Drug-induced acne — acne-like folliculitis without comedones or cysts.

D. Differential diagnosis.
1. Folliculitis.
2. Pseudofolliculitis barbae.
3. Rosacea.
4. Perioral dermatitis.

E. Laboratory and special tests.
1. Hormone workup, if needed, for detecting polycystic ovary syndrome.

III. COMMON THERAPEUTIC MODALITIES

A. Topical therapy.
1. Topical retinoids: apply once daily for comedonal acne to decrease cohesiveness of follicular epithelial cells; side effects include erythema, desquamation, hypo/hyperpigmentation, and sensitization of

skin to sunlight.
a. Tretinoin (Retin A® Micro, 0.1% and 0.04% gel) — oregnancy (category C): not recommended.
b. Adapalene (Differin® 0.1% gel, cream, solution or pledgets) — pregnancy (category C): Not recommended. Less irritating than tretinoin or tazarotene and stable in sunlight.
c. Tazarotene (Tazorac® 0.05% and 0.1% gel or cream) — pregnancy (category X). Women of childbearing potential: Obtain reliable negative pregnancy test within 2 weeks before starting therapy; use effective contraception during therapy; begin therapy during normal menses. Stable in sunlight.
2. Benzoyl peroxide: apply once to twice daily for mixed comedones and inflammatory acne as wash, lotion, cream or gel; side effects include skin irritation, allergic contact dermatitis, and bleaching of clothes. Combining benzoyl peroxide with antibiotics dramatically decreases the incidence of bacterial resistance.
a. Benzoyl peroxide plus erythromycin — pregnancy (category C).
b. Benzoyl peroxide plus clindamycin — pregnancy (category C).
3. Topical antibiotics for inflammatory acne apply once to twice daily as a solution, gel, lotion, or pads; side effects include excessive drying, depending upon vehicle, and emerging bacterial resistance with long-term use.
a. Erythromycin 2% (Emgel®) — pregnancy (category B).
b. Clindamycin 1% (Cleocin T®) — pregnancy (category B).
4. Salicylic acid/glycolic acid for mild comedonal acne apply once to twice daily as a cleanser, gel, lotion, or solution to unplug follicles; side effects include mild local irritation.
5. Azaleic acid (Azelex®) — pregnancy (category B). For comedonal and inflammatory acne apply once to twice daily as an antibacterial of *P. acnes,* to normalize keratinization and for post-inflammatory hyperpigmentation; side effects include mild local irritation.

B. Systemic therapy.
1. Antibiotics for inflammatory acne; take one pill or capsule two times per day for a bactericidal effect; side effects include emerging resistance. Pregnancy, nursing mothers: not recommended.
a. Tetracycline, 250 to 500 mg, bid, inexpensive; side effects include photosensitivity, GI upset, candidiasis, tooth discoloration, and enamel hypoplasia (use only in patients > 8 years old).

b. Doxycycline, 50 to 100 mg, bid, may be taken with food; side effects similar to tetracycline but with greater photosensitivity.

c. Minocycline, 50 to 100 mg bid, rare photosensitivity or GI upset; side effects include blue pigmentation, serum sickness-like reactions and drug-induced lupus.

d. Erythromycin, 250 to 500, mg bid, may be taken during pregnancy; side effects include GI upset.

2. Isotretinoin (Accutane®) 0.5 to 2.0 mg/kg/d for nodulo-cystic acne and inflammatory acne recalcitrant to other modes of treatment to normalize keratinization, decrease sebum production, and deplete *P. acnes*; multiple side effects include teratogenicity, chelitis, conjunctivitis, dry eyes and mouth, pruritus, musculoskeletal pain, and alopecia.

3. Oral contraceptives as an adjunct treatment in female patients for moderate to severe inflammatory acne decrease sebum production; side effects include suppressing growth in patients < 16 years old; contraindicated in males.

IV. COMMON NURSING DIAGNOSES, OUTCOMES, INTERVENTIONS (see Table 1)

V. HOME CARE CONSIDERATIONS AND TREATMENT PEARLS

A. Do not overwash face; two times per day is maximum recommended.

B. Use gentle facial cleanser, not abrasive cleanser.

C. Gently clean with hands only; no washcloth.

D. Allow 15 to 20 minutes after washing before applying medication to decrease burning/stinging.

E. Apply medication to the entire face; benzoyl peroxide may be used as a spot treatment.

F. Certain soaps, creams, lotions, oil, and cosmetics worsen acne; encourage use of noncomedogenic products.

G. Acne often flares when treatment starts.

H. Mild reddening or peeling indicates medication working.

I. No picking; increases post-inflammatory hyperpigmentation; leads to scarring.

J. Keep occlusive hair conditioners off face; hair pomades frequently make acne worse.

K. Keep hands off face after eating oily foods, such as chocolate and potato chips.

ROSACEA
Pearl: think flushers and blushers

I. OVERVIEW

A. Definition: rosacea is a chronic inflammatory disorder involving the flush area of the face associated with diffuse sebaceous gland abnormality and increased reactivity of capillaries that develops over time and is characterized by persistent erythema, papules, tiny pustules, and telangiectasia. There are no blackheads (comedones).

B. Epidemiology.
1. Age: seen between ages 30 to 50 years; peak incidence between 40 and 50.
2. Sex: affects females predominantly; rhinophyma occurs mostly in males.
3. Race: skin phototypes I and II but also in others; rare in people of color.
4. Genetic aspects: familial predisposition.
5. Other factors: (anything that triggers flushing).
   a. Sun exposure.
   b. Stress.
   c. Alcohol and hot or spicy foods or drinks.
   d. Irritating cosmetics.

C. Etiology and pathogenesis.
1. Unknown cause.
2. Erythema results from dilatation of superficial vasculature of face (atrophy of papillary dermis provides for easier visualization of dermal capillaries).
3. Edema develops as result of increased blood flow in superficial vasculature (edema may contribute to late-stage fibroplasia and rhinophyma).

D. Diagnostic hallmarks.
1. Distribution: vertical, central third of face.
2. Lesions: pustules and papules against background of erythema and telangiectasia.

E. Course and prognosis.
1. Chronic disease characterized by periodic exacerbations and remissions.
2. Disease may spontaneously disappear after a few years.

II. ASSESSMENT

A. History.
1. Duration of lesions: days, weeks, and months.
2. Symptoms: episodic facial erythema with increased skin temperature in response to stimuli.

B. Clinical presentation: four stages.
1. Stage I — papules and telangiectasia.
   a. Frequent blushing.
   b. Easy irritation and erythema of facial skin.
   c. Possible ocular inflammation.

2. Stage II — papules and pustules.
   a. Transitory erythema of midfacial areas.
   b. Early telangiectasias, become apparent.
3. Stage III — papules, pustules and nodules.
   a. Permanent, deeper midfacial erythema.
   b. Telangiectasias increase.
   c. Papules and pustules begin to develop.
4. Stage IV — chronic changes.
   a. Tissue hyperplasia.
   b. Rhinophyma.

C. Atypical findings.
   1. Rhinophyma: enlarged nose.
   2. Metophyma: enlarged cushion-like swelling of forehead.
   3. Blepharophyma: swelling of eyelids related to sebaceous gland hyperplasia.
   4. Gnathophyma: swelling of chin.

D. Differential diagnosis.
   1. Acne vulgaris (comedones; no generalized erythema, telangiectasias).
   2. Seborrheic dermatitis, perioral dermatitis, systemic lupus (these conditions will not produce characteristic flushing, telangiectasias, papules, and pustules).
   3. Sarcoidosis (closely mimics with red papules on face, but manifests in other organs as well).

E. Laboratory and special tests.
   1. Bacterial culture if *S. aureus* infection suspected.

III. COMMON THERAPEUTIC MODALITIES

A. Topical therapy.
   1. Topical metronidazole: twice daily (0.75% cream, lotion or gel) or 1.0% formulation, once daily; most common side effect is irritation.
   2. Sulfacetamide wash or lotion; side effects: less irritating than metronidazole; contact dermatitis possible.
   3. Topical retinoic acid applied once daily; side effects include delayed onset of effectiveness, dry skin, erythema, burning/stinging.
   4. Azelaic acid 20% cream applied once daily.
   5. Topical vitamin C antioxidant effect might affect free-radical production that might play role in inflammatory reaction of rosacea.

B. Systemic therapy: once daily doses dramatically increase the development of bacterial resistance so, when possible, use twice daily regimens.
   1. Tetracycline, 1.0 to 1.5 grams per day divided into 2 to 4 daily doses until lesions clear; then gradually reduce to 250 mg, twice daily.
   2. Minocycline, 100 mg, twice daily until lesions clear; then gradually reduce to 50 mg, twice daily.
   3. Doxycycline, monohydrate formulation, 100 mg, once or twice daily, more consistently effective with fewer gastrointestinal side effects than hyclate form.

4. Clarithromycin, 250 mg to 500 mg, twice daily.
5. Oral isotretinoin, 0.1 to 0.2 mg/kg up to 2.0 mg/kg, in individuals with severe disease not responding to antibiotics.

C. Cosmetic surgery.
   1. Residual redness and telangiectasia, after maximum response obtained medically, improves with laser therapy.
   2. Stage IV, involving irreversible fibrotic changes, such as rhinophyma, does not respond well to medical therapy; refer for surgery or laser therapy.

IV. COMMON NURSING DIAGNOSES, OUTCOMES, INTERVENTIONS (see Table 1)

V. HOME CARE CONSIDERATIONS AND TREATMENT PEARLS

A. Avoid triggers (both exposures and situations that can cause a flare-up of the flushing and skin changes in rosacea).
   1. Sun exposure: Always apply nonirritating sun block when outdoors; wear hats.
   2. Stress: autonomic activation increases flushing.
   3. Alcohol consumption: not a cause; aggravates with peripheral vasodilation.
   4. Spicy foods: aggravate through autonomic stimulation.
   5. Cleansers, lotions, cosmetics: use nonirritating, hypoallergenic, noncomedogenic.

B. Avoid rubbing, scrubbing, or massaging face; tends to irritate reddened skin.

C. Avoid applying corticosteroids to skin without health care provider's specific instructions.

D. If exercise results in flushing, exercise in cool environment; don't overheat.

E. Keep diary of flushing episodes and factors.

F. Contact National Rosacea Society, 1-888-NO-BLUSH, 600 S. Northwest Hwy, Suite 200, Barrington, Il 60010.

APOCRINE GLAND DISORDERS: HIDRADENITIS SUPPRATIVA
(Pearl: think boil-like lumps in the groin, under the arms or under the breasts)

I. OVERVIEW

A. Definition: also known as acne inversa, this is a chronic, scarring disease of apocrine gland-bearing skin caused by intense inflammation following follicular obstruction on "inverse" areas of the body (axillae, beneath breasts, groin, upper, inner thighs, and buttocks).

B. Epidemiology.
   1. Race: all races, more severe in people of color.
   2. Age: appears after puberty; most cases in

Table 1.
Nursing Diagnoses, Outcomes, and Interventions

Nursing Diagnosis	Outcome	Interventions
Anxiety disturbance related to disease process.	Patient will verbalize confidence in ability to cope with and manage disease process.	1. Instruct patient regarding management including medications, diet, activity, and routine followup care. 2. Discuss potential exacerbating factors.
Body image disturbance related to presence of lesions or sweating.	Patient will verbalize improved well-being in relation to body image.	1. Assess patient's current perceptions and feelings. 2. Encourage patient to express feelings related to the disease and its impact on self-image and daily life.
Social isolation related to decreased activities due to poor body image.	Patient will continue participation in family, social, and work activities.	1. Assess patient's level of social interactions and activities. 2. Encourage patient to maintain active lifestyle.
Potential for depression related to chronic condition.	Patient will verbalize feelings about condition.	1. Encourage patient to verbalize feelings regarding the condition. 2. Teach patient what he/she can do to control the condition.
Knowledge deficit related to disease diagnosis and therapy modalities.	Patient will verbalize understanding of disease course and treatment options.	1. Assess patient's understanding of disease diagnosis and treatment options. 2. Discuss means to avoid exacerbating factors.

second and third decades of life.

3. Sex: anogenital involvement seen more often in males and axillae involvement seen more often in females.
4. Genetic aspects.
   a. Clustering in families.
   b. Mother-daughter transmission observed.
   c. Genetic predisposition to acne.
5. Other factors.
   a. Obesity.
   b. Apocrine duct obstruction.
   c. Secondary bacterial infection.
C. **Etiology and pathogenesis.**
   1. Unknown cause.
   2. Keratinous plugging of apocrine duct.
   3. Dilatation of apocrine duct and hair follicle.
   4. Severe inflammatory changes limited to single apocrine gland.
   5. Bacterial growth in dilated duct.
   6. Ruptured duct/gland results in extension of inflammation/infection.
   7. Extension of suppuration/tissue destruction.
   8. Ulceration and fibrosis, sinus tract formation.
D. **Diagnostic hallmarks.**
   1. Distribution: axillae, anogenital regions, the scalp, and under female breasts.

2. Lesions: highly characteristic double comedone blackhead with two or more surface openings that communicate under the skin.
   a. Lesions moderately to exquisitely painful.
3. Draining sinus tracts.
E. **Course and prognosis.**
   1. Progressive and relentless.
   2. Course varies from recurrent self-healing tender red nodule to diffuse, painful abscess formation.
   3. Secondary bacterial infection probably major cause of exacerbations.

II. ASSESSMENT

A. **History.**
   1. Intermittent pain.
   2. Marked point tenderness related to abscess formation.
B. **Clinical presentation.**
   1. Initial lesion — inflammatory, tender nodules.
   2. Eventually — abscesses (red, hot, painful, discharging lumps) and sinus tracts with pus drainage.
   3. Finally — fibrosis, hypertrophic, and keloidal scars, and contractures.

C. Associated findings.
1. Cystic acne.
2. Pilonidal sinus.
D. Differential diagnosis.
1. Furuncle/Carbuncle.
2. Lymphadenitis.
3. Ruptured cysts.
4. Cat-scratch disease.
5. Sinus tracts and fistulas associated with ulcerative colitis and regional enteritis.
E. Laboratory and special tests.
1. Cultures may show a variety of pathogens that secondarily infect lesions.

III. COMMON THERAPEUTIC MODALITIES

A. Topical therapy.
1. Drysol®, one to two times per week at bedtime.
2. Tretinoin cream (0.05%) may prevent duct occlusion; side effects include irritation; use only as tolerated.
B. Systemic therapy.
1. Acute painful lesions: injections.
   a. Nodules — intralesional triamcinolone (3 to 5 mg/ml) diluted with lidocaine.
   b. Abscesses — intralesional triamcinolone (3 to 5 mg/ml) diluted with lidocaine followed by incision and drainage of abscess fluid.
2. Chronic low-grade disease: oral antibiotics until lesions resolve and intralesional injections, as above, into early inflammatory lesions to hasten resolution.
   a. Erythromycin — 250 to 500 mg, four times per day.
   b. Tetracycline — 250 to 500 mg, four times per day.
   c. Minocycline — 100 mg, two times per day.
   d. Doxycycline — 50 to 100 mg, two times per day.
3. Oral isotretinoin, 1mg/kg/day for 20 weeks appears useful in early disease with only inflammatory cystic lesions in which undermining sinus tracts have not developed or when combined with surgical excision of individual lesions.
C. Surgical management.
1. Incise and drain abscesses.
2. Excise chronic recurrent, fibrotic nodules or sinus tracts.
3. Complete excision of axilla or involved anogenital area may be required for severe, extensive, chronic disease.

IV. COMMON NURSING DIAGNOSES, OUTCOMES, INTERVENTIONS (see Table 1)

V. HOME CARE CONSIDERATIONS AND TREATMENT PEARLS

A. Wash with antiseptics, antibacterial soaps or acne preparations to reduce skin carriage of bacteria.
B. Avoid roll-on deodorants.
C. Decrease friction and moisture.
D. Avoid constrictive clothing.
E. Lose weight, if obese.
F. Minimize heat buildup and sweat.

ECCRINE GLAND DISORDERS: PRIMARY HYPERHIDROSIS (Pearl: think excess sweating)

I. OVERVIEW

A. Definition: in some people (approximately 1% of the population), the secretion of sweat occurs far higher than needed to keep a constant temperature. This condition is referred to as hyperhidrosis.
B. Epidemiology.
1. Age: up to 0.5% of the population affected; usually appears during 2nd or 3rd decade of life.
2. Sex: not a known factor.
3. Race: not a known factor.
4. Genetic aspects: positive family history in 30% to 50% suggests genetic factor.
5. Other factors: disease is worse in the obese.
C. Etiology and pathogenesis.
1. Cause unknown.
   a. May result from neurogenic overactivity of sweat glands in affected area.
   b. May be secondary to spinal cord injury and some polyneuropathies.
2. Eccrine gland has secretory coil and duct.
   a. Secretion of eccrine sweat involves secretion of ultrafiltrate by secretory coil in response to acetylcholine (released from sympathetic nerve endings) and reabsorption of sodium by ductal portion (surface sweat is hypotonic).
3. Proximal (coiled) duct functionally more active than distal (straight) portion.
D. Diagnostic hallmarks.
1. Distribution: locations.
   a. Palmar (hands).
   b. Axillary (armpits).
   c. Plantar (feet).
   d. Facial (face).
   e. Truncal (trunk).
   f. General (over the whole body).
2. Sweating: can be induced by thermal stimuli and by emotional stress.
   a. Emotional sweating stops during sleep.
   b. Thermal sweating occurs even during sleep.

E. **Course and prognosis.**
1. Persists during lifetime.
2. Exerts negative impact on lives of affected.
3. Triggered by anxiety; rarely associated with psychiatric disorders.
4. Consequences: odor, dehydration, skin maceration, and possible secondary skin infections.

II. ASSESSMENT

A. **History.**
1. Duration: appears suddenly or continuously without any obvious reason.
2. Season: elicited by high outside temperatures.
3. Symptoms: Excessive perspiration; nervousness and anxiety elicit or aggravate sweating; hands not only feel moist, but also cold.

B. **Clinical presentation.**
1. Affected areas often pink or bluish white.
2. Skin, especially on feet, may be macerated.
3. Fissured and scaling

C. **Atypical findings.**
1. Facial hyperhidrosis (forehead).
2. Palmar hyperhidrosis (hands).
3. Axillary hyperhidrosis (armpits).
4. Plantar hyperhidrosis (feet).
5. Other locations.
   a. Trunk.
   b. Thighs.

D. **Differential diagnosis.**
1. Secondary (generalized) disease cause known as part of underlying condition.
   a. Hyperthyroidism or similar endocrine diseases.
   b. Endocrine treatment for prostatic cancer or other types of malignancies.
   c. Severe psychiatric disorders.
   d. Obesity.
   e. Menopause.

E. **Laboratory and special tests.**
1. None specific except to rule out associated conditions.
2. Before Botox® injection, hyperhidrotic field (particularly in axillary hyperhidrosis) may be visualized using the Minor iodine-starch test. In this test, an iodine solution (2 g of iodine in 10 ml of castor oil and alcohol to 100 ml) is painted over the area of the skin to be tested. After it has dried, fine rice or potato starch powder is applied. Sweat causes the mixture to turn dark blue.

III. COMMON THERAPEUTIC MODALITIES

A. **Topical therapy.**
1. Antiperspirants (first measure due to ease of use, time issues, and cost).
   a. Aluminum chloride (20% to 25%) in 70%

to 90% alcohol, qhs, 2 to 3 times/week.
   b. Sufficient in light to moderate cases, repeat regularly.
2. Iontophoresis (time consuming, inefficient at times and expensive).
   a. Low-intensity electric current (15 to 18 mA) supplied by D/C generator, applied to palms or soles immersed in tap water or electrolyte solution.
      (1) 20 minute sessions several times/week to q 1 to 2 weeks.
   b. Results vary; difficult to apply in axillary, and impossible to use in diffuse hyperhidrosis of the face or the trunk/thigh region.

B. **Systemic therapy.**
1. Botulinum toxin type A (BTX-A) (repeat every 7 months).
   a. For axillae, palms, or forehead temporarily blocks release of acetylcholine from cholinergic fibers.
      (1) Inject intradermally at multiple sites of affected area.
         (a) Axillary: inject 10 to 15 sites equally distributed over axilla.
      (2) Palmar: injections 2.5 cm apart over palm and along fingers.

C. **Surgery.**
1. Excision of axillary sweat glands.
2. Sympathectomy to interrupt nerve tracks and nodes (ganglia) which transmit signals to sweat glands.
   a. Endoscopic thoracic sympathectomy (ETS); less invasive than traditional.

IV. COMMON NURSING DIAGNOSES, OUTCOMES, INTERVENTIONS (see Table 1)

V. HOME CARE CONSIDERATIONS AND TREATMENT PEARLS

A. **Lose weight, if obese.**
B. **Stress management (helps with coping and with disrupting anxiety-sweating circle).**

MILIARIA
(Pearl: think sweat rash or prickly heat)

I. OVERVIEW

A. **Definition: itchy rash from inflammation following obstruction and rupture of eccrine sweat ducts.**
B. **Epidemiology.**
1. Age: occurs predominantly in neonates, with a peak in those aged 1 week; but may occur in any age if febrile or recently moved to hot, humid climate.

2. Sex: no sex predilection exists.
3. Race: in all races; Asians produce less sweat, less likely to have miliaria rubra.
4. Other factors.
   a. Wearing synthetic clothing against skin.
   b. Swaddling up in too much clothing.
   c. Sitting too close to fire or heater.
   d. Being hot in bed with electric blanket.
   e. Lying for prolonged periods in bed.

C. **Etiology and pathogenesis.**
   1. Known causes.
      a. Conditions of high heat and humidity that lead to excessive sweating and occlusion of skin, for example, clothing and casts.
      b. Normal skin bacteria, such as *S. epidermidis* and *S. aureus*, thought to play role by producing sticky substance which blocks sweat ducts.
      c. Leakage of sweat through walls of duct behind blocked duct responsible for production of miliaria and for further aggravation.

D. **Diagnostic hallmarks.**
   1. Distribution: skin folds and on body in areas with friction from clothing.
   2. Lesions: minute red papules present in very large numbers.
   3. Characteristic intense discomfort; not so much itching as an unbearable pricking sensation.

E. **Course and prognosis.**
   1. Lasts 5 to 6 weeks despite treatment because plugs formed in sweat duct openings only cast off by outward growth of sweat duct cells, which takes several weeks.

II. ASSESSMENT

A. **History.**
   1. Duration of lesions: 5 to 6 weeks.
   2. Season: worse in hot, humid climate.
   3. Symptoms: characteristic pricking sensation.

B. **Clinical presentation.**
   1. Miliaria crystallina (self-limited).
      a. Clear, superficial vesicles 1 to 2 mm in diameter.
      b. Confluent crops without surrounding erythema.
      c. On head, neck, and upper part of trunk in infants.
      d. On trunk in bedridden, overheated adults.
      e. Lesions rupture easily and resolve with superficial branny desquamation.
   2. Miliaria rubra (prickly heat, heat rash — most common of sweat-retention diseases).
      a. Uniform, small, erythematous papules and vesiculopapules on a background of erythema.
      b. Nonfollicular distribution; do not become

confluent.
      c. On the neck, groin, and axillae in infants.
      d. On covered skin where friction occurs in adults.
         (1) Neck.
         (2) Scalp.
         (3) Upper part of trunk.
         (4) Flexures.
         (5) Face and volar areas spared.
      e. In late stages, anhidrosis observed in affected skin.
   3. Miliaria profunda (in patients who have had several bouts of miliaria rubra).
      a. Firm, flesh-colored, nonfollicular papules that are 1 to 3 mm in diameter.
      b. Primarily on trunk, but can also appear on the extremities.
      c. Transient episodes of sweating.
      d. Affected skin shows diminished or absent sweating.
      e. With heat exhaustion hyperpyrexia and tachycardia observed.

C. **Atypical findings.**
   1. Secondary infection appearing as impetigo or as multiple discrete abscesses.
   2. Heat intolerance most likely to develop in miliaria profunda; recognized by anhidrosis of affected skin, weakness, fatigue, dizziness, and even collapse.

D. **Differential diagnosis.**
   1. Cutaneous candidiasis.
   2. Chickenpox.
   3. Erythema toxicum neonatorum.
   4. Folliculitis.
   5. Herpes simplex.
   6. *Pseudomonas folliculitis.*
   7. Syphilis.
   8. Infantile acne.
   9. Viral exanthem.

E. **Laboratory and special tests.**
   1. Miliaria clinically distinctive; laboratory tests not necessary.

III. COMMON THERAPEUTIC MODALITIES

Note: Miliaria crystallina asymptomatic and self-limited.
Note: Miliaria rubra can cause great discomfort; miliaria profunda may lead to heat exhaustion; treatment of these conditions is warranted.

A. **Topical therapy.**
   1. Lotions containing calamine, boric acid, or menthol.
   2. Cool wet-to-dry compresses.
   3. Frequent showering with soap (although some discourage excessive use of soap).
   4. Topical corticosteroids.
   5. Topical antibiotics, if infection present.

6. Topical application of anhydrous lanolin in patients with miliaria profunda.
B. Systemic therapy.
1. Prophylaxis of miliaria with oral antibiotics is reported.
2. Oral retinoids, vitamin A, and vitamin C have all been used with variable success.

IV. COMMON NURSING DIAGNOSES, OUTCOMES, INTERVENTIONS (see Table 1)

V. HOME CARE CONSIDERATIONS AND TREATMENT PEARLS

A. Control heat and humidity so that sweating is not stimulated.
B. Treat febrile illness.
C. Remove occlusive clothing.
D. Avoid friction from clothing.
E. Shirts and blouses should be high in cotton and low in synthetics.
F. Limit activity.
G. Stay in air conditioning.
H. Do not irritate the skin.
I. Avoid skin irritants.
J. Vitamin C, one gram daily, has been reported to help in some cases.
K. Calamine is probably as effective as anything for relief of discomfort, but because of its drying effect an emollient may subsequently be required.
L. Patients with miliaria profunda are at high risk for heat exhaustion during exertion in hot weather, because ability to dissipate heat by means of evaporation of sweat is impaired.

Bibliography
Freedberg, I.M., Eisen, A.Z., Wolff, K., Austen, K.F., Goldsmith, L.A., Katz, S.I., & Fitzpatrick, T.B. (Eds.). (1999). *Dermatology in general medicine* (5th ed.). New York: McGraw-Hill, Health Professional Division.
Fitzpatrick, T.B., Johnson, R.A., Wolff, K., Polano, M.K., & Suurmond, D. (1997). *Color atlas and synopsis of clinical dermatology* (3rd ed.). New York: McGraw Hill, Health Professional Division.
Habif, T.P. (1996). *Clinical dermatology: A color guide to diagnosis and therapy* (3rd ed.). St. Louis, MO: The CV Mosby Company.
Hill, M. (1992). *Skin disorders*. St. Louis, MO: The CV Mosby Company.
Kawzler, M.H. (2002). *Dermatology core curriculum* (2nd ed.). Dubuque, IA: American Academy of Dermatology.
Lebworhl, M., Heymann, W.R., Berth-Jones, J. & Coulson, I (Eds.). (2002). *Treatment of skin disease*. London: Mosby.
Lynch, P.J. (1994). *Dermatology for the house officer* (3rd ed.). Baltimore, MD: Williams & Wilkins.

STUDY QUESTIONS

Most of the facts below are true. Please circle the false statements.

1. Acne epidemiology:
   a. May affect all ages.
   b. Lower incidence in Asians and blacks.
   c. More severe in males than in females.
   d. No genetic control of sebum excretion.

2. Acne diagnostic hallmarks, course, and prognosis:
   a. Distribution limited to face, neck, upper arms, trunk, and buttocks.
   b. Lesions include comedones, papulopustules, and inflammatory nodules plus cysts.
   c. In women, activity peaks during the week after their menses and may clear up or substantially worsen during pregnancy.
   d. The presence of cysts and a family history of scarring acne are prognostic signs for predicting future severity.

3. Rosacea epidemiology:
   a. Predominantly affects males.
   b. Affects ages 30 to 50, peak incidence between 40 and 50.
   c. Rare in people of color.
   d. Trigger factors: sun exposure, stress, alcohol, spicy foods, and irritating cosmetics.

4. Four stages of rosacea:
   a. Stage I — frequent blushing; easy irritation and erythema of facial skin.
   b. Stage II — transitory erythema of midfacial areas; early telangiectasias; papules and pustules begin to develop.
   c. Stage III — permanent, deeper midfacial erythema; telangiectasias increases.
   d. Stage IV — tissue hyperplasia, rhinophyma, possible ocular inflammation.

5. Rosacea differential diagnoses:
   a. Acne vulgaris.
   b. Perioral dermatitis.
   c. Systemic lupus.
   d. Folliculitis.

6. Hidradenitis suppurativa:
   a. Is a chronic, suppurative, recurring inflammatory disease.
   b. Affects eccrine gland follicles.
   c. Is more common in females and begins after puberty.
   d. Presents in skin that contains apocrine glands with the axilla and groin most frequently involved.

7. Hidradenitis suppurativa clinical presentation, course, and prognosis:
   a. Double comedone, a blackhead with two or sometimes several surface openings that communicate under the skin, is highly characteristic.
   b. Initial lesion: inflammatory, tender nodules.
   c. Disease is chronic but stable.
   d. Secondary bacterial infection probably a major cause of exacerbations.

8. Primary hyperhidrosis epidemiology:
   a. Known cause.
   b. Disease is worse in the obese.
   c. Generally appears localized in one or several locations of the body (most often hands, feet, armpits, or a combination of them).
   d. Positive family history in 30% to 50% of cases suggests a genetic component.

9. Primary hyperhidrosis course and prognosis:
   a. Starts during childhood or adolescence and persists all life.
   b. Exerts negative impact on lives of many who suffer from it.
   c. Anxiety triggers sweating and is associated with psychiatric disorders.
   d. Consequences include dehydration and maceration of the skin, which may result in secondary skin infections.

10. Miliaria diagnostic hallmarks, course, and prognosis:
    a. Distribution: skin folds and on the body in areas of friction from clothing.
    b. Lesions: minute red papules.
    c. Characteristic intense pricking sensation discomfort.
    d. Attack commonly lasts 5 to 6 weeks but can be shortened with treatment.

Answers to Study Questions

1.	d	5.	d	9.	c
2.	c	6.	b	10.	d
3.	a	7.	c		
4.	b	8.	a		

Dermatologic Nursing Essentials: A Core Curriculum 2nd Edition © DNA 2003

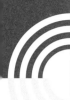

Chapter 24.
Disorders of Glands

Please photocopy this test page and return.

COMPLETE THE FOLLOWING:

Name: _____

Address: _____

City: _____ State: _____ Zip: _____

Preferred telephone: (Home)_____ (Work) _____

State where licensed and license number: _____

CE application fee: DNA member $7.00
                     Nonmember $10.00

POSTTEST INSTRUCTIONS
1. To receive continuing education credit for individual study after reading the article, complete the answer/evaluation form below.
2. Photocopy and send the answer/evaluation form along with a check or money order payable to **Dermatology Nurses' Association** to: **DNA**, East Holly Avenue Box 56, Pitman, NJ 08071-0056.
3. Test returns must be postmarked by December 31, 2008. Upon completion of the answer/evaluation form, a certificate for 1.8 contact hour(s) will be awarded and sent to you.

This chapter was reviewed and formatted for contact hour credit by Marcia J. Hill, MSN, RN, Core Curriculum Editor; and Sally Russell, MN, RN,C, DNA Education Director.

ANSWER FORM

1. Name one new detail (item, issue, or phenomenon) that you learned by completing this activity.

_____

_____

_____

_____

2. How will you apply the information from this learning activity to your practice?
   a. Patient education.
   b. Staff education.
   c. Improve my patient care.
   d. In my education course work.
   e. Other: Please describe _____

_____

Evaluation	Strongly disagree				Strongly agree
3. The offering met the stated objectives.					
a. Identify common dermatology disorders of the sebaceous, apocrine, and eccrine glands.	1	2	3	4	5
b. Recognize the epidemiology, etiology and pathogenesis, diagnostic hallmarks, course and prognosis, clinical presentation, and differential diagnosis for each disease state.	1	2	3	4	5
c. Describe common therapeutic modalities for each disease state.	1	2	3	4	5
d. Specifiy common nursing diagnoses, outcomes, and interventions for each disease state.	1	2	3	4	5
e. List home-care considerations for each disease state.	1	2	3	4	5
4. The content was current and relevant.	1	2	3	4	5
5. The content was presented clearly.	1	2	3	4	5
6. The content was covered adequately.	1	2	3	4	5
7. I am more confident of my abilities since completing this material.	1	2	3	4	5

8. The material was (check one) ☐ new, ☐ review for me.
Comments _____

9. Time required to complete reading assignment: _____ minutes

This independent study is provided by the Dermatology Nurses' Association (DNA) for 1.8 contact hours. DNA is accredited as a provider of continuing education in nursing by the American Nurses Credentialing Center's Commission on Accreditation. DNA is approved as a provider of continuing education by the California Board of Registered Nursing Provider #CEP5708.

Disorders of Oral Mucosa

Lynn A. Babin, MSN, RN, CNS, AAS

OBJECTIVES

At the end of this chapter, the reader will be able to:

- Describe the anatomy and physiology of the mouth as it relates to oral dermatology.
- Differentiate between localized and generalized, ulcerative and white oral mucosal lesions.
- List most common oral diseases and their related etiologies.
- Identify appropriate treatments for various oral lesions.
- Identify the importance of addressing quality of life issues in patients with oral mucosal lesions.
- Identify the relationship between oral lesions and systemic diseases and medical/pharmacological treatments.

KEY POINTS

- Abnormalities of other body systems, as well as medical/pharmacological treatments, can have a significant effect on oral dermatology.
- Examination of the oral cavity should be included in every skin examination.
- Early detection of precancerous/cancerous lesions is of critical importance.
- Appropriate treatment of oral lesion depends upon accurate recognition and diagnosis.
- Biopsy is often necessary for definitive diagnosis of oral lesions.
- Quality of life can be significantly affected by disorders of the oral mucosa and should be appropriately addressed by the practitioner.

Disorders of Oral Mucosa

Lynn A. Babin, MSN, RN, CNS, AAS

OVERVIEW

Studies indicate that oral health problems are increasing in the United States. Examination of the oral cavity should be included in every skin examination, as a wide variety of skin disorders can be accompanied by mucous membrane involvement. Mucosal epithelium varies significantly from the integument. An outer keratinizing layer is made in the absence of disease, adnexal structures are not present, and more rapid epithelialization occurs. The mucosal epithelium is limited in its responses to diseases. Therefore, oral diseases tend to look similar, often making biopsy necessary to support clinical diagnosis. Generalized mucous membrane disorders are divided into two broad categories: (1) erosions and ulcerations and (2) white lesions. Basic anatomy and physiology of the oral cavity and localized lesions will also be discussed.

I. BASIC ANATOMY AND PHYSIOLOGY OF THE MOUTH (ORAL/BUCCAL CAVITY)

A. Any disorder of the oral cavity (and many systemic diseases) can alter its normal functions.

B. Functions of the oral cavity include ingestion, sensory response to food, mastication, chemical digestion, deglutition, and speech.

C. The oral cavity is lined with nonkeratinized stratified squamous epithelium.
1. Except for the dorsum tongue and hard palate, oral membrane possesses neither a granular nor horny layer.

D. Lips.
1. Have superficial nerves and capillaries.
2. Are divided into two regions.
   a. Cutaneous area (mustache area); contains hair and sebaceous glands.
   b. Vermilion (lipstick area); no hair or sebaceous glands.

E. Tongue.
1. Lingual papillae covers surfaces.
2. Nonkeratinized stratified squamous epithelium.
3. Anterior two-thirds is called the "body" and occupies the oral cavity.
4. Posterior one-third is called the "root" and occupies the oropharynx.
5. V-shaped row of vallate papillae and a groove called the terminal sulcus separate the body and root.
6. The body is attached to the mouth floor by the lingual frenulum.
7. Among the muscles are serous and mucous lingual glands that secrete saliva.
8. The lingual tonsils are contained in the root.

F. The palate.
1. Separates the oral and nasal cavities.
2. Anterior portion is known as the hard (bony) palate.
   a. Transverse friction ridges (palatal rugae) aid the tongue in manipulating food.
3. Posterior portion is known as the soft palate.
   a. Spongy texture.
   b. Composed mainly of skeletal muscle and glandular tissue.
4. The small, conical medial process suspended from the medial posterior border of the soft palate is the uvula.

G. Saliva.
1. Functions include moisten mouth, digest small amount of starch and fat, cleanse the teeth, inhibit bacterial growth, dissolve molecules to stimulate taste buds, moisten food, and bind particles together to aid swallowing.
2. Has pH of 6.8 to 7.0; hypotonic solution of 97.0% to 99.5% water.
3. Contains solutes such as salivary amylase, lingual lipase, mucus, lysozyme, IgA, electrolytes.
4. Parasympathetic nervous system (PNS) stimulates the salivary glands to produce abundant thin saliva with a large number of enzymes.
5. Sympathetic stimulation produces less abundant, thick saliva with more mucous making the mouth sticky/dry during stress.
6. Dehydration decreases salivation due to reduced capillary filtration.

II. LOCALIZED LESIONS

A. White patches and plaques.
1. Leukoplakia: a persistent, thickened, white, firmly attached, well-demarcated patch usually occurring on the buccal mucosa. May be idiopathic or caused by external irritants such as tobacco.
   a. Physical exam.
      (1) Begin as localized, sharply demarcated, white waxy patches.
      (2) May develop into thick, leathery plaques.
      (3) Most common on the buccal mucosa, and tongue, but may occur anywhere in mouth and genital mucosa.
      (4) Plaques developing into squamous cell carcinoma (SCC) usually have a red color and may appear warty — erythroplakia.

(5) Induration and ulceration suggestive of carcinoma.

(6) Secondary infection of candidias may occur, but white plaques will not scrape off.

b. History/Symptoms.
(1) Tobacco users.
(2) Asymptomatic.

c. Epidemiology.
(1) Most commonly seen in men.
(2) Middle-aged and elderly adults.

d. Biopsy.
(1) Highly recommended due to risk of SCC.
(2) Benign lesions are leukokeratosis.

e. Laboratory.
(1) Occasional candidias noted on KOH test.

f. Treatment.
(1) Frequently resolves spontaneously if irritant (tobacco) discontinued.
(2) Good dental hygiene.
(3) Persistent lesions have required topical retinoids and surgery.

2. Uncommon causes of localized white patches/plaques.
a. Cheek biting.
b. Genodermatosis.
c. Nicotine stomatitis.
d. Angular cheilitis (perleche — an overgrowth of *Candida albicans*).
e. Wart (check for biting of warts).
f. Lichen planus.

B. Ulcerations.
1. Acute.
a. Recent trauma.
2. Chronic.
a. Biopsy for possible SCC.

C. Nursing considerations: see Table 1 and Figure 1.

III. GENERALIZED ULCERATIONS, EROSIONS, AND VESICLES

A. Aphthous stomatitis: common, recurrent, idiopathic ulcerative, disorder of the mouth. Commonly called "canker sore."
1. Physical exam.
a. Most common on buccal and labial mucosa; occasionally on tongue, soft palate, oropharynx.
b. Ulcers appear punched out.
c. Minor aphthae: 2 to 8 mm round/oval lesions, yellow center, with erythematous rim.
d. Major aphthae: 1 to 3 cm ulceration; similar in appearance to minor aphthae; however, deeper with increased necrosis.
e. Herpetiform: grouped 1-mm erosions that coalesce.

2. History/Symptoms.
a. Previous episodes invariable.
b. Recurrences usually precipitated by trauma or emotional stress.
c. Lesions usually preceded by 1-day prodrome of paresthesia/burning.
d. Pain associated with ulceration may interfere with eating.

3. Epidemiology.
a. Common (20% to 60% in general population).
b. Most common in young adults.

4. Biopsy.
a. Usually not required.

5. Laboratory.
a. Possible CBC to screen for iron, folate, B12 deficiencies.

6. Treatment: usually palliative as highly successful treatment is lacking.
a. Viscous lidocaine or dyclonine hydrochloride may be used 20 minutes prior to meals for less painful eating.
b. Topical steroids.
(1) Flucocinonide gel 0.05%.
(2) Triamcinolone in Orabase®.
c. Tetracycline "swish and swallow."
d. Intralesional trimcinolone sometimes helpful with major aphthous ulcerations.
e. Treat any underlying deficiencies if detected by CBC.
f. Avoid hot, spicy, and acidic foods.
g. Chronic, recurring.

B. Pemphigus vulgaris: intraepidermal autoimmune chronic blistering disease with significant mucosal involvement.
1. Physical exam.
a. Fragile blisters break often forming large (>1cm) coalescent ulcers and erosions.
b. 90% of patients with pemphigus vulgaris have oral involvement.
c. Most common intraoral site is buccal mucosa, but palate, pharynx, larynx, and gingival can be involved.

2. History/Symptoms.
a. Chronic oral involvement.
b. Severe pain and discomfort.
c. Occasionally drug induced.
d. Nikolsky's sign (erosions can be extended with peripheral pressure).

3. Epidemiology.
a. Rare.
b. More common in middle-aged adults.

4. Biopsy.
a. Recommended.

5. Laboratory.
a. Perilesional inflamed skin recommended for direct immunoflorescent studies.
b. Indirect immunofluorescent study.

Table 1.
Nursing Considerations for Patients with Oral Lesions

Nursing Diagnosis	Outcomes	Interventions
Pain related to oral lesions.	Pain is relieved; decreased need for analgesics.	Assess level of discomfort using scale of 0 to 10; intervene appropriately per practitioner orders (topical and/or systemic analgesics/anesthetics); encourage frequent sips of cool water or offer crushed ice; teach patient to avoid commercial mouthwashes and lemon-glycerin swabs; remove dentures. Use a soft toothbrush, toothette, or gauze for oral care every 2 hours. Monitor and record effectiveness of each.
Decreased nutrition related to oral pain.	Patient will maintain adequate nutritional intake as evidenced by weight maintenance and wound healing.	Monitor hydration status for dehydration; assist patient in selecting soft, bland, and nonacidic foods. Apply oral topical anesthetic 15 minutes prior to meals. Add liquid supplements to diet. Monitor daily weight. Refer to nutritionist as needed.
Body image/speech disturbance related to presence of oral lesions.	Patient exhibits improved/positive body image and improved speech.	Assess patient's perception of body image and possible impaired speech; allow verbalization; provide emotional support and positive feedback. Encourage compliance with treatment protocol to decrease edema and appearance of lesions.

6. Treatment.
   a. Oral prednisone.
   b. Immunosuppressents.
   c. Alternate therapies include: topical steroids, cyclosporine, dapsone, parenteral gold, and plasmapheresis.
   d. Current investigation indicating mouthwashes containing 0.05% clobetasol propionate plus 100,000 IU/cc nystatin in aqueous solution may be safe alternative to systemic corticosteroid treatment in patients with severe erosive lesions.
   e. Monitor routinely as disease is chronic.
C. **Herpetic gingivostomatitis: a hepesvirus infection resulting in multiple, painful ulcers on the gums and mucous membranes of the mouth.**
   1. Physical exam/symptoms.
      a. Fever.
      b. Malaise.
      c. Painful erosive stomatitis and pharyngitis resulting in reduced intake.
      d. Lesions usually start in interdental gingival papillae and spread to mucosal surface.
      e. Lesions begin as red macules that vesiculate, and develop into widespread erosions.
      f. Localized lymphadenopathy.
   2. History.
      a. If source known, eruptions begin 2 to 10 days after exposure to HSV.

      b. Immunosuppression.
   3. Epidemiology.
      a. More common in children.
   4. Biopsy.
      a. Not recommended, but can confirm diagnosis by revealing multinucleated giant cells.
   5. Laboratory.
      a. Culture or immunofluorescent tests for herpes to confirm clinical diagnosis.
      b. Tzanck preparation.
   6. Treatment.
      a. Early treatment with antivirals.
         (1) Acyclovir.
         (2) Valacyclovir.
         (3) Famciclovir.
      b. Usually resolves in 1 to 2 weeks without scarring.
D. **Erythema multiforme: a hypersensitivity syndrome characterized by polymorphous eruption of skin and mucous membranes (see Figure 25-1, page 244).**
   1. Physical exam.
      a. Generalized erosions and ulcers.
      b. Entire oral mucosal involved.
      c. Other mucosal surface/glabrous skin involvement common.
      d. Targetoid lesions on skin.
      e. Generalized lymphadenopathy.
   2. History/Symptoms.

Figure 1.
Algorithm for Oral Rashes

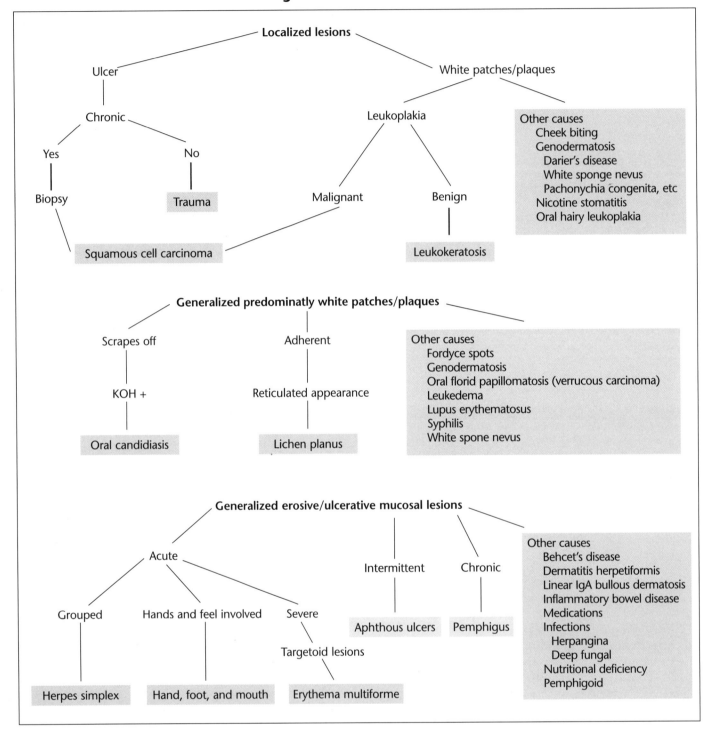

Reprinted from *Atlas of Differential Diagnosis in Dermatology,* Klaus F. Helm & James G. Marks, Jr. (1998). Churchill Livingstone, with permission from Elsevier Science.

a. May have recent URI or other infection.
b. New medications, treatments, environment, foods, and misc. triggers.
c. Difficulty eating/drinking.
d. Pain, discomfort, itching, mild malaise.
e. Erythema multiforme major is defined by mucous membrane involvement and widespread skin involvement (Stevens-Johnson's syndrome).
3. Epidemiology.
a. Most common in young adults.
4. Treatment.
a. Supportive care.
b. Pain medication.
c. Viscous lidocaine 20 minutes prior to meals.
d. Topical dressings to assist in healing of skin lesions.
e. Opthalmologic consultation if eye involvement.
f. Monitor fluids and electrolytes as well as nutrition.
g. Monitor closely for secondary infections.
h. Usually resolves over 4 to 6 weeks with possible scarring.
i. Use of systemic steroids remains controversial.
E. **Differential diagnosis of oral ulcers, erosions, vesicles.**
1. Aphthous stomatitis.
2. Autoimmune blistering.
3. Cytotoxic drugs.
4. Behcet's syndrome.
5. Epidermolysis bullosa.
6. Infections (viruses, syphilis, systemic fungi).
7. Lichen planus.
8. Neoplasia carcinoma.
9. Nutritional deficiency.
10. Trauma.
11. Ulcerative colitis.
12. Vasculitis.
F. **Nursing considerations: see Table 1 and Figure 1.**

IV. GENERALIZED WHITE PATCHES/PLAQUES

A. **Oral candidiasis (oral thrush): also known as acute pseudomembranous candidiasis, is an infection of the oropharyngeal cavity with *Candida albicans,* a yeast.**
1. Physical exam.
a. Infected epithelium appears white, curd-like papules and patches and can be scraped off, leaving an inflamed base.
b. Tongue and buccal mucosa most often affected.
c. Evaluate under dentures.
d. Angles of the mouth may be involved (angular cheilitis) in patients with dentures or orthodontic appliances in whom this

area remains moist.
e. Recent studies suggest that oral candidiasis could be a useful clinical marker for high viral loads and recommend systemic examination of the oral cavity in all medical followups for HIV-infected patients.
2. History/Symptoms.
a. Occasional burning mouth.
b. Immunosuppression from diseases or drugs.
c. Iatrogenic: steroids, antibiotics.
d. Mothers of infected newborns usually have history of vaginal candidiasis in late pregnancy.
3. Epidemiology.
a. Most common in newborns.
b. In adults, most common causes are local or systemic immunosuppression, steroid use, antibiotics, or ill-fitting dentures.
4. Biopsy.
a. Not recommended.
5. Laboratory.
a. Positive KOH.
6. Treatment.
a. Topical therapy.
(1) Infants: nystatin suspension 1 mL (100,000 units) to each side of the mouth QID for 5 to 7 days.
(2) Adults.
(a) Nystatin suspension "swish and swallow" 5 mL (500,000 units) QID.
(b) Clotrimazole troches dissolved in mouth 5 times daily for 1 to 2 weeks.
b. Systemic therapy (adults).
(1) Ketoconazole 200 mg daily for 1 to 2 weeks.
(2) Fluconazole 100 mg daily for 1 to 2 weeks.
c. Candidal colonization of dentures must be treated.
(1) Acrylic dentures can be soaked overnight in a dilute (1:10) sodium hypochlorite solution.
(2) Metal plates can be soaked overnight in a 0.12% chlorhexidine solution.
d. Course and complications.
(1) In newborns, thrush usually clears spontaneously, but is more rapid with treatment.
(2) Immunosuppressed patients can be recurrent and chronic.
(3) Most chronic infections occur with the syndrome of chronic mucocutaneous candidiasis in patients deficient in cellular immunity for *C. albicans.* Recurrences follow cessation of therapy.
(4) Complications are uncommon.

B. **Oral lichen planus: an idiopathic inflammatory dermatitis that may involve both glabrous skin and mucosa (see Figure 25-2, page 244).**
   1. Physical exam.
      a. Most frequently seen on bilateral buccal mucosa, gingival, and tongue.
      b. White, reticulated plaques that do not scrape off.
      c. Three basic clinical classifications.
         (1) Reticular — white lines, plaques, and papules
         (2) Erythematous (atrophic).
         (3) Erosive — including ulcerations and bullae.
      d. Frequent concomitant disease in extraoral sites (for example, genital mucosa).
   2. History/Symptoms.
      a. Reticular disease usually asymptomatic unless tongue involved.
      b. Pain associated with ulcerations.
      c. Occurrence usually associated with stress, cigarettes, spicy/acidic foods, drugs, poor oral hygiene, or trauma.
      d. Secondary candidal infection frequently seen, especially with steroidal treatment.
   3. Epidemiology.
      a. Most frequently seen in adult females.
      b. Familial pattern.
      c. May be early marker of hepatitis in Japanese, Italian, and Spanish populations.
      d. Controversy remains regarding malignant transformation of oral lichen planus.
   4. Biopsy.
      a. Diagnosis usually made clinically; however, biopsy is diagnostic.
   5. Laboratory.
      a. Negative KOH.
      b. Positive KOH if secondary candidal involvement present.
   6. Treatment.
      a. Minimize exacerbative factors such as smoking.
      b. Asymptomatic requires no treatment.
      c. Topical therapy.
         (1) Steroid gel/ointment (monitor for candidias).
         (2) Tretinoin gel.
         (3) Cyclosporine solution.
         (4) Tacrolimus 0.1%.
      d. Intralesional steroids.
      e. Systemic therapy for severe cases.
         (1) Prednisone.
         (2) Acitretin.
         (3) Cyclosporine.
      f. Usually chronic disease.
C. **Differential diagnosis of generalized oral white patches/plaques.**
   1. Lichen planus.

2. Candidiasis
3. Fordyce's spots (enlarged oil glands in the mucous membranes).
4. Leukoplakia.
5. Malignancy.
6. White spongy nevis.
7. Stomatitis.
8. Oral florid papillomatosis.
D. **Nursing considerations: see Table 1 and Figure 1.**

V. **MISCELLANEOUS DISORDERS OF THE ORAL MUCOSA**

A. **Burning mouth syndrome: chronic oral pain, in the absence of any visible mucosal abnormality, psychogenic factors is a possible cause.**
   1. Pain often described as mouth having been burnt.
   2. Discomfort reported to intensify during day.
   3. Tongue most often affected, but may include anterior palate and lips.
   4. Most frequently noted in post-menopausal women.
   5. Recent studies indicate that alpha-lipoic acid may be useful treatment; also suggest that burning mouth syndrome may be neuropathy related to free radical production.
B. **Radiation damage of the oral mucosa: major salivary glands are included in the portal of radiation treatment for many cancers causing irreversible damage, which may lead to xerostomia, mucositis, trismus, dysgeusia, dysphagia, edema, osteoradionecrosis, caries, and periodontal disease.**
   1. Rapid onset of oral dryness is most immediate and common side effect of radiation.
   2. Affects general health and quality of life.
   3. Advances in radiotherapy techniques have led to decreased damage.
   4. Treatment of symptoms.
      a. Moistening agents — salivary substitutes, synthetic salivas, or oral lubricants.
      b. Secretagogues.
         (1) Nonpharmacologic — sugarless gum and nonsucrose candy.
         (2) Pharmacologic — pilocarpine currently only drug approved for radiation-induced xerostomia; other drugs in trial stages.
      c. Other treatments under investigation.
C. **Dry mouth (salivary gland hypofunction): currently no global consensus for terminology; dry mouth relative to oral function and quality of life.**
   1. Xerostomia: subjective sensation of dry mouth; patient-dependent definition with significant impact on quality of life.
      a. Most common etiologic factor is

hyposalivation.
   b. Seen most commonly in women with increasing age.
   c. Possible pharmacotherapy etiology.
   d. Systemic disorders may be related — diabetes mellitus, rheumatoid arthritis, systemic lupus, and HIV.
2. Hyposalivation: reduced saliva flow rate; however, no current standard of measurement for salivation.
   a. Etiologic factors — age, disease, pharmacotherapy, and radiotherapy.
3. Altered saliva composition: alteration of composition alters presumed biological activity. Limited studies exist in this area. Most likely cause is pharmaceuticals.
4. Treatment.
   a. Moistening agents and secretagogues.
   b. Check for possible pharmacologic interactions and alter drug use if possible.
   c. Complete physical exam for possible nondiagnosed underlying systemic disease.
D. **Nursing considerations: see Table 1 and Figure 1.**

Bibliography

Bielan, B. (2000). What's your assessment? *Dermatology Nursing, 12*(2), 113-145.

Campo, J., Del Romero, J., Castilla, J., Garcia, S., Rodriguez, C., & Bascones (2002). Oral candidiasis as a clinical marker related to viral load, CD4 lymphocyte count and CD4 lymphocyte percentage in HIV-infected patients. *Journal of Oral Pathology Medicine, 31,* 5-10.

Eisen, D. (2002). The clinical features, malignant potential, and systemic associations of oral lichen planus: A study of 723 patients. *Journal of the American Academy of Dermatology, 46*(2), 207-214.

Eyeson, J. D., Tenant-Flowers, M., Cooper, D. J., Johnson, N. W., & Warnakulasuriya, K.A.A.S. (2002). Oral manifestations of an HIV positive cohort in the era of hightly active anti-retroviral therapy (HAART) in South London. *Journal of Oral Pathology Medicine, 31,* 169-74.

Femiano, F., & Scully, C. (2002). Burning mouth syndrome (BMS): Double blind controlled study of alpha-lipolic acid (thioctic acid) therapy. *Journal of Oral Pathology Medicine, 31,* 267-9.

Gonzalez-Moles, M.A., Morales, P., Rodriguez-Archilla, A., Isabel, I., & Gonzalez-Moles, S. (2002). Treatment of severe chronic oral erosive leseions with clobetasol propionate in aqueous solution. *Oral Surgery Oral Medicine Oral Pathology, 93*(3), 264-70.

Helm, K.F., & Marks, Jr., J.G. (1998). Oral mucosa. *In Atlas of differential diagnosis in dermatology* (pp. 45-57). Philadelphia: Churchill Livingstone.

Kaliakatsou, F., Hodgson, T.A., Lewsey, J.D., Hegarty, A.M., Murphy, A.G., & Porter, S.R. (2002). Management of recalcitrant ulcerative oral lichen planus with topical tacrolimus. *Journal of the American Academy of Dermatology, 46*(1), 35-41.

Lever, W.F., & Schaumburg-Lever, G. (1990). *Histology of the skin* (7th ed.). Philadelphia: J.B. Lippincott Company.

Lookingbill, D.P., & Marks, J.G. Jr. (2000). *Principles of dermatology* (3rd ed.). Philadelphia: W.B. Saunders Company.

Miller, C.S., Epstein, J. B., Hall, E.H., & Sirois, D. (2001). Changing oral care needs in the United States: The continuing need for oral medicine. *Oral Surgery Oral Medicine Oral Pathology, 91,* 34-44.

Nederfors, T. (2000). Xerostomia and hyosalivation. *Advances in dental research, 14,* 48-56.

O'Connell, A.C., (2000). Natural history and prevention of radiation injury. *Advances in dental research, 14,* 57-61.

Rycroft, R.J., & Robertson, S.J. (1999). *A colour handbook of dermatology.* London: Manson Publishing Ltd.

Saladin, K.S. (2001). *Anatomy and physiology: The unity of form and function.* New York: McGraw-Hill Higher Education.

Wolverton, S.E. (2001). *Comprehensive dermatologic drug therapy.* Philadelphia: W.B. Saunders Company.

1. Examination of the oral mucosa should only be conducted in response to a patient complaint.
   a. True
   b. False

2. A common, recurrent, idiopathic ulcerative disorder of the mouth appearing as a punched out ulcer. Usually occurs on the buccal mucosa. Commonly referred to as a "canker sore."
   a. Leukoplakia.
   b. Phemphigus vulgaris.
   c. Aphthous stomatitis.
   d. Erythema multiforme.

3. Which of the following is *not* a true statement for leukoplakia?
   a. Frequently seen in tobacco uses and usually resolves with discontinuation of use.
   b. May develop into thick leathery plaques.
   c. Is well demarcated.
   d. Biopsy is not recommended.

4. 90% of patients with pemphigus vulgaris have oral involvement.
   a. True
   b. False

5. Herpetic gingivostomatitis:
   a. Is most common in middle-aged adults.
   b. Is accompanied by fever and malaise.
   c. Usually occurs 2 to 10 days after exposure to herpes simplex virus.
   d. Causes painful, erosions and pharyngitis resulting in reduce nutritional intake.
   e. All the above.
   f. b, c, & d only.

6. _____ is most often noted in post-menopausal women, causing oral pain in the absence of any visible mucosal abnormalities.
   a. Burning mouth syndrome.
   b. Fordyces's spots.
   c. Hyposalivation.
   d. Lichen planus.

7. Which of the following is *not* a true statement in regards to oral candidiasis?
   a. It is caused by a yeast, *Candida albicans,* giving a positive KOH test result.
   b. The tongue and buccal mucosa are most often affected.
   c. The white, curd-like papules and patches cannot be scraped off.
   d. Most common in newborns.
   e. In adults, most common causes are immuno-suppression, steroid use, antibiotics, or ill-fitting dentures.

8. Physical exam of a patient with oral lichen planus would reveal which of the following?
   a. Buccal mucosa, gingival, and tongue involvement.
   b. White, reticulated plaques that scrape off easily.
   c. May involve both glabrous skin and oral mucosa.
   d. All the above.
   e. a & c only.

9. Oral lichen planus usually is most frequently seen in adult females.
   a. True
   b. False

10. The most common and immediate side-effect of radiation damage to the salivary glands is:
    a. Dental caries.
    b. Oral dryness.
    c. Osteoradionecrosis.
    d. Periodontal disease.

Answers to Study Questions

1.	b	5.	f	9.	a
2.	c	6.	a	10.	b
3.	d	7.	c		
4.	a	8.	d		

CE Answer/Evaluation Form

Chapter 25.
Disorders of Oral Mucosa

Please photocopy this test page and return.

COMPLETE THE FOLLOWING:

Name: _____

Address: _____

City: _____ State: _____ Zip: _____

Preferred telephone: (Home)_____ (Work) _____

State where licensed and license number: _____

CE application fee: DNA member $7.00
                       Nonmember $10.00

POSTTEST INSTRUCTIONS
1. To receive continuing education credit for individual study after reading the article, complete the answer/evaluation form below.
2. Photocopy and send the answer/evaluation form along with a check or money order payable to **Dermatology Nurses' Association** to: *DNA*, East Holly Avenue Box 56, Pitman, NJ 08071-0056.
3. Test returns must be postmarked by December 31, 2008. Upon completion of the answer/evaluation form, a certificate for 1.6 contact hour(s) will be awarded and sent to you.

This chapter was reviewed and formatted for contact hour credit by Marcia J. Hill, MSN, RN, Core Curriculum Editor; and Sally Russell, MN, RN,C, DNA Education Director.

ANSWER FORM

1. Name one new detail (item, issue, or phenomenon) that you learned by completing this activity.

_____

_____

_____

_____

2. How will you apply the information from this learning activity to your practice?
   a. Patient education.
   b. Staff education.
   c. Improve my patient care.
   d. In my education course work.
   e. Other: Please describe _____

_____

EVALUATION

	Strongly disagree				Strongly agree
3. The offering met the stated objectives.					
a. Describe the anatomy and physiology of the mouth as it relates to oral dermatology.	1	2	3	4	5
b. Differentiate between localized and generalized, ulcerative and white oral mucosal lesions.	1	2	3	4	5
c. List most common oral diseases and their related etiologies.	1	2	3	4	5
d. Identify appropriate treatments for various oral lesions.	1	2	3	4	5
e. Identify the importance of addressing quality of life issues in patients with oral mucosal lesions.	1	2	3	4	5
f. Identify the relationship between oral lesions and systemic diseases and medical/pharmacological treatments.	1	2	3	4	5
4. The content was current and relevant.	1	2	3	4	5
5. The content was presented clearly.	1	2	3	4	5
6. The content was covered adequately.	1	2	3	4	5
7. I am more confident of my abilities since completing this material.	1	2	3	4	5

8. The material was (check one) ☐ new, ☐ review for me.

Comments _____

_____

9. Time required to complete reading assignment: _____ minutes

This independent study is provided by the Dermatology Nurses' Association (DNA) for 1.6 contact hours. DNA is accredited as a provider of continuing education in nursing by the American Nurses Credentialing Center's Commission on Accreditation. DNA is approved as a provider of continuing education by the California Board of Registered Nursing Provider #CEP5708.

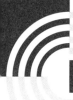

INDEX

Gammabenzene hexachloride (Kwell®), 314, 317

Garamycin, 49

Gastrointestinal disease, wound healing and, 379

Gauze dressings, 392*t,* 394

Gel and Coombs classification, of immune reactions, 417–418

Gels, therapeutic, 45

Genentech, Inc., 491

Generalized pustule psoriasis, assessment, 87

Genetic diseases, of basement membrane zone, 7

Genetic factors
   phototherapy and, 69, 69*t*
   in psoriasis, 85

Genodermatoses
   epidermolysis bullosa, 201–203
   ichthyosis, 198*f,* 199–201

Gianotti-Crosti syndrome (papular acrodermatitis), 211, 212

Glandular disorders, sebaceous, 451–454, 455*t*

Glogau photoaging classification, 260*t*

Glycolic acid, 260

Gnathophyma, 454

Goeckerman regimen, 89

Gottron's papules, 178–179, 423

Graft-versus host disease (GVHD), 164*t*–165*t,* 236*f*–237*f*

Gram stain, 32

Granular cell layer (stratum granulosum), 4, 4*f*

Granulation, 377–378

Granulation tissue, 387–388

Granuloma annulare, 296–297, 299

Griseofulvin, 57, 209

Ground substance, 8

Guidelines, defined, xix

Guttate lesions, 28

Guttate psoriasis
   assessment, 87
   medical interventions, 88–90
   pathophysiology, 86

GVHD (graft-versus host disease), 164*t*–165*t,* 236*f*–237*f*

H

Hair
   anatomy, normal, 341, 342*f*
   assessment, 343
   curly, 325
   diagnostic indicators, 28, 30
   distribution, 11, 341
   embryonic development, 341
   functions, 10
   growth, 341
   in hyperthyroidism, 157
   loss, 331–332, 331*t,* 346*t*
   morphology, 343
   normal findings, 22*t*–23*t*

   nursing diagnoses, outcomes and interventions, 343, 344*t*
   pigmentation, 342–343
   types, 341–342

Hair disorders
   alopecia areata, 343, 344*t,* 345
   hirsutism, 347–349
   trichotillomania, 349–351

Hair pull (pluck), 33

Hairy cell lymphoma, 153

Hallmark sign, 167

Hallucinations, dysmorphic, 433, 434

Halo nevi, 283*t,* 285

Hamilton's classification of male androgenic alopecia, 347*f*–348*f*

H2 antagonists, 293

Harlequin color change, 197

Hashimoto's thyroiditis, 155

H1 blockers, 293

Health care providers, defined, xv

Hemangiomas, 216

Hematoma, 243*f*

Hematopoietic abnormalities, wound healing and, 379

Hemidesmosomes, 7

Hemochromatosis, 158

Hemostasis, 33–34, 377

Henoch-Schonlein purpura, 295, 299

"Herald patch," 95, 227*f*

Herpes simplex virus infections
   assessment, 251
   in children, 211, 212
   eczema herpeticum, 412–413, 413*t*
   in HIV/AIDS, 242*f,* 365
   pathophysiology, 251
   treatment, 251

Herpes viruses, 412

Herpes zoster (shingles), 252, 365, 413

Herpetic gingivostomatitis, 467

Herpetiform lesions, 28

HHV-7 DNA, 95

Hidradenitis suppurativa, 329, 454–456, 455*t*

Hirsutism
   assessment, 343, 348
   drug-related, 350*t*
   etiology/pathophysiology, 347
   nursing considerations, 344*t*
   therapeutic modalities, 349

Hispanics, skin type of, 325

Histiocytes, 9

HIV/AIDS
   assessment, cutaneous, 364
   bacterial infections, 366
   cutaneous manifestations, 367–368
   etiology/pathophysiology, 363*t*
   fungal infections, 366–367
   incidence, 364
   indicator conditions, 363*t,* 364*t*

Kaposi's sarcoma, 133, 134, 231*f,* 364–365
   nursing consideration, 368, 369*t*–370*t*

   post-exposure prophylaxis, 370, 372*t*
   risk factors, 363–364
   universal precautions, 368, 370, 371*t*
   viral infections, 365–366

Hives. *See* Urticaria

HLAs (human leukocyte antigens), 85

Home care considerations. *See under specific conditions*

Homeostasis, skin and, 3

Honeybee, 307–308

Hormones, 5–6, 11

Horn cells, 4

Hornet stings, 308

Horny cell layer (stratum corneum), 4–5, 4*f*

Hot comb alopecia, 331–332, 331*t*

HuM291 (anti-CD3a), 89

Human herpesvirus (HHV-8/KS), 133

Human immunodeficiency virus infection. *See* HIV/AIDS

Human leukocyte antigens (HLAs), 85

Human papilloma virus, 121, 133

Humoral immunity, 13

Hutchinson's papillary psoriasis, 162–163

Hydrocolloid dressing, 392*t,* 393

Hydrogel dressing, 392*t,* 393–394

Hydroquinone, 282

Hylan B gels, 260–261

Hymenoptera, hypersensitivity reactions, 307, 307*t*

Hyperhidrosis, primary, 455*t,* 456–457

Hyperpigmentation
   acquired, 277
   chemically induced, 279*t,* 282, 284
   diffuse brown, 277
   melasma, 279*t,* 281–282

Hyperplasia, sebaceous, 146

Hypersensitivity reactions
   dermatologic emergencies, 415–417, 416*t*
   to hymenoptera, 307, 307*t*
   morphologic classifications, 298–299
   nursing considerations, 293*t*
   types, 13–14, 291
   urticaria. *See* Urticaria
   vasculitides, 294–296. *See also specific vasculitides*

Hypertrichosis, 30

Hypertrichosis lanuginosa, 156*t*

Hypertrophic scars, 144–145, 145*t,* 244*f,* 330

Hyponychium, 351, 352*t*

Hypopigmentation
   acquired, 277–280
   albinism, 280
   congenital, 277
   piebaldism, 279*t,* 280–281
   tuberous sclerosis, 279*t,* 281
   vitiligo, 277–280

Hypotension, wound healing and, 379

Hypothyroidism, 155, 157–158

Hypotrichosis, 30

Hypoxia, wound healing and, 380

Dermatologic Nursing Essentials: A Core Curriculum 2nd Edition © DNA 2003

X

Y

Z

The Dermatology Nurses' Association thanks the following companies for their generous financial support of Dermatologic Nursing Essentials: A Core Curriculum (2nd edition)

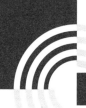

AMGEN®

Amgen
One Amgen Center Drive
Thousand Oaks, CA   91320
Telephone: 805-447-1000
Web site: www.amgen.com

Description of Company:

Amgen, the world's largest biotechnology company, uses science and innovation to dramatically improve people's lives. Amgen researchers harness the powerful tools of cellular and molecular biology and medicinal chemistry to discover, develop and commercialize naturally occurring proteins, antibodies and small molecules, with the goal of extending the reach of science to unleash the body's own powerful therapeutic responses.

Beiersdorf Inc.

Beiersdorf Inc.
187 Danbury Road
Wilton, CT   06897
Telephone: 203-563-5800
Web site: www.eucerin.com

Description of Company:

Since its beginnings at the turn of the 19th century in Germany, Beiersdorf has made its mark as a forerunner in the development of advanced and unique medical and cosmetic skin care products. In addition to its original headquarters in Hamburg, Germany, Beiersdorf currently has subsidiaries in over fifty countries throughout the world. Its skin care products, which include the Eucerin and Aquaphor product lines, are widely recognized and recommended by health care professionals.

Description/Brand Names of Main Dermatology Products:

Eucerin

For over 50 years, medical professionals have recommended Eucerin to patients with even the driest and most sensitive skin. Eucerin sensitive skin formulations are non-irritating, fragrance-free and contain no potentially sensitizing colorings or additives. And Eucerin has been proven safe over years of use in a variety of specialties and skin conditions, on a variety of patient types. Today, there's a full line of Eucerin products to fit all your patients' needs, from cleansing to moisturizing to sun protection, for both body and face.

Aquaphor

Health care professionals have known for years that Aquaphor provides ideal daily therapy for cracked, dry or damaged skin on the body or face. Aquaphor's highly occlusive formulation creates a moist, protective, yet semi-permeable environment that allows the passage of fluids and air. Aquaphor is clinically proven to accelerate healing time and is hypoallergenic, non-comedogenic, and contains no preservatives or fragrances.

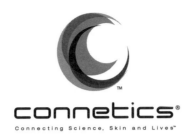

Connetics Corporation
3290 West Bayshore Road
Palo Alto, CA   94043
Telephone: 650-843-2800
Web site: www.connetics.com

Description of Company:

Connetics Corporation (NASDAQ: CNCT) is a specialty pharmaceutical company focused on the development and commercialization of innovative therapeutics for the $4 billion U.S. prescription dermatology market. This market has been projected to grow to $10 billion U.S. by 2010 (Adis International; POV® Report, Dermatological Therapeutics; February 2002). The Company's marketed products - sold through its highly specialized sales force - include Luxíq® (betamethasone valerate) Foam, 0.12% for treating mild-to-moderate scalp dermatoses and OLUX® (clobetasol propionate) Foam, 0.05% for short-term topical treatment of the inflammatory and pruritic manifestations of moderate to severe corticosteroid-responsive dermatoses of the scalp, and for short-term topical treatment of mild to moderate plaque-type psoriasis of non-scalp regions excluding the face and intertriginous areas. Connetics' drug delivery subsidiary, Connetics Australia Pty Ltd., formerly Soltec Research Pty Ltd., provides a portfolio of patented topical drug-delivery technologies, including those used in its marketed products. In 2002, Connetics granted an exclusive global license for its Liquipatch™ technology to Novartis Consumer Health for Lamisil®, their antifungal application, and licensed its foam delivery technology to Pharmacia for use in Rogaine®. Connetics recently in-licensed Velac® gel, a combination clindamycin/tretinoin acne drug, from Yamanouchi Europe. Phase III clinical trials are underway for two products: a foam formulation of ketoconazole under the brand name Extina™ and a foam formulation of clindamycin under the brand name Actiza™

Description/Brand Names of Main Dermatology Products:

Luxíq®

In April 1999, Connetics' introduced Luxíq®, a medium potency topical corticosteroid indicated for treating inflammatory and pruritic manifestations of corticosteroid-responsive dermatoses of the scalp, such as psoriasis, eczema, and seborrheic dermatitis. The most frequent side effects associated with the use of Luxíq® are mild and transient burning, stinging, or itching at the application site. Luxíq® is a 0.12% foam formulation of betamethasone valerate, which has been commonly prescribed for more than 20 years as a treatment for various skin dermatoses.

OLUX®

In 2000, OLUX® was approved for the short-term topical treatment of the inflammatory and pruritic manifestations of moderate to severe corticosteroid-responsive dermatoses of the scalp including psoriasis. In December 2002, OLUX® received expanded FDA approval for short-term topical treatment of mild to moderate plaque-type psoriasis of non-scalp regions excluding the face and intertriginous areas.

Treatment with OLUX® Foam beyond 2 consecutive weeks is not recommended, and the total dosage should not exceed 50g per week because of the potential for the drug to suppress the hypothalamic-pituitary-adrenal (HPA) axis. OLUX® Foam is not recommended for use in children under 12 years of age. The most common adverse events that occurred in patients treated with OLUX® Foam included application site burning, application site dryness and other application site reactions.

DERMIK®

Dermik Laboratories
1050 Westlakes Drive
Berwyn, PA   19312
Telephone: 484-595-2700
Web site: www.dermik.com

Description of Company:

Dermik Laboratories has built a strong, ongoing relationship with the dermatology community by providing a wide range of products and support services.

Description/Brand Names of Main Dermatology Products:

Key products include BenzaClin®, Benzamycin Pak® and Klaron® for acne; Carac® for actinic keratosis; Penlac™ for onychomycosis; Noritate™ for rosacea; and the topical steroids Dermatop-e® and Psorcon-e® for psoriasis.

Additional Services:

Dermik supports a textbook distribution service, publication of acne case reports, and many worthy organizations' requests for financial and educational grants. Over the years, we have established a reputation as one of the very best companies in the industry, demonstrated in the quality of our products and by the dedicated efforts of Dermik employees around the world.

⊞ Fujisawa Healthcare, Inc.

Fujisawa Healthcare
Three Parkway North
Deerfield, IL   60015-2548
Telephone: 800-888-7704 or 847-317-8800
Web site: www.protopic.com

Description of Company:

Fujisawa Healthcare, Inc., manufactures cutting-edge prescription medications in dermatology and conducts long-term, large-scale research projects with dermatologists and investigators around the world, seeking to discover new treatments for skin diseases.

Our focus on dermatology can be seen most clearly in our field-dedicated R&D division, which has become an ideal environment to generate and publish key information on dermatologic advances. In fact, Fujisawa has conducted some of the world's largest clinical trials in dermatology, with more than 15,000 patients involved.

Description/Brand Names of Main Dermatology Products:

Fujisawa's dermatology product portfolio includes:
- Protopic®, Aristocort®, and Cyclocort®.
- Protopic (tacrolimus) ointment introduced a new drug class, the topical immunomodulators.
- Aristocort (triamcinolone) cream and ointment are topical corticosteroid preparations.
- Cyclocort (amcinonide) cream, lotion, and ointment are topical corticosteroid preparations.

Additional Services:

Fujisawa services and resources include:
- EczemaNet - An on-line resource to living with and treating eczema. Presented in partnership with the American Academy of Dermatology and sponsored by an educational grant from Fujisawa.
- Fujisawa Medical Information - A department dedicated to answering questions from healthcare professionals and consumers and providing resources, including educational slide kits discussing the safety and efficacy of products and patient guides to dermatology and cardiology. Contact Fujisawa Medical Information at 1-800-727-7003, or by e-mail at Medical_Information@fujisawa.com.
- *Under My Skin* - A booklet serving child's guide to atopic dermatitis.
- Protopic.com - Web site with both consumer and healthcare professional areas providing important disease state, treatment, and product information.

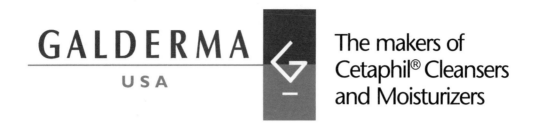

Galderma Laboratories, L.P.
14501 North Freeway
Fort Worth, TX   76177
Telephone: 817-961-5000
Web site: www.galdermaus.com

Mission Statement:

Galderma Laboratories is dedicated to being the leading company worldwide in the marketing of dermatological products to meet the needs of dermatologists and their patients. We will constantly strive to set new standards of service, professionalism, and commitment to the specialty.

Galderma has always focused on a single field of science: dermatology. While other companies choose to develop and promote their products and services to multiple specialties, Galderma has emerged as the only major pharmaceutical group whose concentration is firmly centered on dermatology.

Description/Brand Names of Main Dermatology Products:
   Capex® Shampoo
   Cetaphil® Cleansers and Moisturizers
   Clindagel®
   Differin®
   MetroGel®
   Rosanil®
   Solage®
   Tri-Luma®

Additional Services:
Online Services for the Dermatology Professional and Patient:

   www.capexshampoo.com
   www.cetaphil.com
   www.clindagel.com
   www.differin.com
   www.metrogel.com
   www.rosanil.com
   www.solage.com
   www.triluma.com
   www.dermquest.com
   www.galdermaUSA.com

Genentech

Genentech, Inc.
1 DNA Way
South San Francisco, CA   94080
Telephone: 650-225-1000
Web site: www.gene.com

Description of Company:

Genentech is a leading biotechnology company that discovers, develops, manufactures and commercializes biotherapeutics for significant unmet medical needs. Genentech and XOMA Ltd. are co-developing Raptiva™ (efalizumab), a therapeutic antibody in Phase III clinical trials for the treatment of moderate-to-severe plaque psoriasis. The company has headquarters in South San Francisco, California and is located online at www.gene.com.

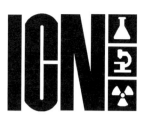

ICN Pharmaceuticals, Inc.
3300 Hyland Avenue
Costa Mesa, CA   92626
Telephone: 714-545-0100
Web site: www.icnpharm.com

Description of Company:

ICN Pharmaceuticals offers a wide range of products to dermatologists and plastic surgeons. Efudex® (Fluorouracil) is supplied in a 5% cream or solution and a 2% solution. GLYQUIN XM™ (Hydroquinone USP, 4%) cream contains 10% glycolic acid, vitamins C and E, SPF 15 and hyaluronic acid. Cosmetic products available include Kinerase (N6-furfuryladenine), which helps photodamaged skin without the side effects of topical retinoids, and the GlyDerm line of esterified glycolic acid products. Also available is Oxsoralen-Ultra® and 8-MOP® (Methoxsalen USP, 10 mg), Oxsoralen® Lotion (1% Methoxsalen USP) for phototherapy.

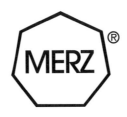

Merz Pharmaceuticals
4215 Tudor Lane
Greensboro, NC   27410
Telephone: 336-856-2003
Web site: www.merzusa.com

Description of Company:

Merz Pharmaceuticals, LLC is a specialty pharmaceuticals company that is dedicated to addressing unmet medical needs with innovative health care solutions that improve self-esteem and quality of life.

The Merz mission focuses our efforts on addressing the unmet medical needs of dermatology health care professionals who trust us to introduce high quality products that provide the solutions they need. Merz is pleased to be an active supporter of dermatology nurses and we appreciate the opportunity to be a part of the DNA mission to educate nurses and support dermatology patients.

Merz Pharmaceuticals is a subsidiary of Merz Pharmaceuticals of Germany, a leader in the development of prescription and over the counter products. Merz Pharmaceuticals GmbH has established subsidiaries and operations in more than 90 countries. For more information about Merz, call 1-888-MERZ-USA (637-9872) or visit www.merzusa.com.

Description/Brand Names of Main Dermatology Products:

One of the ways Merz addresses unmet medical needs is with a number of products that focus on the needs of health care professionals.

Merz offers Naftin®, the only prescription allylamine offered in a cream, quick-drying gel, and multi-pack (Naftin®-MP™). Naftin® offers physicians increased prescribing flexibility in treating fungal infections.

Our newest member to our dermatology portfolio, Appearex™, is a once-daily oral therapy that promotes strong, healthy nail growth from within. The active ingredient in Appearex™, 2.5mg biotin, has been clinically proven to strengthen weak, brittle fingernails.

Merz also produces Aqua Glycolic®, an alphahydroxy acid-based line of skin care products. Aqua Glycolic® contains the high percentage of glycolic compound (10-14%) available at retail, and has a balanced pH of 4.4.

And, Mederma® Skin Care for Scars™, is an invisible gel that helps both new and existing scars appear softer, smoother and less noticeable. Mederma® is available at all major pharmacy chains and is also available for distribution in dermatology offices.

For additional information and for full prescribing information on Naftin®, visit the Merz Web site at www.merzusa.com.

CORPORATE SPONSORS

OrthoNeutrogena

Ortho Neutrogena
5760 West 96th Street
Los Angeles, CA 90045
Telephone: 310-642-1150
Web site: www.neutrogena.com

Description of Company:

Ortho Dermatological has been in the business of healthy skin for over 25 years and Neutrogena has been a partner with dermatology for over 30 years. Both have been committed to advancing the treatment of dermatologic conditions. Now, Ortho Dermatological and Neutrogena have combined efforts and resources with the formation of OrthoNeutrogena. Through continuous support of the dermatologic community, we seek to advance the science of skin and hair care. We are committed to the development of clinically sound products that fulfill the skin and hair care needs of physicians, nurses and their patients.

Description/Brand Names of Main Dermatology Products:

Products in the OrthoNeutrogena prescription drug line include RETIN-A® Micro™ (tretinoin gel) microsphere, 0.1%, RETIN-A® Micro™ (tretinoin gel) 0.04%, RENOVA® (tretinoin emollient cream) 0.05%, RENOVA® (tretinoin emollient cream) 0.02%, SPECTAZOLE® (econazole nitrate 1%) Cream, Grifulvin V® (griseofulvin tablets) microsize and Grifulvin V® (griseofulvin oral suspension) microsize.

In addition, OrthoNeutrogena also provides nurses and physicians with a full over-the-counter portfolio, which includes Neutrogena's acne cleansers and treatments, body cleansers and moisturizers, facial cleansers and moisturizers, hair care, men's skin care, suncare, and cosmetics.

493